MW01178510

QUICK LOOK
DRUG BOOK

QUICK LOOK DRUG BOOK

1998

Leonard L. Lance, RPh
Senior Editor
Pharmacist
Lexi-Comp Inc.
Hudson, Ohio

Charles Lacy, RPh, PharmD
Editor
Drug Information Pharmacist
Cedars-Sinai Medical Center
Los Angeles, California

Morton P. Goldman, PharmD
Associate Editor
Infectious Diseases Pharmacist
Cleveland Clinic Foundation
Cleveland, Ohio

Williams & Wilkins

BALTIMORE • PHILADELPHIA • HONG KONG
LONDON • MUNICH • SYDNEY • TOKYO

A WAVERLY COMPANY

NOTICE

This handbook is intended to serve the user as a handy quick reference and not as a complete drug information resource. It does not include information on every therapeutic agent available. The publication covers 1439 commonly used drugs and is specifically designed to present certain important aspects of drug data in a more concise format than is generally found in medical literature or product material supplied by manufacturers.

Although great care was taken to ensure the accuracy of the handbook's content when it went to press, the editors, contributors, and publisher cannot be responsible for the continued accuracy of the supplied information due to ongoing research and new developments in the field. Further, the *Quick Look Drug Book* is not offered as a guide to dosing. The reader, herewith, is advised that information shown under the heading **Usual Dosage** is provided only as an indication of the amount of the drug typically given or taken during therapy. Actual dosing amount for any specific drug should be based on an in-depth evaluation of the individual patient's therapy requirement and strong consideration given to such issues as contraindications, warnings, precautions, adverse reactions, along with the interaction of other drugs. The manufacturers most current product information or other standard recognized references should always be consulted for such detailed information prior to drug use.

The editors and contributors have written this book in their private capacities. No official support or endorsement by any federal agency or pharmaceutical company is intended or inferred.

This manual was produced using the FormuLex™ Program —
a complete publishing service of Lexi-Comp Inc.

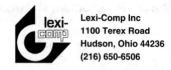

Lexi-Comp Inc
1100 Terex Road
Hudson, Ohio 44236
(216) 650-6506

TABLE OF CONTENTS

ABOUT THE AUTHORS

Leonard L. Lance, RPh

Leonard L. (Bud) Lance has been directly involved in the pharmaceutical industry since receiving his bachelor's degree in pharmacy from Ohio Northern University in 1970. Upon graduation from ONU, Mr Lance spent four years as a navy pharmacist in various military assignments and was instrumental in the development and operation of the first whole hospital I.V. admixture program in a military (Portsmouth Naval Hospital) facility.

After completing his military service, he entered the retail pharmacy field and has managed both an independent and a home I.V. franchise pharmacy operation. Since the late 1970s, Mr Lance has focused much of his interest on using computers to improve pharmacy service and to advance the dissemination of drug information to practitioners and other health care professionals.

As a result of his strong publishing interest, he serves in the capacity of pharmacy editor and technical advisor as well as pharmacy (information) database coordinator for Lexi-Comp. Along with the *Quick Look Drug Book*, he provides technical support to Lexi-Comp's Clinical Reference Library™ publications. Mr Lance has also assisted over 100 major hospitals in producing their own formulary (pharmacy) publications through Lexi-Comp's custom publishing service.

L. Lance is a member and past president (1984) of the Summit County Pharmaceutical Association (SCPA). He is also a member of the Ohio Pharmacists Association (OPA), the American Pharmaceutical Association (APhA), and the American Society of Health-System Pharmacists (ASHP).

Charles F. Lacy, PharmD

Dr Lacy received his doctorate from the University of Southern California School of Pharmacy. With over 15 years of clinical experience at one of the nation's largest teaching hospitals, he has developed a reputation as an acknowledged expert in drug information and critical care drug therapy.

In his current capacity as Drug Information Specialist at Cedar-Sinai Medical Center in Los Angeles, Dr Lacy plays an active role in the education and training of the medical, pharmacy, and nursing staff. He coordinates the Drug Information Center, the Medical Center's Intern Pharmacist Clinical Training Program, the Department's Continuing Education Program for pharmacists; maintains the Medical Center formulary program; and is editor of the Medical Center's *Drug Formulary Handbook* and the drug information newsletter — *Prescription*.

Presently, Dr Lacy holds teaching affiliations with the University of Southern California School of Pharmacy, the University of California at San Francisco School of Pharmacy, the University of the Pacific School of Pharmacy and the University of Alberta at Edmonton, School of Pharmacy and Health Sciences.

Dr Lacy is an active member of numerous professional associations including the American Society of Health-System Pharmacists (ASHP), the California Society of Hospital Pharmacists (CSHP), and the American College of Clinical Pharmacy (ACCP).

Morton P. Goldman, PharmD

Dr Goldman received his bachelor's degree in pharmacy from the University of Pittsburgh in 1983 and his doctorate from the University of Cincinnati. He completed his residency at the V.A. Medical Center in Cincinnati and subsequently began pharmacy practice at several prominent Cleveland medical centers concentrating in the area of infectious diseases.

In his capacity as infectious disease pharmacist at the Cleveland Clinic Foundation, Dr Goldman is actively involved in the continuing education of the medical and pharmacy staff. He is an editor of the foundation's *Guideline for Antibiotic Use* and has coordinated their Renal Dose Monitoring Program. Dr Goldman has authored numerous journal articles and lectures locally and nationally on the topic of infectious diseases and current drug therapies. He is currently a coauthor of the *Infectious Diseases Handbook* produced by Lexi-Comp Inc. He also provides technical support to Lexi-Comp's Clinical Reference Library™ publications.

Dr Goldman is an active member of the Society of Infectious Disease Pharmacists, American College of Clinical Pharmacy and the American Society of Health-System Pharmacists.

EDITORIAL ADVISORY PANEL

PREFACE

Working with clinical pharmacists, hospital pharmacy and therapeutics committees, and hospital drug information centers, our editors have assisted in developing hospital-specific formulary manuals for major medical institutions in the United States and Canada. These manuals provide pertinent details on medications used within the hospital, office and other clinical settings. The most current information on drugs and medications has been reviewed, coalesced, and cross-referenced to form the *Quick Look Drug Book*.

The Indication/Therapeutic Category Index is an expedient mechanism for locating the medication of choice along with its classification. This index helps the user to, with knowledge of the disease state, identify medications which are most commonly used in treatment. All disease states are cross-referenced to a varying number of medications with the most likely or best medications noted.

All generic names and synonyms appear in lower case, whereas the brand names appear in upper/lower case with the proper trademark information. These three items appear as individual entries in the alphabetical listing of drugs. Thus, there is no alphabetical index of drugs.

This handbook gives the user quick access to data on 1439 medications. A standard, concise format was developed to ensure consistent presentation of information. Selection of medications included in this handbook was based on an analysis of medications offered in a wide range of hospital formularies.

— L.L. Lance

ACKNOWLEDGMENTS

The *Quick Look Drug Book* exists in its present form as the result of the concerted efforts of the following individuals: the publisher and president of Lexi-Comp Inc, Robert D. Kerscher; senior director of programming and publications, James P. Caro, American Pharmaceutical Association (APhA); and Lynn D. Coppinger, managing editor.

Other members of the Lexi-Comp staff whose contributions deserve special mention include Diane Harbart, MT (ASCP), medical editor; Barbara F. Kerscher, production manager; Jeanne Wilson, Leslie Ruggles, and Julie Katzen, project managers; Alexandra Hart, composition specialist; Jennifer Harbart, and Jackie Mizer, production assistants; Brian B. Vossler, Marc L. Long, and Jerry M. Reeves, sales managers; Tracey J. Reinecke, graphics; Jay L. Katzen, product manager; Kenneth J. Hughes, manager of authoring systems; Kristin M. Thompson, Matthew C. Kerscher, Tina L. Collins, and Mary M. Murphy, sales and marketing representatives; Edmund A. Harbart, vice-president, custom publishing division; Jack L. Stones, vice-president, reference publishing division; Dennis P. Smithers, David C. Marcus, and Sean Conrad, system analysts; and Thury L. O'Connor, vice-president of technology.

USE OF THE HANDBOOK

The *Quick Look Drug Book* is organized into a drug information section, an appendix, and indication/therapeutic category index.

The drug information section of the handbook, wherein all drugs are listed alphabetically, details information pertinent to each drug. Extensive cross referencing is provided by brand name and synonyms.

Drug information is presented in a consistent format and for quick reference will provide the following:

Generic Name	U.S. adopted name
Pronunciation Guide	
Brand Names	Common trade names
Synonyms	
Therapeutic Category	
Use	Information pertaining to appropriate use of the drug
Usual Dosage	The amount of the drug to be typically given or taken during therapy
Dosage Forms	Information with regard to form, strength and availability of the drug

Appendix

The appendix offers a compilation of tables, guidelines and conversion information which can often be helpful when considering patient care.

Indication/Therapeutic Category Index

This index provides a listing of accepted drugs for various disease states thus focusing attention on selection of medications most frequently prescribed in relation to a clinical diagnosis. Diseases may have other nonofficial drugs for their treatment and this indication/therapeutic category index should not be used by itself to determine the appropriateness of a particular therapy. The listed indications may encompass varying degrees of severity and, since certain medications may not be appropriate for a given degree of severity, it should not be assumed that the agents listed for specific indications are interchangeable. Also included as a valuable reference is each medication's therapeutic category.

SAFE WRITING

Health professionals and their support personnel frequently produce handwritten copies of information they see in print; therefore, such information is subjected to even greater possibilities for error or misinterpretation on the part of others. Thus, particular care must be given to how drug names and strengths are expressed when creating written health care documents.

The following are a few examples of safe writing rules suggested by the Institute for Safe Medication Practices, Inc.*

1. There should be a space between a number and its units as it is easier to read. There should be no periods after the abbreviations mg or mL.

Correct	Incorrect
10 mg	10mg
100 mg	100mg

2. Never place a decimal and a zero after a whole number (2 mg is correct and 2.0 mg is incorrect). If the decimal point is not seen because it falls on a line or because individuals are working from copies where the decimal point is not seen, this causes a tenfold overdose.

3. Just the opposite is true for numbers less than one. Always place a zero before a naked decimal (0.5 mL is correct, .5 mL is **in**correct).

4. Never abbreviate the word "unit." The handwritten U or u, looks like a 0 (zero), and may cause a tenfold overdose error to be made.

5. Q.D. is not a safe abbreviation for once daily, as when the Q is followed by a sloppy dot, it looks like QID which means four times daily.

6. O.D. is not a safe abbreviation for once daily, as it is properly interpreted as meaning "right eye" and has caused liquid medications such as saturated solution of potassium iodide and lugol's solution to be administered incorrectly. There is no safe abbreviation for once daily. It must be written out in full.

7. Do not use chemical names such as 6-mercaptopurine or 6-thioguanine, as 6 fold overdoses have been given when these were not recognized as chemical names. The proper names of these drugs are mercaptopurine or thioguanine.

8. Do not abbreviate drug names (5FC, 6MP, 5-ASA, MTX, HCTZ CPZ, PBZ, etc) as they are misinterpreted and cause error.

9. Do not use the apothecary system or symbols.

10. Do not abbreviate microgram as μg; instead use mcg as there is less likelihood of misinterpretation.

11. When writing an outpatient prescription, write a complete prescription. A complete prescription can prevent the prescriber, the pharmacist, and/or the

---

*From "Safe Writing" by Davis NM, PharmD and Cohen MR, MS, Lecturers and Consultants for Safe Medication Practices, 1143 Wright Drive, Huntingdon Valley, PA 19006. Phone: (215) 947-7566.

patient from making a mistake and can eliminate the need for further clarification. The legible prescriptions should contain:

a. patient's full name

b. for pediatric or geriatric patients: their age (or weight where applicable)

c. drug name, dosage form and strength; if a drug is new or rarely prescribed, print this information

d. number or amount to be dispensed

e. complete instructions for the patient, including the purpose of the medication

f. when there are recognized contraindications for a prescribed drug, indicate to the pharmacist that you are aware of this fact (ie, when prescribing a potassium salt for a patient receiving an ACE inhibitor, write "K serum leveling being monitored")

SELECTED REFERENCES

AMA Drug Evaluations Subscription, American Medical Association, Department of Drugs, Division of Drugs and Toxicology, Spring, 1990.

Drug Interaction Facts, St Louis, MO: J.B. Lippincott Co (Facts and Comparisons Division), 1996.

Facts and Comparisons, St Louis, MO: J.B. Lippincott Co (Facts and Comparisons Division), 1996.

Handbook of Nonprescription Drugs, 10th ed, Washington, DC: American Pharmaceutical Association, 1996.

Isada CM, Kasten BL, Goldman MP, et al, *Infectious Diseases Handbook*, 2nd ed, Hudson, OH: Lexi-Comp Inc, 1997.

Jacobs DS, DeMott WR, Finley PR, et al, *Laboratory Test Handbook with Key Word Index*, 4th ed, Hudson, OH: Lexi-Comp Inc, 1996.

Lacy CF, Armstrong LL, Lipsy RJ, and Lance LL, *Drug Information Handbook*, 4th ed, Hudson, OH: Lexi-Comp Inc, 1997.

Leikin JB and Paloucek FP, *Poisoning & Toxicology Handbook*, 1st ed, Hudson, OH: Lexi-Comp Inc, 1997.

McEvoy GK and Litvak K, *AHFS Drug Information*, Bethesda, MD: American Society of Health-System Pharmacists, 1996.

Physician's Desk Reference, 50th ed, Oradell, NJ: Medical Economics Books, 1996.

Semla TP, Beizer JL, and Higbee MD, *Geriatric Dosage Handbook*, 2nd ed, Hudson, OH: Lexi-Comp Inc, 1997.

Taketomo CK, Hodding JH, and Kraus DM, *Pediatric Dosage Handbook*, 4th ed, Hudson, OH: Lexi-Comp Inc, 1997.

United States Pharmacopeia Dispensing Information (USP DI), 15th ed, Rockville, MD: United States Pharmacopeial Convention, Inc, 1996.

Wynn RL, Meiller TF, and Crossley HL, *Drug Information Handbook for Dentistry,* 3rd ed, Hudson, OH: Lexi-Comp Inc, 1997.

ALPHABETICAL LISTING OF DRUGS

A-200™ Shampoo [OTC] *see* pyrethrins *on page 452*

A and D™ Ointment [OTC] *see* vitamin a and vitamin d *on page 552*

Abbokinase® Injection *see* urokinase *on page 543*

abciximab (ab SIK si mab)
Synonyms c7E3
Brand Names ReoPro™
Therapeutic Category Platelet Aggregation Inhibitor
Use Adjunct to percutaneous transluminal coronary angioplasty or atherectomy (PTCA) for the prevention of acute cardiac ischemic complications in patients at high risk for abrupt closure of the treated coronary vessel
Usual Dosage I.V.: 0.25 mg/kg bolus followed by an infusion of 10 mcg/minute for 12 hours
Dosage Forms Injection: 2 mg/mL (5 mL)

Abelcet™ Injection *see* amphotericin b lipid complex *on page 32*

ABLC *see* amphotericin b lipid complex *on page 32*

absorbable cotton *see* cellulose, oxidized *on page 102*

absorbable gelatin sponge *see* gelatin, absorbable *on page 238*

Absorbine® Antifungal [OTC] *see* tolnaftate *on page 523*

Absorbine® Antifungal Foot Powder [OTC] *see* miconazole *on page 348*

Absorbine® Jock Itch [OTC] *see* tolnaftate *on page 523*

Absorbine Jr.® Antifungal [OTC] *see* tolnaftate *on page 523*

acarbose (AY car bose)
Brand Names Precose®
Therapeutic Category Antidiabetic Agent (Oral)
Use Treatment of noninsulin-dependent diabetes mellitus (NIDDM); as monotherapy or in combination with a sulfonylurea when diet plus acarbose or a sulfonylurea does not result in adequate glycemic control
Usual Dosage Adults: Oral: Dosage must be individualized on the basis of effectiveness and tolerance while not exceeding the maximum recommended dose of 100 mg 3 times/day

Initial dose: 25 mg 3 times/day with the first bite of each main meal
Maintenance dose: Should be adjusted at 4- to 8-week intervals based on 1-hour postprandial glucose levels and tolerance. Dosage may be increased from 25 mg 3 times/day to 50 mg 3 times/day; some patients may benefit from increasing the dose to 100 mg 3 times/day; maintenance dose ranges: 50-100 mg 3 times/day.
Maximum dose:
≤60 kg: 50 mg 3 times/day
>60 kg: 100 mg 3 times/day
Dosage Forms Tablet: 50 mg, 100 mg

Accolate® *see* zafirlukast *on page 558*

Accupril® *see* quinapril *on page 455*

Accutane® *see* isotretinoin *on page 292*

acebutolol (a se BYOO toe lole)
Synonyms acebutolol hydrochloride
Brand Names Sectral®
Therapeutic Category Antiarrhythmic Agent, Class II; Beta-Adrenergic Blocker
Use Treatment of hypertension; ventricular arrhythmias; angina
Usual Dosage Adults: Oral: 400-800 mg/day in 2 divided doses
Dosage Forms Capsule, as hydrochloride: 200 mg, 400 mg

acebutolol hydrochloride *see* acebutolol *on previous page*

Acel-Imune® *see* diphtheria, tetanus toxoids, and acellular pertussis vaccine *on page 175*

Aceon® *see* perindopril erbumine *on page 406*

Acephen® **[OTC]** *see* acetaminophen *on this page*

Aceta® **[OTC]** *see* acetaminophen *on this page*

acetaminophen (a seet a MIN oh fen)

Synonyms apap; n-acetyl-p-aminophenol; paracetamol

Brand Names Acephen® [OTC]; Aceta® [OTC]; Apacet® [OTC]; Arthritis Foundation® Pain Reliever, Aspirin Free [OTC]; Aspirin Free Anacin® Maximum Strength [OTC]; Children's Dynafed® Jr [OTC]; Children's Silapap® [OTC]; Extra Strength Dynafed® E.X. [OTC]; Feverall™ [OTC]; Feverall™ Sprinkle Caps [OTC]; Genapap® [OTC]; Halenol® Childrens [OTC]; Infants Feverall™ [OTC]; Infants' Silapap® [OTC]; Junior Strength Panadol® [OTC]; Liquiprin® [OTC]; Mapap® [OTC]; Maranox® [OTC]; Neopap® [OTC]; Panadol® [OTC]; Redutemp® [OTC]; Ridenol® [OTC]; Tempra® [OTC]; Tylenol® [OTC]; Tylenol® Extended Relief [OTC]; Uni-Ace® [OTC]

Therapeutic Category Analgesic, Non-narcotic; Antipyretic

Use Treatment of mild to moderate pain and fever; does not have antirheumatic or systemic anti-inflammatory effects

Usual Dosage Oral, rectal (if fever not controlled with acetaminophen alone, administer with full doses of aspirin on an every 4- to 6-hour schedule, if aspirin is not otherwise contraindicated):

Children <12 years: 10-15 mg/kg/dose every 4-6 hours as needed; do **not** exceed 5 doses (2.6 g) in 24 hours

Adults: 325-650 mg every 4-6 hours or 1000 mg 3-4 times/day; do **not** exceed 4 g/day

Dosage Forms

Caplet: 160 mg, 325 mg, 500 mg

Extended: 650 mg

Capsule: 80 mg

Drops: 48 mg/mL (15 mL); 60 mg/0.6 mL (15 mL); 80 mg/0.8 mL (15 mL); 100 mg/mL (15 mL, 30 mL)

Elixir: 80 mg/5 mL, 120 mg/5 mL, 160 mg/5 mL, 167 mg/5 mL, 325 mg/5 mL

Liquid, oral: 160 mg/5 mL, 500 mg/15 mL

Solution: 100 mg/mL (15 mL); 120 mg/2.5 mL

Suppository, rectal: 80 mg, 120 mg, 125 mg, 300 mg, 325 mg, 650 mg

Suspension, oral: 160 mg/5 mL

Oral drops: 80 mg/0.8 mL

Tablet: 325 mg, 500 mg, 650 mg

Chewable: 80 mg, 160 mg

acetaminophen and butalbital compound *see* butalbital compound and acetaminophen *on page 78*

acetaminophen and codeine (a seet a MIN oh fen & KOE deen)

Synonyms codeine and acetaminophen

Brand Names Capital® and Codeine; Phenaphen® With Codeine; Tylenol® With Codeine

Therapeutic Category Analgesic, Narcotic

Controlled Substance C-III; C-V

Use Relief of mild to moderate pain

Usual Dosage Doses should be adjusted according to severity of pain and response of the patient. Adult doses ≥60 mg codeine fail to give commensurate relief of pain but merely prolong analgesia and are associated with an appreciably increased incidence of side effects. Oral:

(Continued)

acetaminophen and codeine *(Continued)*

Children:
Analgesic: 0.5-1 mg codeine/kg/dose every 4-6 hours
Acetaminophen: 10-15 mg/kg/dose every 4 hours up to a maximum of 2.6 g/24 hours for children <12 years
3-6 years: 5 mL 3-4 times/day as needed of elixir
7-12 years: 10 mL 3-4 times/day as needed of elixir
>12 years: 15 mL every 4 hours as needed of elixir
Adults:
Antitussive: Based on codeine (15-30 mg/dose) every 4-6 hours
Analgesic: Based on codeine (30-60 mg/dose) every 4-6 hours
1-2 tablets every 4 hours to a maximum of 12 tablets/24 hours

Dosage Forms
Capsule:
#2: Acetaminophen 325 mg and codeine phosphate 15 mg (C-III)
#3: Acetaminophen 325 mg and codeine phosphate 30 mg (C-III)
#4: Acetaminophen 325 mg and codeine phosphate 60 mg (C-III)
Elixir: Acetaminophen 120 mg and codeine phosphate 12 mg per 5 mL with alcohol 7% (C-V)
Suspension, oral, alcohol free: Acetaminophen 120 mg and codeine phosphate 12 mg per 5 mL (C-V)
Tablet: Acetaminophen 500 mg and codeine phosphate 30 mg (C-III); acetaminophen 650 mg and codeine phosphate 30 mg (C-III)
Tablet:
#1: Acetaminophen 300 mg and codeine phosphate 7.5 mg (C-III)
#2: Acetaminophen 300 mg and codeine phosphate 15 mg (C-III)
#3: Acetaminophen 300 mg and codeine phosphate 30 mg (C-III)
#4: Acetaminophen 300 mg and codeine phosphate 60 mg (C-III)

acetaminophen and dextromethorphan

(a seet a MIN oh fen & dex troe meth OR fan)
Brand Names Bayer® Select® Chest Cold Caplets [OTC]; Drixoral® Cough & Sore Throat Liquid Caps [OTC]
Therapeutic Category Antitussive/Analgesic
Use Treatment of mild to moderate pain; symptomatic relief of coughs caused by minor viral upper respiratory tract infections or inhaled irritants; most effective for a chronic nonproductive cough
Usual Dosage Oral:
Children: 10-15 mg/kg/dose every 4-6 hours as needed; do **not** exceed 5 doses in 24 hours
Adults: 325-650 mg every 4-6 hours or 1000 mg 3-4 times/day; do **not** exceed 4 g/day
Dosage Forms
Caplet: Acetaminophen 500 and dextromethorphan hydrobromide 15 mg
Capsule: Acetaminophen 325 and dextromethorphan hydrobromide 15 mg

acetaminophen and diphenhydramine

(a seet a MIN oh fen & dye fen HYE dra meen)
Brand Names Excedrin® P.M. [OTC]; Midol® PM [OTC]
Therapeutic Category Analgesic, Non-narcotic
Use Relief of mild to moderate pain or sinus headache
Usual Dosage Oral:
Children <12 years: Not recommended
Adults: 2 caplets or 5 mL of liquid at bedtime or as directed by physician; do not exceed recommended dosage
Dosage Forms
Caplet:
Excedrin® P.M.: Acetaminophen 500 mg and diphenhydramine citrate 30 mg

Midol® PM: Acetaminophen 500 mg and diphenhydramine 25 mg
Liquid (wild berry flavor) (Excedrin® P.M.): Acetaminophen 1000 mg and diphenhydramine hydrochloride 50 mg per 30 mL (180 mL)

acetaminophen and hydrocodone *see* hydrocodone and acetaminophen *on page 266*

acetaminophen and oxycodone *see* oxycodone and acetaminophen *on page 390*

acetaminophen and phenyltoloxamine

(a seet a MIN oh fen & fen il to LOKS a meen)
Brand Names Percogesic® [OTC]
Therapeutic Category Analgesic, Non-narcotic
Use Relief of mild to moderate pain
Usual Dosage Adults: Oral: 1-2 tablets every 4 hours
Dosage Forms Tablet: Acetaminophen 325 mg and phenyltoloxamine citrate 30 mg

acetaminophen and pseudoephedrine

(a seet a MIN oh fen & soo doe e FED rin)
Synonyms pseudoephedrine and acetaminophen
Brand Names Allerest® No Drowsiness [OTC]; Bayer® Select Head Cold Caplets [OTC]; Coldrine® [OTC]; Dristan® Cold Caplets [OTC]; Dynafed®, Maximum Strength [OTC]; Ornex® No Drowsiness [OTC]; Sinarest®, No Drowsiness [OTC]; Sine-Aid®, Maximum Strength [OTC]; Sine-Off® Maximum Strength No Drowsiness Formula [OTC]; Sinus Excedrin® Extra Strength [OTC]; Sinus-Relief® [OTC]; Sinutab® Without Drowsiness [OTC]; Tylenol® Sinus, Maximum Strength [OTC]
Therapeutic Category Decongestant/Analgesic
Usual Dosage Adults: Oral: 2 tablets every 4-6 hours
Dosage Forms Tablet:
Allerest® No Drowsiness; Coldrine®, Tylenol® Sinus, Maximum Strength; Ornex® No Drowsiness, Sinus-Relief®: Acetaminophen 325 mg and pseudoephedrine hydrochloride 30 mg
Bayer® Select Head Cold; Dristan® Cold; Dynafed®, Maximum Strength; Sinarest®, No Drowsiness; Sine-Aid®, Maximum Strength; Sine-Off® Maximum Strength No Drowsiness Formula; Sinus Excedrin® Extra Strength; Sinutab® Without Drowsiness; Tylenol® Sinus, Maximum Strength: Acetaminophen 500 mg and pseudoephedrine hydrochloride 30 mg

acetaminophen, aspirin, and caffeine

(a seet a MIN oh fen, AS pir in, & KAF een)
Brand Names Excedrin®, Extra Strength [OTC]; Gelpirin® [OTC]; Goody's® Headache Powders
Therapeutic Category Analgesic, Non-narcotic
Use Relief of mild to moderate pain or fever
Usual Dosage Adults: Oral: 1-2 tablets or powders every 2-6 hours as needed for pain
Dosage Forms
Geltab: Acetaminophen 250 mg, aspirin 250 mg, and caffeine 65 mg
Powder: Acetaminophen 250 mg, aspirin 520 mg, and caffeine 32.5 mg per dose
Tablet: Acetaminophen 125 mg, aspirin 240 mg, and caffeine 32 mg; acetaminophen 250 mg, aspirin 250 mg, and caffeine 65 mg

acetaminophen, chlorpheniramine, and pseudoephedrine

(a seet a MIN oh fen, klor fen IR a meen, & soo doe e FED rin)
Brand Names Alka-Seltzer® Plus Cold Liqui-Gels Capsules [OTC]; Aspirin-Free Bayer® Select® Allergy Sinus Caplets [OTC]; Co-Hist® [OTC]; Sinutab® Tablets [OTC]
Therapeutic Category Antihistamine/Decongestant/Analgesic
Use Temporary relief of sinus symptoms
(Continued)

acetaminophen, chlorpheniramine, and pseudoephedrine
(Continued)
Usual Dosage Adults: Oral: 2 caplets/capsules/tablets every 6 hours
Dosage Forms
Caplet: Acetaminophen 500 mg, chlorpheniramine maleate 2 mg, and pseudoephedrine hydrochloride 30 mg
Capsule: Acetaminophen 250 mg, chlorpheniramine maleate 2 mg, and pseudoephedrine hydrochloride 30 mg
Tablet: Acetaminophen 325 mg, chlorpheniramine maleate 2 mg, and pseudoephedrine hydrochloride 30 mg

acetaminophen, dextromethorphan, and pseudoephedrine
(a seet a MIN oh fen, deks troe meth OR fan, & soo doe e FED rin)
Synonyms dextromethorphan, acetaminophen, and pseudoephedrine; pseudoephedrine, acetaminophen, and dextromethorphan; pseudoephedrine, dextromethorphan, and acetaminophen
Brand Names Alka-Seltzer® Plus Flu & Body Aches Non-Drowsy Liqui-Gels [OTC]; Comtrex® Maximum Strength Non-Drowsy [OTC]; Sudafed® Severe Cold [OTC]; Theraflu® Non-Drowsy Formula Maximum Strength [OTC]; Tylenol® Cold No Drowsiness [OTC]; Tylenol® Flu Maximum Strength [OTC]
Therapeutic Category Cold Preparation
Usual Dosage Adults: Oral: 2 tablets every 6 hours
Dosage Forms Tablet:
Alka-Seltzer® Plus Flu & Body Aches Non-Drowsy: Acetaminophen 500 mg, dextromethorphan hydrobromide 10 mg, and pseudoephedrine hydrochloride 30 mg
Comtrex® Maximum Strength Non-Drowsy; Sudafed® Severe Cold; Theraflu® Non-Drowsy Formula Maximum Strength; Tylenol® Flu Maximum Strength: Acetaminophen 500 mg, dextromethorphan hydrobromide 15 mg, and pseudoephedrine hydrochloride 30 mg
Tylenol® Cold No Drowsiness: Acetaminophen 325 mg, dextromethorphan hydrobromide 15 mg, and pseudoephedrine hydrochloride 30 mg

acetaminophen, isometheptene, and dichloralphenazone
(a seet a MIN oh fen, eye soe me THEP teen, & dye KLOR al FEN a zone)
Brand Names Isocom®; Isopap®; Midchlor®; Midrin®; Migratine®
Therapeutic Category Analgesic, Non-narcotic
Use Relief of migraine and tension headache
Usual Dosage Adults: Oral: 2 capsules at first sign of headache, followed by 1 capsule every 60 minutes until relieved, up to 5 capsules in a 12-hour period
Dosage Forms Capsule: Acetaminophen 326 mg, isometheptene mucate 65 mg, dichloralphenazone 100 mg

Acetasol® HC Otic *see* acetic acid, propylene glycol diacetate, and hydrocortisone
on next page

acetazolamide (a set a ZOLE a mide)
Brand Names Diamox®; Diamox Sequels®
Therapeutic Category Anticonvulsant; Carbonic Anhydrase Inhibitor
Use Reduce elevated intraocular pressure in glaucoma, a diuretic, an adjunct to the treatment of refractory seizures and acute altitude sickness; centrencephalic epilepsies
Usual Dosage
Children:
Glaucoma:
Oral: 8-30 mg/kg/day divided every 6-8 hours
I.M., I.V.: 20-40 mg/kg/day divided every 6 hours
Edema: Oral, I.M., I.V.: 5 mg/kg or 150 mg/m^2 once every day or every other day
Epilepsy: Oral: 8-30 mg/kg/day in 2-4 divided doses, not to exceed 1 g/day

Adults:
Glaucoma:
Oral: 250 mg 1-4 times/day or 500 mg sustained release capsule twice daily
I.M., I.V.: 250-500 mg, may repeat in 2-4 hours
Edema: Oral, I.M., I.V.: 250-375 mg once daily
Epilepsy: Oral: 8-30 mg/kg/day in 1-4 divided doses
Altitude sickness: Oral: 250 mg every 8-12 hours
Dosage Forms
Capsule, sustained release: 500 mg
Injection: 500 mg
Tablet: 125 mg, 250 mg

acetic acid (a SEE tik AS id)
Synonyms ethanoic acid
Brand Names Aci-jel® Vaginal; VōSol® Otic
Therapeutic Category Antibacterial, Otic; Antibacterial, Topical
Use Continuous or intermittent irrigation of the bladder; treatment of superficial bacterial infections of the external auditory canal and vagina
Usual Dosage
Irrigation: For continuous irrigation of the urinary bladder with 0.25% acetic acid irrigation, the rate of administration will approximate the rate of urine flow; usually 500-1500 mL/24 hours; for periodic irrigation of an indwelling urinary catheter to maintain patency, approximately 50 mL of 0.25% acetic acid irrigation is required. (Note: Dosage of an irrigating solution depends on the capacity or surface area of the structure being irrigated.)
Otic: Insert saturated wick, keep moist 24 hours; remove wick and instill 5 drops 3-4 times/day
Vaginal: One applicatorful morning and evening
Dosage Forms
Jelly, vaginal (Aci-jel®): 0.921% with oxyquinolone sulfate 0.025%, ricinoleic acid 0.7%, and glycerin 5% (85 g)
Solution:
Irrigation: 0.25% (1000 mL)
Otic (VōSol®): Acetic acid 2% in propylene glycol (15 mL, 30 mL, 60 mL)

acetic acid and aluminum acetate otic *see* aluminum acetate and acetic acid
on page 20

acetic acid, propylene glycol diacetate, and hydrocortisone
(a SEE tik AS id, PRO pa leen GLY kole dye AS e tate, & hye droe KOR ti sone)
Brand Names Acetasol® HC Otic; VōSol® HC Otic
Therapeutic Category Antibiotic/Corticosteroid, Otic
Use Treatment of superficial infections of the external auditory canal caused by organisms susceptible to the action of the antimicrobial, complicated by inflammation
Usual Dosage Adults: Otic: Instill 4 drops in ear(s) 3-4 times/day
Dosage Forms Solution, otic: Acetic acid 2%, propylene glycol diacetate 3%, and hydrocortisone 1% (10 mL)

acetohexamide (a set oh HEKS a mide)
Brand Names Dymelor®
Therapeutic Category Antidiabetic Agent (Oral)
Use Adjunct to diet for the management of mild to moderately severe, stable, noninsulin-dependent (type II) diabetes mellitus
Usual Dosage Adults: Oral: 250 mg to 1.5 g/day in 1-2 divided doses
Dosage Forms Tablet: 250 mg, 500 mg

acetohydroxamic acid (a SEE toe hye droks am ik AS id)
Synonyms aha
Brand Names Lithostat®
Therapeutic Category Urinary Tract Product
Use Adjunctive therapy in chronic urea-splitting urinary infection
Usual Dosage Oral:
  Children: Initial: 10 mg/kg/day
  Adults: 250 mg 3-4 times/day for a total daily dose of 10-15 mg/kg/day
Dosage Forms Tablet: 250 mg

acetophenazine (a set oh FEN a zeen)
Synonyms acetophenazine maleate
Therapeutic Category Phenothiazine Derivative
Use Management of manifestations of psychotic disorders
Usual Dosage Adults: Oral: 20 mg 3 times/day up to 40-80 mg/day

  Hospitalized schizophrenic patients may require doses as high as 400-600 mg/day
Dosage Forms Tablet, as maleate: 20 mg

acetophenazine maleate *see* acetophenazine *on this page*

acetoxymethylprogesterone *see* medroxyprogesterone acetate *on page 326*

acetylcholine (a se teel KOE leen)
Synonyms acetylcholine chloride
Brand Names Miochol-E®
Therapeutic Category Cholinergic Agent
Use Produces complete miosis in cataract surgery, keratoplasty, iridectomy and other anterior segment surgery where rapid miosis is required
Usual Dosage Adults: Intraocular: 0.5-2 mL of 1% injection (5-20 mg) instilled into anterior chamber before or after securing one or more sutures
Dosage Forms Powder, intraocular, as chloride: 1:100 [10 mg/mL] (2 mL, 15 mL)

acetylcholine chloride *see* acetylcholine *on this page*

acetylcysteine (a se teel SIS teen)
Synonyms acetylcysteine sodium; mercapturic acid; NAC; N-acetylcysteine; N-acetyl-L-cysteine
Brand Names Mucomyst®; Mucosil™
Therapeutic Category Mucolytic Agent
Use Adjunctive therapy in patients with abnormal or viscid mucous secretions in bronchopulmonary diseases, pulmonary complications of surgery, and cystic fibrosis; diagnostic bronchial studies; antidote for acute acetaminophen toxicity; enema to treat bowel obstruction due to meconium ileus or its equivalent
Usual Dosage
  Acetaminophen poisoning: Children and Adults: Oral: 140 mg/kg; followed by 17 doses of 70 mg/kg every 4 hours; repeat dose if emesis occurs within 1 hour of administration; therapy should continue until all doses are administered even though the acetaminophen plasma level has dropped below the toxic range
  Inhalation: Acetylcysteine 10% and 20% solution (Mucomyst®) (dilute 20% solution with sodium chloride or sterile water for inhalation); 10% solution may be used undiluted
  Infants: 1-2 mL of 20% solution or 2-4 mL 10% solution until nebulized administered 3-4 times/day
  Children: 3-5 mL of 20% solution or 6-10 mL of 10% solution until nebulized administered 3-4 times/day
  Adolescents: 5-10 mL of 10% to 20% solution until nebulized administered 3-4 times/day
  Note: Patients should receive an aerosolized bronchodilator 10-15 minutes prior to acetylcysteine

Meconium ileus equivalent: Children and Adults: 100-300 mL of 4% to 10% solution by irrigation or orally

Dosage Forms Solution, as sodium: 10% [100 mg/mL] (4 mL, 10 mL, 30 mL); 20% [200 mg/mL] (4 mL, 10 mL, 30 mL, 100 mL)

acetylcysteine sodium *see* acetylcysteine *on previous page*

acetylsalicylic acid *see* aspirin *on page 44*

Achromycin® Ophthalmic *see* tetracycline *on page 510*

Achromycin® Topical *see* tetracycline *on page 510*

aciclovir *see* acyclovir *on next page*

acidulated phosphate fluoride *see* fluoride *on page 228*

Aci-jel® Vaginal *see* acetic acid *on page 7*

Aclovate® Topical *see* alclometasone *on page 14*

acrivastine and pseudoephedrine (AK ri vas teen & soo doe e FED rin)

Synonyms pseudoephedrine and acrivastine

Brand Names Semprex-D®

Therapeutic Category Antihistamine/Decongestant Combination

Use Temporary relief of nasal congestion, decongest sinus openings, running nose, itching of nose or throat, and itchy, watery eyes due to hay fever or other upper respiratory allergies

Usual Dosage Adults: 1 capsule 3-4 times/day

Dosage Forms Capsule: Acrivastine 8 mg and pseudoephedrine hydrochloride 60 mg

act *see* dactinomycin *on page 147*

ACT® [OTC] *see* fluoride *on page 228*

Actagen-C® *see* triprolidine, pseudoephedrine, and codeine *on page 537*

Actagen® Syrup [OTC] *see* triprolidine and pseudoephedrine *on page 536*

Actagen® Tablet [OTC] *see* triprolidine and pseudoephedrine *on page 536*

acth *see* corticotropin *on page 138*

Acthar® *see* corticotropin *on page 138*

Actidose-Aqua® [OTC] *see* charcoal *on page 105*

Actidose® With Sorbitol [OTC] *see* charcoal *on page 105*

Actifed® Allergy Tablet (Day) [OTC] *see* pseudoephedrine *on page 449*

Actifed® Allergy Tablet (Night) [OTC] *see* diphenhydramine and pseudoephedrine *on page 173*

Actigall™ *see* ursodiol *on page 544*

Actimmune® *see* interferon gamma-1b *on page 286*

Actinex® Topical *see* masoprocol *on page 322*

actinomycin d *see* dactinomycin *on page 147*

Activase® Injection *see* alteplase *on page 19*

activated carbon *see* charcoal *on page 105*

activated dimethicone *see* simethicone *on page 480*

activated ergosterol *see* ergocalciferol *on page 197*

activated methylpolysiloxane *see* simethicone *on page 480*

Actron® [OTC] *see* ketoprofen *on page 297*

ACU-dyne® [OTC] *see* povidone-iodine *on page 431*

Acular® Ophthalmic *see* ketorolac tromethamine *on page 297*

Acutrim® 16 Hours [OTC] *see* phenylpropanolamine *on page 413*

Acutrim® II, Maximum Strength [OTC] *see* phenylpropanolamine *on page 413*

Acutrim® Late Day [OTC] *see* phenylpropanolamine *on page 413*

acv *see* acyclovir *on this page*

acycloguanosine *see* acyclovir *on this page*

acyclovir (ay SYE kloe veer)

Synonyms aciclovir; acv; acycloguanosine

Brand Names Zovirax®

Therapeutic Category Antiviral Agent

Use Treatment of initial and prophylaxis of recurrent mucosal and cutaneous herpes simplex (HSV-1 and HSV-2) infections; herpes simplex encephalitis; herpes zoster infections; varicella-zoster infections in healthy, nonpregnant persons >13 years of age, children >12 months of age who have a chronic skin or lung disorder or are receiving long-term aspirin therapy, and immunocompromised patients

Usual Dosage

Children and Adults: I.V.:

Mucocutaneous HSV infection: 750 mg/m^2/day divided every 8 hours or 15 mg/kg/day divided every 8 hours for 5-10 days

HSV encephalitis: 1500 mg/m^2/day divided every 8 hours or 30 mg/kg/day divided every 8 hours for 10 days

Varicella-zoster virus infection: 1500 mg/m^2/day divided every 8 hours or 30 mg/kg/day divided every 8 hours for 5-10 days

Adults:

Oral: Initial: 200 mg every 4 hours while awake (5 times/day); prophylaxis: 200 mg 3-4 times/day or 400 mg twice daily. Prophylaxis of varicella or herpes zoster in HIV positive patients: 400 mg 5 times/day

Topical: 1/2" ribbon of ointment every 3 hours (6 times/day)

Herpes zoster in immunocompromised patients:

Children: Oral: 250-600 mg/m^2/dose 4-5 times/day

Adults: Oral: 800 mg every 4 hours (5 times/day) for 7-10 days

Children and Adults: I.V.: 7.5 mg/kg/dose every 8 hours

Varicella-zoster infections: Oral:

Children: 10-20 mg/kg/dose (up to 800 mg) 4 times/day

Adults: 600-800 mg/dose 5 times/day for 7-10 days or 1000 mg every 6 hours for 5 days

Prophylaxis of bone marrow transplant recipients: Children and Adults: I.V.:

Autologous patients who are HSV seropositive: 150 mg/m^2/dose every 12 hours; with clinical symptoms of herpes simplex: 150 mg/m^2/dose every 8 hours

Autologous patients who are CMV seropositive: 500 mg/m^2/dose every 8 hours; for clinically symptomatic CMV infection, ganciclovir should be used in place of acyclovir

Dosage Forms

Capsule: 200 mg

Powder for Injection: 500 mg (10 mL); 1000 mg (20 mL)

Ointment, topical: 5% [50 mg/g] (3 g, 15 g)

Suspension, oral (banana flavor): 200 mg/5 mL

Tablet: 400 mg, 800 mg

Adagen™ *see* pegademase (bovine) *on page 398*

Adalat® *see* nifedipine *on page 374*

Adalat® CC *see* nifedipine *on page 374*

adamantanamine hydrochloride *see* amantadine *on page 22*

adapalene (a DAP a leen)

Brand Names Differin®

Therapeutic Category Acne Products

Use Topical treatment of acne vulgaris

Usual Dosage Adults: Topical: Apply once daily, before retiring, in a thin film to affected areas after washing; not recommended in children
Dosage Forms Gel, topical (alcohol free): 0.1% (15 g, 45 g)

Adapin® **Oral** *see* doxepin *on page 183*

Adderall® *see* dextroamphetamine and amphetamine *on page 160*

Adeflor® *see* vitamin, multiple (pediatric) *on page 554*

adenine arabinoside *see* vidarabine *on page 549*

Adenocard® *see* adenosine *on this page*

adenosine (a DEN oh seen)
Synonyms 9-beta-D-ribofuranosyladenine
Brand Names Adenocard®
Therapeutic Category Antiarrhythmic Agent, Miscellaneous
Use Treatment of paroxysmal supraventricular tachycardia (PSVT)
Usual Dosage
Children: Initial: Rapid I.V.: 0.05 mg/kg; if not effective within 2 minutes, increase dose in 0.05 mg/kg increments every 2 minutes to a maximum dose of 0.25 mg/kg or until termination of PSVT; median dose required: 0.15 mg/kg; do not exceed adult doses
Adults: Rapid I.V. push: 6 mg, if the dose is not effective within 1-2 minutes, a rapid I.V. dose of 12 mg may be administered; may repeat 12 mg bolus if needed
Dosage Forms Injection, preservative free: 3 mg/mL (2 mL)

Adlone® **Injection** *see* methylprednisolone *on page 343*

adr *see* doxorubicin *on page 183*

Adrenalin® *see* epinephrine *on page 195*

adrenaline *see* epinephrine *on page 195*

adrenocorticotropic hormone *see* corticotropin *on page 138*

Adriamycin PFS™ *see* doxorubicin *on page 183*

Adriamycin RDF™ *see* doxorubicin *on page 183*

Adrucil® **Injection** *see* fluorouracil *on page 229*

Adsorbocarpine® **Ophthalmic** *see* pilocarpine *on page 417*

Adsorbonac® **Ophthalmic [OTC]** *see* sodium chloride *on page 483*

Adsorbotear® **Ophthalmic Solution [OTC]** *see* artificial tears *on page 42*

Advanced Formula Oxy® **Sensitive Gel [OTC]** *see* benzoyl peroxide *on page 61*

Advil® **[OTC]** *see* ibuprofen *on page 278*

Advil® **Cold & Sinus Caplets [OTC]** *see* pseudoephedrine and ibuprofen *on page 450*

Aeroaid® **[OTC]** *see* thimerosal *on page 515*

AeroBid®**-M Oral Aerosol Inhaler** *see* flunisolide *on page 226*

AeroBid® **Oral Aerosol Inhaler** *see* flunisolide *on page 226*

Aerodine® **[OTC]** *see* povidone-iodine *on page 431*

Aerolate III® *see* theophylline *on page 511*

Aerolate JR® *see* theophylline *on page 511*

Aerolate SR® *see* theophylline *on page 511*

Aeroseb-Dex® *see* dexamethasone *on page 156*

Aeroseb-HC® *see* hydrocortisone *on page 268*

AeroZoin® **[OTC]** *see* benzoin *on page 61*

Afrin® **Children's Nose Drops [OTC]** *see* oxymetazoline *on page 390*

Afrin® Saline Mist [OTC] *see* sodium chloride *on page 483*

Afrin® Sinus [OTC] *see* oxymetazoline *on page 390*

Afrin® Tablet [OTC] *see* pseudoephedrine *on page 449*

Aftate® for Athlete's Foot [OTC] *see* tolnaftate *on page 523*

Aftate® for Jock Itch [OTC] *see* tolnaftate *on page 523*

AgNO₃ *see* silver nitrate *on page 479*

Agrylin® *see* anagrelide *on page 34*

aha *see* acetohydroxamic acid *on page 8*

ahf *see* antihemophilic factor (human) *on page 37*

A-hydroCort® *see* hydrocortisone *on page 268*

Airet® *see* albuterol *on page 14*

Akarpine® Ophthalmic *see* pilocarpine *on page 417*

AKBeta® *see* levobunolol *on page 304*

AK-Chlor® Ophthalmic *see* chloramphenicol *on page 108*

AK-Cide® Ophthalmic *see* sulfacetamide sodium and prednisolone *on page 497*

AK-Con® Ophthalmic *see* naphazoline *on page 364*

AK-Dex® Ophthalmic *see* dexamethasone *on page 156*

AK-Dilate® Ophthalmic Solution *see* phenylephrine *on page 411*

AK-Fluor® Injection *see* fluorescein sodium *on page 227*

AK-Homatropine® Ophthalmic *see* homatropine *on page 261*

Akineton® *see* biperiden *on page 67*

AK-NaCl® [OTC] *see* sodium chloride *on page 483*

AK-Nefrin® Ophthalmic Solution *see* phenylephrine *on page 411*

Akne-Mycin® Topical *see* erythromycin, topical *on page 201*

AK-Neo-Dex® Ophthalmic *see* neomycin and dexamethasone *on page 368*

AK-Pentolate® *see* cyclopentolate *on page 143*

AK-Poly-Bac® Ophthalmic *see* bacitracin and polymyxin b *on page 53*

AK-Pred® Ophthalmic *see* prednisolone *on page 434*

AKPro® Ophthalmic *see* dipivefrin *on page 176*

AK-Spore H.C.® Ophthalmic Ointment *see* bacitracin, neomycin, polymyxin b, and hydrocortisone *on page 53*

AK-Spore H.C.® Ophthalmic Suspension *see* neomycin, polymyxin b, and hydrocortisone *on page 369*

AK-Spore H.C.® Otic *see* neomycin, polymyxin b, and hydrocortisone *on page 369*

AK-Spore® Ophthalmic Ointment *see* bacitracin, neomycin, and polymyxin b *on page 53*

AK-Spore® Ophthalmic Solution *see* neomycin, polymyxin b, and gramicidin *on page 369*

AK-Sulf® Ophthalmic *see* sulfacetamide sodium *on page 496*

AK-Taine® *see* proparacaine *on page 444*

AKTob® Ophthalmic *see* tobramycin *on page 521*

AK-Tracin® Ophthalmic *see* bacitracin *on page 52*

AK-Trol® *see* neomycin, polymyxin b, and dexamethasone *on page 369*

Akwa Tears® Solution [OTC] *see* artificial tears *on page 42*

Ala-Cort® *see* hydrocortisone *on page 268*

Ala-Scalp® *see* hydrocortisone *on page 268*

Albalon-A® **Ophthalmic** *see* naphazoline and antazoline *on page 365*

Albalon® **Liquifilm**® **Ophthalmic** *see* naphazoline *on page 364*

albendazole (al BEN da zole)

Brand Names Albenza®

Therapeutic Category Anthelmintic

Use Treatment of parenchymal neurocysticercosis and cystic hydatid disease of the liver, lung, and peritoneum; albendazole may also be useful in the treatment of ascariasis, trichuriasis, enterobiasis, hook worm, strongyloidiasis, giardiasis, and microsporidiosis in AIDS

Usual Dosage Oral:

Children ≤2 years:

Neurocysticercosis: 15 mg/kg for 8 days; repeat as necessary

Hookworm, pinworm, roundworm: 200 mg as a single dose; may be repeated in 3 weeks

Strongyloidiasis and tapeworm: 200 mg/day for 3 days; may repeat in 3 weeks

Children >2 years and Adults:

Hydatid cyst: 400 mg twice daily with meals for 3 cycles (each cycle consists of 28 days of dosing followed by a 14-day albendazole-free interval)

Neurocysticercosis: 400 mg twice daily for 8-30 days

Roundworm, pinworm, hookworm: 400 mg as a single dose; treatment may be repeated in 3 weeks

Giardiasis: Strongyloidiasis and tapeworm: 400 mg/day for 3 days; treatment may be repeated in 3 weeks (giardiasis is a single course)

Dosage Forms Tablet: 200 mg

Albenza® *see* albendazole *on this page*

albumin (al BYOO min)

Synonyms albumin (human)

Brand Names Albuminar®; Albumisol®; Albunex®; Albutein®; Buminate®; Plasbumin®

Therapeutic Category Blood Product Derivative

Use Treatment of hypovolemia; plasma volume expansion and maintenance of cardiac output in the treatment of certain types of shock or impending shock; hypoproteinemia resulting in generalized edema or decreased intravascular volume (eg, hypoproteinemia associated with acute nephrotic syndrome, premature infants)

Usual Dosage 5% should be used in hypovolemic patients; 25% should be used in patients in whom fluid and sodium intake must be minimized

Children: Emergency initial dose: 25 g; nonemergencies: 25% to 50% of the adult dose

Adults: Depends on condition of patient, usual adult dose is 25 g; no more than 250 g should be administered within 48 hours

Hypoproteinemia: I.V.: 0.5-1 g/kg/dose; repeat every 1-2 days as calculated to replace ongoing losses

Hypovolemia: I.V.: 0.5-1 g/kg/dose; repeat as needed; maximum dose: 6 g/kg/day

Dosage Forms Injection, as human: 5% [50 mg/mL] (50 mL, 250 mL, 500 mL, 1000 mL); 25% [250 mg/mL] (10 mL, 20 mL, 50 mL, 100 mL)

Albuminar® *see* albumin *on this page*

albumin (human) *see* albumin *on this page*

Albumisol® *see* albumin *on this page*

Albunex® *see* albumin *on this page*

Albutein® *see* albumin *on this page*

albuterol (al BYOO ter ole)

Synonyms salbutamol
Brand Names Airet®; Proventil®; Proventil® HFA; Ventolin®; Ventolin® Rotocaps®; Volmax®
Therapeutic Category Adrenergic Agonist Agent
Use Bronchodilator in reversible airway obstruction due to asthma or COPD
Usual Dosage
Oral:
2-6 years: 0.1-0.2 mg/kg/dose 3 times/day; maximum dose not to exceed 12 mg/day (divided doses)
6-12 years: 2 mg/dose 3-4 times/day; maximum dose not to exceed 24 mg/day (divided doses)
>12 years: 2-4 mg/dose 3-4 times/day; maximum dose not to exceed 32 mg/day (divided doses)
Inhalation MDI: 90 mcg/spray:
<12 years: 1-2 inhalations 4 times/day using a tube spacer
≥12 years: 1-2 inhalations every 4-6 hours
Exercise-induced bronchospasm: 2 inhalations 15 minutes before exercising
Inhalation: Nebulization: 2.5 mg = 0.5 mL of the 0.5% inhalation solution to be diluted in 1-2.5 mL of NS
<5 years: 1.25-2.5 mg every 4-6 hours as needed
>5 years: 2.5-5 mg every 4-6 hours
Dosage Forms
Aerosol (Proventil®, Ventolin®): 90 mcg/dose (17 g) [200 doses]
Chlorofluorocarbon free (Proventil® HFA): 90 mcg/dose (17 g)
Capsule for oral inhalation (Ventolin® Rotocaps®): 200 mcg [to be used with Rotahaler® inhalation device]
Solution, inhalation: 0.083% (3 mL); 0.5% (20 mL)
Airet®: 0.083%
Proventil®: 0.083% (3 mL); 0.5% (20 mL)
Ventolin®: 0.5% (20 mL)
Syrup, as sulfate: 2 mg/5 mL (480 mL)
Proventil®, Ventolin®: 2 mg/5 mL (480 mL)
Tablet, as sulfate: 2 mg, 4 mg
Proventil®, Ventolin®: 2 mg, 4 mg
Tablet, extended release:
Proventil® Repetabs®: 4 mg
Volmax®: 4 mg, 8 mg

Alcaine® *see* proparacaine *on page 444*

alclometasone (al kloe MET a sone)

Synonyms alclometasone dipropionate
Brand Names Aclovate® Topical
Therapeutic Category Corticosteroid, Topical
Use Inflammation of corticosteroid-responsive dermatosis
Usual Dosage Topical: Apply a thin film to the affected area 2-3 times/day
Dosage Forms
Cream, as dipropionate: 0.05% (15 g, 45 g, 60 g)
Ointment, topical, as dipropionate: 0.05% (15 g, 45 g, 60 g)

alclometasone dipropionate *see* alclometasone *on this page*

alcohol, ethyl (AL koe hol, ETH il)

Synonyms ethanol
Brand Names Lavacol® [OTC]
Therapeutic Category Intravenous Nutritional Therapy; Pharmaceutical Aid

Use Topical anti-infective; pharmaceutical aid; an antidote for ethylene glycol overdose; an antidote for methanol overdose

Usual Dosage

I.V.: Doses of 100-125 mg/kg/hour to maintain blood levels of 100 mg/dL are recommended after a loading dose of 0.6 g/kg; maximum dose: 400 mL of a 5% solution within 1 hour

Topical: Use as needed

Dosage Forms

Injection, absolute: 2 mL

Liquid, topical, denatured: 70% (473 mL)

Solution, inhalation: 20%, 40%

Alconefrin® Nasal Solution [OTC] *see* phenylephrine *on page 411*

Aldactazide® *see* hydrochlorothiazide and spironolactone *on page 265*

Aldactone® *see* spironolactone *on page 491*

Aldara® *see* imiquimod *on page 281*

aldesleukin (al des LOO kin)

Synonyms interleukin-2

Brand Names Proleukin®

Therapeutic Category Biological Response Modulator

Use Primarily investigated in tumors known to have a response to immunotherapy, such as melanoma and renal cell carcinoma; has been used in conjunction with LAK cells, TIL cells, IL-1, and interferon

Usual Dosage All orders should be written in million International units (million IU) (refer to individual protocols)

Adults: Metastatic renal cell carcinoma:

Treatment consists of two 5-day treatment cycles separated by a rest period. 600,000 units/kg (0.037 mg/kg)/dose administered every 8 hours by a 15-minute I.V. infusion for a total of 14 doses; following 9 days of rest, the schedule is repeated for another 14 doses, for a maximum of 28 doses per course.

Investigational regimen: I.V. continuous infusion: 4.5 million units/m²/day in 250-1000 mL of D_5W for 5 days

Dose modification: Hold or interrupt a dose rather than reducing dose; refer to protocol

Retreatment: Patients should be evaluated for response ~4 weeks after completion of a course of therapy and again immediately prior to the scheduled start of the next treatment course. Additional courses of treatment may be administered to patients only if there is some tumor shrinkage following the last course and retreatment is not contraindicated. Each treatment course should be separated by a rest period of at least 7 weeks from the date of hospital discharge. Tumors have continued to regress up to 12 months following the initiation of therapy.

Dosage Forms Powder for injection, lyophilized: 22×10^6 IU [18 million IU/mL = 1.1 mg/mL when reconstituted]

Aldoclor® *see* chlorothiazide and methyldopa *on page 111*

Aldomet® *see* methyldopa *on page 341*

Aldoril® *see* methyldopa and hydrochlorothiazide *on page 341*

alendronate (a LEN droe nate)

Synonyms alendronate sodium

Brand Names Fosamax®

Therapeutic Category Bisphosphonate Derivative

Use Symptomatic treatment of Paget's disease and heterotopic ossification due to spinal cord injury or after total hip replacement, hypercalcemia associated with malignancy

(Continued)

15

alendronate *(Continued)*

Usual Dosage Oral:
Adults: Patients with osteoporosis or Paget's disease should receive supplemental calcium and vitamin D if dietary intake is inadequate
Osteoporosis in postmenopausal women: 10 mg once daily. Safety of treatment for >4 years has not been studied (extension studies are ongoing).
Paget's disease of bone: 40 mg once daily for 6 months
Retreatment: Relapses during the 12 months following therapy occurred in 9% of patients who responded to treatment. Specific retreatment data are not available. Retreatment with alendronate may be considered, following a 6-month post-treatment evaluation period, in patients who have relapsed based on increases in serum alkaline phosphatase, which should be measured periodically. Retreatment may also be considered in those who failed to normalize their serum alkaline phosphatase.
Elderly: No dosage adjustment is necessary
Dosage Forms Tablet, as sodium: 10 mg, 40 mg

alendronate sodium *see alendronate on previous page*

Alesse® *see ethinyl estradiol and levonorgestrel on page 208*

Aleve® [OTC] *see naproxen on page 365*

Alfenta® Injection *see alfentanil on this page*

alfentanil (al FEN ta nil)

Synonyms alfentanil hydrochloride
Brand Names Alfenta® Injection
Therapeutic Category Analgesic, Narcotic; General Anesthetic
Controlled Substance C-II
Use Analgesia; analgesia adjunct; anesthetic agent
Usual Dosage Doses should be titrated to appropriate effects; wide range of doses is dependent upon desired degree of analgesia/anesthesia

Children <12 years: Dose not established
Adults: Anesthesia of ≤30 minutes: Initial (induction): 8-20 mcg/kg, then 3-5 mcg/kg/dose or 0.5-1 mcg/kg/minute for maintenance; total dose: 8-40 mcg/kg; higher doses used for longer anesthesia required procedures
Dosage Forms Injection, preservative free, as hydrochloride: 500 mcg/mL (2 mL, 5 mL, 10 mL, 20 mL)

alfentanil hydrochloride *see alfentanil on this page*

Alferon® N *see interferon alfa-n3 on page 286*

alglucerase (al GLOO ser ase)

Synonyms glucocerebrosidase
Brand Names Ceredase®
Therapeutic Category Enzyme
Use Long-term enzyme replacement in patients with confirmed Type I Gaucher's disease who exhibit one or more of the following conditions: Moderate to severe anemia; thrombocytopenia and bleeding tendencies; bone disease; hepatomegaly or splenomegaly
Usual Dosage I.V. infusion: Administer 20-60 units/kg with a frequency ranging from 3 times/week to once every 2 weeks
Dosage Forms Injection: 10 units/mL (5 mL); 80 units/mL (5 mL)

Alkaban-AQ® *see vinblastine on page 550*

Alka-Mints® [OTC] *see calcium carbonate on page 82*

Alka-Seltzer® Plus Cold Liqui-Gels Capsules [OTC] *see acetaminophen, chlorpheniramine, and pseudoephedrine on page 5*

Alka-Seltzer® Plus Flu & Body Aches Non-Drowsy Liqui-Gels [OTC] *see* acetaminophen, dextromethorphan, and pseudoephedrine *on page 6*

Alkeran® *see* melphalan *on page 327*

Allbee® With C [OTC] *see* vitamin b complex with vitamin c *on page 553*

Allegra® *see* fexofenadine *on page 222*

Aller-Chlor® [OTC] *see* chlorpheniramine *on page 113*

Allercon® Tablet [OTC] *see* triprolidine and pseudoephedrine *on page 536*

Allerest® 12 Hour Capsule [OTC] *see* chlorpheniramine and phenylpropanolamine *on page 114*

Allerest® 12 Hour Nasal Solution [OTC] *see* oxymetazoline *on page 390*

Allerest® Eye Drops [OTC] *see* naphazoline *on page 364*

Allerest® Maximum Strength [OTC] *see* chlorpheniramine and pseudoephedrine *on page 114*

Allerest® No Drowsiness [OTC] *see* acetaminophen and pseudoephedrine *on page 5*

Allerfrin® Syrup [OTC] *see* triprolidine and pseudoephedrine *on page 536*

Allerfrin® Tablet [OTC] *see* triprolidine and pseudoephedrine *on page 536*

Allerfrin® w/Codeine *see* triprolidine, pseudoephedrine, and codeine *on page 537*

Allergan® Ear Drops *see* antipyrine and benzocaine *on page 38*

AllerMax® Oral [OTC] *see* diphenhydramine *on page 173*

Allerphed Syrup [OTC] *see* triprolidine and pseudoephedrine *on page 536*

allopurinol (al oh PURE i nole)

Brand Names Zyloprim®

Therapeutic Category Xanthine Oxidase Inhibitor

Use Prevention of attacks of gouty arthritis and nephropathy; also used to treat secondary hyperuricemia which may occur during treatment of tumors or leukemia; prevent recurrent calcium oxalate calculi

Usual Dosage Oral:

Children: 10 mg/kg/day in 2-3 divided doses or 200-300 mg/m^2/day in 2-4 divided doses, maximum: 600 mg/24 hours

Alternative:

<6 years: 150 mg/day in 3 divided doses

6-10 years: 300 mg/day in 2-3 divided doses

Children >10 years and Adults: Daily doses >300 mg should be administered in divided doses

Myeloproliferative neoplastic disorders: 600-800 mg/day in 2-3 divided doses for prevention of acute uric acid nephropathy for 2-3 days starting 1-2 days before chemotherapy

Gout: 200-300 mg/day (mild); 400-600 mg/day (severe)

Maximum dose: 800 mg/day

Dosage Forms Tablet: 100 mg, 300 mg

All-*trans*-Retinoic Acid *see* tretinoin (oral) *on page 527*

Alomide® Ophthalmic *see* lodoxamide tromethamine *on page 312*

Alor® 5/500 *see* hydrocodone and aspirin *on page 266*

Alora® Transdermal *see* estradiol *on page 202*

alpha$_1$-PI *see* alpha$_1$-proteinase inhibitor *on next page*

17

alpha₁-proteinase inhibitor (al fa won PRO tee in ase in HI bi tor)

Synonyms alpha₁-PI
Brand Names Prolastin® Injection
Therapeutic Category Antitrypsin Deficiency Agent
Use Congenital alpha₁-antitrypsin deficiency
Usual Dosage Adults: I.V.: 60 mg/kg once weekly
Dosage Forms Injection (human): 500 mg alpha₁-PI (20 mL diluent); 1000 mg alpha ₁-PI (40 mL diluent)

Alphagan® *see* brimonidine *on page 71*

Alphamul® [OTC] *see* castor oil *on page 95*

AlphaNine® SD *see* factor ix complex (human) *on page 215*

Alphatrex® *see* betamethasone *on page 64*

alprazolam (al PRAY zoe lam)

Brand Names Xanax®
Therapeutic Category Benzodiazepine
Controlled Substance C-IV
Use Treatment of anxiety; adjunct in the treatment of depression; management of panic attacks
Usual Dosage Oral:
Children <18 years: Dose not established
Adults: 0.25-0.5 mg 2-3 times/day, titrate dose upward; maximum: 4 mg/day (anxiety); 10 mg/day (panic attacks)
Dosage Forms Tablet: 0.25 mg, 0.5 mg, 1 mg, 2 mg

alprostadil (al PROS ta dill)

Synonyms pge₁; prostaglandin e₁
Brand Names Caverject® Injection; Edex® Injection; Muse® Pellet; Prostin VR Pediatric® Injection
Therapeutic Category Prostaglandin
Use Temporary maintenance of patency of ductus arteriosus in neonates with ductal-dependent congenital cyanotic or acyanotic heart disease until surgery can be performed; these defects include cyanotic (eg, pulmonary atresia, pulmonary stenosis, tricuspid atresia, Fallot's tetralogy, transposition of the great vessels) and acyanotic (eg, interruption of aortic arch, coarctation of aorta, hypoplastic left ventricle) heart disease. Alprostadil has also been used investigationally for the treatment of pulmonary hypertension in infants and children with congenital heart defects with left-to-right shunts and primary graft nonfunction following liver transplant. Used in penile erectile dysfunction
Usual Dosage
Patent ductus arteriosus (Prostin VR Pediatric®):
I.V. continuous infusion into a large vein, or alternatively through an umbilical artery catheter placed at the ductal opening: 0.05-0.1 mcg/kg/minute with therapeutic response, rate is reduced to lowest effective dosage; with unsatisfactory response, rate is increased gradually; maintenance: 0.01-0.4 mcg/kg/minute

Alprostadil

Add 1 Ampul (500 mcg) to:	Concentration (mcg/mL)	Infusion Rate	
		mL/min/kg Needed to Infuse 0.1 mcg/kg/min	mL/kg/24 h
250 mL	2	0.05	72
100 mL	5	0.02	28.8
50 mL	10	0.01	14.4
25 mL	20	0.005	7.2

PGE_1 is usually given at an infusion rate of 0.1 mcg/kg/minute, but it is often possible to reduce the dosage to $\frac{1}{2}$ or even $\frac{1}{10}$ without losing the therapeutic effect. The mixing schedule is shown in the table.

Therapeutic response is indicated by increased pH in those with acidosis or by an increase in oxygenation (pO_2) usually evident within 30 minutes

Erectile dysfunction:

Caverject®:

Vasculogenic, psychogenic, or mixed etiology: Individualize dose by careful titration; usual dose: 2.5-60 mcg (doses >60 mcg are not recommended); initiate dosage titration at 2.5 mcg, increasing by 2.5 mcg to a dose of 5 mcg and then in increments of 5-10 mcg depending on the erectile response until the dose produces an erection suitable for intercourse, not lasting >1 hour; if there is absolutely no response to initial 2.5 mcg dose, the second dose may increased to 7.5 mcg, followed by increments of 5-10 mcg

Neurogenic etiology (eg, spinal cord injury): Initiate dosage titration at 1.25 mcg, increasing to a doses of 2.5 mcg and then 5 mcg; increase further in increments 5 mcg until the dose is reached that produces an erection suitable for intercourse, not lasting >1 hour

Note: Patient must stay in the physician's office until complete detumescence occurs; if there is no response, then the next higher dose may be given within 1 hour; if there is still no response, a 1-day interval before giving the next dose is recommended; increasing the dose or concentration in the treatment of impotence results in increasing pain and discomfort

Muse® Pellet: Intraurethral: Administer as needed to achieve an erection; duration of action: ~30-60 minutes; use only two systems per 24-hour period

Dosage Forms

Injection:

Caverject®: 5 mcg, 10 mcg, 20 mcg

Edex® Injection: 5 mcg, 10 mcg, 20 mcg, 40 mcg

Prostin VR Pediatric®: 500 mcg/mL (1 mL)

Pellet, urethral: 125 mcg, 250 mcg, 500 mcg, 1000 mcg

AL-R® [OTC] *see* chlorpheniramine *on page 113*

Altace™ *see* ramipril *on page 459*

alteplase (AL te plase)

Synonyms alteplase, recombinant; tissue plasminogen activator, recombinant; t-PA

Brand Names Activase® Injection

Therapeutic Category Thrombolytic Agent

Use Management of acute myocardial infarction for the lysis of thrombi in coronary arteries; management of acute massive pulmonary embolism (PE) in adults

Usual Dosage

Coronary artery thrombi: I.V.: Front loading dose: Total dose is 100 mg over 1.5 hours (for patients who weigh <65 kg, use 1.25 mg/kg/total dose). Add this dose to a 100 mL bag of 0.9% sodium chloride for a total volume of 200 mL. Infuse 15 mg (30 mL) over 1-2 minutes; infuse 50 mg (100 mL) over 30 minutes. Begin heparin 5000-10,000 unit bolus followed by continuous infusion of 1000 units/hour. Infuse 35 mg/hour (70 mL) for next 2 hours.

Acute pulmonary embolism: 100 mg over 2 hours

Dosage Forms Powder for injection, lyophilized (recombinant): 20 mg [11.6 million units] (20 mL); 50 mg [29 million units] (50 mL); 100 mg [58 million units] (100 mL)

alteplase, recombinant *see* alteplase *on this page*

ALternaGEL® [OTC] *see* aluminum hydroxide *on page 21*

altretamine (al TRET a meen)
Synonyms hexamethylmelamine
Brand Names Hexalen®
Therapeutic Category Antineoplastic Agent
Use Palliative treatment of persistent or recurrent ovarian cancer
Usual Dosage Adults: Oral (refer to protocol): 4-12 mg/kg/day in 3-4 divided doses for 21-90 days
Alternatively: 240-320 mg/m^2/day in 3-4 divided doses for 21 days, repeated every 6 weeks
Alternatively: 260 mg/m^2/day for 14-21 days of a 28-day cycle in 4 divided doses
Dosage Forms Capsule: 50 mg

Alu-Cap® [OTC] *see* aluminum hydroxide *on next page*

Aludrox® [OTC] *see* aluminum hydroxide and magnesium hydroxide *on next page*

aluminum acetate and acetic acid
(a LOO mi num AS e tate & a SEE tik AS id)
Synonyms acetic acid and aluminum acetate otic; Burow's otic
Brand Names Otic Domeboro®
Therapeutic Category Otic Agent, Anti-infective
Use Treatment of superficial infections of the external auditory canal
Usual Dosage Otic: Instill 4-6 drops in ear(s) every 2-3 hours
Dosage Forms Solution, otic: Aluminum acetate 10% and acetic acid 2% (60 mL)

aluminum acetate and calcium acetate
(a LOO mi num SUL fate & KAL see um AS e tate)
Brand Names Bluboro® [OTC]; Boropak® [OTC]; Domeboro® Topical [OTC]; Pedi-Boro® [OTC]
Therapeutic Category Topical Skin Product
Use Astringent wet dressing for relief of inflammatory conditions of the skin and to reduce weeping that may occur in dermatitis
Usual Dosage Topical: Soak affected area in the solution 2-4 times/day for 15-30 minutes or apply wet dressing soaked in the solution 2-4 times/day for 30-minute treatment periods; rewet dressing with solution every few minutes to keep it moist
Dosage Forms
Powder, to make topical solution: 1 packet/pint of water [1:40 solution]
Tablet, effervescent: 1 tablet/pint [1:40 dilution]

aluminum carbonate (a LOO mi num KAR bun ate)
Brand Names Basaljel® [OTC]
Therapeutic Category Antacid
Use Hyperacidity; hyperphosphatemia
Usual Dosage Adults: Oral:
Antacid: 2 tablets/capsules or 10 mL of suspension every 2 hours, up to 12 times/day
Hyperphosphatemia: 2 tablets/capsules or 12 mL of suspension with meals
Dosage Forms
Capsule: Equivalent to 500 mg aluminum hydroxide
Suspension: Equivalent to 400 mg/5 mL aluminum hydroxide
Tablet: Equivalent to 500 mg aluminum hydroxide

aluminum chloride hexahydrate
(a LOO mi num KLOR ide heks a HYE drate)
Brand Names Drysol™
Therapeutic Category Topical Skin Product
Use Astringent in the management of hyperhidrosis

Usual Dosage Adults: Topical: Apply at bedtime
Dosage Forms Solution, topical: 20% in SD alcohol 40 (35 mL, 37.5 mL)

aluminum hydroxide (a LOO mi num hye DROKS ide)
Brand Names ALternaGEL® [OTC]; Alu-Cap® [OTC]; Alu-Tab® [OTC]; Amphojel® [OTC]; Dialume® [OTC]; Nephrox Suspension [OTC]
Therapeutic Category Antacid
Use Hyperacidity; hyperphosphatemia
Usual Dosage Oral:
Peptic ulcer disease:
Children: 5-15 mL/dose every 3-6 hours or 1 and 3 hours after meals and at bedtime
Adults: 15-45 mL every 3-6 hours or 1 and 3 hours after meals and at bedtime
Prophylaxis against gastrointestinal bleeding:
Infants: 2-5 mL/dose every 1-2 hours
Children: 5-15 mL/dose every 1-2 hours
Adults: 30-60 mL/dose every hour
Titrate to maintain the gastric pH >5
Hyperphosphatemia:
Children: 50 mg to 150 mg/kg/24 hours in divided doses every 4-6 hours, titrate dosage to maintain serum phosphorus within normal range
Adults: 500-1800 mg, 3-6 times/day, between meals and at bedtime

Antacid: Adults: 30 mL 1 and 3 hours postprandial and at bedtime
Dosage Forms
Capsule:
Alu-Cap®: 400 mg
Dialume®: 500 mg
Liquid: 600 mg/5 mL
ALternaGEL®: 600 mg/5 mL
Suspension, oral: 320 mg/5 mL; 450 mg/5 mL; 675 mg/5 mL
Amphojel®: 320 mg/5 mL
Tablet:
Amphojel®: 300 mg, 600 mg
Alu-Tab®: 500 mg

aluminum hydroxide and magnesium carbonate
(a LOO mi num hye DROKS ide & mag NEE zhum KAR bun nate)
Brand Names Gaviscon® Liquid [OTC]
Therapeutic Category Antacid
Use Temporary relief of symptoms associated with gastric acidity
Usual Dosage Adults: Oral: 15-30 mL 4 times/day after meals and at bedtime
Dosage Forms Liquid: Aluminum hydroxide 95 mg and magnesium carbonate 358 mg per 15 mL

aluminum hydroxide and magnesium hydroxide
(a LOO mi num hye DROKS ide & mag NEE zhum hye DROK side)
Synonyms magnesium hydroxide and aluminum hydroxide
Brand Names Aludrox® [OTC]; Maalox® [OTC]; Maalox® Therapeutic Concentrate [OTC]
Therapeutic Category Antacid
Use Antacid, hyperphosphatemia in renal failure
Usual Dosage Adults: Oral: 5-10 mL or 1-2 tablets 4-6 times/day, between meals and at bedtime; may be used every hour for severe symptoms
Dosage Forms
Suspension:
Aludrox®: Aluminum hydroxide 307 mg and magnesium hydroxide 103 mg per 5 mL
Maalox®: Aluminum hydroxide 225 mg and magnesium hydroxide 200 mg per 5 mL
(Continued)

aluminum hydroxide and magnesium hydroxide *(Continued)*

High potency (Maalox® TC): Aluminum hydroxide 600 mg and magnesium hydroxide 300 mg per 5 mL

Tablet, chewable (Maalox®): Aluminum hydroxide 600 mg and magnesium hydroxide 300 mg

aluminum hydroxide and magnesium trisilicate

(a LOO mi num hye DROKS ide & mag NEE zhum trye SIL i kate)

Brand Names Gaviscon®-2 Tablet [OTC]; Gaviscon® Tablet [OTC]

Therapeutic Category Antacid

Use Temporary relief of hyperacidity

Usual Dosage Adults: Oral: Chew 2-4 tablets 4 times/day or as directed by physician

Dosage Forms Tablet, chewable:

Gaviscon®: Aluminum hydroxide 80 mg and magnesium trisilicate 20 mg

Gaviscon®-2: Aluminum hydroxide 160 mg and magnesium trisilicate 40 mg

aluminum hydroxide, magnesium hydroxide, and simethicone

(a LOO mi num hye DROKS ide, mag NEE zhum hye DROKS ide, & sye METH i kone)

Brand Names Di-Gel® [OTC]; Gas-Ban DS® [OTC]; Gelusil® [OTC]; Maalox® Plus [OTC]; Magalox Plus® [OTC]; Mylanta®-II [OTC]; Mylanta® [OTC]

Therapeutic Category Antacid; Antiflatulent

Use Temporary relief of hyperacidity associated with gas; may also be used for indications associated with other antacids

Usual Dosage Adults: Oral: 15-30 mL or 2-4 tablets 4-6 times/day between meals and at bedtime; may be used every hour for severe symptoms

Dosage Forms

Liquid:

Mylanta®: Aluminum hydroxide 200 mg, magnesium hydroxide, 200 mg, and simethicone 20 mg per 5 mL

Maalox® Plus: Aluminum hydroxide 225 mg, magnesium hydroxide 200 mg, and simethicone 25 mg per 5 mL (30 mL, 180 mL)

Mylanta®-II: Aluminum hydroxide 400 mg, magnesium hydroxide 400 mg, and simethicone 40 mg per 5 mL (150 mL, 360 mL)

Tablet, chewable:

Magalox Plus®: Aluminum hydroxide 200 mg, magnesium hydroxide 200 mg, and simethicone 25 mg

Mylanta®: Aluminum hydroxide 200 mg, magnesium hydroxide 200 mg, and simethicone 20 mg

Gas-Ban DS®, Mylanta®-II: Aluminum hydroxide 400 mg, magnesium hydroxide 400 mg, and simethicone 40 mg

aluminum sucrose sulfate, basic *see* sucralfate *on page 494*

Alupent® *see* metaproterenol *on page 332*

Alu-Tab® [OTC] *see* aluminum hydroxide *on previous page*

amantadine (a MAN ta deen)

Synonyms adamantanamine hydrochloride; amantadine hydrochloride

Brand Names Symmetrel®

Therapeutic Category Anti-Parkinson's Agent; Antiviral Agent

Use Prophylaxis and treatment of influenza A viral infection; symptomatic and adjunct treatment of parkinsonism

Usual Dosage Oral:

Children:

1-9 years: 4.4-8.8 mg/kg/day in 1-2 divided doses to a maximum of 150 mg/day

9-12 years: 100-200 mg/day in 1-2 divided doses

After first influenza A virus vaccine dose, amantadine prophylaxis may be administered for up to 6 weeks or until 2 weeks after the second dose of vaccine
Adults:
Parkinson's disease: 100 mg twice daily
Influenza A viral infection: 200 mg/day in 1-2 divided doses
Prophylaxis: Minimum 10-day course of therapy following exposure or continue for 2-3 weeks after influenza A virus vaccine is administered
Elderly patients should administer the drug in 2 daily doses rather than a single dose to avoid adverse neurologic reactions
Dosage Forms
Capsule, as hydrochloride: 100 mg
Syrup, as hydrochloride: 50 mg/5 mL (480 mL)

amantadine hydrochloride *see* amantadine *on previous page*
Amaphen® *see* butalbital compound and acetaminophen *on page 78*
Amaryl® *see* glimepiride *on page 241*

ambenonium (am be NOE nee um)
Synonyms ambenonium chloride
Brand Names Mytelase® Caplets®
Therapeutic Category Cholinergic Agent
Use Treatment of myasthenia gravis
Usual Dosage Adults: Oral: 5-25 mg 3-4 times/day
Dosage Forms Tablet, as chloride: 10 mg

ambenonium chloride *see* ambenonium *on this page*
Ambenyl® **Cough Syrup** *see* bromodiphenhydramine and codeine *on page 72*
Ambi 10® **[OTC]** *see* benzoyl peroxide *on page 61*
Ambien™ *see* zolpidem *on page 562*
Ambi® **Skin Tone [OTC]** *see* hydroquinone *on page 272*

amcinonide (am SIN oh nide)
Brand Names Cyclocort® Topical
Therapeutic Category Corticosteroid, Topical
Use Relief of the inflammatory and pruritic manifestations of corticosteroid-responsive dermatoses
Usual Dosage Adults: Topical: Apply in a thin film 2-3 times/day
Dosage Forms
Cream: 0.1% (15 g, 30 g, 60 g)
Lotion: 0.1% (20 mL, 60 mL)
Ointment, topical: 0.1% (15 g, 30 g, 60 g)

Amcort® *see* triamcinolone *on page 528*
Amen® **Oral** *see* medroxyprogesterone acetate *on page 326*
Americaine [OTC] *see* benzocaine *on page 59*
A-methaPred® **Injection** *see* methylprednisolone *on page 343*
amethocaine hydrochloride *see* tetracaine *on page 509*
amethopterin *see* methotrexate *on page 338*
amfepramone *see* diethylpropion *on page 166*
Amgenal® **Cough Syrup** *see* bromodiphenhydramine and codeine *on page 72*
Amicar® *see* aminocaproic acid *on page 25*
Amidate® **Injection** *see* etomidate *on page 213*

amifostine (am i FOS teen)
Synonyms ethiofos; gammaphos
Brand Names Ethyol®
Therapeutic Category Antidote
Use Protection against cisplatin-induced nephrotoxicity in advanced ovarian cancer patients; it may also provide protection from cisplatin-induced peripheral neuropathy
Usual Dosage I.V.: 910 mg/m^2 beginning 30 minutes before starting chemotherapy; dose adjustment is recommended for subsequent doses if the previous dose was interrupted, and not able to be resumed; secondary to hypotension, the recommended dose for subsequent administration is 740 mg/m^2
Dosage Forms Injection: 500 mg

amikacin (am i KAY sin)
Synonyms amikacin sulfate
Brand Names Amikin® Injection
Therapeutic Category Aminoglycoside (Antibiotic)
Use Treatment of documented gram-negative enteric infection resistant to gentamicin and tobramycin; documented infection of mycobacterial organisms susceptible to amikacin
Usual Dosage I.M., I.V.:
Infants and Children: 15-20 mg/kg/day divided every 8 hours
Adults: 15 mg/kg/day divided every 8-12 hours
Dosage Forms Injection, as sulfate: 50 mg/mL (2 mL, 4 mL); 250 mg/mL (2 mL, 4 mL)

amikacin sulfate *see* amikacin *on this page*

Amikin® Injection *see* amikacin *on this page*

amiloride (a MIL oh ride)
Synonyms amiloride hydrochloride
Brand Names Midamor®
Therapeutic Category Diuretic, Potassium Sparing
Use Counteract potassium loss induced by other diuretics in the treatment of hypertension or edematous conditions including CHF, hepatic cirrhosis and hypoaldosteronism; usually used in conjunction with a more potent diuretic such as thiazides or loop diuretics
Usual Dosage Oral:
Children: Although safety and efficacy have not been established by the FDA in children, a dosage of 0.625 mg/kg/day has been used in children weighing 6-20 kg
Adults: 5-10 mg/day (up to 20 mg)
Dosage Forms Tablet, as hydrochloride: 5 mg

amiloride and hydrochlorothiazide
(a MIL oh ride & hye droe klor oh THYE a zide)
Synonyms hydrochlorothiazide and amiloride
Brand Names Moduretic®
Therapeutic Category Diuretic, Combination
Use Antikaliuretic diuretic, antihypertensive
Usual Dosage Adults: Oral: Start with 1 tablet/day, then may be increased to 2 tablets/day if needed; usually administered in a single dose
Dosage Forms Tablet: Amiloride hydrochloride 5 mg and hydrochlorothiazide 50 mg

amiloride hydrochloride *see* amiloride *on this page*

Amin-Aid® [OTC] *see* enteral nutritional products *on page 194*

2-amino-6-mercaptopurine *see* thioguanine *on page 515*

2-amino-6-trifluoromethoxy-benzothiazole *see* riluzole *on page 466*

aminobenzylpenicillin *see* ampicillin *on page 33*

aminocaproic acid (a mee noe ka PROE ik AS id)
Brand Names Amicar®
Therapeutic Category Hemostatic Agent
Use Treatment of excessive bleeding resulting from systemic hyperfibrinolysis and urinary fibrinolysis
Usual Dosage In the management of acute bleeding syndromes, oral dosage regimens are the same as the I.V. dosage regimens in adults and children

Chronic bleeding: Oral, I.V.: 5-30 g/day in divided doses at 3- to 6-hour intervals
Acute bleeding syndrome:
Children: Oral, I.V.: 100 mg/kg or 3 g/m^2 during the first hour, followed by continuous infusion at the rate of 33.3 mg/kg/hour or 1 g/m^2/hour; total dosage should not exceed 18 g/m^2/24 hours
Adults:
Oral: For elevated fibrinolytic activity, administer 5 g during first hour, followed by 1-1.25 g/hour for approximately 8 hours or until bleeding stops
I.V.: Administer 4-5 g in 250 mL of diluent during first hour followed by continuous infusion at the rate of 1-1.25 g/hour in 50 mL of diluent, continue for 8 hours or until bleeding stops
Dosage Forms
Injection: 250 mg/mL (20 mL, 96 mL, 100 mL)
Syrup: 1.25 g/5 mL (480 mL)
Tablet: 500 mg

Amino-Cerv™ Vaginal Cream *see* urea *on page 542*

aminoglutethimide (a mee noe gloo TETH i mide)
Brand Names Cytadren®
Therapeutic Category Antineoplastic Agent
Use Suppression of adrenal function in selected patients with Cushing's syndrome; also used successfully in postmenopausal patients with advanced breast carcinoma and in patients with metastatic prostate carcinoma
Usual Dosage Adults: Oral: 250 mg every 6 hours, may be increased at 1- to 2-week intervals to a total of 2 g/day; administer in divided doses 2-3 times/day to reduce incidence of nausea and vomiting
Dosage Forms Tablet, scored: 250 mg

Amino-Opti-E® [OTC] *see* vitamin e *on page 553*

aminophylline (am in OFF i lin)
Synonyms theophylline ethylenediamine
Brand Names Phyllocontin®; Truphylline®
Therapeutic Category Theophylline Derivative
Use Bronchodilator in reversible airway obstruction due to asthma or COPD; increase diaphragmatic contractility; neonatal idiopathic apnea of prematurity
Usual Dosage
Neonates: Apnea of prematurity:
Loading dose: 5 mg/kg for one dose
Maintenance: I.V.:
0-24 days: Begin at 2 mg/kg/day divided every 12 hours and titrate to desired levels and effects
>24 days: 3 mg/kg/day divided every 12 hours; increased dosages may be indicated as liver metabolism matures (usually >30 days of life); monitor serum levels to determine appropriate dosages
Theophylline levels should be initially drawn after 3 days of therapy; repeat levels are indicated 3 days after each increase in dosage or weekly if on a stabilized dosage
(Continued)

aminophylline *(Continued)*

Treatment of acute bronchospasm:
Loading dose (in patients not currently receiving aminophylline or theophylline): 6 mg/kg (based on aminophylline) administered I.V. over 20-30 minutes; administration rate should not exceed 25 mg/minute (aminophylline)

Approximate I.V. maintenance dosages are based upon **continuous infusions**; bolus dosing (often used in children <6 months of age) may be determined by multiplying the hourly infusion rate by 24 hours and dividing by the desired number of doses/day
6 weeks to 6 months: 0.5 mg/kg/hour
6 months to 1 year: 0.6-0.7 mg/kg/hour
1-9 years: 1-1.2 mg/kg/hour
9-12 years and young adult smokers: 0.9 mg/kg/hour
12-16 years: 0.7 mg/kg/hour
Adults (healthy, nonsmoking): 0.7 mg/kg/hour
Older patients and patients with cor pulmonale, patients with congestive heart failure or liver failure: 0.25 mg/kg/hour
Dosage should be adjusted according to serum level measurements during the first 12- to 24-hour period; avoid using suppositories due to erratic, unreliable absorption.

Rectal: Adults: 500 mg 3 times/day
Dosage Forms
Injection, I.V.: 25 mg/mL (10 mL, 20 mL)
Liquid, oral: 105 mg/5 mL (240 mL)
Suppository, rectal (Truphylline®): 250 mg, 500 mg
Tablet: 100 mg, 200 mg
Controlled release [12 hours] (Phyllocontin®): 225 mg

aminophylline, amobarbital, and ephedrine

(am in OFF i lin, am oh BAR bi tal, & e FED rin)
Therapeutic Category Theophylline Derivative
Use Symptomatic relief of asthma
Usual Dosage Adults: Oral: 1 capsule every 6 hours
Dosage Forms Capsule: Aminophylline 130 mg, amobarbital 24 mg, and ephedrine sulfate 24 mg

aminosalicylate sodium (a MEE noe sa LIS i late SOW dee um)

Synonyms para-aminosalicylate sodium; PAS
Therapeutic Category Nonsteroidal Anti-Inflammatory Agent (NSAID)
Use Treatment of tuberculosis with combination drugs
Usual Dosage Oral:
Children: 150-300 mg/kg/day in 3-4 equally divided doses
Adults: 150 mg/kg/day in 2-3 equally divided doses (usually 12-14 g/day)
Dosage Forms Tablet: 500 mg

5-aminosalicylic acid *see* mesalamine *on page 331*

amiodarone (a MEE oh da rone)

Synonyms amiodarone hydrochloride
Brand Names Cordarone®
Therapeutic Category Antiarrhythmic Agent, Class III
Use Management of resistant, life-threatening ventricular arrhythmias unresponsive to conventional therapy with less toxic agents; also used for treatment of supraventricular arrhythmias unresponsive to conventional therapy; injectable available from manufacturer via orphan drug status or compassionate use for acute treatment and prophylaxis of life-threatening ventricular tachycardia or ventricular fibrillation (see Dosage Forms)
Usual Dosage Children <1 year should be dosed as calculated by body surface area
Children: Loading dose: 10-15 mg/kg/day or 600-800 mg/1.73 m^2/day for 4-14 days or until adequate control of arrhythmia or prominent adverse effects occur (this loading

dose may be administered in 1-2 divided doses/day); dosage should then be reduced to 5 mg/kg/day or 200-400 mg/1.73 m^2/day administered once daily for several weeks; if arrhythmia does not recur reduce to lowest effective dosage possible; usual daily minimal dose: 2.5 mg/kg; maintenance doses may be administered for 5 of 7 days/week

Adults: Ventricular arrhythmias: 800-1600 mg/day in 1-2 doses for 1-3 weeks, then 600-800 mg/day in 1-2 doses for 1 month; maintenance: 400 mg/day; lower doses are recommended for supraventricular arrhythmias, usually 100-400 mg/day

Dosage Forms
Injection, as hydrochloride: 50 mg/mL with benzyl alcohol (3 mL)
Tablet, scored, as hydrochloride: 200 mg

amiodarone hydrochloride *see* amiodarone *on previous page*
Ami-Tex LA® *see* guaifenesin and phenylpropanolamine *on page 249*
Amitone® [OTC] *see* calcium carbonate *on page 82*

amitriptyline (a mee TRIP ti leen)
Synonyms amitriptyline hydrochloride
Brand Names Elavil®
Therapeutic Category Antidepressant, Tricyclic (Tertiary Amine)
Use Treatment of various forms of depression, often in conjunction with psychotherapy; analgesic for certain chronic and neuropathic pain; migraine prophylaxis
Usual Dosage
Children <12 years: Not recommended
Adolescents: Oral: Initial: 25-50 mg/day; may administer in divided doses; increase gradually to 100 mg/day in divided doses
Adults:
Oral: 30-100 mg/day single dose at bedtime or in divided doses; dose may be gradually increased up to 300 mg/day; once symptoms are controlled, decrease gradually to lowest effective dose
I.M.: 20-30 mg 4 times/day
Dosage Forms
Injection, as hydrochloride: 10 mg/mL (10 mL)
Tablet, as hydrochloride: 10 mg, 25 mg, 50 mg, 75 mg, 100 mg, 150 mg

amitriptyline and chlordiazepoxide
(a mee TRIP ti leen & klor dye az e POKS ide)
Synonyms chlordiazepoxide and amitriptyline
Brand Names Limbitrol® DS 10-25
Therapeutic Category Antidepressant, Tricyclic (Tertiary Amine)
Controlled Substance C-IV
Use Treatment of moderate to severe anxiety and/or agitation and depression
Usual Dosage Oral: Initial: 3-4 tablets in divided doses; this may be increased to 6 tablets/day as required; some patients respond to smaller doses and can be maintained on 2 tablets
Dosage Forms Tablet:
5-12.5: Amitriptyline hydrochloride 12.5 mg and chlordiazepoxide 5 mg
10-25: Amitriptyline hydrochloride 25 mg and chlordiazepoxide 10 mg

amitriptyline and perphenazine (a mee TRIP ti leen & per FEN a zeen)
Synonyms perphenazine and amitriptyline
Brand Names Etrafon®; Triavil®
Therapeutic Category Antidepressant/Phenothiazine
Use Treatment of patients with moderate to severe anxiety and depression
Usual Dosage Oral: 1 tablet 2-4 times/day
Dosage Forms Tablet:
2-10: Amitriptyline hydrochloride 10 mg and perphenazine 2 mg
(Continued)

amitriptyline and perphenazine *(Continued)*
4-10: Amitriptyline hydrochloride 10 mg and perphenazine 4 mg
2-25: Amitriptyline hydrochloride 25 mg and perphenazine 2 mg
4-25: Amitriptyline hydrochloride 25 mg and perphenazine 4 mg
4-50: Amitriptyline hydrochloride 50 mg and perphenazine 4 mg

amitriptyline hydrochloride *see* amitriptyline *on previous page*

amlexanox (am LEKS an oks)
Brand Names Aphthasol®
Therapeutic Category Anti-inflammatory, Locally Applied
Use Treating signs a symptoms of canker sores (minor aphthous ulcers)
Usual Dosage Administer directly on ulcers 4 times/day following oral hygiene, after meals, and before going to bed
Dosage Forms Paste: 5%

amlodipine (am LOE di peen)
Brand Names Norvasc®
Therapeutic Category Calcium Channel Blocker
Use Treatment of hypertension alone or in combination with antihypertensives; chronic stable angina alone or with other antianginal agents; vasospastic angina alone or in combination with other agents
Usual Dosage Oral:
Adults: 2.5-10 mg once daily
Elderly: 2.5 mg once daily; increase by 2.5 mg increments at 7- to 14-day intervals; maximum recommended dose: 10 mg/day
Dosage Forms Tablet: 2.5 mg, 5 mg, 10 mg

amlodipine and benazepril (am LOE di peen & ben AY ze pril)
Brand Names Lotrel™
Therapeutic Category Antihypertensive, Combination
Use Treatment of hypertension
Usual Dosage Adults: Oral: 1 capsule daily
Dosage Forms Capsule:
Amlodipine 2.5 mg and benazepril hydrochloride 10 mg
Amlodipine 5 mg and benazepril hydrochloride 10 mg
Amlodipine 5 mg and benazepril hydrochloride 20 mg

Ammonapse *see* sodium phenylbutyrate *on page 486*

ammonia spirit, aromatic (a MOE nee ah SPEAR it, air oh MAT ik)
Synonyms smelling salts
Brand Names Aromatic Ammonia Aspirols®
Therapeutic Category Respiratory Stimulant
Use Respiratory and circulatory stimulant; treatment of fainting
Usual Dosage Used as "smelling salts" to treat or prevent fainting
Dosage Forms
Inhalant, crushable glass perles: 0.33 mL, 0.4 mL
Solution: 30 mL, 60 mL, 120 mL

ammonium chloride (a MOE nee um KLOR ide)
Therapeutic Category Electrolyte Supplement
Use Diuretic or systemic and urinary acidifying agent; treatment of hypochloremic states
Usual Dosage
Children: Oral, I.V.: 75 mg/kg/day in 4 divided doses for urinary acidification; maximum daily dose: 6 g

Adults:
Oral: 2-3 g every 6 hours
I.V.: 1.5 g/dose every 6 hours
Dosage Forms
Injection: 26.75% [5 mEq/mL] (20 mL)
Tablet: 500 mg
Enteric coated: 500 mg

ammonium lactate *see* lactic acid with ammonium hydroxide *on page 300*

Amnipaque® *see* radiological/contrast media (non-ionic) *on page 459*

amobarbital (am oh BAR bi tal)

Synonyms amylobarbitone
Brand Names Amytal®
Therapeutic Category Barbiturate
Controlled Substance C-II
Use
Oral: Hypnotic in short-term treatment of insomnia, to reduce anxiety and provide sedation preoperatively
I.M., I.V.: Used to control status epilepticus or acute seizure episodes; also used in catatonic, negativistic, or manic reactions and in "Amytal® Interviewing" for narcoanalysis
Usual Dosage
Children: Oral:
Insomnia: 2 mg/kg or 70 mg/m^2/day in 4 equally divided doses
Hypnotic: 2-3 mg/kg
Adults:
Insomnia: Oral: 65-200 mg at bedtime
Sedation: Oral: 30-50 mg 2-3 times/day
Preanesthetic: Oral: 200 mg 1-2 hours before surgery
Hypnotic:
Oral: 65-200 mg at bedtime
I.M.: 65-500 mg, should not exceed 500 mg
I.V.: 65-500 mg, should not exceed 1000 mg
Dosage Forms
Capsule, as sodium: 65 mg, 200 mg
Injection, as sodium: 250 mg, 500 mg
Tablet: 30 mg, 50 mg, 100 mg

amobarbital and secobarbital (am oh BAR bi tal & see koe BAR bi tal)

Synonyms secobarbital and amobarbital
Brand Names Tuinal®
Therapeutic Category Barbiturate
Controlled Substance C-II
Use Short-term treatment of insomnia
Usual Dosage Adults: Oral: 1-2 capsules at bedtime
Dosage Forms Capsule:
100: Amobarbital 50 mg and secobarbital 50 mg
200: Amobarbital 100 mg and secobarbital 100 mg

AMO Vitrax® *see* sodium hyaluronate *on page 485*

amoxapine (a MOKS a peen)

Brand Names Asendin®
Therapeutic Category Antidepressant, Tricyclic (Secondary Amine)
Use Treatment of neurotic and endogenous depression and mixed symptoms of anxiety and depression
(Continued)

amoxapine *(Continued)*

Usual Dosage Oral (once symptoms are controlled, decrease gradually to lowest effective dose):

Children <16 years: Dose not established
Adolescents: Initial: 25-50 mg/day; increase gradually to 100 mg/day; may administer as divided doses or as a single dose at bedtime
Adults: Initial: 25 mg 2-3 times/day, if tolerated, dosage may be increased to 100 mg 2-3 times/day; may be administered in a single bedtime dose when dosage <300 mg/day
Maximum daily dose:
Outpatient: 400 mg
Inpatient: 600 mg
Dosage Forms Tablet: 25 mg, 50 mg, 100 mg, 150 mg

amoxicillin (a moks i SIL in)

Synonyms amoxicillin trihydrate; amoxycillin; *p*-hydroxyampicillin
Brand Names Amoxil®; Biomox®; Polymox®; Trimox®; Wymox®
Therapeutic Category Penicillin
Use Treatment of otitis media, sinusitis, and infections involving the respiratory tract, skin, and urinary tract due to susceptible *H. influenzae*, *N. gonorrhoeae*, *E. coli*, *P. mirabilis*, *E. faecalis*, streptococci, and nonpenicillinase-producing staphylococci; prophylaxis of bacterial endocarditis
Usual Dosage Oral:
Children: 25-50 mg/kg/day in divided doses every 8 hours
Uncomplicated gonorrhea: ≥2 years: 50 mg/kg plus probenecid 25 mg/kg in a single dose; do not use this regimen in children <2 years of age, probenecid is contraindicated in this age group
SBE prophylaxis: 50 mg/kg 1 hour before procedure and 25 mg/kg 6 hours later; not to exceed adult dosage
Adults: 250-500 mg every 8 hours; maximum dose: 2-3 g/day
Uncomplicated gonorrhea: 3 g plus probenecid 1 g in a single dose
Endocarditis prophylaxis: 3 g 1 hour before procedure and 1.5 g 6 hours later
Dosage Forms
Capsule, as trihydrate: 250 mg, 500 mg
Powder for oral suspension:
As trihydrate: 125 mg/5 mL (5 mL, 80 mL, 100 mL, 150 mL, 200 mL); 250 mg/5 mL (5 mL, 80 mL, 100 mL, 150 mL, 200 mL)
Drops, as trihydrate: 50 mg/mL (15 mL, 30 mL)
Tablet, chewable, as trihydrate: 125 mg, 250 mg

amoxicillin and clavulanate potassium

(a moks i SIL in & klav yoo LAN ate poe TASS ee um)
Synonyms amoxicillin and clavulanic acid
Brand Names Augmentin®
Therapeutic Category Penicillin
Use Infections caused by susceptible organisms involving the lower respiratory tract, otitis media, sinusitis, skin and skin structure, and urinary tract; spectrum same as amoxicillin in addition to beta-lactamase producing *B. catarrhalis*, *H. influenzae*, *N. gonorrhoeae*, and *S. aureus* (not MRSA)
Usual Dosage Oral:
Children ≤40 kg: 20-40 mg (amoxicillin)/kg/day in divided doses every 8 hours
Children >40 kg and Adults: 250-500 mg every 8 hours or 875 mg every 12 hours
Dosage Forms
Suspension, oral:
125 (banana flavor): Amoxicillin trihydrate 125 mg and clavulanate potassium 31.25 mg per 5 mL (75 mL, 150 mL)
200: Amoxicillin 200 mg and clavulanate potassium 28.5 mg per 5 mL (50 mL, 75 mL, 100 mL)

250 (orange flavor): Amoxicillin trihydrate 250 mg and clavulanate potassium 62.5 mg per 5 mL (75 mL, 150 mL)
400: Amoxicillin 400 mg and clavulanate potassium 57 mg per 5 mL (50 mL, 75 mL, 100 mL)
Tablet:
250: Amoxicillin trihydrate 250 mg and clavulanate potassium 125 mg
500: Amoxicillin trihydrate 500 mg and clavulanate potassium 125 mg
875: Amoxicillin trihydrate 875 mg and clavulanate potassium 125 mg
Tablet, chewable:
125: Amoxicillin trihydrate 125 mg and clavulanate potassium 31.25 mg
200: Amoxicillin trihydrate 200 mg and clavulanate potassium 28.5 mg
250: Amoxicillin trihydrate 250 mg and clavulanate potassium 62.5 mg
400: Amoxicillin trihydrate 400 mg and clavulanate potassium 57 mg

amoxicillin and clavulanic acid *see* amoxicillin and clavulanate potassium *on previous page*

amoxicillin trihydrate *see* amoxicillin *on previous page*

Amoxil® *see* amoxicillin *on previous page*

amoxycillin *see* amoxicillin *on previous page*

amphetamine (am FET a meen)
Synonyms amphetamine sulfate
Therapeutic Category Amphetamine
Controlled Substance C-II
Use Narcolepsy; exogenous obesity; abnormal behavioral syndrome in children (minimal brain dysfunction); attention deficit hyperactive disorder (ADHD)
Usual Dosage Oral:
Narcolepsy:
Children:
6-12 years: 5 mg/day, increase by 5 mg at weekly intervals
>12 years: 10 mg/day, increase by 10 mg at weekly intervals
Adults: 5-60 mg/day in divided doses
Minimal brain dysfunction: Children:
3-5 years: 2.5 mg/day, increase by 2.5 mg at weekly intervals
>6 years: 5 mg/day, increase by 5 mg at weekly intervals
Short-term adjunct to exogenous obesity: Children >12 years and Adults: 10 mg or 15 mg long-acting capsule daily, up to 30 mg/day; or 5-30 mg/day in divided doses (immediate release tablets only)
Dosage Forms Tablet, as sulfate: 5 mg, 10 mg

amphetamine sulfate *see* amphetamine *on this page*

ampho *see* amphotericin B *on this page*

Amphojel® [OTC] *see* aluminum hydroxide *on page 21*

Amphotec® *see* amphotericin B colloidal dispersion *on next page*

amphotericin B (am foe TER i sin bee)
Synonyms ampho
Brand Names Fungizone®
Therapeutic Category Antifungal Agent
Use Treatment of severe systemic infections and meningitis caused by susceptible fungi such as *Candida* species, *Histoplasma capsulatum*, *Cryptococcus neoformans*, *Aspergillus* species, *Blastomyces dermatitidis*, *Torulopsis glabrata*, and *Coccidioides immitis*; fungal peritonitis; irrigant for bladder fungal infections; and topically for cutaneous and mucocutaneous candidal infections
(Continued)

amphotericin B *(Continued)*

Usual Dosage

I.V.:

Infants and Children:

Test dose (not required): I.V.: 0.1 mg/kg/dose to a maximum of 1 mg; infuse over 30-60 minutes

Initial therapeutic dose: 0.25 mg/kg gradually increased, usually in 0.25 mg/kg increments on each subsequent day, until the desired daily dose is reached

Maintenance dose: 0.25-1 mg/kg/day given once daily; infuse over 2-6 hours. Once therapy has been established, amphotericin B can be administered on an every other day basis at 1-1.5 mg/kg/dose; cumulative dose: 1.5-2 g over 6-10 week

Adults:

Test dose (not required): 1 mg infused over 20-30 minutes

Initial dose: 0.25 mg/kg administered over 2-6 hours, gradually increased on subsequent days to the desired level by 0.25 mg/kg increments per day; in critically ill patients, may initiate with 1-1.5 mg/kg/day with close observation

Maintenance dose: 0.25-1 mg/kg/day or 1.5 mg/kg over 4-6 hours every other day; do not exceed 1.5 mg/kg/day; cumulative dose: 1-4 g over 4-10 weeks

Duration of therapy varies with nature of infection: Histoplasmosis, *Cryptococcus*, or blastomycosis may be treated with total dose of 2-4 g

I.T.:

Children.: 25-100 mcg every 48-72 hours; increase to 500 mcg as tolerated

Adults: 25-300 mcg every 48-72 hours; increase to 500 mcg to 1 mg as tolerated

Oral: 1 mL (100 mg) 4 times daily

Topical: Apply to affected areas 2-4 times/day for 1-4 weeks of therapy depending on nature and severity of infection

Administration in dialysate: Children and Adults: 1-2 mg/L of peritoneal dialysis fluid either with or without low-dose I.V. amphotericin B (a total dose of 2-10 mg/kg given over 7-14 days)

Administration via bladder irrigation: Children and Adults: 50 mg/day in 1 L of sterile water irrigation solution instilled over 24 hours for 2-7 days or until cultures are clear

Dosage Forms

Cream: 3% (20 g)

Lotion: 3% (30 mL)

Ointment, topical: 3% (20 g)

Powder for injection, lyophilized: 50 mg

Suspension, oral: 100 mg/mL (24 mL with dropper)

amphotericin B colloidal dispersion

(am foe TER i sin bee koe LOY dal dis PER shun)

Brand Names Amphotec®

Therapeutic Category Antifungal Agent

Use Effective in the treatment of invasive mycoses in patient refractory to or intolerant of conventional amphotericin B

Usual Dosage Children and Adults: 3-4 mg/kg/day I.V. (infusion of 1 mg/kg/hour); maximum: 7.5 mg/kg/day; duration of therapy is often <6 weeks

Dosage Forms Suspension for injection: 5 mg/mL (20 mL)

amphotericin b lipid complex (am foe TER i sin bee LIP id KOM pleks)

Synonyms ABLC

Brand Names Abelcet™ Injection

Therapeutic Category Antifungal Agent

Use Treatment of aspergillosis in patients who are refractory to or intolerant of conventional amphotericin B therapy. This indication is based on results obtained primarily from emergency use studies for the treatment of aspergillosis; orphan drug status for cryptococcal meningitis

Usual Dosage Children and Adults: I.V.: 2.5-5 mg/kg/day as a single infusion **Note:** Significantly higher dose of ABLC are tolerated; it appears that attaining higher doses with ABLC produce more rapid fungicidal activity *in vivo* than standard amphotericin B preparations

Dosage Forms Injection: 5 mg (20 mL)

ampicillin (am pi SIL in)

Synonyms aminobenzylpenicillin; ampicillin sodium; ampicillin trihydrate

Brand Names Marcillin®; Omnipen®; Omnipen®-N; Polycillin®; Polycillin-N®; Principen®; Totacillin®; Totacillin®-N

Therapeutic Category Penicillin

Use Treatment of susceptible bacterial infections caused by streptococci, pneumococci, nonpenicillinase-producing staphylococci, *Listeria*, meningococci; some strains of *H. influenzae*, *Salmonella*, *Shigella*, *E. coli*, *Enterobacter*, and *Klebsiella*

Usual Dosage

Infants and Children:

Oral: 50-100 mg/kg/day divided every 6 hours; maximum dose: 2-3 g/day

I.M., I.V.: 100-200 mg/kg/day in 4-6 divided doses; meningitis: 200-400 mg/kg/day in 4-6 divided doses; maximum dose: 12 g/day

Adults:

Oral: 250-500 mg every 6 hours

I.M., I.V.: 8-12 g/day in 4-6 divided doses

Dosage Forms

Capsule:

As anhydrous: 250 mg, 500 mg

As trihydrate: 250 mg, 500 mg

Powder:

For injection, as sodium: 125 mg, 250 mg, 500 mg, 1 g, 2 g, 10 g

For oral suspension, as trihydrate: 125 mg/5 mL (5 mL unit dose, 80 mL, 100 mL, 150 mL, 200 mL); 250 mg/5 mL (5 mL unit dose, 80 mL, 100 mL, 150 mL, 200 mL); 500 mg/5 mL (5 mL unit dose, 100 mL)

For oral suspension, drops, as trihydrate: 100 mg/mL (20 mL)

ampicillin and probenecid (am pi SIL in & proe BEN e sid)

Brand Names Polycillin-PRB®; Probampacin®

Therapeutic Category Penicillin

Use Uncomplicated infections caused by susceptible strains of *Neisseria gonorrhoeae* in adults

Usual Dosage Oral: Administer entire contents of bottle as a single one-time dose

Dosage Forms Powder for oral suspension: Ampicillin 3.5 g and probenecid 1 g per bottle

ampicillin and sulbactam (am pi SIL in & SUL bak tam)

Synonyms sulbactam and ampicillin

Brand Names Unasyn®

Therapeutic Category Penicillin

Use Treatment of susceptible bacterial infections involved with skin and skin structure, intra-abdominal infections, gynecological infections; spectrum is that of ampicillin plus organisms producing beta-lactamases such as *S. aureus*, *H. influenzae*, *E. coli*, *Klebsiella*, *Acinetobacter*, *Enterobacter* and anaerobes

Usual Dosage Unasyn® (ampicillin/sulbactam) is a combination product. Each 3 g vial contains 2 g of ampicillin and 1 g of sulbactam. Sulbactam has very little antibacterial activity by itself, but effectively extends the spectrum of ampicillin to include beta-lactamase producing strains that are resistant to ampicillin alone. Therefore, dosage recommendations for Unasyn® are based on the ampicillin component. (Continued)

ampicillin and sulbactam *(Continued)*

I.M., I.V.:

Children: 100-200 mg ampicillin/kg/day (150-300 mg Unasyn®) divided every 6 hours; maximum dose: 8 g ampicillin/day (12 g Unasyn®)

Adults: 1-2 g ampicillin (1.5-3 g Unasyn®) every 6-8 hours; maximum dose: 8 g ampicillin/day (12 g Unasyn®)

Dosage Forms Powder for injection: 1.5 g [ampicillin sodium 1 g and sulbactam sodium 0.5 g]; 3 g [ampicillin sodium 2 g and sulbactam sodium 1 g]

ampicillin sodium *see* ampicillin *on previous page*

ampicillin trihydrate *see* ampicillin *on previous page*

AMPT *see* metyrosine *on page 347*

amrinone (AM ri none)

Synonyms amrinone lactate

Brand Names Inocor®

Therapeutic Category Adrenergic Agonist Agent

Use Treatment of low cardiac output states (sepsis, congestive heart failure); adjunctive therapy of pulmonary hypertension

Usual Dosage Dosage is based on clinical response. **Note:** Dose should not exceed 10 mg/kg/24 hours.

Children: 0.75 mg/kg I.V. bolus over 2-3 minutes followed by maintenance infusion 5-10 mcg/kg/minute; I.V. bolus may need to be repeated in 30 minutes

Adults: 0.75 mg/kg I.V. bolus over 2-3 minutes followed by maintenance infusion of 5-10 mcg/kg/minute

Dosage Forms Injection, as lactate: 5 mg/mL (20 mL)

amrinone lactate *see* amrinone *on this page*

Amvisc® *see* sodium hyaluronate *on page 485*

Amvisc® Plus *see* sodium hyaluronate *on page 485*

amyl nitrite (AM il NYE trite)

Synonyms isoamyl nitrite

Therapeutic Category Vasodilator

Use Coronary vasodilator in angina pectoris; an adjunct in treatment of cyanide poisoning; also used to produce changes in the intensity of heart murmurs

Usual Dosage 1-6 inhalations from 1 capsule are usually sufficient to produce the desired effect

Dosage Forms Inhalant, crushable glass perles: 0.18 mL, 0.3 mL

amylobarbitone *see* amobarbital *on page 29*

Amytal® *see* amobarbital *on page 29*

Anabolin® Injection *see* nandrolone *on page 364*

Anacin® [OTC] *see* aspirin *on page 44*

Anadrol® *see* oxymetholone *on page 391*

Anafranil® *see* clomipramine *on page 129*

anagrelide (an AG gre lide)

Synonyms anagrelide hydrochloride

Brand Names Agrylin®

Therapeutic Category Platelet Aggregation Inhibitor

Use Agent for essential thrombocythemia (ET)

Usual Dosage Adults: Oral: 0.5 mg 4 times/day or 1 mg twice daily, maintain for ≥1 week, then adjust to the lowest effective dose to reduce and maintain platelet count <600,000 μL ideally to the normal range
Dosage Forms Capsule: 0.5 mg, 1 mg

anagrelide hydrochloride *see* anagrelide *on previous page*

Ana-Kit® *see* insect sting kit *on page 284*

Anamine® Syrup [OTC] *see* chlorpheniramine and pseudoephedrine *on page 114*

Anaplex® Liquid [OTC] *see* chlorpheniramine and pseudoephedrine *on page 114*

Anaprox® *see* naproxen *on page 365*

Anaspaz® *see* hyoscyamine *on page 275*

anastrozole (an AS troe zole)
Brand Names Arimidex®
Therapeutic Category Antineoplastic Agent
Use Treatment of advanced breast cancer in postmenopausal women with disease progression following tamoxifen therapy. Patients with ER-negative disease and patients who did not respond to tamoxifen therapy rarely responded to anastrozole.
Usual Dosage Breast cancer: Adults: Oral (refer to individual protocols): 1 mg once daily
Dosage Forms Tablet: 1 mg

Anatrast® *see* radiological/contrast media (ionic) *on page 457*

Anatuss® [OTC] *see* guaifenesin, phenylpropanolamine, and dextromethorphan *on page 251*

Anatuss® DM [OTC] *see* guaifenesin, pseudoephedrine, and dextromethorphan *on page 252*

Anbesol® [OTC] *see* benzocaine *on page 59*

Anbesol® Maximum Strength [OTC] *see* benzocaine *on page 59*

Ancef® *see* cefazolin *on page 96*

Ancobon® *see* flucytosine *on page 225*

Androderm® Transdermal System *see* testosterone *on page 507*

Andro/Fem® Injection *see* estradiol and testosterone *on page 203*

Android® *see* methyltestosterone *on page 343*

Andro-L.A.® Injection *see* testosterone *on page 507*

Androlone®-D Injection *see* nandrolone *on page 364*

Androlone® Injection *see* nandrolone *on page 364*

Andropository® Injection *see* testosterone *on page 507*

Anectine® Chloride Injection *see* succinylcholine *on page 494*

Anectine® Flo-Pack® *see* succinylcholine *on page 494*

Anergan® *see* promethazine *on page 441*

Anestacon® *see* lidocaine *on page 307*

aneurine hydrochloride *see* thiamine *on page 514*

Anexsia® *see* hydrocodone and acetaminophen *on page 266*

Angio Conray® *see* radiological/contrast media (ionic) *on page 457*

Angiovist® *see* radiological/contrast media (ionic) *on page 457*

anisotropine (an iss oh TROE peen)
Synonyms anisotropine methylbromide
Therapeutic Category Anticholinergic Agent
(Continued)

anisotropine *(Continued)*

Use Adjunctive treatment of peptic ulcer
Usual Dosage Adults: Oral: 50 mg 3 times/day
Dosage Forms Tablet, as methylbromide: 50 mg

anisotropine methylbromide *see anisotropine on previous page*

anisoylated plasminogen streptokinase activator complex *see anistreplase on this page*

anistreplase (a NISS tre plase)

Synonyms anisoylated plasminogen streptokinase activator complex; apsac
Brand Names Eminase®
Therapeutic Category Thrombolytic Agent
Use Management of acute myocardial infarction (AMI) in adults; lysis of thrombi obstructing coronary arteries, reduction of infarct size; and reduction of mortality associated with AMI
Usual Dosage Adults: I.V.: 30 units injected over 2-5 minutes as soon as possible after onset of symptoms
Dosage Forms Powder for injection, lyophilized: 30 units

Anodynos-DHC® *see hydrocodone and acetaminophen on page 266*

Anoquan® *see butalbital compound and acetaminophen on page 78*

Ansaid® Oral *see flurbiprofen on page 231*

ansamycin *see rifabutin on page 465*

Antabuse® *see disulfiram on page 178*

Antazoline-V® Ophthalmic *see naphazoline and antazoline on page 365*

Anthra-Derm® *see anthralin on this page*

anthralin (AN thra lin)

Synonyms dithranol
Brand Names Anthra-Derm®; Drithocreme®; Drithocreme® HP 1%; Dritho-Scalp®; Micanol® Cream
Therapeutic Category Keratolytic Agent
Use Treatment of psoriasis
Usual Dosage Adults: Topical: Generally, apply once daily or as directed. The irritant potential of anthralin is directly related to the strength being used and each patient's individual tolerance. Always commence treatment for at least one week using the lowest strength possible.

Skin application: Apply sparingly only to psoriatic lesions and rub gently and carefully into the skin until absorbed. Avoid applying an excessive quantity which may cause unnecessary soiling and staining of the clothing or bed linen.
Scalp application: Comb hair to remove scalar debris and, after suitably parting, rub cream well into the lesions, taking care to prevent the cream from spreading onto the forehead
Remove by washing or showering; optimal period of contact will vary according to the strength used and the patient's response to treatment. Continue treatment until the skin is entirely clear (ie, when there is nothing to feel with the fingers and the texture is normal)
Dosage Forms
Cream: 0.1% (50 g, 65 g); 0.2% (65 g); 0.25% (50 g); 0.4% (65 g); 0.5% (50 g); 1% (50 g, 65 g)
Ointment, topical: 0.1% (42.5 g); 0.25% (42.5 g); 0.4% (60 g); 0.5% (42.5 g); 1% (42.5 g)

AntibiOtic® Otic *see neomycin, polymyxin b, and hydrocortisone on page 369*

antidigoxin fab fragments *see* digoxin immune fab *on page 169*
antidiuretic hormone *see* vasopressin *on page 547*

antihemophilic factor (human) (an tee hee moe FIL ik FAK tor HYU man)
Synonyms ahf; factor viii
Brand Names Hemofil® M; Humate-P®; Koāte®-HP; Koāte®-HS; Monoclate-P®; Profilate® OSD; Profilate® SD
Therapeutic Category Blood Product Derivative
Use Management of hemophilia A in patients whom a deficiency in factor VIII has been demonstrated
Usual Dosage I.V.: Individualize dosage based on coagulation studies performed prior to and during treatment at regular intervals. One AHF unit is the activity present in 1 mL of normal pooled human plasma; dosage should be adjusted to actual vial size currently stocked in the pharmacy.

Hospitalized patients: 20-50 units/kg/dose; may be higher for special circumstances; dose can be administered every 12-24 hours and more frequently in special circumstances
Dosage Forms Injection: 10 mL, 20 mL, 30 mL

antihemophilic factor (recombinant)
(an tee hee moe FIL ik FAK tor ree KOM be nant)
Synonyms factor VIII recombinant
Brand Names Bioclate®; Helixate®; Kogenate®; Recombinate®
Therapeutic Category Blood Product Derivative
Use Management of hemophilia A in patients whom a deficiency in factor VIII has been demonstrated
Usual Dosage I.V.: Individualize dosage based on coagulation studies performed prior to and during treatment at regular intervals. One AHF unit is the activity present in 1 mL of normal pooled human plasma; dosage should be adjusted to actual vial size currently stocked in the pharmacy.

Hospitalized patients: 20-50 units/kg/dose; may be higher for special circumstances; dose can be administered every 12-24 hours and more frequently in special circumstances
Dosage Forms Injection: 250 units, 500 units, 1000 units

Antihist-1® **[OTC]** *see* clemastine *on page 126*
Antihist-D® *see* clemastine and phenylpropanolamine *on page 127*

anti-inhibitor coagulant complex
(an tee-in HI bi tor coe AG yoo lant KOM pleks)
Synonyms coagulant complex inhibitor
Brand Names Autoplex T®; Feiba VH Immuno®
Therapeutic Category Hemophilic Agent
Use Patients with factor VIII inhibitors who are to undergo surgery or those who are bleeding
Usual Dosage Dosage range: I.V.: 25-100 factor VIII correctional units per kg depending on the severity of hemorrhage
Dosage Forms Injection:
Autoplex T®, with heparin 2 units: Each bottle is labeled with correctional units of Factor VIII
Feiba VH Immuno®, heparin free: Each bottle is labeled with correctional units of Factor VIII

Antilirium® *see* physostigmine *on page 416*
Antiminth® **[OTC]** *see* pyrantel pamoate *on page 451*

antipyrine and benzocaine (an tee PYE reen & BEN zoe kane)

Synonyms benzocaine and antipyrine
Brand Names Allergan® Ear Drops; Auralgan®; Auroto®; Otocalm® Ear
Therapeutic Category Otic Agent, Analgesic; Otic Agent, Cerumenolytic
Use Temporary relief of pain and reduction of inflammation associated with acute congestive and serous otitis media, swimmer's ear, otitis externa; facilitates ear wax removal
Usual Dosage Otic: Fill ear canal; moisten cotton pledget, place in external ear, repeat every 1-2 hours until pain and congestion is relieved; for ear wax removal instill drops 3-4 times/day for 2-3 days
Dosage Forms Solution, otic: Antipyrine 5.4% and benzocaine 1.4% (10 mL, 15 mL)

antirabies serum (equine) (an tee RAY beez SEER um EE kwine)

Synonyms ars
Therapeutic Category Serum
Use Rabies prophylaxis
Usual Dosage I.M.: 1000 units/55 lb in a single dose, infiltrate up to 50% of dose around the wound
Dosage Forms Injection: 125 units/mL (8 mL)

Antispas® Injection *see* dicyclomine *on page 165*

antithrombin III (an tee THROM bin three)

Synonyms ATIII; heparin cofactor I
Brand Names ATnativ®; Thrombate III™
Therapeutic Category Blood Product Derivative
Use Agent for hereditary antithrombin III deficiency
Usual Dosage After first dose of antithrombin III, level should increase to 120% of normal; thereafter maintain at levels >80%. Generally, achieved by administration of maintenance doses once every 24 hours; initially and until patient is stabilized, measure antithrombin III level at least twice daily, thereafter once daily and always immediately before next infusion.

Initial dosage (units) = [desired AT-III level % - baseline AT-III level %] x body weight (kg) divided by 1%/units/kg

Measure antithrombin III preceding and 30 minutes after dose to calculate *in vivo* recovery rate; maintain level within normal range for 2-8 days depending on type of surgery or procedure
Dosage Forms Powder for injection: 500 units (50 mL)

antithymocyte globulin (equine) *see* lymphocyte immune globulin *on page 316*

Anti-Tuss® Expectorant [OTC] *see* guaifenesin *on page 247*

antivenin (*Crotalidae*) polyvalent
(an tee VEN in (kroe TAL ih die) pol i VAY lent)

Synonyms crotaline antivenin, polyvalent; North and South American antisnake-bite serum; pit vipers antivenin; snake (pit vipers) antivenin
Therapeutic Category Antivenin
Use Neutralization of venoms of North and South American crotalids: rattlesnake, copperhead, cottonmouth, tropical moccasins, fer-de-lance, bushmaster
Usual Dosage Initial intradermal sensitivity test. The entire initial dose of antivenin should be administered as soon as possible to be most effective (within 4 hours after the bite).

Children and Adults: I.V.: Minimal envenomation: 20-40 mL; moderate envenomation: 50-90 mL; severe envenomation: 100-150 mL

Additional doses of antivenin is based on clinical response to the initial dose. If swelling continues to progress, symptoms increase in severity, hypotension occurs, or decrease in hematocrit appears, an additional 10-50 mL should be administered.

For I.V. infusion: 1:1-1:10 dilution of reconstituted antivenin in normal saline or D_5W should be prepared. Infuse the initial 5-10 mL of diluted antivenin over 3-5 minutes monitoring closely for signs of sensitivity reactions.

Dosage Forms Injection: Lyophilized serum, diluent (10 mL); one vacuum vial to yield 10 mL of serum

antivenin (*Latrodectus mactans*) (an tee VEN in lak tro DUK tus MAK tans)

Synonyms black widow spider antivenin (*Latrodectus mactans*); *Latrodectus mactans* antivenin

Therapeutic Category Antivenin

Use Treat patients with symptoms of black widow spider bites

Usual Dosage
Children <12 years (severe or shock): I.V.: 2.5 mL in 10-50 mL over 15 minutes
Children and Adults: I.M.: 2.5 mL

Dosage Forms Powder for injection: 6000 antivenin units (2.5 mL)

antivenin (*Micrurus fulvius*) (an tee VEN in mye KRU rus FUL vee us)

Synonyms North American coral snake antivenin

Therapeutic Category Antivenin

Use Neutralize the venom of Eastern coral snake and Texas coral snake but does not neutralize venom of Arizona or Sonoran coral snake

Usual Dosage I.V.: 3-5 vials by slow injection

Dosage Forms Injection: One vial antivenin and one vial diluent

Antivert® *see* meclizine *on page 324*

Antrizine® *see* meclizine *on page 324*

Anturane® *see* sulfinpyrazone *on page 499*

Anucort-HC® **Suppository** *see* hydrocortisone *on page 268*

Anuprep HC® **Suppository** *see* hydrocortisone *on page 268*

Anusol® **HC 1 [OTC]** *see* hydrocortisone *on page 268*

Anusol® **HC 2.5% [OTC]** *see* hydrocortisone *on page 268*

Anusol-HC® **Suppository** *see* hydrocortisone *on page 268*

Anusol® **Ointment [OTC]** *see* pramoxine *on page 432*

Anxanil® *see* hydroxyzine *on page 275*

Apacet® **[OTC]** *see* acetaminophen *on page 3*

apap *see* acetaminophen *on page 3*

Apatate® **[OTC]** *see* vitamin b complex *on page 553*

Aphrodyne™ *see* yohimbine *on page 558*

Aphthasol® *see* amlexanox *on page 28*

A.P.L.® *see* chorionic gonadotropin *on page 122*

Aplisol® *see* tuberculin tests *on page 539*

Aplitest® *see* tuberculin tests *on page 539*

appg *see* penicillin g procaine *on page 401*

apraclonidine (a pra KLOE ni deen)

Synonyms apraclonidine hydrochloride

Brand Names Iopidine®

Therapeutic Category Alpha$_2$-Adrenergic Agonist Agent, Ophthalmic
(Continued)

apraclonidine *(Continued)*

Use 1%: Prevention and treatment of postsurgical intraocular pressure elevation; 0.5%: Short-term adjunctive therapy in patients on maximally tolerated medical therapy who require additional redirection of intraocular pressure

Usual Dosage Adults: Ophthalmic: Instill 1 drop in operative eye 1 hour prior to laser surgery, second drop in eye upon completion of procedure

Dosage Forms Solution, ophthalmic, as hydrochloride: 0.5% (5 mL); 1% (0.1 mL, 0.25 mL)

apraclonidine hydrochloride *see* apraclonidine *on previous page*

Apresazide® *see* hydralazine and hydrochlorothiazide *on page 264*

Apresoline® *see* hydralazine *on page 263*

Aprodine® **Syrup [OTC]** *see* triprolidine and pseudoephedrine *on page 536*

Aprodine® **Tablet [OTC]** *see* triprolidine and pseudoephedrine *on page 536*

Aprodine® **w/C** *see* triprolidine, pseudoephedrine, and codeine *on page 537*

aprotinin (a proe TYE nin)

Brand Names Trasylol®

Therapeutic Category Hemostatic Agent

Use Reduction or prevention of blood loss in patients undergoing coronary artery bypass surgery when a high index of suspicion of excessive bleeding potential exists; this includes open heart reoperation, pre-existing coagulopathy, operations on the great vessels, and patients whose religious beliefs prohibit blood transfusions

Usual Dosage Test dose: **All** patients should receive a 1 mL I.V. test dose at least 10 minutes prior to the loading dose to assess the potential for allergic reactions

Regimen A (standard dose):
2 million units (280 mg) loading dose I.V. over 20-30 minutes
2 million units (280 mg) into pump prime volume
500,000 units/hour (70 mg/hour) I.V. during operation
Regimen B (low dose):
1 million units (140 mg) loading dose I.V. over 20-30 minutes
1 million units (140 mg) into pump prime volume
250,000 units/hour (35 mg/hour) I.V. during operation

Dosage Forms Injection: 1.4 mg/mL [10,000 units/mL] (100 mL, 200 mL)

apsac *see* anistreplase *on page 36*

Aquacare® **Topical [OTC]** *see* urea *on page 542*

Aquachloral® **Supprettes**® *see* chloral hydrate *on page 107*

AquaMEPHYTON® **Injection** *see* phytonadione *on page 416*

Aquaphyllin® *see* theophylline *on page 511*

AquaSite® **Ophthalmic Solution [OTC]** *see* artificial tears *on page 42*

Aquasol A® *see* vitamin a *on page 552*

Aquasol E® **[OTC]** *see* vitamin e *on page 553*

AquaTar® **[OTC]** *see* coal tar *on page 132*

Aquatensen® *see* methyclothiazide *on page 340*

aqueous procaine penicillin g *see* penicillin g procaine *on page 401*

aqueous testosterone *see* testosterone *on page 507*

Aquest® *see* estrone *on page 205*

ara-a *see* vidarabine *on page 549*

arabinofuranosyladenine *see* vidarabine *on page 549*

arabinosylcytosine *see* cytarabine *on page 146*

ara-c *see* cytarabine *on page 146*

Aralen® Phosphate *see* chloroquine phosphate *on page 111*

Aralen® Phosphate With Primaquine Phosphate *see* chloroquine and primaquine *on page 110*

Aramine® *see* metaraminol *on page 333*

ardeoarin sodium *see* ardeparin *on this page*

ardeparin (ar dee PA rin)
Synonyms ardeoarin sodium
Brand Names Normiflo®
Therapeutic Category Anticoagulant
Use Prevention of deep vein thrombosis (DVT) which may lead to pulmonary embolism following knee replacement surgery
Usual Dosage Adults: S.C.: 50 anti-Xa units every 12 hours
Dosage Forms Injection, as sodium: Anti-Xa units 5000 (0.5 mL); Anti-Xa units 10,000 (0.5 mL)

Arduan® *see* pipecuronium *on page 418*

Aredia™ *see* pamidronate *on page 393*

Arfonad® Injection *see* trimethaphan camsylate *on page 534*

Argesic®-SA *see* salsalate *on page 473*

arginine (AR ji neen)
Synonyms arginine hydrochloride
Brand Names R-Gene®
Therapeutic Category Diagnostic Agent
Use Pituitary function test (growth hormone); management of severe, uncompensated, metabolic alkalosis (pH ≥7.55) **after** optimizing therapy with sodium, potassium, or ammonium chloride supplements
Usual Dosage I.V.:
Growth hormone (pituitary function) reserve test:
Children: 500 mg (5 mL) kg/dose administered over 30 minutes
Adults: 30 g (300 mL) administered over 30 minutes
Metabolic alkalosis: Children and Adults: Usual dose: 10 g/hour
Acid required (mEq) =
[1] 0.2 (L/kg) x wt (kg) x [103 - serum chloride] (mEq/L) **or**
[2] 0.3 (L/kg) x wt (kg) x base excess (mEq/L) **or**
[3] 0.5 (L/kg) x wt (kg) x [serum HCO_3 - 24] (mEq/L)
Administer 1/2 to 2/3 of calculated dose and re-evaluate

Note: Arginine hydrochloride should never be used as an alternative to chloride supplementation but used in the patient who is unresponsive to sodium chloride or potassium chloride supplementation
Dosage Forms Injection, as hydrochloride: 10% [100 mg/mL = 950 mOsm/L] (500 mL)

arginine hydrochloride *see* arginine *on this page*

8-arginine vasopressin *see* vasopressin *on page 547*

Aricept® *see* donepezil *on page 181*

Arimidex® *see* anastrozole *on page 35*

Aristocort® *see* triamcinolone *on page 528*

Aristocort® A *see* triamcinolone *on page 528*

Aristocort® Forte *see* triamcinolone *on page 528*

Aristocort® Intralesional *see* triamcinolone *on page 528*

Aristospan® Intra-Articular *see* triamcinolone *on page 528*

Aristospan® Intralesional *see* triamcinolone *on page 528*

Arm-a-Med® Isoetharine *see* isoetharine *on page 289*

Arm-a-Med® Isoproterenol *see* isoproterenol *on page 291*

Arm-a-Med® Metaproterenol *see* metaproterenol *on page 332*

A.R.M.® Caplet [OTC] *see* chlorpheniramine and phenylpropanolamine *on page 114*

Armour® Thyroid *see* thyroid *on page 518*

Aromatic Ammonia Aspirols® *see* ammonia spirit, aromatic *on page 28*

Arrestin® *see* trimethobenzamide *on page 534*

ars *see* antirabies serum (equine) *on page 38*

Artane® *see* trihexyphenidyl *on page 533*

Artha-G® *see* salsalate *on page 473*

Arthritis Foundation® Pain Reliever [OTC] *see* aspirin *on page 44*

Arthritis Foundation® Pain Reliever, Aspirin Free [OTC] *see* acetaminophen *on page 3*

Arthropan® [OTC] *see* choline salicylate *on page 121*

Articulose-50® Injection *see* prednisolone *on page 434*

artificial tears (ar ti FISH il tears)

Synonyms polyvinyl alcohol

Brand Names Adsorbotear® Ophthalmic Solution [OTC]; Akwa Tears® Solution [OTC]; AquaSite® Ophthalmic Solution [OTC]; Bion® Tears Solution [OTC]; Comfort® Tears Solution [OTC]; Dakrina® Ophthalmic Solution [OTC]; Dry Eye® Therapy Solution [OTC]; Dry Eyes® Solution [OTC]; Dwelle® Ophthalmic Solution [OTC]; Eye-Lube-A® Solution [OTC]; HypoTears PF Solution [OTC]; HypoTears Solution [OTC]; Isopto® Plain Solution [OTC]; Isopto® Tears Solution [OTC]; Just Tears® Solution [OTC]; Lacril® Ophthalmic Solution [OTC]; Liquifilm® Tears Solution [OTC]; Liquifilm® Forte Solution [OTC]; LubriTears® Solution [OTC]; Moisture® Ophthalmic Drops [OTC]; Murine® Solution [OTC]; Murocel® Ophthalmic Solution [OTC]; Nature's Tears® Solution [OTC]; Nu-Tears® Solution [OTC]; Nu-Tears® II Solution [OTC]; OcuCoat® Ophthalmic Solution [OTC]; OcuCoat® PF Ophthalmic Solution [OTC]; Puralube® Tears Solution [OTC]; Refresh® Ophthalmic Solution [OTC]; Refresh® Plus Ophthalmic Solution [OTC]; Tear Drop® Solution [OTC]; TearGard® Ophthalmic Solution [OTC]; Teargen® Ophthalmic Solution [OTC]; Tearisol® Solution [OTC]; Tears Naturale® Free Solution [OTC]; Tears Naturale® II Solution [OTC]; Tears Naturale® Solution [OTC]; Tears Plus® Solution [OTC]; Tears Renewed® Solution [OTC]; Ultra Tears® Solution [OTC]; Viva-Drops® Solution [OTC]

Therapeutic Category Ophthalmic Agent, Miscellaneous

Use Ophthalmic lubricant; relief of dry eyes and eye irritation

Usual Dosage Ophthalmic: Use as needed to relieve symptoms, 1-2 drops into eye(s) 3-4 times/day

Dosage Forms Solution, ophthalmic: 15 mL and 30 mL with dropper

asa *see* aspirin *on page 44*

A.S.A. [OTC] *see* aspirin *on page 44*

5-asa *see* mesalamine *on page 331*

Asacol® Oral *see* mesalamine *on page 331*

ascorbic acid (a SKOR bik AS id)

Synonyms vitamin c

Brand Names Ascorbicap® [OTC]; C-Crystals® [OTC]; Cebid® Timecelles® [OTC]; Cecon® [OTC]; Cevalin® [OTC]; Cevi-Bid® [OTC]; Ce-Vi-Sol® [OTC]; Dull-C® [OTC]; Flavorcee® [OTC]; N'ice® Vitamin C Drops [OTC]; Vita-C® [OTC]

Therapeutic Category Vitamin, Water Soluble

Use Prevention and treatment of scurvy; urinary acidification; dietary supplementation; prevention and reduction in the severity of colds

Usual Dosage Oral, I.M., I.V., S.C.:

Recommended daily allowance (RDA):
<6 months: 30 mg
6 months to 1 year: 35 mg
1-3 years: 40 mg
4-10 years: 45 mg
11-14 years: 50 mg
>14 years and Adults: 60 mg

Children:
Scurvy: 100-300 mg/day in divided doses for at least 2 weeks
Urinary acidification: 500 mg every 6-8 hours
Dietary supplement: 35-100 mg/day
Adults:
Scurvy: 100-250 mg 1-2 times/day for at least 2 weeks
Urinary acidification: 4-12 g/day in 3-4 divided doses
Prevention and treatment of colds: 1-3 g/day
Dietary supplement: 50-200 mg/day

Dosage Forms

Capsule, timed release: 500 mg
Crystals: 4 g/teaspoonful (100 g, 500 g); 5 g/teaspoonful (180 g)
Injection: 250 mg/mL (2 mL, 30 mL); 500 mg/mL (2 mL, 50 mL)
Liquid, oral: 35 mg/0.6 mL (50 mL)
Lozenges: 60 mg
Powder: 4 g/teaspoonful (100 g, 500 g)
Solution, oral: 100 mg/mL (50 mL)
Syrup: 500 mg/5 mL (5 mL, 10 mL, 120 mL, 480 mL)
Tablet: 25 mg, 50 mg, 100 mg, 250 mg, 500 mg, 1000 mg
Chewable: 100 mg, 250 mg, 500 mg
Timed release: 500 mg, 1000 mg, 1500 mg

ascorbic acid and ferrous sulfate *see* ferrous salt and ascorbic acid *on page 220*

Ascorbicap® **[OTC]** *see* ascorbic acid *on previous page*

Ascriptin® **[OTC]** *see* aspirin *on next page*

Asendin® *see* amoxapine *on page 29*

Asmalix® *see* theophylline *on page 511*

asparaginase (a SPIR a ji nase)

Synonyms colaspase

Brand Names Elspar®; Erwiniar®

Therapeutic Category Antineoplastic Agent

Use Treatment of acute lymphocytic leukemia, lymphoma; used for induction therapy

Usual Dosage Refer to individual protocols; the manufacturer recommends performing intradermal sensitivity testing before the initial dose

Children and Adults:
I.M. (preferred route): 6000 units/m^2 3 times/week for 3 weeks for combination therapy
I.V.: 1000 units/kg/day for 10 days for combination therapy or 200 units/kg/day for 28 days if combination therapy is inappropriate

Dosage Forms Injection: 10,000 units/vial

A-Spas® **S/L** *see* hyoscyamine *on page 275*

Aspergum® **[OTC]** *see* aspirin *on next page*

aspirin (AS pir in)

Synonyms acetylsalicylic acid; asa

Brand Names Anacin® [OTC]; Arthritis Foundation® Pain Reliever [OTC]; A.S.A. [OTC]; Ascriptin® [OTC]; Aspergum® [OTC]; Asprimox® [OTC]; Bayer® Aspirin [OTC]; Bayer® Buffered Aspirin [OTC]; Bayer® Low Adult Strength [OTC]; Bufferin® [OTC]; Buffex® [OTC]; Cama® Arthritis Pain Reliever [OTC]; Easprin®; Ecotrin® [OTC]; Ecotrin® Low Adult Strength [OTC]; Empirin® [OTC]; Extra Strength Adprin-B® [OTC]; Extra Strength Bayer® Enteric 500 Aspirin [OTC]; Extra Strength Bayer® Plus [OTC]; Halfprin® 81® [OTC]; Heartline® [OTC]; Regular Strength Bayer® Enteric 500 Aspirin [OTC]; St Joseph® Adult Chewable Aspirin [OTC]; ZORprin®

Therapeutic Category Analgesic, Non-narcotic; Antiplatelet Agent; Antipyretic; Nonsteroidal Anti-Inflammatory Agent (NSAID)

Use Treatment of mild to moderate pain, inflammation and fever; adjunctive treatment of Kawasaki disease; may be used for prophylaxis of myocardial infarction and transient ischemic attacks (TIA)

Usual Dosage

Children:

Analgesic and antipyretic: Oral, rectal: 10-15 mg/kg/dose every 4-6 hours

Anti-inflammatory: Oral: Initial: 60-90 mg/kg/day in divided doses; usual maintenance: 80-100 mg/kg/day divided every 6-8 hours; monitor serum concentrations

Kawasaki disease: Oral: 100 mg/kg/day divided every 6 hours; after fever resolves: 8-10 mg/kg/day once daily; monitor serum concentrations

Adults:

Analgesic and antipyretic: Oral, rectal: 325-1000 mg every 4-6 hours up to 4 g/day

Anti-inflammatory: Oral: Initial: 2.4-3.6 g/day in divided doses; usual maintenance: 3.6-5.4 g/day; monitor serum concentrations

Transient ischemic attack: Oral: 1.3 g/day in 2-4 divided doses

Myocardial infarction prophylaxis: 160-325 mg/day

Dosage Forms

Capsule: 356.4 mg and caffeine 30 mg

Suppository, rectal: 60 mg, 120 mg, 125 mg, 130 mg, 195 mg, 200 mg, 300 mg, 325 mg, 600 mg, 650 mg, 1.2 g

Tablet: 65 mg, 75 mg, 81 mg, 325 mg, 500 mg

Tablet: 400 mg and caffeine 32 mg

Tablet:

Buffered: 325 mg and magnesium-aluminum hydroxide 150 mg; 325 mg, magnesium hydroxide 75 mg, aluminum hydroxide 75 mg, buffered with calcium carbonate; 325 mg and magnesium-aluminum hydroxide 75 mg

Chewable: 81 mg

Controlled release: 800 mg

Delayed release: 81 mg

Enteric coated: 81 mg, 325 mg, 500 mg, 650 mg, 975 mg

Gum: 227.5 mg

Timed release: 650 mg

aspirin and codeine (AS pir in & KOE deen)

Synonyms codeine and aspirin

Brand Names Empirin® With Codeine

Therapeutic Category Analgesic, Narcotic

Controlled Substance C-III

Use Relief of mild to moderate pain

Usual Dosage Oral:

Children:

Aspirin: 10 mg/kg/dose every 4 hours

Codeine: 0.5-1 mg/kg/dose every 4 hours

Adults: 1-2 tablets every 4-6 hours as needed for pain

Dosage Forms Tablet:

#2: Aspirin 325 mg and codeine phosphate 15 mg

#3: Aspirin 325 mg and codeine phosphate 30 mg
#4: Aspirin 325 mg and codeine phosphate 60 mg

aspirin and meprobamate (AS pir in & me proe BA mate)
Synonyms meprobamate and aspirin
Brand Names Equagesic®
Therapeutic Category Skeletal Muscle Relaxant
Controlled Substance C-IV
Use Adjunct to treatment of skeletal muscular disease in patients exhibiting tension and/
or anxiety
Usual Dosage Oral: 1 tablet 3-4 times/day
Dosage Forms Tablet: Aspirin 325 mg and meprobamate 200 mg

Aspirin Free Anacin® Maximum Strength [OTC] *see* acetaminophen *on
page 3*

Aspirin-Free Bayer® Select® Allergy Sinus Caplets [OTC] *see* acetaminophen, chlorpheniramine, and pseudoephedrine *on page 5*

Asprimox® [OTC] *see* aspirin *on previous page*

Astelin® *see* azelastine *on page 50*

astemizole (a STEM mi zole)
Brand Names Hismanal®
Therapeutic Category Antihistamine
Use Perennial and seasonal allergic rhinitis and other allergic symptoms including urti-
caria
Usual Dosage Oral:
Children:
<6 years: 0.2 mg/kg/day
6-12 years: 5 mg/day
Children >12 years and Adults: 10-30 mg/day; administer 30 mg on first day, 20 mg on
second day, then 10 mg/day in a single dose
Dosage Forms Tablet: 10 mg

AsthmaHaler® *see* epinephrine *on page 195*

Astramorph™ PF Injection *see* morphine sulfate *on page 356*

Atarax® *see* hydroxyzine *on page 275*

atenolol (a TEN oh lole)
Brand Names Tenormin®
Therapeutic Category Beta-Adrenergic Blocker
Use Treatment of hypertension, alone or in combination with other agents; management
of angina pectoris; antiarrhythmic; postmyocardial infarction patients; acute alcohol
withdrawal
Usual Dosage
Oral:
Children: 1-2 mg/kg/dose administered daily
Adults:
Hypertension: 50 mg once daily, may increase to 100 mg/day; doses >100 mg are
unlikely to produce any further benefit
Angina pectoris: 50 mg once daily, may increase to 100 mg/day; some patients may
require 200 mg/day
Postmyocardial infarction: Follow I.V. dose with 100 mg/day or 50 mg twice daily for 6-
9 days postmyocardial infarction
I.V.: Postmyocardial infarction: Early treatment: 5 mg slow I.V. over 5 minutes; may
repeat in 10 minutes; if both doses are tolerated, may start oral atenolol 50 mg every
12 hours or 100 mg/day for 6-9 days postmyocardial infarction
(Continued)

atenolol *(Continued)*

Dosage Forms
Injection: 0.5 mg/mL (10 mL)
Tablet: 25 mg, 50 mg, 100 mg

atenolol and chlorthalidone (a TEN oh lole & klor THAL i done)

Brand Names Tenoretic®
Therapeutic Category Antihypertensive, Combination
Use Treatment of hypertension with a cardioselective beta-blocker and a diuretic
Usual Dosage Adults: Oral: Initial: 1 tablet (50) once daily, then individualize dose until optimal dose is achieved
Dosage Forms Tablet:
50: Atenolol 50 mg and chlorthalidone 25 mg
100: Atenolol 100 mg and chlorthalidone 25 mg

atg *see* lymphocyte immune globulin *on page 316*

Atgam® *see* lymphocyte immune globulin *on page 316*

ATIII *see* antithrombin III *on page 38*

Ativan® *see* lorazepam *on page 314*

ATnativ® *see* antithrombin III *on page 38*

Atolone® *see* triamcinolone *on page 528*

atorvastatin (a TORE va sta tin)

Brand Names Lipitor®
Therapeutic Category HMG-CoA Reductase Inhibitor
Use Adjunct to diet for the reduction of elevated total and LDL-cholesterol levels in patients with hypercholesterolemia (Type IIa, IIb, and IIc); used in hypercholesterolemic patients without clinically evident heart disease to reduce the risk of myocardial infarction, to reduce the risk for revascularization, and reduce the risk of death due to cardiovascular causes with no increase in death from noncardiovascular diseases
Usual Dosage Adults: Oral: Initial: 10 mg/day, with a range of 10-80 mg/day, administered as a single dose at any time of day, with or without food
Dosage Forms Tablet: 10 mg, 20 mg, 40 mg

atovaquone (a TOE va kwone)

Brand Names Mepron™
Therapeutic Category Antiprotozoal
Use Acute oral treatment of mild to moderate *Pneumocystis carinii* pneumonia (PCP) in patients who are intolerant to co-trimoxazole
Usual Dosage Adults: Oral: 750 mg twice daily with food for 21 days
Dosage Forms Suspension, oral (citrus flavor): 750 mg/5 mL (210 mL)

atracurium (a tra KYOO ree um)

Synonyms atracurium besylate
Brand Names Tracrium®
Therapeutic Category Skeletal Muscle Relaxant
Use Eases endotracheal intubation as an adjunct to general anesthesia and relaxes skeletal muscle during surgery or mechanical ventilation
Usual Dosage I.V.:
Children 1 month to 2 years: Initial: 0.3-0.4 mg/kg followed by maintenance doses of 0.08-0.1 mg/kg as needed to maintain neuromuscular blockade
Children >2 years to Adults: Initial: 0.4-0.5 mg/kg then 0.08-0.1 mg/kg every 20-45 minutes after initial dose to maintain neuromuscular block

Continuous infusion: 0.4-0.8 mg/kg/hour

Dosage Forms Injection:
As besylate: 10 mg/mL (5 mL, 10 mL)
Preservative-free, as besylate: 10 mg/mL (5 mL)

atracurium besylate *see* atracurium *on previous page*

Atrohist® Plus *see* chlorpheniramine, phenylephrine, phenylpropanolamine, and belladonna alkaloids *on page 116*

Atromid-S® *see* clofibrate *on page 129*

Atropair® *see* atropine *on this page*

atropine (A troe peen)

Synonyms atropine sulfate
Brand Names Atropair®; Atropine-Care®; Atropisol®; Isopto® Atropine; I-Tropine®
Therapeutic Category Anticholinergic Agent
Use Preoperative medication to inhibit salivation and secretions; treatment of sinus bradycardia; management of peptic ulcer; treatment of exercise-induced bronchospasm; antidote for organophosphate pesticide poisoning; used to produce mydriasis and cycloplegia for examination of the retina and optic disk and accurate measurement of refractive errors; treatment of uveitis
Usual Dosage
Preanesthesia: I.M., I.V., S.C.:
Infants:
<5 kg: 0.04 mg/kg/dose repeated every 4-6 hours as needed
>5 kg: 0.03 mg/kg/dose repeated every 4-6 hours as needed
Children: 0.01 mg/kg/dose up to a maximum of 0.4 mg/dose; repeat every 4-6 hours as needed
Adults: 0.5 mg/dose repeated every 4-6 hours as needed

Bronchodilation:
Children:
Oral: 0.02 mg/kg/dose 3 times/day
Inhalation: 0.03-0.05 mg/kg/dose 3-4 times/day
Adults: Inhalation: 0.025-0.05 mg/kg/dose over 10 minutes, repeated every 4-5 hours as needed
Cardiopulmonary resuscitation (bradycardia): I.T., I.V.:
Infants: 0.02-0.04 mg/kg/dose; repeat every 2-5 minutes, if needed, up to 2-3 times
Children: 0.01-0.02 mg/kg/dose; repeat every 2-5 minutes, if needed, up to 2-3 times; minimum dose should be 0.1 mg (smaller doses may cause paradoxic bradycardia); maximum total dose is 1 mg (2 mg for adolescents)
Adults: 0.5 mg/dose; repeat every 5 minutes, if needed, up to 2-3 times for a maximum total dose of 2 mg
Organophosphate or carbamate poisoning: I.V.:
Children: 0.02-0.05 mg/kg/dose every 10-20 minutes until atropine effect (dry flushed skin, tachycardia, mydriasis, fever) is observed, then every 1-4 hours to maintain atropine effect for at least 24 hours
Children >12 years and Adults: 1-2 mg/dose every 10-20 minutes until atropine effect (see above) is observed, then 1-3 mg/dose every 1-4 hours, as needed to maintain atropine effect for at least 24 hours
Neuromuscular blockade reversal: I.V.:
Before neostigmine: Administer 25-30 mcg/kg (0.025-0.03 mg/kg) 30 seconds before neostigmine (0.07-0.08 mg/kg)
Before edrophonium: 10 mcg/kg (0.01 mg/kg) 30 seconds before edrophonium (1 mg/kg)

Note: May contain benzyl alcohol as a preservative; administration of benzyl alcohol in doses ranging from 99-234 mg/kg has been associated with a fatal gasping syndrome in neonates; clinical signs of this syndrome include metabolic acidosis, hypotension, CNS depression, and cardiovascular collapse
(Continued)

atropine *(Continued)*

Dosage Forms
Injection, as sulfate: 0.1 mg/mL (5 mL, 10 mL); 0.3 mg/mL (1 mL, 30 mL); 0.4 mg/mL (1 mL, 20 mL, 30 mL); 0.5 mg/mL (1 mL, 5 mL, 30 mL); 0.8 mg/mL (0.5 mL, 1 mL); 1 mg/mL (1 mL, 10 mL)
Ointment, ophthalmic, as sulfate: 0.5%, 1% (3.5 g)
Solution, ophthalmic, as sulfate: 0.5% (1 mL, 5 mL); 1% (1 mL, 2 mL, 5 mL, 15 mL); 2% (1 mL, 2 mL); 3% (5 mL)
Tablet, as sulfate: 0.4 mg

atropine and diphenoxylate *see* diphenoxylate and atropine *on page 174*

Atropine-Care® *see* atropine *on previous page*

atropine sulfate *see* atropine *on previous page*

Atropisol® *see* atropine *on previous page*

Atrovent® *see* ipratropium *on page 288*

A/T/S® Topical *see* erythromycin, topical *on page 201*

attapulgite (at a PULL gite)

Brand Names Children's Kaopectate® [OTC]; Diasorb® [OTC]; Kaopectate® Advanced Formula [OTC]; Kaopectate® Maximum Strength Caplets; Rheaban® [OTC]
Therapeutic Category Antidiarrheal
Use Treatment of uncomplicated diarrhea
Usual Dosage Oral:
Children:
<3 years: Not recommended
3-6 years: 750 mg/dose up to 2250 mg/24 hours
6-12 years: 1200-1500 mg/dose up to 4500 mg/24 hours
Adults: 1200-1500 mg after each loose bowel movement or every 2 hours; 15-30 mL up to 8 times/day, up to 9000 mg/24 hours
Dosage Forms
Liquid, oral concentrate: 600 mg/15 mL (180 mL, 240 mL, 360 mL, 480 mL); 750 mg/15 mL (120 mL)
Tablet: 750 mg
Chewable: 300 mg, 600 mg

Attenuvax® *see* measles virus vaccine, live *on page 323*

Augmentin® *see* amoxicillin and clavulanate potassium *on page 30*

Auralgan® *see* antipyrine and benzocaine *on page 38*

auranofin (au RANE oh fin)

Brand Names Ridaura®
Therapeutic Category Gold Compound
Use Management of active stage of classic or definite rheumatoid or psoriatic arthritis in patients that do not respond to or tolerate other agents
Usual Dosage Oral:
Children: Initial: 0.1 mg/kg/day divided daily; usual maintenance: 0.15 mg/kg/day in 1-2 divided doses; maximum: 0.2 mg/kg/day in 1-2 divided doses
Adults: 6 mg/day in 1-2 divided doses; after 3 months may be increased to 9 mg/day in 3 divided doses; if still no response after 3 months at 9 mg/day, discontinue drug
Dosage Forms Capsule: 3 mg [gold 29%]

Aureomycin® *see* chlortetracycline *on page 120*

Auro® Ear Drops [OTC] *see* carbamide peroxide *on page 90*

Aurolate® *see* gold sodium thiomalate *on page 244*

aurothioglucose (aur oh thye oh GLOO kose)
Brand Names Solganal®
Therapeutic Category Gold Compound
Use Management of active stage of classic or definite rheumatoid or psoriatic arthritis in patients that do not respond to or tolerate other agents
Usual Dosage I.M. (doses should initially be administered at weekly intervals):
Children 6-12 years: Initial: 0.25 mg/kg/dose first week; increment at 0.25 mg/kg/dose increasing with each weekly dose; maintenance: 0.75-1 mg/kg/dose weekly not to exceed 25 mg/dose to a total of 20 doses, then every 2-4 weeks
Adults: 10 mg first week; 25 mg second and third week; then 50 mg/week until 800 mg to 1 g cumulative dose has been administered - if improvement occurs without adverse reactions, administer 25-50 mg every 2-3 weeks, then every 3-4 weeks
Dosage Forms Injection, suspension: 50 mg/mL [gold 50%] (10 mL)

Auroto® *see* antipyrine and benzocaine *on page 38*

Autoplex T® *see* anti-inhibitor coagulant complex *on page 37*

AVC™ Cream *see* sulfanilamide *on page 498*

AVC™ Suppository *see* sulfanilamide *on page 498*

Aveeno® Cleansing Bar [OTC] *see* sulfur and salicylic acid *on page 499*

Aventyl® Hydrochloride *see* nortriptyline *on page 379*

Avita® *see* tretinoin (topical) *on page 528*

Avitene® *see* microfibrillar collagen hemostat *on page 349*

Avlosulfon® *see* dapsone *on page 149*

Avonex® *see* interferon beta-1a *on page 286*

Axid® *see* nizatidine *on page 377*

Axid® AR [OTC] *see* nizatidine *on page 377*

Aygestin® *see* norethindrone *on page 378*

Ayr® Saline [OTC] *see* sodium chloride *on page 483*

azacitidine (ay za SYE ti deen)
Synonyms aza-cr; 5-azacytidine; 5-azc; ladakamycin
Brand Names Mylosar®
Therapeutic Category Antineoplastic Agent
Use Refractory acute lymphocytic and myelogenous leukemia
Usual Dosage Children and Adults: I.V.: 200-300 mg/m²/day for 5-10 days, repeated at 2- to 3-week intervals
Dosage Forms Injection: 100 mg

aza-cr *see* azacitidine *on this page*

Azactam® *see* aztreonam *on page 51*

5-azacytidine *see* azacitidine *on this page*

azatadine (a ZA ta deen)
Synonyms azatadine maleate
Brand Names Optimine®
Therapeutic Category Antihistamine
Use Treatment of perennial and seasonal allergic rhinitis and chronic urticaria
Usual Dosage Children >12 years and Adults: Oral: 1-2 mg twice daily
Dosage Forms Tablet, as maleate: 1 mg

azatadine and pseudoephedrine (a ZA ta deen & soo doe e FED rin)
Synonyms pseudoephedrine and azatadine
Brand Names Trinalin®
Therapeutic Category Antihistamine/Decongestant Combination
Use Perennial and seasonal allergic rhinitis and other allergic symptoms including urticaria
Dosage Forms Tablet: Azatadine maleate 1 mg and pseudoephedrine sulfate 120 mg

azatadine maleate *see* azatadine *on previous page*

azathioprine (ay za THYE oh preen)
Synonyms azathioprine sodium
Brand Names Imuran®
Therapeutic Category Immunosuppressant Agent
Use Adjunct with other agents in prevention of transplant rejection; also used as an immunosuppressant in a variety of autoimmune diseases such as systemic lupus erythematosus, severe rheumatoid arthritis unresponsive to other agents, and nephrotic syndrome
Usual Dosage
Children and Adults: Renal transplantation: Oral, I.V.: Initial: 3-5 mg/kg/day; maintenance: 1-3 mg/kg/day
Adults: Rheumatoid arthritis: Oral: 1 mg/kg/day for 6-8 weeks; increase by 0.5 mg/kg every 4 weeks until response or up to 2.5 mg/kg/day I.V. dose is equivalent to oral dose
Dosage Forms
Injection, as sodium: 100 mg (20 mL)
Tablet (scored): 50 mg

azathioprine sodium *see* azathioprine *on this page*

5-azc *see* azacitidine *on previous page*

Azdone® *see* hydrocodone and aspirin *on page 266*

azelaic acid (a zeh LAY ik AS id)
Brand Names Azelex®
Therapeutic Category Topical Skin Product
Use Treatment of mild to moderate acne vulgaris
Usual Dosage Adults: Topical: After skin is thoroughly washed and patted dry, gently but thoroughly massage a thin film of azelaic acid cream into the affected areas twice daily, in the morning and evening. The duration of use can vary and depends on the severity of the acne. In the majority of patients with inflammatory lesions, improvement of the condition occurs within 4 weeks.
Dosage Forms Cream: 20% (30 g)

azelastine (a ZEL as teen)
Synonyms Azelastine Hydrochloride
Brand Names Astelin®
Therapeutic Category Antihistamine
Use Seasonal allergic rhinitis
Usual Dosage Children ≥12 years and Adults: Nasal: 2 sprays in each nostril twice daily
Dosage Forms Spray, nasal: 137 mcg/actuation [100 actuations/bottle]

Azelastine Hydrochloride *see* azelastine *on this page*

Azelex® *see* azelaic acid *on this page*

azidothymidine *see* zidovudine *on page 559*

azithromycin (az ith roe MYE sin)

Synonyms azithromycin dihydrate

Brand Names Zithromax™

Therapeutic Category Macrolide (Antibiotic)

Use

Children: Treatment of acute otitis media due to *H. influenzae, M. catarrhalis* or *S. pneumoniae*; pharyngitis/tonsillitis due to *S. pyogenes*

Adults:

Treatment of mild to moderate upper and lower respiratory tract infections, infections of the skin and skin structure, and sexually transmitted diseases due to susceptible strains of *C. trachomatis, M. catarrhalis, H. influenzae, S. aureus, S. pneumoniae, Mycoplasma pneumoniae,* and *C. psittaci*; community-acquired pneumonia, pelvic inflammatory disease (PID)

For preventing or delaying the onset of infection with *Mycobacterium avium* complex (MAC)

Usual Dosage Oral:

Children:

Acute otitis media: 10 mg/kg on day 1 (not to exceed 500 mg/day) followed by 5 mg/kg/day once daily on days 2-5 (not to exceed 250 mg/day)

Pharyngitis/tonsillitis: 12 mg/kg/day for 5 days (not to exceed 500 mg/day)

Adolescents ≥16 years and Adults:

Mild to moderate respiratory tract, skin, and soft tissue infections: 500 mg in a single dose on day 1; 250 mg in a single dose on days 2-5

Nongonococcal urethritis and cervicitis: 1 g in a single dose

Chancroid and *Chlamydia*: 1 g in a single dose

I.V.: Adults:

Community-acquired pneumonia: 500 mg as a single dose for at least 2 days, follow I.V. therapy by the oral route with a single daily dose of 500 mg to complete a 7- to 10-day course of therapy

Pelvic inflammatory disease (PID): 500 mg as a single dose for 1-2 days, follow I.V. therapy by the oral route with a single daily dose of 250 mg to complete a 7-day course of therapy

Dosage Forms

Capsule, as dihydrate: 250 mg

Powder:

For injection: 500 mg

For oral suspension, as dihydrate: 100 mg/5 mL (15 mL); 200 mg/5 mL (15 mL, 22.5 mL); 1 g (single-dose packet)

Tablet, as dihydrate: 250 mg, 600 mg

azithromycin dihydrate *see* azithromycin *on this page*

Azmacort™ *see* triamcinolone *on page 528*

Azo-Standard® [OTC] *see* phenazopyridine *on page 408*

azt *see* zidovudine *on page 559*

AZT + 3TC *see* zidovudine and lamivudine *on page 560*

azthreonam *see* aztreonam *on this page*

aztreonam (AZ tree oh nam)

Synonyms azthreonam

Brand Names Azactam®

Therapeutic Category Antibiotic, Miscellaneous

Use Treatment of patients with documented multidrug resistant aerobic gram-negative infection in which beta-lactam therapy is contraindicated; used for urinary tract infection, lower respiratory tract infections, septicemia, skin/skin structure infections, intra-abdominal infections and gynecological infections caused by susceptible *Enterobacteriaceae, H. influenzae,* and *P. aeruginosa*

(Continued)

aztreonam *(Continued)*

Usual Dosage
Children >1 month: I.M., I.V.: 90-120 mg/kg/day divided every 6-8 hours
Cystic fibrosis: 50 mg/kg/dose every 6-8 hours (ie, up to 200 mg/kg/day); maximum: 6-8 g/day
Adults:
Urinary tract infection: I.M., I.V.: 500 mg to 1 g every 8-12 hours
Moderately severe systemic infections: 1 g I.V. or I.M. or 2 g I.V. every 8-12 hours
Severe systemic or life-threatening infections (especially caused by *Pseudomonas aeruginosa*): I.V.: 2 g every 6-8 hours; maximum: 8 g/day
Dosage Forms Powder for injection: 500 mg (15 mL, 100 mL); 1 g (15 mL, 100 mL); 2 g (15 mL, 100 mL)

Azulfidine® *see* sulfasalazine *on page 498*

Azulfidine® EN-tabs® *see* sulfasalazine *on page 498*

Babee Teething® [OTC] *see* benzocaine *on page 59*

bac *see* benzalkonium chloride *on page 59*

bacampicillin (ba kam pi SIL in)
Synonyms bacampicillin hydrochloride; carampicillin hydrochloride
Brand Names Spectrobid®
Therapeutic Category Penicillin
Use Treatment of susceptible bacterial infections involving the urinary tract, skin structure, upper and lower respiratory tract; activity is identical to that of ampicillin
Usual Dosage Oral:
Children: 25-50 mg/kg/day in divided doses every 12 hours
Adults: 400-800 mg every 12 hours
Dosage Forms
Powder for oral suspension, as hydrochloride: 125 mg/5 mL [chemically equivalent to ampicillin 87.5 mg per 5 mL] (70 mL)
Tablet, as hydrochloride: 400 mg [chemically equivalent to ampicillin 280 mg]

bacampicillin hydrochloride *see* bacampicillin *on this page*

Bacid® [OTC] *see Lactobacillus acidophilus* and *Lactobacillus bulgaricus* on page 300

Baciguent® Topical [OTC] *see* bacitracin *on this page*

Baci-IM® Injection *see* bacitracin *on this page*

Bacillus Calmette-Guérin (BCG) Live *see* bcg vaccine *on page 55*

bacitracin (bas i TRAY sin)
Brand Names AK-Tracin® Ophthalmic; Baciguent® Topical [OTC]; Baci-IM® Injection
Therapeutic Category Antibiotic, Ophthalmic; Antibiotic, Topical; Antibiotic, Miscellaneous
Use Treatment of pneumonia and emphysema caused by susceptible staphylococci; prevention or treatment of superficial skin infections or infections of the eye caused by susceptible organisms; due to its toxicity, use of bacitracin systemically or as an irrigant should be limited to situations where less toxic alternatives would not be effective; treatment of antibiotic-associated colitis
Usual Dosage I.M. recommended; **do not administer I.V.:**
Infants:
<2.5 kg: 900 units/kg/day in 2-3 divided doses
>2.5 kg: 1000 units/kg/day in 2-3 divided doses
Children: 800-1200 units/kg/day divided every 8 hours
Adults: 10,000-25,000 units/dose every 6 hours; not to exceed 100,000 units/day

Topical: Apply 1-5 times/day

Ophthalmic ointment: ¼" to ½" ribbon every 3-4 hours to conjunctival sac for acute infections or 2-3 times/day for mild to moderate infections for 7-10 days

Irrigation, solution: 50-100 units/mL in normal saline, lactated Ringer's, or sterile water for irrigation; soak sponges in solution for topical compresses 1-5 times/day or as needed during surgical procedures

Dosage Forms
Injection: 50,000 units
Ointment:
  Ophthalmic: 500 units/g (3.5 g, 3.75 g)
  AK-Tracin®: 500 units/g (3.5 g)
  Topical: 500 units/g (1.5 g, 3.75 g, 15 g, 30 g, 120 g, 454 g)

bacitracin and polymyxin b (bas i TRAY sin & pol i MIKS in bee)

Brand Names AK-Poly-Bac® Ophthalmic; Betadine® First Aid Antibiotics + Moisturizer [OTC]; Polysporin® Ophthalmic; Polysporin® Topical

Therapeutic Category Antibiotic, Ophthalmic; Antibiotic, Topical

Use Treatment of superficial infections involving the conjunctiva and/or cornea caused by susceptible organisms; prevent infection in minor cuts, scrapes and burns

Usual Dosage
Ophthalmic: Apply ½" ribbon to the affected eye(s) every 3-4 hours
Topical: Apply to affected area 1-3 times/day; may cover with sterile bandage if needed

Dosage Forms
Ointment:
  Ophthalmic: Bacitracin 500 units and polymyxin B sulfate 10,000 units per g (3.5 g)
  Topical: Bacitracin 500 units and polymyxin B sulfate 10,000 units per g in white petrolatum (15 g, 30 g)
Powder: Bacitracin 500 units and polymyxin B sulfate 10,000 units per g (10 g)

bacitracin, neomycin, and polymyxin b

(bas i TRAY sin, nee oh MYE sin & pol i MIKS in bee)

Brand Names AK-Spore® Ophthalmic Ointment; Medi-Quick® Topical Ointment [OTC]; Mycitracin® Topical [OTC]; Neomixin® Topical [OTC]; Neosporin® Ophthalmic Ointment; Neosporin® Topical Ointment [OTC]; Ocutricin® Topical Ointment; Septa® Topical Ointment [OTC]; Triple Antibiotic® Topical

Therapeutic Category Antibiotic, Ophthalmic; Antibiotic, Topical

Use Help prevent infection in minor cuts, scrapes and burns; short-term treatment of superficial external ocular infections caused by susceptible organisms

Usual Dosage Children and Adults:
Ophthalmic ointment: Instill into the conjunctival sac one or more times/day every 3-4 hours for 7-10 days
Topical: Apply 1-3 times/day

Dosage Forms Ointment:
Ophthalmic: Bacitracin 400 units, neomycin sulfate 3.5 mg, and polymyxin B sulfate 10,000 units and per g
Topical: Bacitracin 400 units, neomycin sulfate 3.5 mg, and polymyxin B sulfate 5000 units per g

bacitracin, neomycin, polymyxin b, and hydrocortisone

(bas i TRAY sin, nee oh MYE sin, pol i MIKS in bee & hye droe KOR ti sone)

Brand Names AK-Spore H.C.® Ophthalmic Ointment; Cortisporin® Ophthalmic Ointment; Cortisporin® Topical Ointment; Neotricin HC® Ophthalmic Ointment

Therapeutic Category Antibiotic/Corticosteroid, Ophthalmic; Antibiotic/Corticosteroid, Topical

Use Prevention and treatment of susceptible superficial topical infections

Usual Dosage
Ophthalmic ointment: Apply ½" ribbon to inside of lower lid every 3-4 hours until improvement occurs
Topical: Apply sparingly 2-4 times/day
(Continued)

bacitracin, neomycin, polymyxin b, and hydrocortisone
(Continued)
Dosage Forms Ointment:
Ophthalmic: Bacitracin 400 units, neomycin sulfate 3.5 mg, polymyxin B sulfate 10,000 units, and hydrocortisone 10 mg per g (3.5 g)
Topical: Bacitracin 400 units, neomycin sulfate 3.5 mg, polymyxin B sulfate 10,000 units, and hydrocortisone 10 mg per g (15 g)

bacitracin, neomycin, polymyxin B, and lidocaine
(bas i TRAY sin, nee oh MYE sin, pol i MIKS in bee & LYE doe kane)
Brand Names Clomycin® [OTC]
Therapeutic Category Antibiotic, Topical
Use Prevention and treatment of susceptible superficial topical infections
Usual Dosage Adults: Topical: Apply 1-4 times/day to infected areas; cover with sterile bandage if needed
Dosage Forms Ointment, topical: Bacitracin 500 units, neomycin base 3.5 g, polymyxin B sulfate 5000 units, and lidocaine 40 mg per g (28.35 g)

baclofen (BAK loe fen)
Brand Names Lioresal®
Therapeutic Category Skeletal Muscle Relaxant
Use Treatment of reversible spasticity associated with multiple sclerosis or spinal cord lesions; intrathecal use for the management of spasticity in patients who are unresponsive to oral baclofen or experience intolerable CNS side effects; treatment of trigeminal neuralgia; adjunctive treatment of tardive dyskinesia
Usual Dosage
Oral:
Children:
2-7 years: Initial: 10-15 mg/24 hours divided every 8 hours; titrate dose every 3 days in increments of 5-15 mg/day to a maximum of 40 mg/day
≥8 years: Maximum: 60 mg/day in 3 divided doses
Adults: 5 mg 3 times/day, may increase 5 mg/dose every 3 days to a maximum of 80 mg/day
Intrathecal:
Test dose: 50-100 mcg, doses >50 mcg should be administered in 25 mcg increments, separated by 24 hours
Maintenance: After positive response to test dose, a maintenance intrathecal infusion can be administered via an implanted intrathecal pump. Initial dose via pump: Infusion at a 24-hourly rate dosed at twice the test dose.
Dosage Forms
Injection, intrathecal, preservative free: 500 mcg/mL (20 mL); 2000 mcg/mL (5 mL)
Tablet: 10 mg, 20 mg

Bactocill® *see* oxacillin *on page 387*

BactoShield® Topical [OTC] *see* chlorhexidine gluconate *on page 109*

Bactrim™ *see* co-trimoxazole *on page 140*

Bactrim™ DS *see* co-trimoxazole *on page 140*

Bactroban® *see* mupirocin *on page 358*

Bactroban® Nasal *see* mupirocin *on page 358*

Baker's P&S Topical [OTC] *see* phenol *on page 410*

baking soda *see* sodium bicarbonate *on page 483*

bal *see* dimercaprol *on page 171*

balanced salt solution (BAL anced salt soe LOO shun)
Brand Names BSS® Ophthalmic
Therapeutic Category Ophthalmic Agent, Miscellaneous
Use Intraocular irrigating solution; also used to soothe and cleanse the eye in conjunction with hard contact lenses
Usual Dosage Use as needed for foreign body removal, gonioscopy, and other general ophthalmic office procedures
Dosage Forms Ophthalmic:
Drops: 15 mL
Solution, sterile: 500 mL

Baldex® *see* dexamethasone *on page 156*

BAL in Oil® *see* dimercaprol *on page 171*

Balnetar® [OTC] *see* coal tar, lanolin, and mineral oil *on page 133*

Bancap® *see* butalbital compound and acetaminophen *on page 78*

Bancap HC® *see* hydrocodone and acetaminophen *on page 266*

Banophen® Decongestant Capsule [OTC] *see* diphenhydramine and pseudoephedrine *on page 173*

Banophen® Oral [OTC] *see* diphenhydramine *on page 173*

Banthine® *see* methantheline *on page 335*

Barbidonna® *see* hyoscyamine, atropine, scopolamine, and phenobarbital *on page 276*

Barbita® *see* phenobarbital *on page 409*

Barc™ Liquid [OTC] *see* pyrethrins *on page 452*

Baricon® *see* radiological/contrast media (ionic) *on page 457*

Baridium® [OTC] *see* phenazopyridine *on page 408*

Barobag® *see* radiological/contrast media (ionic) *on page 457*

Baro-CAT® *see* radiological/contrast media (ionic) *on page 457*

Baroflave® *see* radiological/contrast media (ionic) *on page 457*

Barosperse® *see* radiological/contrast media (ionic) *on page 457*

Bar-Test® *see* radiological/contrast media (ionic) *on page 457*

Basaljel® [OTC] *see* aluminum carbonate *on page 20*

Baycol® *see* cerivastatin *on page 104*

Bayer® Aspirin [OTC] *see* aspirin *on page 44*

Bayer® Buffered Aspirin [OTC] *see* aspirin *on page 44*

Bayer® Low Adult Strength [OTC] *see* aspirin *on page 44*

Bayer® Select® Chest Cold Caplets [OTC] *see* acetaminophen and dextromethorphan *on page 4*

Bayer® Select Head Cold Caplets [OTC] *see* acetaminophen and pseudoephedrine *on page 5*

Bayer® Select® Pain Relief Formula [OTC] *see* ibuprofen *on page 278*

bcg vaccine (bee see jee vak SEEN)
Synonyms Bacillus Calmette-Guérin (BCG) Live
Brand Names TheraCys™; TICE® BCG
Therapeutic Category Biological Response Modulator
Use BCG vaccine is no longer recommended for adults at high risk for tuberculosis in the United States. BCG vaccination may be considered for infants and children who are skin test-negative to 5 tuberculin units of tuberculin and who cannot be given isoniazid preventive therapy but have close contact with untreated or ineffectively treated active
(Continued)

bcg vaccine *(Continued)*

tuberculosis patients or who belong to groups which other control measures have not been successful.

In the United States, tuberculosis control efforts are directed toward early identification, treatment of cases, and preventive therapy with isoniazid.

Usual Dosage Intravesical treatment and prophylaxis for carcinoma *in situ* of the urinary bladder: Begin between 7-14 days after biopsy or transurethral resection. Administer a dose of 3 vials of BCG live intravesically under aseptic conditions once weekly for 6 weeks (induction therapy). Each dose (3 reconstituted vials) is further diluted in an additional 50 mL sterile, preservative free saline for a total of 53 mL. A urethral catheter is inserted into the bladder under aseptic conditions, the bladder is drained, and then the 53 mL suspension is instilled slowly by gravity, following which the catheter is withdrawn. If the bladder catheterization has been traumatic, BCG live should not be administered, and there must be a treatment delay of at least 1 week. Resume subsequent treatment; follow the induction therapy by one treatment administered 3, 6, 12, 18 and 24 months following the initial treatment.

Dosage Forms Freeze-dried suspension for reconstitution
Injection: 50 mg (2 mL)
Injection, intravesical: 27 mg (3 vials)

bcnu *see* carmustine *on page 93*

B-D Glucose® [OTC] *see* glucose, instant *on page 242*

Because® [OTC] *see* nonoxynol 9 *on page 377*

beclomethasone (be kloe METH a sone)

Synonyms beclomethasone dipropionate
Brand Names Beclovent® Oral Inhaler; Beconase AQ® Nasal Inhaler; Beconase® Nasal Inhaler; Vancenase® AQ Inhaler; Vancenase® Nasal Inhaler; Vanceril® Oral Inhaler
Therapeutic Category Adrenal Corticosteroid
Use
Oral inhalation: Treatment of bronchial asthma in patients who require chronic administration of corticosteroids
Nasal aerosol: Symptomatic treatment of seasonal or perennial rhinitis and nasal polyposis
Usual Dosage
Inhalation:
Children 6-12 years: 1-2 inhalations 3-4 times/day, not to exceed 10 inhalations/day
Adults: 2-4 inhalations twice daily, not to exceed 20 inhalations/day
Aerosol inhalation (nasal):
Children 6-12 years: 1 spray each nostril 3 times/day
Adults: 2-4 sprays each nostril twice daily
Aqueous inhalation (nasal): 1-2 sprays each nostril twice daily
Dosage Forms
Nasal, as dipropionate:
Inhalation: (Beconase®, Vancenase®): 42 mcg/inhalation [200 metered doses] (16.8 g)
Spray, as dipropionate (Vancenase® AQ Nasal): 0.084% [120 actuations] (19 g)
Spray, aqueous, nasal, as dipropionate (Beconase AQ®, Vancenase® AQ): 42 mcg/inhalation [≥200 metered doses] (25 g); 84 mcg/inhalation [≥200 metered doses] (25 g)
Oral: Inhalation, as dipropionate:
Beclovent®, Vanceril®: 42 mcg/inhalation [200 metered doses] (16.8 g)
Vanceril® Double Strength: 84 mcg/inhalation (5.4 g - 40 metered doses, 12.2 g - 120 metered doses)

beclomethasone dipropionate *see* beclomethasone *on this page*

Beclovent® Oral Inhaler *see* beclomethasone *on this page*

Beconase AQ® **Nasal Inhaler** *see* beclomethasone *on previous page*

Beconase® **Nasal Inhaler** *see* beclomethasone *on previous page*

Becotin® **Pulvules®** *see* vitamins, multiple (oral, adult) *on page 556*

Beepen-VK® *see* penicillin v potassium *on page 402*

Belix® **Oral [OTC]** *see* diphenhydramine *on page 173*

belladonna (bel a DON a)

Therapeutic Category Anticholinergic Agent

Use Decrease gastrointestinal activity in functional bowel disorders and to delay gastric emptying as well as decrease gastric secretion

Usual Dosage Tincture: Oral:

Children: 0.03 mL/kg 3 times/day

Adults: 0.6-1 mL 3-4 times/day

Dosage Forms Tincture: Belladonna alkaloids (principally hyoscyamine and atropine) 0.3 mg/mL with alcohol 65% to 70% (120 mL, 480 mL, 3780 mL)

belladonna and opium (bel a DON a & OH pee um)

Synonyms opium and belladonna

Brand Names B&O Supprettes®

Therapeutic Category Analgesic, Narcotic

Controlled Substance C-II

Use Relief of moderate to severe pain associated with rectal or bladder tenesmus that may occur in postoperative states and neoplastic situations; pain associated with ureteral spasms not responsive to non-narcotic analgesics and to space intervals between injections of opiates

Usual Dosage Rectal:

Children: Dose not established

Adults: 1 suppository 1-2 times/day, up to 4 doses/day

Dosage Forms Suppository:

#15 A: Belladonna extract 15 mg and opium 30 mg

#16 A: Belladonna extract 15 mg and opium 60 mg

belladonna, phenobarbital, and ergotamine tartrate

(bel a DON a, fee noe BAR bi tal, & er GOT a meen TAR trate)

Brand Names Bellergal-S®; Bel-Phen-Ergot S®; Phenerbel-S®

Therapeutic Category Ergot Alkaloid

Use Management and treatment of menopausal disorders, gastrointestinal disorders and recurrent throbbing headache

Usual Dosage Oral: 1 tablet each morning and evening

Dosage Forms Tablet, sustained release: l-alkaloids of belladonna 0.2 mg, phenobarbital 40 mg, and ergotamine tartrate 0.6 mg

Bellergal-S® *see* belladonna, phenobarbital, and ergotamine tartrate *on this page*

Bel-Phen-Ergot S® *see* belladonna, phenobarbital, and ergotamine tartrate *on this page*

Benadryl® **Decongestant Allergy Tablet [OTC]** *see* diphenhydramine and pseudoephedrine *on page 173*

Benadryl® **Injection** *see* diphenhydramine *on page 173*

Benadryl® **Oral [OTC]** *see* diphenhydramine *on page 173*

Benadryl® **Topical** *see* diphenhydramine *on page 173*

Ben-Allergin-50® **Injection** *see* diphenhydramine *on page 173*

Ben-Aqua® **[OTC]** *see* benzoyl peroxide *on page 61*

benazepril (ben AY ze pril)

Synonyms benazepril hydrochloride

Brand Names Lotensin®

Therapeutic Category Angiotensin-Converting Enzyme (ACE) Inhibitors

Use Treatment of hypertension, either alone or in combination with other antihypertensive agents

Usual Dosage Adults: Oral: 20-40 mg/day as a single dose or 2 divided doses

Dosage Forms Tablet, as hydrochloride: 5 mg, 10 mg, 20 mg, 40 mg

benazepril and hydrochlorothiazide

(ben AY ze pril & hye droe klor oh THYE a zide)

Brand Names Lotensin HCT®

Therapeutic Category Antihypertensive, Combination

Use Treatment of hypertension

Usual Dosage Dose is individualized

Dosage Forms Tablet: Benazepril 5 mg and hydrochlorothiazide 6.25 mg; benazepril 10 mg and hydrochlorothiazide 12.5 mg; benazepril 20 mg and hydrochlorothiazide 12.5 mg; benazepril 20 mg and hydrochlorothiazide 25 mg

benazepril hydrochloride see benazepril on this page

bendroflumethiazide (ben droe floo meth EYE a zide)

Brand Names Naturetin®

Therapeutic Category Diuretic, Thiazide

Use Management of mild to moderate hypertension, edema associated with congestive heart failure, pregnancy, or nephrotic syndrome; reportedly does not alter serum electrolyte concentrations appreciably at recommended doses

Usual Dosage Oral:

Children: Initial: 0.1-0.4 mg/kg in 1-2 doses; maintenance dose: 0.05-0.1 mg/kg/day in 1-2 doses

Adults: 2.5-20 mg/day or twice daily in divided doses

Dosage Forms Tablet: 5 mg, 10 mg

Benoquin® see monobenzone on page 355

Benoxyl® see benzoyl peroxide on page 61

bentiromide (ben TEER oh mide)

Synonyms btpaba

Brand Names Chymex®

Therapeutic Category Diagnostic Agent

Use Screening test for pancreatic exocrine insufficiency

Usual Dosage Oral:

Children <12 years: 14 mg/kg followed with 8 oz of water

Children >12 years and Adults: Administer following an overnight fast and morning void, single 500 mg dose and follow with 8 oz of water

Dosage Forms Solution, oral: 500 mg [PABA 170 mg] in propylene glycol 40% (7.5 mL)

bentoquatam (ben to KWA tam)

Brand Names IvyBlock®

Therapeutic Category Protectant, Topical

Use To protect the skin from rash due to exposure to poison sumac, poison ivy or poison oak

Usual Dosage Topical: Apply to exposed skin at least 15 minutes before potential contact and reapply every 4 hours

Dosage Forms Lotion: 5% (120 mL)

Bentyl® **Hydrochloride Injection** see dicyclomine on page 165

Bentyl® Hydrochloride Oral *see* dicyclomine *on page 165*

Benylin® Cough Syrup [OTC] *see* diphenhydramine *on page 173*

Benylin DM® [OTC] *see* dextromethorphan *on page 160*

Benylin® Expectorant [OTC] *see* guaifenesin and dextromethorphan *on page 248*

Benylin® Pediatric [OTC] *see* dextromethorphan *on page 160*

Benza® [OTC] *see* benzalkonium chloride *on this page*

Benzac AC® Gel *see* benzoyl peroxide *on page 61*

Benzac AC® Wash *see* benzoyl peroxide *on page 61*

Benzac W® Gel *see* benzoyl peroxide *on page 61*

Benzac W® Wash *see* benzoyl peroxide *on page 61*

5-Benzagel® *see* benzoyl peroxide *on page 61*

10-Benzagel® *see* benzoyl peroxide *on page 61*

benzalkonium chloride (benz al KOE nee um KLOR ide)

Synonyms bac

Brand Names Benza® [OTC]; Zephiran® [OTC]

Therapeutic Category Antibacterial, Topical

Use Surface antiseptic and germicidal preservative

Usual Dosage Thoroughly rinse anionic detergents and soaps from the skin or other areas prior to use of solutions because they reduce the antibacterial activity of BAC; to protect metal instruments stored in BAC solution, add crushed Anti-Rust Tablets, 4 tablets per quart, to antiseptic solution, change solution at least once weekly; not to be used for storage of aluminum or zinc instruments, instruments with lenses fastened by cement, lacquered catheters or some synthetic rubber goods

Dosage Forms

Concentrate, topical: 17% (500 mL, 4000 mL)

Solution, aqueous: 1:750 (60 mL, 120 mL, 240 mL)

Tincture: 1:750 (30 mL, 960 mL)

Spray: 1:750 (30 g, 180 g)

Tissue: 1:750 (packets)

Benzamycin® *see* erythromycin and benzoyl peroxide *on page 200*

Benzashave® Cream *see* benzoyl peroxide *on page 61*

benzathine benzylpenicillin *see* penicillin g benzathine *on page 400*

benzathine penicillin g *see* penicillin g benzathine *on page 400*

benzazoline hydrochloride *see* tolazoline *on page 523*

Benzedrex® [OTC] *see* propylhexedrine *on page 447*

benzene hexachloride *see* lindane *on page 309*

benzhexol hydrochloride *see* trihexyphenidyl *on page 533*

benzocaine (BEN zoe kane)

Synonyms ethyl aminobenzoate

Brand Names Americaine [OTC]; Anbesol® [OTC]; Anbesol® Maximum Strength [OTC]; Babee Teething® [OTC]; Benzocol® [OTC]; Benzodent® [OTC]; Chiggertox® [OTC]; Cylex® [OTC]; Dermoplast® [OTC]; Foille® [OTC]; Foille® Medicated First Aid [OTC]; Hurricaine®; Lanacane® [OTC]; Maximum Strength Anbesol® [OTC]; Maximum Strength Orajel® [OTC]; Mycinettes® [OTC]; Numzitdent® [OTC]; Numzit Teething® [OTC]; Orabase®-B [OTC]; Orabase®-O [OTC]; Orajel® Brace-Aid Oral Anesthetic [OTC]; Orajel® Maximum Strength [OTC]; Orajel® Mouth-Aid [OTC]; Orasept® [OTC]; Orasol® [OTC]; Rhulicaine® [OTC]; Rid-A-Pain® [OTC]; Slim-Mint® [OTC]; Solarcaine® [OTC]; Spec-T® [OTC]; Tanac® [OTC]; Trocaine® [OTC]; Unguentine® [OTC]; Vicks Children's (Continued)

benzocaine *(Continued)*

Chloraseptic® [OTC]; Vicks Chloraseptic® Sore Throat [OTC]; Zilactin-B® Medicated [OTC]; ZilaDent® [OTC]

Therapeutic Category Local Anesthetic

Use Temporary relief of pain associated with pruritic dermatosis, pruritus, minor burns, toothache, minor sore throat pain, canker sores, hemorrhoids, rectal fissures; anesthetic lubricant for passage of catheters and endoscopic tubes

Usual Dosage

Children and Adults:

Mucous membranes: Dosage varies depending on area to be anesthetized and vascularity of tissues

Oral mouth/throat preparations: Do not administer for >2 days or in children <2 years of age, unless directed by a physician; refer to specific package labeling

Topical: Apply to affected area as needed

Adults: Nonprescription diet aid: 6-15 mg just prior to food consumption, not to exceed 45 mg/day

Dosage Forms

Mouth/throat preparations:

Cream: 5% (10 g)

Gel: 6.3% (7.5 g); 7.5% (7.2 g, 9.45 g, 14.1 g); 10% (6 g, 9.45 g, 10 g, 15 g); 15% (10.5 g); 20% (9.45 g, 14.1 g)

Liquid: (3.7 mL); 5% (8.8 mL); 6.3% (9 mL, 22 mL, 14.79 mL); 10% (13 mL); 20% (13.3 mL)

Lotion: 0.2% (15 mL); 2.5% (15 mL)

Lozenges: 5 mg, 6 mg, 10 mg, 15 mg

Ointment: 20% (30 g)

Paste: 20% (5 g, 15 g)

Nonprescription diet aid:

Candy: 6 mg

Gum: 6 mg

Topical for mucous membranes:

Gel: 6% (7.5 g); 20% (2.5 g, 3.75 g, 7.5 g, 30 g)

Liquid: 20% (3.75 mL, 9 mL, 13.3 mL, 30 mL)

Topical for skin disorders:

Aerosol, external use: 5% (92 mL, 105 g); 20% (82.5 mL, 90 mL, 92 mL, 150 mL)

Cream: (30 g, 60 g); 5% (30 g, 1 lb); 6% (28.4 g)

Lotion: (120 mL); 8% (90 mL)

Ointment: 5% (3.5 g, 28 g)

Spray: 5% (97.5 mL); 20% (20 g, 60 g, 120 g, 13.3 mL, 120 mL)

benzocaine and antipyrine *see* antipyrine and benzocaine *on page 38*

benzocaine and cetylpyridinium chloride *see* cetylpyridinium and benzocaine *on page 105*

benzocaine, butyl aminobenzoate, tetracaine, and benzalkonium chloride

(BEN zoe kane, BYOO til a meen oh BENZ oh ate, TET ra kane, & benz al KOE nee um KLOR ide)

Brand Names Cetacaine®

Therapeutic Category Local Anesthetic

Use Topical anesthetic to control pain or gagging

Usual Dosage Topical: Apply to affected area for approximately 1 second or less

Dosage Forms Aerosol: Benzocaine 14%, butyl aminobenzoate 2%, tetracaine 2%, and benzalkonium chloride 0.5% (56 g)

benzocaine, gelatin, pectin, and sodium carboxymethylcellulose

(BEN zoe kane, JEL a tin, PEK tin, & SOW dee um kar box ee meth il SEL yoo lose)

Brand Names Orabase® With Benzocaine [OTC]

Therapeutic Category Local Anesthetic

Use Topical anesthetic and emollient for oral lesions

Usual Dosage Topical: Apply 2-4 times/day

Dosage Forms Paste: Benzocaine 20%, gelatin, pectin, and sodium carboxymethylcellulose (15 g, 5 g)

Benzocol® [OTC] *see* benzocaine *on page 59*

Benzodent® [OTC] *see* benzocaine *on page 59*

benzoic acid and salicylic acid (ben ZOE ik AS id & sal i SIL ik AS id)

Synonyms salicylic acid and benzoic acid

Brand Names Whitfield's Ointment [OTC]

Therapeutic Category Antifungal Agent

Use Treatment of athlete's foot and ringworm of the scalp

Usual Dosage Topical: Apply 1-4 times/day

Dosage Forms
Lotion, topical:
Full strength: Benzoic acid 12% and salicylic acid 6% with isopropyl alcohol 70% (240 mL)
Half strength: Benzoic acid 6% and salicylic acid 3% with isopropyl alcohol 70% (240 mL)
Ointment, topical: Benzoic acid 12% and salicylic acid 6% in anhydrous lanolin and petrolatum (30 g, 454 g)

benzoin (BEN zoyn)

Synonyms gum benjamin

Brand Names AeroZoin® [OTC]; TinBen® [OTC]; TinCoBen® [OTC]

Therapeutic Category Pharmaceutical Aid; Protectant, Topical

Use Protective application for irritations of the skin; sometimes used in boiling water as steam inhalants for their expectorant and soothing action

Usual Dosage Topical: Apply 1-2 times/day

Dosage Forms
Spray, as compound tincture: 40% (105 mL)
Tincture: 79% (480 mL)
As compound tincture: 20% (60 mL); 25% (120 mL)

benzonatate (ben ZOE na tate)

Brand Names Tessalon® Perles

Therapeutic Category Antitussive

Use Symptomatic relief of nonproductive cough

Usual Dosage Oral:
Children <10 years: 8 mg/kg in 3-6 divided doses
Children >10 years and Adults: 100 mg 3 times/day up to 600 mg/day

Dosage Forms Capsule: 100 mg

benzoyl peroxide (BEN zoe il peer OKS ide)

Brand Names Advanced Formula Oxy® Sensitive Gel [OTC]; Ambi 10® [OTC]; Ben-Aqua® [OTC]; Benoxyl®; Benzac AC® Gel; Benzac AC® Wash; Benzac W® Gel; Benzac W® Wash; 5-Benzagel®; 10-Benzagel®; Benzashave® Cream; BlemErase® Lotion [OTC]; Brevoxyl® Gel; Clear By Design® Gel [OTC]; Clearsil® Maximum Strength [OTC]; Del Aqua-5® Gel; Del Aqua-10® Gel; Desquam-E® Gel; Desquam-X® Gel; Desquam-X® Wash; Dryox® Gel [OTC]; Dryox® Wash [OTC]; Exact® Cream [OTC]; Fostex® 10% (Continued)

benzoyl peroxide *(Continued)*

BPO Gel [OTC]; Fostex® 10% Wash [OTC]; Fostex® Bar [OTC]; Loroxide® [OTC]; Neutrogena® Acne Mask [OTC]; Oxy-5® Advanced Formula for Sensitive Skin [OTC]; Oxy-5® Tinted [OTC]; Oxy-10® Advanced Formula for Sensitive Skin [OTC]; Oxy 10® Wash [OTC]; PanOxyl®-AQ; PanOxyl® Bar [OTC]; Perfectoderm® Gel [OTC]; Peroxin A5®; Peroxin A10®; Persa-Gel®; Theroxide® Wash [OTC]; Vanoxide® [OTC]

Therapeutic Category Acne Products

Use Adjunctive treatment of mild to moderate acne vulgaris

Usual Dosage Children and Adults:

Cleansers: Wash once or twice daily; control amount of drying or peeling by modifying dose frequency or concentration

Topical: Apply sparingly once daily; gradually increase to 2-3 times/day if needed. If excessive dryness or peeling occurs, reduce dose frequency or concentration; if excessive stinging or burning occurs, remove with mild soap and water; resume use the next day.

Dosage Forms

Bar: 5% (113 g); 10% (106 g, 113 g)

Cream: 5% (18 g, 113.4 g); 10% (18 g, 28 g, 113.4 g)

Gel: 2.5% (30 g, 42.5 g, 45 g, 57 g, 60 g, 90 g, 113 g); 5% (42.5 g, 45 g, 60 g, 80 g, 90 g, 113.4 g); 10% (30 g, 42.5 g, 45 g, 56.7 g, 60 g, 90 g, 113.4 g, 120 g); 20% (30 g, 60 g)

Liquid: 5% (120 mL, 150 mL, 240 mL); 10% (120 mL, 150 mL, 240 mL)

Lotion: 5% (25 mL, 30 mL); 5.5% (25 mL); 10% (12 mL, 29 mL, 30 mL, 60 mL)

Mask: 5% (30 mL, 60 mL, 60 g)

benzoyl peroxide and hydrocortisone

(BEN zoe il peer OKS ide & hye droe KOR ti sone)

Brand Names Vanoxide-HC®

Therapeutic Category Acne Products

Use Treatment of acne vulgaris and oily skin

Usual Dosage Topical: Shake well; apply thin film 1-3 times/day, gently massage into skin

Dosage Forms Lotion: Benzoyl peroxide 5% and hydrocortisone alcohol 0.5% (25 mL)

benzphetamine (benz FET a meen)

Synonyms benzphetamine hydrochloride

Brand Names Didrex®

Therapeutic Category Anorexiant

Controlled Substance C-III

Use Short-term adjunct in exogenous obesity

Usual Dosage Adults: Oral: 25-50 mg 2-3 times/day, preferably twice daily, midmorning and midafternoon

Dosage Forms Tablet, as hydrochloride: 25 mg, 50 mg

benzphetamine hydrochloride *see* benzphetamine *on this page*

benzthiazide (benz THYE a zide)

Brand Names Exna®

Therapeutic Category Diuretic, Thiazide

Use Management of mild to moderate hypertension; treatment of edema in congestive heart failure and nephrotic syndrome

Usual Dosage Adults: Oral: 50-200 mg/day

Dosage Forms Tablet: 50 mg

benztropine (BENZ troe peen)

Synonyms benztropine mesylate

Brand Names Cogentin®

Therapeutic Category Anticholinergic Agent; Anti-Parkinson's Agent

Use Adjunctive treatment of parkinsonism; also used in treatment of drug-induced extra-pyramidal effects (except tardive dyskinesia) and acute dystonic reactions

Usual Dosage Titrate dose in 0.5 mg increments at 5- to 6-day intervals

Extrapyramidal reaction, drug induced: Oral, I.M., I.V.:

Children >3 years: 0.02-0.05 mg/kg/dose 1-2 times/day

Adults: 1-4 mg/dose 1-2 times/day

Parkinsonism: Oral: 0.5-6 mg/day in 1-2 divided doses; if one dose is greater, administer at bedtime

Dosage Forms

Injection, as mesylate: 1 mg/mL (2 mL)

Tablet, as mesylate: 0.5 mg, 1 mg, 2 mg

benztropine mesylate *see* benztropine *on previous page*

benzylpenicillin benzathine *see* penicillin g benzathine *on page 400*

benzylpenicillin potassium *see* penicillin g, parenteral, aqueous *on page 401*

benzylpenicillin sodium *see* penicillin g, parenteral, aqueous *on page 401*

benzylpenicilloyl-polylysine (BEN zil pen i SIL oyl pol i LIE seen)

Synonyms penicilloyl-polylysine; ppl

Brand Names Pre-Pen®

Therapeutic Category Diagnostic Agent

Use As an adjunct in assessing the risk of administering penicillin (penicillin or benzylpenicillin) in patients with a history of clinical penicillin hypersensitivity

Usual Dosage

Use scratch technique with a 20-gauge needle to make 3-5 mm scratch on epidermis, apply a small drop of solution to scratch, rub in gently with applicator or toothpick

A positive reaction consists of a pale wheal surrounding the scratch site which develops within 10 minutes and ranges from 5-15 mm or more in diameter

If the scratch test is negative an intradermal test may be performed

Intradermal test: Use intradermal test with a tuberculin syringe with a 26- to 30-gauge short bevel needle; a dose of 0.01-0.02 mL is injected intradermally. A control of 0.9% sodium chloride should be injected at least 1½" from the PPL test site. Most skin responses to the intradermal test will develop within 5-15 minutes.

(-) = no reaction or increase in size compared to control

(±) = wheal slightly larger with or without erythematous flare and larger than control site

(+) = itching and increase in size of original bleb may exceed 20 mm in diameter

Dosage Forms Solution: 0.25 mL

bepridil (BE pri dil)

Synonyms bepridil hydrochloride

Brand Names Vascor®

Therapeutic Category Calcium Channel Blocker

Use Treatment of chronic stable angina; only approved indication is hypertension, but may be used for congestive heart failure; doses should not be adjusted for at least 10 days after beginning therapy

Usual Dosage Adults: Oral: Initial: 200 mg/day, then adjust dose until optimal response is achieved; maximum daily dose: 400 mg

Dosage Forms Tablet, as hydrochloride: 200 mg, 300 mg, 400 mg

bepridil hydrochloride *see* bepridil *on this page*

beractant (ber AKT ant)

Synonyms bovine lung surfactant; natural lung surfactant

Brand Names Survanta®

Therapeutic Category Lung Surfactant

(Continued)

beractant *(Continued)*

Use Prevention and treatment of respiratory distress syndrome (RDS) in premature infants

Prophylactic therapy: Infants with body weight <1250 g who are at risk for developing or with evidence of surfactant deficiency

Rescue therapy: Treatment of infants with RDS confirmed by x-ray and requiring mechanical ventilation

Usual Dosage Intratracheal:

Prophylactic treatment: Administer 4 mL/kg as soon as possible; as many as 4 doses may be administered during the first 48 hours of life, no more frequently than 6 hours apart. The need for additional doses is determined by evidence of continuing respiratory distress; if the infant is still intubated and requiring at least 30% inspired oxygen to maintain a PaO_2 ≤80 torr.

Rescue treatment: Administer 4 mL/kg as soon as the diagnosis of RDS is made

Dosage Forms Suspension: 200 mg (8 mL)

Berocca® *see* vitamin b complex with vitamin c and folic acid *on page 553*

Beta-2® *see* isoetharine *on page 289*

beta-carotene (BAY tah KARE oh teen)

Brand Names Provatene® [OTC]; Solatene®

Therapeutic Category Vitamin, Fat Soluble

Use Reduce the severity of photosensitivity reactions in patients with erythropoietic protoporphyria (EPP)

Usual Dosage Oral:

Children <14 years: 30-150 mg/day

Adults: 30-300 mg/day

Dosage Forms Capsule: 15 mg, 30 mg

Betachron E-R® Capsule *see* propranolol *on page 446*

Betadine® [OTC] *see* povidone-iodine *on page 431*

Betadine® 5% Sterile Ophthalmic Prep Solution *see* povidone-iodine *on page 431*

Betadine® First Aid Antibiotics + Moisturizer [OTC] *see* bacitracin and polymyxin b *on page 53*

9-beta-D-ribofuranosyladenine *see* adenosine *on page 11*

Betagan® Liquifilm® *see* levobunolol *on page 304*

Betagen [OTC] *see* povidone-iodine *on page 431*

betaine anhydrous (BAY tayne an HY drus)

Brand Names Cystadane®

Therapeutic Category Urinary Tract Product

Use Treatment of homocystinuria

Usual Dosage Oral: 6 g/day, usually given in two 3 g doses

Dosage Forms Powder: 1 g/1.7 mL (180 g)

betamethasone (bay ta METH a sone)

Synonyms betamethasone dipropionate; betamethasone dipropionate, augmented; betamethasone sodium phosphate; betamethasone valerate; flubenisolone

Brand Names Alphatrex®; Betatrex®; Beta-Val®; Celestone®; Celestone® Soluspan®; Cel-U-Jec®; Diprolene®; Diprolene® AF; Diprosone®; Maxivate®; Teladar®; Valisone®

Therapeutic Category Adrenal Corticosteroid; Corticosteroid, Topical

Use Anti-inflammatory; immunosuppressant agent; corticosteroid replacement therapy

Topical: Inflammatory dermatoses such as psoriasis, seborrheic or atopic dermatitis, neurodermatitis, inflammatory phase of xerosis, late phase of allergic dermatitis or irritant dermatitis

Usual Dosage Children and Adults:
I.M.: Betamethasone sodium phosphate and betamethasone acetate: 0.5-9 mg/day ($\frac{1}{3}$ to $\frac{1}{2}$ of oral dose)
Intrabursal, intra-articular: 0.5-2 mL
Oral: 0.6-7.2 mg/day
Topical: Apply thin film 2-4 times/day

Dosage Forms
Base (Celestone®), Oral:
  Syrup: 0.6 mg/5 mL (118 mL)
  Tablet: 0.6 mg
Dipropionate (Diprosone®)
  Aerosol: 0.1% (85 g)
  Cream: 0.05% (15 g, 45 g)
  Lotion: 0.05% (20 mL, 30 mL, 60 mL)
  Ointment: 0.05% (15 g, 45 g)
Dipropionate augmented (Diprolene®)
  Cream: 0.05% (15 g, 45 g)
  Gel: 0.05% (15 g, 45 g)
  Lotion: 0.05% (30 mL, 60 mL)
  Ointment, topical: 0.05% (15 g, 45 g)
Valerate (Betatrex®, Valisone®)
  Cream: 0.01% (15 g, 60 g); 0.1% (15 g, 45 g, 110 g, 430 g)
  Lotion: 0.1% (20 mL, 60 mL)
  Ointment: 0.1% (15 g, 45 g)
Valerate (Beta-Val®)
  Cream: 0.01% (15 g, 60 g); 0.1% (15 g, 45 g, 110 g, 430 g)
  Lotion: 0.1% (20 mL, 60 mL)
Injection: Sodium phosphate (Celestone Phosphate®, Cel-U-Jec®): 4 mg betamethasone phosphate/mL (equivalent to 3 mg betamethasone/mL) (5 mL)
Injection, suspension: Sodium phosphate and acetate (Celestone® Soluspan®): 6 mg/mL (3 mg of betamethasone sodium phosphate and 3 mg of betamethasone acetate per mL) (5 mL)

betamethasone and clotrimazole
(bay ta METH a sone & kloe TRIM a zole)
Brand Names Lotrisone®
Therapeutic Category Antifungal/Corticosteroid
Use Topical treatment of various dermal fungal infections
Usual Dosage Topical: Apply twice daily
Dosage Forms Cream: Betamethasone dipropionate 0.05% and clotrimazole 1% (15 g, 45 g)

betamethasone dipropionate see betamethasone on previous page

betamethasone dipropionate, augmented see betamethasone on previous page

betamethasone sodium phosphate see betamethasone on previous page

betamethasone valerate see betamethasone on previous page

Betapace® see sotalol on page 490

Betapen®-VK see penicillin v potassium on page 402

Betasept® [OTC] see chlorhexidine gluconate on page 109

Betaseron® see interferon beta-1b on page 286

Betatrex® see betamethasone on previous page

Beta-Val® see betamethasone on previous page

betaxolol (be TAKS oh lol)
Synonyms betaxolol hydrochloride
Brand Names Betoptic® Ophthalmic; Betoptic® S Ophthalmic; Kerlone® Oral
Therapeutic Category Beta-Adrenergic Blocker
Use Treatment of chronic open-angle glaucoma, ocular hypertension; management of hypertension
Usual Dosage Adults:
Ophthalmic: Instill 1 drop twice daily
Oral: 10 mg/day; may increase dose to 20 mg/day after 7-14 days if desired response is not achieved; initial dose in elderly patients: 5 mg/day
Dosage Forms
Solution, ophthalmic, as hydrochloride (Betoptic®): 0.5% (2.5 mL, 5 mL, 10 mL)
Suspension, ophthalmic, as hydrochloride (Betoptic® S): 0.25% (2.5 mL, 10 mL, 15 mL)
Tablet, as hydrochloride (Kerlone®): 10 mg, 20 mg

betaxolol hydrochloride *see* betaxolol *on this page*

bethanechol (be THAN e kole)
Synonyms bethanechol chloride
Brand Names Duvoid®; Myotonachol™; Urecholine®
Therapeutic Category Cholinergic Agent
Use Treatment of nonobstructive urinary retention and retention due to neurogenic bladder; gastroesophageal reflux
Usual Dosage
Children:
Oral:
Abdominal distention or urinary retention: 0.6 mg/kg/day divided 3-4 times/day
Gastroesophageal reflux: 0.1-0.2 mg/kg/dose administered 30 minutes to 1 hour before each meal to a maximum of 4 times/day
S.C.: 0.15-0.2 mg/kg/day divided 3-4 times/day
Adults:
Oral: 10-50 mg 2-4 times/day
S.C.: 2.5-5 mg 3-4 times/day, up to 7.5-10 mg every 4 hours for neurogenic bladder
Dosage Forms
Injection, as chloride: 5 mg/mL (1 mL)
Tablet, as chloride: 5 mg, 10 mg, 25 mg, 50 mg

bethanechol chloride *see* bethanechol *on this page*

Betimol® Ophthalmic *see* timolol *on page 520*

Betoptic® Ophthalmic *see* betaxolol *on this page*

Betoptic® S Ophthalmic *see* betaxolol *on this page*

Bexophene® *see* propoxyphene and aspirin *on page 446*

Biavax® II *see* rubella and mumps vaccines, combined *on page 471*

Biaxin™ *see* clarithromycin *on page 126*

bicalutamide (bye ka LOO ta mide)
Brand Names Casodex®
Therapeutic Category Androgen
Use Combination therapy with a luteinizing hormone-releasing hormone (LHRH) analog for the treatment of advanced prostate cancer
Usual Dosage Adults: Oral: 50 mg once daily (morning or evening), with or without food, in combination with a LHRH analog
Dosage Forms Tablet: 50 mg

Bicillin® C-R 900/300 Injection *see* penicillin g benzathine and procaine combined *on page 401*

Bicillin® C-R Injection *see* penicillin g benzathine and procaine combined *on page 401*

Bicillin® L-A *see* penicillin g benzathine *on page 400*

BiCNU® *see* carmustine *on page 93*

Bilopaque® *see* radiological/contrast media (ionic) *on page 457*

Biltricide® *see* praziquantel *on page 433*

Biocef *see* cephalexin *on page 103*

Bioclate® *see* antihemophilic factor (recombinant) *on page 37*

Biodine [OTC] *see* povidone-iodine *on page 431*

Biohist-LA® *see* carbinoxamine and pseudoephedrine *on page 91*

Biomox® *see* amoxicillin *on page 30*

Bion® Tears Solution [OTC] *see* artificial tears *on page 42*

Bio-Tab® Oral *see* doxycycline *on page 184*

Biozyme-C® *see* collagenase *on page 136*

biperiden (bye PER i den)

Synonyms biperiden hydrochloride; biperiden lactate
Brand Names Akineton®
Therapeutic Category Anticholinergic Agent; Anti-Parkinson's Agent
Use Treatment of all forms of Parkinsonism including drug induced type (extrapyramidal symptoms)
Usual Dosage Adults:
  Parkinsonism: Oral: 2 mg 3-4 times/day
  Extrapyramidal:
   Oral: 2-6 mg 2-3 times/day
   I.M., I.V.: 2 mg every 30 minutes up to 4 doses or 8 mg/day
Dosage Forms
  Injection, as lactate: 5 mg/mL (1 mL)
  Tablet, as hydrochloride: 2 mg

biperiden hydrochloride *see* biperiden *on this page*

biperiden lactate *see* biperiden *on this page*

Bisac-Evac® [OTC] *see* bisacodyl *on this page*

bisacodyl (bis a KOE dil)

Brand Names Bisac-Evac® [OTC]; Bisacodyl Uniserts®; Bisco-Lax® [OTC]; Carter's Little Pills® [OTC]; Clysodrast®; Dacodyl® [OTC]; Deficol® [OTC]; Dulcolax® [OTC]; Fleet® Laxative [OTC]
Therapeutic Category Laxative
Use Treatment of constipation; colonic evacuation prior to procedures or examination
Usual Dosage
  Children:
   Oral: >6 years: 5-10 mg (0.3 mg/kg) at bedtime or before breakfast
   Rectal suppository:
   <2 years: 5 mg as a single dose
   >2 years: 10 mg
  Adults:
   Oral: 5-15 mg as single dose (up to 30 mg when complete evacuation of bowel is required)
   Rectal suppository: 10 mg as single dose
   Tannex:
   Enema: 2.5 g in 1000 mL warm water
   Barium enema: 2.5-5 g in 1000 mL barium suspension
   Do not administer >10 g within a 72-hour period
(Continued)

bisacodyl *(Continued)*
Dosage Forms
Powder, as tannex: 2.5 g packets (50 packet/box)
Suppository, rectal: 5 mg, 10 mg
Tablet, enteric coated: 5 mg

Bisacodyl Uniserts® *see bisacodyl on previous page*
Bisco-Lax® **[OTC]** *see bisacodyl on previous page*
bishydroxycoumarin *see dicumarol on page 165*
Bismatrol® **[OTC]** *see bismuth subsalicylate on this page*

bismuth subgallate (BIZ muth sub GAL ate)
Brand Names Devrom® [OTC]
Therapeutic Category Gastrointestinal Agent, Miscellaneous
Use Symptomatic treatment of mild, nonspecific diarrhea
Usual Dosage Oral: 1-2 tablets 3 times/day with meals
Dosage Forms Tablet, chewable: 200 mg

bismuth subsalicylate (BIZ muth sub sa LIS i late)
Brand Names Bismatrol® [OTC]; Pepto-Bismol® [OTC]
Therapeutic Category Gastrointestinal Agent, Miscellaneous
Use Symptomatic treatment of mild, nonspecific diarrhea including traveler's diarrhea; chronic infantile diarrhea
Usual Dosage Oral:
Nonspecific diarrhea:
Children: Up to 8 doses/24 hours:
3-6 years: $^1/_3$ tablet or 5 mL every 30 minutes to 1 hour as needed
6-9 years: $^2/_3$ tablet or 10 mL every 30 minutes to 1 hour as needed
9-12 years: 1 tablet or 15 mL every 30 minutes to 1 hour as needed
Adults: 2 tablets or 30 mL every 30 minutes to 1 hour as needed up to 8 doses/24 hours
Prevention of traveler's diarrhea: 2.1 g/day or 2 tablets 4 times/day before meals and at bedtime
Dosage Forms
Caplet, swallowable: 262 mg
Liquid: 262 mg/15 mL (120 mL, 240 mL, 360 mL, 480 mL); 524 mg/15 mL (120 mL, 240 mL, 360 mL)
Tablet, chewable: 262 mg

bisoprolol (bis OH proe lol)
Synonyms bisoprolol fumarate
Brand Names Zebeta®
Therapeutic Category Beta-Adrenergic Blocker
Use Treatment of hypertension, alone or in combination with other agents
Usual Dosage Adults: Oral: 5 mg once daily, may be increased to 10 mg, and then up to 20 mg once daily, if necessary
Dosage Forms Tablet, as fumarate: 5 mg, 10 mg

bisoprolol and hydrochlorothiazide
(bis OH proe lol & hye droe klor oh THYE a zide)
Brand Names Ziac™
Therapeutic Category Antihypertensive, Combination
Use Treatment of hypertension
Usual Dosage Adults: Oral: Dose is individualized, administered once daily

Dosage Forms Tablet: Bisoprolol fumarate 2.5 mg and hydrochlorothiazide 6.25 mg; bisoprolol fumarate 5 mg and hydrochlorothiazide 6.25 mg; bisoprolol fumarate 10 mg and hydrochlorothiazide 6.25 mg

bisoprolol fumarate *see* bisoprolol *on previous page*

bistropamide *see* tropicamide *on page 538*

bitolterol (bye TOLE ter ole)
Synonyms bitolterol mesylate
Brand Names Tornalate®
Therapeutic Category Adrenergic Agonist Agent
Use Prevent and treat bronchial asthma and bronchospasm
Usual Dosage Children >12 years and Adults:
Bronchospasm: 2 inhalations at an interval of at least 1-3 minutes, followed by a third inhalation if needed
Prevention of bronchospasm: 2 inhalations every 8 hours
Dosage Forms
Aerosol, oral, as mesylate: 0.8% [370 mcg/metered spray, 300 inhalations] (15 mL)
Solution, inhalation, as mesylate: 0.2% (10 mL, 30 mL, 60 mL)

bitolterol mesylate *see* bitolterol *on this page*

Black Draught® [OTC] *see* senna *on page 477*

black widow spider antivenin (*Latrodectus mactans*) *see* antivenin (*Latrodectus mactans*) *on page 39*

BlemErase® Lotion [OTC] *see* benzoyl peroxide *on page 61*

Blenoxane® *see* bleomycin *on this page*

bleomycin (blee oh MYE sin)
Synonyms bleomycin sulfate; blm
Brand Names Blenoxane®
Therapeutic Category Antineoplastic Agent
Use Palliative treatment of squamous cell carcinoma, testicular carcinoma, germ cell tumors, and the following lymphomas: Hodgkin's, lymphosarcoma and reticulum cell sarcoma; sclerosing agent to control malignant effusions
Usual Dosage Refer to individual protocol
Children and Adults:
Test dose for lymphoma patients: I.M., I.V., S.C.: 1-2 units of bleomycin for the first 2 doses; monitor vital signs every 15 minutes; wait a minimum of 1 hour before administering remainder of dose
I.M., I.V., S.C.: 10-20 units/m^2 (0.25-0.5 units/kg) 1-2 times/week in combination regimens
I.V. continuous infusion: 15-20 units/m^2/day for 4-5 days
Adults: Intracavitary injection for pleural effusion: 15-240 units have been administered
Dosage Forms Powder for injection, as sulfate: 15 units

bleomycin sulfate *see* bleomycin *on this page*

Bleph®-10 Ophthalmic *see* sulfacetamide sodium *on page 496*

Blephamide® Ophthalmic *see* sulfacetamide sodium and prednisolone *on page 497*

Blis-To-Sol® [OTC] *see* tolnaftate *on page 523*

blm *see* bleomycin *on this page*

Blocadren® Oral *see* timolol *on page 520*

Bluboro® [OTC] *see* aluminum acetate and calcium acetate *on page 20*

Bonine® [OTC] *see* meclizine *on page 324*

boric acid (BOR ik AS id)
Brand Names Borofax® Topical [OTC]; Dri-Ear® Otic [OTC]; Swim-Ear® Otic [OTC]
Therapeutic Category Pharmaceutical Aid
Use
Ophthalmic: Mild antiseptic used for inflamed eyelids
Otic: Prophylaxis of swimmer's ear
Topical ointment: Temporary relief of chapped, chafed, or dry skin, diaper rash, abrasions, minor burns, sunburn, insect bites, and other skin irritations
Usual Dosage
Ophthalmic: Apply to lower eyelid 1-2 times/day
Otic: Place 2-4 drops in ears
Topical: Apply as needed
Dosage Forms
Ointment:
Ophthalmic: 5% (3.5 g); 10% (3.5 g)
Topical: 5% (52.5 g); 10% (28 g)
Topical (Borofax®): 5% boric acid and lanolin (1³/₄ oz)
Solution, otic: 2.75% with isopropyl alcohol (30 mL)

Borofax® Topical [OTC] *see* boric acid *on this page*

Boropak® [OTC] *see* aluminum acetate and calcium acetate *on page 20*

B&O Supprettes® *see* belladonna and opium *on page 57*

Botox® *see* botulinum toxin type A *on this page*

botulinum toxin type A (BOT yoo lin num TOKS in type aye)
Brand Names Botox®
Therapeutic Category Ophthalmic Agent, Toxin
Use Treatment of strabismus and blepharospasm
Usual Dosage
Strabismus: 1.25-5 units (0.05-0.15 mL) injected into any one muscle
Subsequent doses for residual/recurrent strabismus: Re-examine patients 7-14 days after each injection to assess the effect of that dose. Subsequent doses for patients experiencing incomplete paralysis of the target may be increased up to two fold the previously administered dose. Maximum recommended dose as a single injection for any one muscle is 25 units.
Blepharospasm: 1.25-2.5 units (0.05-0.10 mL) injected into the orbicularis oculi muscle
Subsequent doses: Each treatment lasts approximately 3 months. At repeat treatment sessions, the dose may be increased up to twofold if the response from the initial treatment is considered insufficient (usually defined as an effect that does not last >2 months). There appears to be little benefit obtainable from injecting >5 units per site. Some tolerance may be found if treatments are administered any more frequently than every 3 months.
The cumulative dose should not exceed 200 units in a 30-day period
Dosage Forms Injection: 100 units *Clostridium botulinum* toxin type A

bovine lung surfactant *see* beractant *on page 63*

Breathe Free® [OTC] *see* sodium chloride *on page 483*

Breezee® Mist Antifungal [OTC] *see* miconazole *on page 348*

Breezee® Mist Antifungal [OTC] *see* tolnaftate *on page 523*

Breonesin® [OTC] *see* guaifenesin *on page 247*

Brethaire® *see* terbutaline *on page 505*

Brethine® *see* terbutaline *on page 505*

bretylium (bre TIL ee um)

Synonyms bretylium tosylate
Therapeutic Category Antiarrhythmic Agent, Class III
Use Ventricular tachycardia or ventricular fibrillation; other serious ventricular arrhythmias resistant to lidocaine
Usual Dosage
Children:
I.M.: 2-5 mg/kg as a single dose
I.V.: Initial: 5 mg/kg, then attempt electrical defibrillation; repeat with 10 mg/kg if ventricular fibrillation persists
Maintenance dose: I.M., I.V.: 5 mg/kg every 6-8 hours
Adults:
Immediate life-threatening ventricular arrhythmias; ventricular fibrillation; unstable ventricular tachycardia. **Note**: Patients should undergo defibrillation/cardioversion before and after bretylium doses as necessary:
Initial dose: I.V.: 5 mg/kg (undiluted) over 1 minute; if arrhythmia persists, administer 10 mg/kg (undiluted) over 1 minute and repeat as necessary (usually at 15- to 30-minute intervals) up to a total dose of 30 mg/kg
Other life-threatening ventricular arrhythmias:
Initial dose: I.M., I.V.: 5-10 mg/kg, may repeat every 1-2 hours if arrhythmia persist; administer I.V. dose (diluted) over 10-30 minutes
Maintenance dose: I.M.: 5-10 mg/kg every 6-8 hours; I.V. (diluted): 5-10 mg/kg every 6 hours; I.V. infusion (diluted): 1-2 mg/minute (little experience with doses >40 mg/kg/day)
Dosage Forms Injection:
As tosylate: 50 mg/mL (10 mL, 20 mL)
As tosylate, premixed in D_5W: 1 mg/mL (500 mL); 2 mg/mL (250 mL); 4 mg/mL (250 mL, 500 mL)

bretylium tosylate *see* bretylium *on this page*

Brevibloc® Injection *see* esmolol *on page 201*

Brevicon® *see* ethinyl estradiol and norethindrone *on page 209*

Brevital® Sodium *see* methohexital *on page 337*

Brevoxyl® Gel *see* benzoyl peroxide *on page 61*

Bricanyl® *see* terbutaline *on page 505*

brimonidine (bri MOE ni deen)

Synonyms brimonidine tartrate
Brand Names Alphagan®
Therapeutic Category Alpha$_2$-Adrenergic Agonist Agent, Ophthalmic
Use Lowering of intraocular pressure in patients with open-angle glaucoma or ocular hypertension
Usual Dosage Adults: Ophthalmic: 1 drop in affected eye(s) 3 times/day (approximately every 8 hours)
Dosage Forms Solution, ophthalmic, as tartrate: 0.2% (5 mL, 10 mL)

brimonidine tartrate *see* brimonidine *on this page*

British anti-lewisite *see* dimercaprol *on page 171*

Brofed® Elixir [OTC] *see* brompheniramine and pseudoephedrine *on page 74*

Bromaline® Elixir [OTC] *see* brompheniramine and phenylpropanolamine *on page 73*

Bromanate DC® *see* brompheniramine, phenylpropanolamine, and codeine *on page 74*

Bromanate® Elixir [OTC] *see* brompheniramine and phenylpropanolamine *on page 73*

Bromanyl® Cough Syrup *see* bromodiphenhydramine and codeine *on this page*

Bromarest® [OTC] *see* brompheniramine *on next page*

Bromatapp® [OTC] *see* brompheniramine and phenylpropanolamine *on next page*

Brombay® [OTC] *see* brompheniramine *on next page*

Bromfed® Syrup [OTC] *see* brompheniramine and pseudoephedrine *on page 74*

Bromfed® Tablet [OTC] *see* brompheniramine and pseudoephedrine *on page 74*

bromfenac (BROME fen ak)

Synonyms bromfenac sodium
Brand Names Duract™
Therapeutic Category Analgesic, Non-narcotic
Use Short-term (generally less than 10 days) management of pain; not indicated for such conditions as osteoarthritis or rheumatoid arthritis
Usual Dosage Adults: Oral: Short-term (generally <10 days) management of pain: one capsule (25 mg) every 6-8 hours as needed, except when taken with high-fat food, when a 50 mg dose may be needed; maximum daily dose: 150 mg (6 capsules/day)
Dosage Forms Capsule, as sodium: 25 mg

bromfenac sodium *see* bromfenac *on this page*

Bromfenex® *see* brompheniramine and pseudoephedrine *on page 74*

Bromfenex® PD *see* brompheniramine and pseudoephedrine *on page 74*

bromocriptine (broe moe KRIP teen)

Synonyms bromocriptine mesylate
Brand Names Parlodel®
Therapeutic Category Anti-Parkinson's Agent; Ergot Alkaloid
Use Treatment of parkinsonism in patients unresponsive or allergic to levodopa; also used in conditions associated with hyperprolactinemia and to suppress lactation
Usual Dosage Oral:
  Parkinsonism: 1.25 mg twice daily, increased by 2.5 mg/day in 2- to 4-week intervals (usual dose range: 30-90 mg/day in 3 divided doses)
  Hyperprolactinemia and postpartum lactation: 2.5 mg 2-3 times/day
Dosage Forms
  Capsule, as mesylate: 5 mg
  Tablet, as mesylate: 2.5 mg

bromocriptine mesylate *see* bromocriptine *on this page*

bromodiphenhydramine and codeine
(brome oh dye fen HYE dra meen & KOE deen)
Synonyms codeine and bromodiphenhydramine
Brand Names Ambenyl® Cough Syrup; Amgenal® Cough Syrup; Bromanyl® Cough Syrup; Bromotuss® w/Codeine Cough Syrup
Therapeutic Category Antihistamine/Antitussive
Controlled Substance C-V
Use Relief of upper respiratory symptoms and cough associated with allergies or common cold
Usual Dosage Oral: 5-10 mL every 4-6 hours
Dosage Forms Liquid: Bromodiphenhydramine hydrochloride 12.5 mg and codeine phosphate 10 mg per 5 mL

Bromotuss® w/Codeine Cough Syrup *see* bromodiphenhydramine and codeine *on previous page*

Bromphen® [OTC] *see* brompheniramine *on this page*

Bromphen DC® w/Codeine *see* brompheniramine, phenylpropanolamine, and codeine *on next page*

brompheniramine (brome fen IR a meen)

Synonyms brompheniramine maleate; parabromdylamine

Brand Names Bromarest® [OTC]; Brombay® [OTC]; Bromphen® [OTC]; Brotane® [OTC]; Chlorphed® [OTC]; Cophene-B®; Diamine T.D.® [OTC]; Dimetane® Extentabs® [OTC]; Nasahist B®; ND-Stat®

Therapeutic Category Antihistamine

Use Perennial and seasonal allergic rhinitis and other allergic symptoms including urticaria

Usual Dosage
Oral:
  Children:
    <6 years: 0.125 mg/kg/dose administered every 6 hours; maximum: 6-8 mg/day
    6-12 years: 2-4 mg every 6-8 hours; maximum: 12-16 mg/day
    Adults: 4 mg every 4-6 hours or 8 mg of sustained release form every 8-12 hours or 12 mg of sustained release every 12 hours; maximum: 24 mg/day
  I.M., I.V., S.C.:
    Children <12 years: 0.5 mg/kg/24 hours divided every 6-8 hours
    Adults: 5-50 mg every 4-12 hours, maximum: 40 mg/24 hours

Dosage Forms
  Elixir, as maleate: 2 mg/5 mL with 3% alcohol (120 mL, 480 mL, 4000 mL)
  Injection, as maleate: 10 mg/mL (10 mL)
  Tablet, as maleate: 4 mg, 8 mg, 12 mg
  Sustained release: 8 mg, 12 mg

brompheniramine and phenylephrine
(brome fen IR a meen & fen il EF rin)

Brand Names Dimetane® Decongestant Elixir [OTC]

Therapeutic Category Antihistamine/Decongestant Combination

Use Temporary relief of symptoms of seasonal and perennial allergic rhinitis, and vasomotor rhinitis, including nasal obstruction

Usual Dosage Children >12 years and Adults: Oral: 10 mL every 4 hours

Dosage Forms Elixir: Brompheniramine maleate 4 mg and phenylephrine hydrochloride 5 mg per 5 mL

brompheniramine and phenylpropanolamine
(brome fen IR a meen & fen il proe pa NOLE a meen)

Synonyms phenylpropanolamine and brompheniramine

Brand Names Bromaline® Elixir [OTC]; Bromanate® Elixir [OTC]; Bromatapp® [OTC]; Bromphen® Tablet [OTC]; Cold & Allergy® Elixir [OTC]; Dimaphen® Elixir [OTC]; Dimaphen® Tablets [OTC]; Dimetapp® 4-Hour Liqui-Gel Capsule [OTC]; Dimetapp® Elixir [OTC]; Dimetapp® Extentabs® [OTC]; Dimetapp® Tablet [OTC]; Genatap® Elixir [OTC]; Tamine® [OTC]; Vicks® DayQuil® Allergy Relief 4 Hour Tablet [OTC]

Therapeutic Category Antihistamine/Decongestant Combination

Use Temporary relief of nasal congestion, running nose, sneezing, and itchy, watery eyes

Usual Dosage Oral:
  Children:
    1-6 months: 1.25 mL 3-4 times/day
    7-24 months: 2.5 mL 3-4 times/day
    2-4 years: 3.75 mL 3-4 times/day
    4-12 years: 5 mL 3-4 times/day
(Continued)

brompheniramine and phenylpropanolamine *(Continued)*

Adults: 5-10 mL 3-4 times/day or regular capsule or tablet 3-4 times daily or 1 sustained release tablet twice daily

Dosage Forms

Capsule (Dimetapp® 4-Hour Liqui-Gel): Brompheniramine maleate 4 mg and phenylpropanolamine hydrochloride 25 mg

Liquid (Bromaline®, Bromanate®, Cold & Allergy®, Dimaphen®, Dimetapp®, Genatap®): Brompheniramine maleate 2 mg and phenylpropanolamine hydrochloride 12.5 mg per 5 mL

Tablet (Dimaphen®, Dimetapp®, Vicks® DayQuil® Allergy Relief 4 Hour): Brompheniramine maleate 4 mg and phenylpropanolamine hydrochloride 25 mg

Tablet, sustained release: Brompheniramine maleate 12 mg and phenylpropanolamine hydrochloride 75 mg

brompheniramine and pseudoephedrine

(brome fen IR a meen & soo doe e FED rin)

Brand Names Brofed® Elixir [OTC]; Bromfed® Syrup [OTC]; Bromfed® Tablet [OTC]; Bromfenex®; Bromfenex® PD; Drixoral® Syrup [OTC]; Iofed®; Iofed® PD

Therapeutic Category Antihistamine/Decongestant Combination

Use Temporary relief of symptoms of seasonal and perennial allergic rhinitis, and vasomotor rhinitis, including nasal obstruction

Usual Dosage Oral:

Children 6-12 years: 5-10 mL 3-4 times/day

Children >12 years and Adults: 1 or 2 capsules every 12 hours or 1 or 2 tablets 3-4 times/day or 5-10 mL 3-4 times/day

Dosage Forms

Capsule, extended release:

Bromfenex® PD, Iofed® PD: Brompheniramine maleate 6 mg and pseudoephedrine hydrochloride 60 mg

Bromfenex®, Iofed®: Brompheniramine maleate 12 mg and pseudoephedrine hydrochloride 120 mg

Elixir:

Brofed®: Brompheniramine maleate 4 mg and pseudoephedrine hydrochloride 30 mg per 5 mL

Bromfed®: Brompheniramine maleate 2 mg and pseudoephedrine hydrochloride 30 mg per 5 mL

Drixoral®: Brompheniramine maleate 2 mg and pseudoephedrine sulfate 30 mg per 5 mL

Tablet (Bromfed®): Brompheniramine maleate 4 mg and pseudoephedrine hydrochloride 60 mg

brompheniramine maleate *see* brompheniramine *on previous page*

brompheniramine, phenylpropanolamine, and codeine

(brome fen IR a meen, fen il proe pa NOLE a meen, & KOE deen)

Brand Names Bromanate DC®; Bromphen DC® w/Codeine; Dimetane®-DC; Myphetane DC®; Poly-Histine CS®

Therapeutic Category Antihistamine/Decongestant/Antitussive

Controlled Substance C-V

Use Relief of coughs and upper respiratory symptoms, including nasal congestion, associated with allergy or the common cold

Usual Dosage Oral:

Children:

2-6 years: 2.5 mL every 4 hours

6-12 years: 5 mL every 4 hours

Children >12 years and Adults: 10 mL every 4 hours

Dosage Forms Liquid: Brompheniramine maleate 2 mg, phenylpropanolamine hydrochloride 12.5 mg, and codeine phosphate 10 mg per 5 mL with alcohol 0.95% (480 mL)

Bromphen® **Tablet [OTC]** *see* brompheniramine and phenylpropanolamine *on page 73*

Bronchial® *see* theophylline and guaifenesin *on page 512*

Bronitin® *see* epinephrine *on page 195*

Bronkaid® **Mist [OTC]** *see* epinephrine *on page 195*

Bronkodyl® *see* theophylline *on page 511*

Bronkometer® *see* isoetharine *on page 289*

Bronkosol® *see* isoetharine *on page 289*

Brontex® **Liquid** *see* guaifenesin and codeine *on page 247*

Brontex® **Tablet** *see* guaifenesin and codeine *on page 247*

Brotane® **[OTC]** *see* brompheniramine *on page 73*

BSS® **Ophthalmic** *see* balanced salt solution *on page 55*

btpaba *see* bentiromide *on page 58*

Bucladin®**-S Softab**® *see* buclizine *on this page*

buclizine (BYOO kli zeen)

Synonyms buclizine hydrochloride
Brand Names Bucladin®-S Softab®
Therapeutic Category Antihistamine
Use Prevention and treatment of motion sickness; symptomatic treatment of vertigo
Usual Dosage Adults: Oral:
  Motion sickness (prophylaxis): 50 mg 30 minutes prior to traveling; may repeat 50 mg after 4-6 hours
  Vertigo: 50 mg twice daily, up to 150 mg/day
Dosage Forms Tablet, chewable, as hydrochloride: 50 mg

buclizine hydrochloride *see* buclizine *on this page*

budesonide (byoo DES oh nide)

Brand Names Pulmicort® Turbuhaler®; Rhinocort®
Therapeutic Category Adrenal Corticosteroid
Use
  Children and Adults: Management of symptoms of seasonal or perennial rhinitis
  Adults: Nonallergic perennial rhinitis
Usual Dosage Children ≥6 years and Adults: 256 mcg/day, administered as either 2 sprays in each nostril in the morning and evening or as 4 sprays in each nostril in the morning
Dosage Forms
  Aerosol, nasal: 32 mcg per actuation (7 g)
  Powder (dry) for inhalation: 200 mcg per metered dose

Bufferin® **[OTC]** *see* aspirin *on page 44*

Buffex® **[OTC]** *see* aspirin *on page 44*

bumetanide (byoo MET a nide)

Brand Names Bumex®
Therapeutic Category Diuretic, Loop
Use Management of edema secondary to congestive heart failure or hepatic or renal disease including nephrotic syndrome; may also be used alone or in combination with antihypertensives in the treatment of hypertension
Usual Dosage
  Children:
  <6 months: Dose not established
(Continued)

bumetanide *(Continued)*

>6 months:
  Oral: Initial: 0.015 mg/kg/dose once daily or every other day; maximum dose: 0.1 mg/kg/day
  I.M., I.V.: Dose not established
Adults:
  Oral: 0.5-2 mg/dose (maximum: 10 mg/day) 1-2 times/day
  I.M., I.V.: 0.5-1 mg/dose (maximum: 10 mg/day)
Dosage Forms
  Injection: 0.25 mg/mL (2 mL, 4 mL, 10 mL)
  Tablet: 0.5 mg, 1 mg, 2 mg

Bumex® *see* bumetanide *on previous page*

Buminate® *see* albumin *on page 13*

Bupap® *see* butalbital compound and acetaminophen *on page 78*

Buphenyl® *see* sodium phenylbutyrate *on page 486*

bupivacaine (byoo PIV a kane)

Synonyms bupivacaine hydrochloride
Brand Names Marcaine®; Sensorcaine®; Sensorcaine®-MPF
Therapeutic Category Local Anesthetic
Use Local anesthetic (injectable) for peripheral nerve block, infiltration, sympathetic block, caudal or epidural block, retrobulbar block
Usual Dosage Dose varies with procedure, depth of anesthesia, vascularity of tissues, duration of anesthesia and condition of patient

Caudal block (with or without epinephrine):
  Children: 1-3.7 mg/kg
  Adults: 15-30 mL of 0.25% or 0.5%
Epidural block (other than caudal block):
  Children: 1.25 mg/kg/dose
  Adults: 10-20 mL of 0.25% or 0.5%
Peripheral nerve block: 5 mL dose of 0.25% or 0.5% (12.5-25 mg); maximum: 2.5 mg/kg (plain); 3 mg/kg (with epinephrine); up to a maximum of 400 mg/day
Sympathetic nerve block: 20-50 mL of 0.25% (no epinephrine) solution
Dosage Forms Injection:
  As hydrochloride: 0.25% (10 mL, 20 mL, 30 mL, 50 mL); 0.5% (10 mL, 20 mL, 30 mL, 50 mL); 0.75% (2 mL, 10 mL, 20 mL, 30 mL)
  As hydrochloride, with epinephrine (1:200,000): 0.25% (10 mL, 30 mL, 50 mL); 0.5% (1.8 mL, 3 mL, 5 mL, 10 mL, 30 mL, 50 mL); 0.75% (30 mL)

bupivacaine hydrochloride *see* bupivacaine *on this page*

Buprenex® *see* buprenorphine *on this page*

buprenorphine (byoo pre NOR feen)

Synonyms buprenorphine hydrochloride
Brand Names Buprenex®
Therapeutic Category Analgesic, Narcotic
Controlled Substance C-V
Use Management of moderate to severe pain
Usual Dosage Adults: I.M., slow I.V.: 0.3-0.6 mg every 6 hours as needed
Dosage Forms Injection, as hydrochloride: 0.3 mg/mL (1 mL)

buprenorphine hydrochloride *see* buprenorphine *on this page*

bupropion (byoo PROE pee on)
Brand Names Wellbutrin®; Wellbutrin® SR; Zyban®
Therapeutic Category Antidepressant, Aminoketone
Use Treatment of depression; as an aid to smoking cessation treatment
Usual Dosage Oral:
Adults:
Depression: 100 mg 3 times/day; begin at 100 mg twice daily; may increase to a maximum dose of 450 mg/day
Smoking cessation: Initiate with 150 mg once daily for 3 days; increase to 150 mg twice daily; treatment should continue for 7-12 weeks
Elderly: Depression: 50-100 mg/day, increase by 50-100 mg every 3-4 days as tolerated; there is evidence that the elderly respond at 150 mg/day in divided doses, but some may require a higher dose
Dosage Forms
Tablet (Wellbutrin®): 75 mg, 100 mg
Sustained release (Wellbutrin® SR, Zyban®): 100 mg, 150 mg

Burow's otic *see* aluminum acetate and acetic acid *on page 20*

BuSpar® *see* buspirone *on this page*

buspirone (byoo SPYE rone)
Synonyms buspirone hydrochloride
Brand Names BuSpar®
Therapeutic Category Antianxiety Agent, Miscellaneous
Use Management of anxiety
Usual Dosage Adults: Oral: 15 mg/day (5 mg 3 times/day); may increase to a maximum of 60 mg/day
Dosage Forms Tablet, as hydrochloride: 5 mg, 10 mg

buspirone hydrochloride *see* buspirone *on this page*

busulfan (byoo SUL fan)
Brand Names Myleran®
Therapeutic Category Antineoplastic Agent
Use Chronic myelogenous leukemia; component of marrow-ablative conditioning regimen prior to bone marrow transplantation
Usual Dosage Oral (refer to individual protocols):
Children:
Remission induction of chronic myelogenous leukemia: 0.06-0.12 mg/kg/day or 1.8-4.6 mg/m²/day; titrate dose to maintain leukocyte count about 20,000/mm³
BMT marrow-ablative conditioning regimen: 1 mg/kg/dose every 6 hours for 16 doses
Adults: Remission induction of chronic myelogenous leukemia: 4-8 mg/day; maintenance dose: controversial, range from 1-4 mg/day to 2 mg/week
Dosage Forms Tablet: 2 mg

butabarbital sodium (byoo ta BAR bi tal SOW dee um)
Brand Names Butalan®; Buticaps®; Butisol Sodium®
Therapeutic Category Barbiturate
Controlled Substance C-III
Use Sedative, hypnotic
Usual Dosage
Children: Preop: 2-6 mg/kg/dose; maximum: 100 mg
Adults:
Sedative: 15-30 mg 3-4 times/day
Hypnotic: 50-100 mg
Preop: 50-100 mg 1-1½ hours before surgery
(Continued)

butabarbital sodium *(Continued)*

Dosage Forms
Capsule: 15 mg, 30 mg
Elixir, with alcohol 7%: 30 mg/5 mL (480 mL, 3780 mL); 33.3 mg/5 mL (480 mL, 3780 mL)
Tablet: 15 mg, 30 mg, 50 mg, 100 mg

Butalan® *see* butabarbital sodium *on previous page*

butalbital compound and acetaminophen

(byoo TAL bi tal KOM pound & a seet a MIN oh fen)

Synonyms acetaminophen and butalbital compound

Brand Names Amaphen®; Anoquan®; Bancap®; Bupap®; Endolor®; Esgic®; Esgic-Plus®; Femcet®; Fioricet®; G-1®; Medigesic®; Phrenilin®; Phrenilin Forte®; Repan®; Sedapap-10®; Triapin®; Two-Dyne®

Therapeutic Category Barbiturate/Analgesic

Controlled Substance C-III

Use Relief of the symptomatic complex of tension or muscle contraction headache

Usual Dosage Adults: Oral: 1-2 tablets or capsules every 4 hours; not to exceed 6/day

Dosage Forms
Capsule:
  Amaphen®, Anoquan®, Butace®, Endolor®, Esgic®, Femcet®, G-1®, Medigesic®, Repan®, Two-Dyne®: Butalbital 50 mg, caffeine 40 mg, and acetaminophen 325 mg
  Bancap®, Triapin®: Butalbital 50 mg and acetaminophen 325 mg
  Phrenilin Forte®: Butalbital 50 mg and acetaminophen 650 mg
Tablet:
  Esgic®, Fioricet®, Repan®: Butalbital 50 mg, caffeine 40 mg, and acetaminophen 325 mg
  Phrenilin®: Butalbital 50 mg and acetaminophen 325 mg
  Sedapap-10®: Butalbital 50 mg and acetaminophen 650 mg

butalbital compound and aspirin (byoo TAL bi tal KOM pound & AS pir in)

Brand Names Fiorgen PF®; Fiorinal®; Isollyl® Improved; Lanorinal®

Therapeutic Category Barbiturate/Analgesic

Controlled Substance C-III (Fiorinal®)

Use Relief of the symptomatic complex of tension or muscle contraction headache

Usual Dosage Adults: Oral: 1-2 tablets or capsules every 4 hours; not to exceed 6/day

Dosage Forms
Capsule: (Fiorgen PF®, Fiorinal®, Isollyl Improved®, Lanorinal®, Marnal®): Butalbital 50 mg, caffeine 40 mg, and aspirin 325 mg
Tablet:
  B-A-C®: Butalbital 50 mg, caffeine 40 mg, and aspirin 650 mg
  Fiorinal®, Isollyl Improved®, Lanorinal®, Marnal®: Butalbital 50 mg, caffeine 40 mg, and aspirin 325 mg

butalbital compound and codeine

(byoo TAL bi tal KOM pound & KOE deen)

Synonyms codeine and butalbital compound

Brand Names Fiorinal® With Codeine

Therapeutic Category Analgesic, Narcotic; Barbiturate

Controlled Substance C-III

Use Mild to moderate pain when sedation is needed

Usual Dosage Adults: Oral: 1-2 capsules every 4 hours as needed for pain; up to 6/day

Dosage Forms Capsule: Butalbital 50 mg, caffeine 40 mg, aspirin 325 mg and codeine phosphate 30 mg

butenafine (byoo TEN a fine)
Synonyms butenafine hydrochloride
Brand Names Mentax®
Therapeutic Category Antifungal Agent
Use Topical treatment of inter-digital tinea pedis (athlete's foot) due to *Epidermophyton floccosum*, *Trichophyton mentagrophytes*, or *Trichophyton rubrum*
Usual Dosage Adults: Topical: Apply cream to the affected area and surrounding skin once daily for 4 weeks
Dosage Forms Cream, as hydrochloride: 1% (2 g, 15 g, 30 g)

butenafine hydrochloride see butenafine on this page

Buticaps® see butabarbital sodium on page 77

Butisol Sodium® see butabarbital sodium on page 77

butoconazole (byoo toe KOE na zole)
Synonyms butoconazole nitrate
Therapeutic Category Antifungal Agent
Use Local treatment of vulvovaginal candidiasis
Usual Dosage Adults:
Nonpregnant: Insert 1 applicatorful (~5 g) intravaginally at bedtime for 3 days, may extend for up to 6 days if necessary
Pregnant: **Use only during second or third trimesters**
Dosage Forms Cream, vaginal, as nitrate: 2% with applicator (28 g)

butoconazole nitrate see butoconazole on this page

butorphanol (byoo TOR fa nole)
Synonyms butorphanol tartrate
Brand Names Stadol®; Stadol® NS
Therapeutic Category Analgesic, Narcotic
Use Management of moderate to severe pain
Usual Dosage Adults:
I.M.: 1-4 mg every 3-4 hours as needed
I.V.: 0.5-2 mg every 3-4 hours as needed
Nasal: Initial: 1 mg (1 spray in one nostril), allow 60-90 minutes to elapse before deciding whether a second 1 mg dose is needed; this 2-dose sequence may be repeated in 3-4 hours if needed
Dosage Forms
Injection, as tartrate: 1 mg/mL (1 mL); 2 mg/mL (1 mL, 2 mL, 10 mL)
Spray, nasal, as tartrate: 10 mg/mL [14-15 doses] (2.5 mL)

butorphanol tartrate see butorphanol on this page

Byclomine® Injection see dicyclomine on page 165

Bydramine® Cough Syrup [OTC] see diphenhydramine on page 173

c7E3 see abciximab on page 2

c8-cck see sincalide on page 480

cabergoline (ca BER go leen)
Brand Names Dostinex®
Therapeutic Category Ergot-like Derivative
Use Treatment of hyperprolactinemia
Usual Dosage Adults: Oral: 0.25 mg twice weekly; dosage may be increased by 0.25 mg twice weekly to a dose of up to 1 mg twice weekly (according to the patient's prolactin level)
Dosage Forms Tablet: 0.5 mg

Cafatine® *see* ergotamine *on page 198*

Cafergot® *see* ergotamine *on page 198*

Cafetrate® *see* ergotamine *on page 198*

caffeine and sodium benzoate (KAF een & SOW dee um BEN zoe ate)
Synonyms sodium benzoate and caffeine
Therapeutic Category Diuretic, Miscellaneous
Use Emergency stimulant in acute circulatory failure; as a diuretic; and to relieve spinal puncture headache
Usual Dosage
Children: I.M., I.V., S.C.: 8 mg/kg every 4 hours as needed
Adults: I.M., I.V.: 500 mg, maximum single dose: 1 g
Dosage Forms Injection: Caffeine 125 mg and sodium benzoate 125 mg per mL (2 mL)

caffeine, citrated (KAF een, SIT rated)
Therapeutic Category Respiratory Stimulant
Use Central nervous system stimulant; used in the treatment of idiopathic apnea of prematurity
Usual Dosage Apnea of prematurity: Oral:
Loading dose: 10-20 mg/kg as caffeine citrate (5-10 mg/kg as caffeine base). If theophylline has been administered to the patient within the previous 5 days, a full or modified loading dose (50% to 75% of a loading dose) may be administered at the discretion of the physician.
Maintenance dose: 5-10 mg/kg/day as caffeine citrate (2.5-5 mg/kg/day as caffeine base) once daily starting 24 hours after the loading dose. Maintenance dose is adjusted based on patient's response, (efficacy and adverse effects), and serum caffeine concentrations.
Dosage Forms
Solution, oral: 20 mg/mL [anhydrous caffeine 10 mg/mL]
Tablet: 65 mg [anhydrous caffeine 32.5 mg]

Calan® *see* verapamil *on page 548*

Calan® **SR** *see* verapamil *on page 548*

Cal Carb-HD® **[OTC]** *see* calcium carbonate *on page 82*

Calcibind® *see* cellulose sodium phosphate *on page 102*

Calci-Chew™ **[OTC]** *see* calcium carbonate *on page 82*

Calciday-667® **[OTC]** *see* calcium carbonate *on page 82*

calcifediol (kal si fe DYE ole)
Synonyms 25-d_3; 25-hydroxycholecalciferol; 25-hydroxyvitamin d_3
Brand Names Calderol®
Therapeutic Category Vitamin D Analog
Use Treatment and management of metabolic bone disease associated with chronic renal failure
Usual Dosage Hepatic osteodystrophy: Oral:
Infants: 5-7 mcg/kg/day
Children and Adults: 20-100 mcg/day or every other day; titrate to obtain normal serum calcium/phosphate levels
Dosage Forms Capsule: 20 mcg, 50 mcg

Calciferol™ **Injection** *see* ergocalciferol *on page 197*

Calciferol™ **Oral** *see* ergocalciferol *on page 197*

Calcijex™ *see* calcitriol *on next page*

Calcimar® **Injection** *see* calcitonin *on next page*

Calci-Mix™ [OTC] *see* calcium carbonate *on next page*

calcipotriene (kal si POE try een)
Brand Names Dovonex®
Therapeutic Category Antipsoriatic Agent
Use Treatment of plaque psoriasis
Usual Dosage Topical: Apply to skin lesions twice daily
Dosage Forms
Cream: 0.005% (30 g, 60 g, 100 g)
Ointment, topical: 0.005% (30 g, 60 g, 100 g)
Solution, topical: 0.005%

calcitonin (kal si TOE nin)
Synonyms calcitonin (human); calcitonin (salmon)
Brand Names Calcimar® Injection; Cibacalcin® Injection; Miacalcin® Injection; Miacalcin® Nasal Spray; Osteocalcin® Injection; Salmonine® Injection
Therapeutic Category Polypeptide Hormone
Use
Calcitonin (salmon): Treatment of Paget's disease of bone and as adjunctive therapy for hypercalcemia; also used in postmenopausal osteoporosis and osteogenesis imperfecta
Calcitonin (human): Treatment of Paget's disease of bone
Usual Dosage Dosage for calcitonin salmon is expressed in international units (IU); dosage of calcitonin human is expressed in mg
Calcitonin salmon:
Skin test: 1 IU/0.1 mL intracutaneously on the inner aspect of the forearm
The skin test is 0.1 mL of 10 IU dilution of calcitonin (must be prepared) injected intradermally; observe injection site for 15 minutes for wheal or significant erythema
Paget's disease: S.C.: 100 IU/day
Postmenopause osteoporosis:
I.M., S.C.: 100 IU/day (concomitant therapy with supplemental calcium and vitamin D is recommended)
Nasal: 50-400 IU daily, usually 200 IU per day
Hypercalcemia: I.M., S.C.: 4 IU/kg every 12 hours. If response is unsatisfactory, may increase at 2 day intervals to 8 IU/kg every 12 hours then to maximum of 8 IU/kg every 6 hours
Calcitonin human: Paget's disease: S.C.: 0.5 mg/day initially; some patients require as little as 0.25 mg or 0.5 mg 2-3 times/week; some patients require up to 0.5 mg twice daily
Nasal: Postmenopausal osteoporosis: 200 IU/day, alternating nostrils daily
Dosage Forms
Injection:
Human (Cibacalcin®): 0.5 mg/vial
Salmon: 200 units/mL (2 mL)
Spray, nasal: 200 units/activation (0.09 mL/dose) (2 mL glass bottle with pump)

calcitonin (human) *see* calcitonin *on this page*

calcitonin (salmon) *see* calcitonin *on this page*

calcitriol (kal si TRYE ole)
Synonyms 1,25 dihydroxycholecalciferol
Brand Names Calcijex™; Rocaltrol®
Therapeutic Category Vitamin D Analog
Use Management of hypocalcemia in patients on chronic renal dialysis; reduce elevated parathyroid hormone levels
Usual Dosage Individualize dosage to maintain calcium levels of 9-10 mg/dL
(Continued)

calcitriol *(Continued)*

Renal failure: Oral:
Children: Initial: 15 ng/kg/day; maintenance: 30-60 ng/kg/day
Adults: 0.25 mcg/day or every other day (may require 0.5-1 mcg/day)

Unlabeled dose:
Renal failure: I.V.: Adults: 0.5 mcg (0.01 mcg/kg) 3 times/week; most doses in the range of 0.5-3 mcg (0.01-0.05 mcg/kg) 3 times/week
Hypoparathyroidism/pseudohypoparathyroidism: Oral:
Children 1-5 years: 0.25-0.75 mcg/day
Children >6 years and Adults: 0.5-2 mcg/day

Dosage Forms
Capsule: 0.25 mcg, 0.5 mcg
Injection: 1 mcg/mL (1 mL); 2 mcg/mL (1 mL)

calcium acetate (KAL see um AS e tate)

Brand Names Calphron®; PhosLo®
Therapeutic Category Electrolyte Supplement
Use Control of hyperphosphatemia in end stage renal failure and does not promote aluminum absorption
Usual Dosage Adults: Oral: 2 tablets with each meal; dosage may be increased to bring serum phosphate value to <6 mg/dL; most patients require 3-4 tablets with each meal
Dosage Forms Elemental calcium listed in brackets
Capsule (Phos-Ex® 125): 500 mg [125 mg]
Tablet:
Calphron®: 667 mg [169 mg]
PhosLo®: 667 mg [169 mg]

calcium carbonate (KAL see um KAR bun ate)

Brand Names Alka-Mints® [OTC]; Amitone® [OTC]; Cal Carb-HD® [OTC]; Calci-Chew™ [OTC]; Calciday-667® [OTC]; Calci-Mix™ [OTC]; Cal-Plus® [OTC]; Caltrate® 600 [OTC]; Caltrate, Jr.® [OTC]; Chooz® [OTC]; Dicarbosil® [OTC]; Equilet® [OTC]; Florical® [OTC]; Gencalc® 600 [OTC]; Mallamint® [OTC]; Nephro-Calci® [OTC]; Os-Cal® 500 [OTC]; Oyst-Cal 500 [OTC]; Oystercal® 500; Rolaids® Calcium Rich [OTC]; Tums® [OTC]; Tums® E-X Extra Strength Tablet [OTC]; Tums® Extra Strength Liquid [OTC]
Therapeutic Category Antacid; Electrolyte Supplement
Use Treatment and prevention of calcium depletion; relief of acid indigestion, heartburn
Usual Dosage Dosage is in terms of elemental calcium
Recommended daily allowance (RDA): Oral:
<6 months: 360 mg/day
6-12 months: 540 mg/day
1-10 years: 800 mg/day
10-18 years: 1200 mg/day
Adults: 800 mg/day
Hypocalcemia (dose depends on clinical condition and serum calcium level):
Children: 20-65 mg/kg/day in 4 divided doses
Adults: 1-2 g or more per day
Dosage Forms Elemental calcium listed in brackets
Capsule: 1500 mg [600 mg]
Calci-Mix™: 1250 mg [500 mg]
Florical®: 364 mg [145.6 mg] with sodium fluoride 8.3 mg
Liquid (Tums® Extra Strength): 1000 mg/5 mL (360 mL)
Lozenge (Mylanta® Soothing Antacids): 600 mg [240 mg]
Powder (Cal Carb-HD®): 6.5 g/packet [2.6 g]
Suspension, oral: 1250 mg/5 mL [500 mg]
Tablet: 650 mg [260 mg], 1500 mg [600 mg]
Calciday-667®: 667 mg [267 mg]
Os-Cal® 500, Oyst-Cal® 500, Oystercal® 500: 1250 mg [500 mg]

Cal-Plus®, Caltrate® 600, Gencalc® 600, Nephro-Calci®: 1500 mg [600 mg]
Chewable:
 Alka-Mints®: 850 mg [340 mg]
 Amitone®: 350 mg [140 mg]
 Caltrate, Jr.®: 750 mg [300 mg]
 Calci-Chew™, Os-Cal®: 750 mg [300 mg]
 Chooz®, Dicarbosil®, Equilet®, Tums®: 500 mg [200 mg]
 Mallamint®: 420 mg [168 mg]
 Rolaids® Calcium Rich: 550 mg [220 mg]
 Tums® E-X Extra Strength: 750 mg [300 mg]
 Tums® Ultra®: 1000 mg [400 mg]
 Florical®: 364 mg [145.6 mg]with sodium fluoride 8.3 mg

calcium carbonate and magnesium carbonate
(KAL see um KAR bun ate & mag NEE zhum KAR bun ate)
Brand Names Mylanta® Gelcaps®
Therapeutic Category Antacid
Use Hyperacidity
Dosage Forms Capsule: Calcium carbonate 311 mg and magnesium carbonate 232 mg

calcium carbonate and simethicone
(KAL see um KAR bun ate & sye METH i kone)
Synonyms simethicone and calcium carbonate
Brand Names Titralac® Plus Liquid [OTC]
Therapeutic Category Antacid; Antiflatulent
Use Relief of acid indigestion, heartburn, peptic esophagitis, hiatal hernia, and gas
Usual Dosage Oral: 0.5-2 g 4-6 times/day
Dosage Forms Elemental calcium listed in brackets
 Liquid: Calcium carbonate 500 mg [200 mg] and simethicone 20 mg per 5 mL

calcium chloride (KAL see um KLOR ide)
Therapeutic Category Electrolyte Supplement
Use Emergency treatment of hypocalcemic tetany; treatment of hypermagnesemia; cardiac disturbances of hyperkalemia, hypocalcemia or calcium channel blocking agent toxicity
Usual Dosage I.V.:
 Cardiac arrest in the presence of hyperkalemia or hypocalcemia, magnesium toxicity, or calcium antagonist toxicity:
 Infants and Children: 10-20 mg/kg; may repeat in 10 minutes if necessary
 Adults: 1.5-4 mg/kg/dose or 2.5-5 mL/dose every 10 minutes
 Hypocalcemia:
 Infants and Children: 10-20 mg/kg/dose, repeat every 4-6 hours if needed
 Adults: 500 mg to 1 g at 1- to 3-day intervals
 Exchange transfusion: 0.45 mEq after each 100 mL of blood exchanged I.V.
 Hypocalcemia secondary to citrated blood transfusion: Administer 0.45 mEq **elemental** calcium for each 100 mL citrated blood infused
 Tetany:
 Infants and Children: 10 mg/kg over 5-10 minutes; may repeat after 6 hours or follow with an infusion with a maximum dose of 200 mg/kg/day
 Adults: 1 g over 10-30 minutes; may repeat after 6 hours
Dosage Forms Elemental calcium listed in brackets
 Injection: 10% = 100 mg/mL [27.2 mg/mL] (10 mL)

calcium citrate (KAL see um SIT rate)
Brand Names Citracal® [OTC]
Therapeutic Category Electrolyte Supplement
(Continued)

calcium citrate *(Continued)*

Use Adjunct in prevention of postmenopausal osteoporosis, treatment and prevention of calcium depletion

Usual Dosage Oral (dosage is in terms of elemental calcium): Adults: Oral: 1-2 g/day

Recommended daily allowance (RDA):
<6 months: 360 mg/day
6-12 months: 540 mg/day
1-10 years: 800 mg/day
10-18 years: 1200 mg/day
Adults: 800 mg/day

Dosage Forms Elemental calcium listed in brackets
Tablet: 950 mg [200 mg]
Effervescent: 2376 mg [500 mg]

Calcium Disodium Versenate® *see* edetate calcium disodium *on page 189*

calcium edta *see* edetate calcium disodium *on page 189*

calcium glubionate (KAL see um gloo BYE oh nate)

Brand Names Neo-Calglucon® [OTC]

Therapeutic Category Electrolyte Supplement

Use Treatment and prevention of calcium depletion

Usual Dosage Oral (syrup is a hyperosmolar solution; dosage is in terms of calcium glubionate):

Neonatal hypocalcemia: 1200 mg/kg/day in 4-6 divided doses
Maintenance: Infants and Children: 600-2000 mg/kg/day in 4 divided doses up to a maximum of 9 g/day
Adults: 6-18 g/day in divided doses

Recommended daily allowance (RDA):
<6 months: 360 mg/day
6-12 months: 540 mg/day
1-10 years: 800 mg/day
10-18 years: 1200 mg/day
Adults: 800 mg/day

Dosage Forms Elemental calcium listed in brackets
Syrup: 1.8 g/5 mL [115 mg/5 mL] (480 mL)

calcium gluceptate (KAL see um gloo SEP tate)

Therapeutic Category Electrolyte Supplement

Use Emergency treatment of hypocalcemia; treatment of hypermagnesemia; cardiac disturbances of hyperkalemia, hypocalcemia, or calcium channel blocker toxicity

Usual Dosage I.V.:
Cardiac resuscitation in the presence of hypocalcemia, hyperkalemia, or calcium channel blocker toxicity:
Children: 110 mg/kg/dose or 0.5 mL/kg/dose every 10 minutes
Adults: 5 mL every 10 minutes
Hypocalcemia:
Children: 200-500 mg/kg/day divided every 6 hours
Adults: 500 mg to 1.1 g/dose as needed
Exchange transfusion: 0.45 mEq (0.5 mL) after each 100 mL of blood exchanged
After citrated blood administration: Children and Adults: 0.4 mEq/100 mL blood infused

Dosage Forms Elemental calcium listed in brackets
Injection: 220 mg/mL [18 mg/mL] (5 mL, 50 mL)

calcium gluconate (KAL see um GLOO koe nate)

Brand Names Kalcinate®

Therapeutic Category Electrolyte Supplement

Use Treatment and prevention of hypocalcemia, hypermagnesemia, cardiac disturbances of hyperkalemia, hypocalcemia, or calcium channel blocker toxicity

Usual Dosage Dosage is in terms of elemental calcium

Recommended daily allowance (RDA):
<6 months: 360 mg/day
6-12 months: 540 mg/day
1-10 years: 800 mg/day
10-18 years: 1200 mg/day
Adults: 800 mg/day

Calcium gluconate electrolyte requirement in newborn period:
Premature: 200-1000 mg/kg/24 hours
Term:
0-24 hours: 0-500 mg/kg/24 hours
24-48 hours: 200-500 mg/kg/24 hours
48-72 hours: 200-600 mg/kg/24 hours
>3 days: 200-800 mg/kg/24 hours

Hypocalcemia:
I.V.:
Infants and Children: 200-1000 mg/kg/day as a continuous infusion or in 4 divided doses
Adults: 2-15 g/24 hours as a continuous infusion or in divided doses
Oral:
Children: 200-500 mg/kg/day divided every 6 hours
Adults: 500 mg to 2 g 2-4 times/day

Calcium antagonist toxicity, magnesium intoxication; cardiac arrest in the presence of hyperkalemia or hypocalcemia: I.V.:
Infants and Children: 100 mg/kg/dose
Adults: 1-3 g

Tetany: I.V.: doses or as an infusion
Infants and Children: 100-200 mg/kg/dose over 5-10 minutes; may repeat after 6 hours or follow with an infusion of 500 mg/kg/day
Adults: 1-3 g may be administered until therapeutic response occurs

Cardiac resuscitation: I.V.:
Infants and Children: 100 mg/kg/dose (1 mL/kg/dose) every 10 minutes
Adults: 500-800 mg/dose (5-8 mL) every 10 minutes

Hypocalcemia secondary to citrated blood infusion; administer 0.45 mEq **elemental** calcium for each 100 mL citrated blood infused

Exchange transfusion:
Adults: 300 mg/100 mL of citrated blood exchanged

Maintenance electrolyte requirements for total parenteral nutrition: I.V.: Daily requirements: Adults: 10-20 mEq/1000 kcals/24 hours

Dosage Forms Elemental calcium listed in brackets
Injection: 10% = 100 mg/mL [9 mg/mL] (10 mL, 50 mL, 100 mL, 200 mL)
Tablet: 500 mg [45 mg], 650 mg [58.5 mg], 975 mg [87.75 mg], 1 g [90 mg]

calcium lactate (KAL see um LAK tate)

Therapeutic Category Electrolyte Supplement

Use Treatment and prevention of calcium depletion

Usual Dosage Oral:
Infants: 400-500 mg/kg/day divided every 4-6 hours
Children: 500 mg/kg/day divided every 6-8 hours; maximum daily dose: 9 g
Adults: 1.5-3 g divided every 8 hours

Dosage Forms Elemental calcium listed in brackets
Tablet: 325 mg [42.25 mg], 650 mg [84.5 mg]

calcium leucovorin *see* leucovorin *on page 302*

calcium pantothenate *see* pantothenic acid *on page 395*

calcium phosphate, dibasic (KAL see um FOS fate tri BAY sik)
Synonyms dicalcium phosphate
Brand Names Posture® [OTC]
Therapeutic Category Electrolyte Supplement
Use Adjunct in prevention of postmenopausal osteoporosis, treatment and prevention of calcium depletion
Usual Dosage Oral:
Children: 45-65 mg/kg/day
Adults: 1-2 g/day (doses in g of elemental calcium)
Dosage Forms Elemental calcium listed in brackets
Tablet, sugar free: 1565.2 mg [600 mg]

calcium polycarbophil (KAL see um pol i KAR boe fil)
Brand Names Equalactin® Chewable Tablet [OTC]; Fiberall® Chewable Tablet [OTC]; FiberCon® Tablet [OTC]; Fiber-Lax® Tablet [OTC]; Mitrolan® Chewable Tablet [OTC]
Therapeutic Category Gastrointestinal Agent, Miscellaneous; Laxative
Use Treatment of constipation or diarrhea by restoring a more normal moisture level and providing bulk in the patient's intestinal tract; calcium polycarbophil is supplied as the approved substitute whenever a bulk-forming laxative is ordered in a tablet, capsule, wafer, or other oral solid dosage form
Usual Dosage Oral:
Children:
2-6 years: 500 mg 1-2 times/day, up to 1.5 g/day
6-12 years: 500 mg 1-3 times/day, up to 3 g/day
Adults: 1 g 4 times/day, up to 6 g/day
Dosage Forms Tablet:
Sodium free:
Fiber-Lax®: 625 mg
FiberCon®: 500 mg
Chewable:
Equalactin®, Mitrolan®: 500 mg
Fiberall®: 1250 mg

Caldecort® *see* hydrocortisone *on page 268*
Caldecort® Anti-Itch Spray *see* hydrocortisone *on page 268*
Calderol® *see* calcifediol *on page 80*
Caldesene® Topical [OTC] *see* undecylenic acid and derivatives *on page 541*
Calm-X® Oral [OTC] *see* dimenhydrinate *on page 171*
Calphron® *see* calcium acetate *on page 82*
Cal-Plus® [OTC] *see* calcium carbonate *on page 82*
Caltrate® 600 [OTC] *see* calcium carbonate *on page 82*
Caltrate, Jr.® [OTC] *see* calcium carbonate *on page 82*
Cama® Arthritis Pain Reliever [OTC] *see* aspirin *on page 44*
Campho-Phenique® [OTC] *see* camphor and phenol *on this page*

camphor and phenol (KAM for & FEE nole)
Brand Names Campho-Phenique® [OTC]
Therapeutic Category Topical Skin Product
Use Relief of pain and for minor infections
Usual Dosage Topical: Apply as needed
Dosage Forms Liquid: Camphor 10.8% and phenol 4.7%

camphorated tincture of opium *see* paregoric *on page 397*

camphor, menthol, and phenol (KAM for, MEN thol, & FEE nole)
Brand Names Sarna [OTC]
Therapeutic Category Topical Skin Product
Use Relief of dry, itching skin
Usual Dosage Topical: Apply as needed for dry skin
Dosage Forms Lotion, topical: Camphor 0.5%, menthol 0.5%, and phenol 0.5% in emollient base (240 mL)

Camptosar® *see* irinotecan *on page 288*

Candida albicans (*Monilia*) (KAN dee da AL bi kans mo NIL ya)
Synonyms *Monilia* skin test
Brand Names Dermatophytin-O
Therapeutic Category Diagnostic Agent
Use Screen for detection of nonresponsiveness to antigens in immunocompromised individuals
Usual Dosage Intradermal: 0.1 mL, examine reaction site in 24-48 hours; induration of ≥5 mm in diameter is a positive reaction
Dosage Forms Injection:
Intradermal: 1:100 (5 mL)
Scratch: 1:10 (5 mL)

Cantil® *see* mepenzolate *on page 328*

Capastat® **Sulfate** *see* capreomycin *on this page*

Capital® **and Codeine** *see* acetaminophen and codeine *on page 3*

Capitrol® *see* chloroxine *on page 112*

Capoten® *see* captopril *on next page*

Capozide® *see* captopril and hydrochlorothiazide *on next page*

capreomycin (kap ree oh MYE sin)
Synonyms capreomycin sulfate
Brand Names Capastat® Sulfate
Therapeutic Category Antibiotic, Miscellaneous
Use In conjunction with at least one other antituberculosis agent in the treatment of tuberculosis
Usual Dosage Adults: I.M.: 15 mg/kg/day up to 1 g/day for 60-120 days
Dosage Forms Injection, as sulfate: 100 mg/mL (10 mL)

capreomycin sulfate *see* capreomycin *on this page*

capsaicin (kap SAY sin)
Brand Names Capsin® [OTC]; Capzasin-P® [OTC]; Dolorac® [OTC]; No Pain-HP® [OTC]; R-Gel® [OTC]; Zostrix® [OTC]; Zostrix-® HP [OTC]
Therapeutic Category Analgesic, Topical
Use FDA approved for the topical treatment of pain associated with postherpetic neuralgia, rheumatoid arthritis, osteoarthritis, diabetic neuropathy, and postsurgical pain

Unlabeled uses: Treatment of pain associated with psoriasis, chronic neuralgias unresponsive to other forms of therapy, and intractable pruritus
Usual Dosage Children >2 years and Adults: Topical: Apply to area up to 3-4 times/day only
Dosage Forms
Cream:
Capzasin-P®, Zostrix®: 0.025% (45 g, 90 g)
Dolorac®: 0.25% (28 g)
Zostrix-® HP: 0.075% (30 g, 60 g)
(Continued)

capsaicin *(Continued)*
Gel (R-Gel®): 0.025% (15 g, 30 g)
Lotion (Capsin®): 0.025% (59 mL); 0.075% (59 mL)
Roll-on (No Pain-HP®): 0.075% (60 mL)

Capsin® [OTC] *see* capsaicin *on previous page*

captopril (KAP toe pril)
Brand Names Capoten®
Therapeutic Category Angiotensin-Converting Enzyme (ACE) Inhibitors
Use Management of hypertension and treatment of congestive heart failure; in postmyo-cardial infarction, improves survival in clinically stable patients with left-ventricular dysfunction
Usual Dosage Note: Dosage must be titrated according to patient's response; use lowest effective dose. Oral:

Infants: Initial: 0.15-0.3 mg/kg/dose; titrate dose upward to maximum of 6 mg/kg/day in 1-4 divided doses; usual required dose: 2.5-6 mg/kg/day

Children: Initial: 0.5 mg/kg/dose; titrate upward to maximum of 6 mg/kg/day in 2-4 divided doses

Older Children: Initial: 6.25-12.5 mg/dose every 12-24 hours; titrate upward to maximum of 6 mg/kg/day

Adolescents and Adults: Initial: 12.5-25 mg/dose administered every 8-12 hours; increase by 25 mg/dose to maximum of 450 mg/day

Note: Smaller dosages administered every 8-12 hours are indicated in patients with renal dysfunction. Renal function and leukocyte count should be carefully monitored during therapy.
Dosage Forms Tablet: 12.5 mg, 25 mg, 50 mg, 100 mg

captopril and hydrochlorothiazide
(KAP toe pril & hye droe klor oh THYE a zide)
Brand Names Capozide®
Therapeutic Category Antihypertensive, Combination
Use Management of hypertension and treatment of congestive heart failure
Usual Dosage Adults: Oral:
Hypertension: Initial: 25 mg 2-3 times/day; may increase at 1- to 2-week intervals up to 150 mg 3 times/day (captopril dosages)
Congestive heart failure: 6.25-25 mg 3 times/day (maximum: 450 mg/day) (captopril dosages)
Dosage Forms Tablet:
25/15: Captopril 25 mg and hydrochlorothiazide 15 mg
25/25: Captopril 25 mg and hydrochlorothiazide 25 mg
50/15: Captopril 50 mg and hydrochlorothiazide 15 mg
50/25: Captopril 50 mg and hydrochlorothiazide 25 mg

Capzasin-P® [OTC] *see* capsaicin *on previous page*

Carafate® *see* sucralfate *on page 494*

caramiphen and phenylpropanolamine
(kar AM i fen & fen il proe pa NOLE a meen)
Synonyms phenylpropanolamine and caramiphen
Brand Names Ordrine AT® Extended Release Capsule; Rescaps-D® S.R. Capsule; Tuss-Allergine® Modified T.D. Capsule; Tussogest® Extended Release Capsule
Therapeutic Category Antihistamine/Decongestant Combination
Use Symptomatic relief of cough and nasal congestion associated with the common cold

Usual Dosage Oral:
Children:
2-6 years: $\frac{1}{2}$ teaspoonful every 4 hours
6-12 years: 1 teaspoonful every 4 hours
Children >12 years and Adults: 1 capsule every 12 hours or 2 teaspoonfuls every 4 hours

Dosage Forms
Capsule, timed release: Caramiphen edisylate 40 mg and phenylpropanolamine hydrochloride 75 mg
Liquid: Caramiphen edisylate 6.7 mg and phenylpropanolamine hydrochloride 12.5 mg per 5 mL

carampicillin hydrochloride *see bacampicillin on page 52*

carbachol (KAR ba kole)

Synonyms carbacholine; carbamylcholine chloride
Brand Names Carbastat® Ophthalmic; Carboptic® Ophthalmic; Isopto® Carbachol Ophthalmic; Miostat® Intraocular
Therapeutic Category Cholinergic Agent
Use Lower intraocular pressure in the treatment of glaucoma; to cause miosis during surgery
Usual Dosage Adults:
Intraocular: 0.5 mL instilled into anterior chamber before or after securing sutures
Ophthalmic: Instill 1-2 drops up to 4 times/day
Dosage Forms Solution:
Intraocular (Carbastat®, Miostat®): 0.01% (1.5 mL)
Topical, ophthalmic:
Carboptic®: 3% (15 mL)
Isopto® Carbachol: 0.75% (15 mL, 30 mL); 1.5% (15 mL, 30 mL); 2.25% (15 mL); 3% (15 mL, 30 mL)

carbacholine *see carbachol on this page*

carbamazepine (kar ba MAZ e peen)

Brand Names Epitol®; Tegretol®; Tegretol-XR®
Therapeutic Category Anticonvulsant
Use Prophylaxis of generalized tonic-clonic, partial (especially complex partial), and mixed partial or generalized seizure disorder; may be used to relieve pain in trigeminal neuralgia or diabetic neuropathy; has been used to treat bipolar disorders
Usual Dosage Oral (dosage must be adjusted according to patient's response and serum concentrations):
Children:
<6 years: Initial: 5 mg/kg/day; dosage may be increased every 5-7 days to 10 mg/kg/day; then up to 20 mg/kg/day if necessary; administer in 2-4 divided doses/day
6-12 years: Initial: 100 mg twice daily or 10 mg/kg/day in 2 divided doses; increase by 100 mg/day depending upon response; usual maintenance: 15-30 mg/kg/day in 2-4 divided doses/day; maximum: 1000 mg/24 hours
Children >12 years and Adults: 200 mg twice daily to start, increase by 200 mg/day at weekly intervals until therapeutic levels achieved; usual dose: 800-1200 mg/day in 3-4 divided doses; some patients have required up to 1.6-2.4 g/day
Dosage Forms
Suspension, oral (citrus-vanilla flavor): 100 mg/5 mL (450 mL)
Tablet: 200 mg
Chewable: 100 mg
Extended release: 100 mg, 200 mg, 400 mg

carbamide *see urea on page 542*

carbamide peroxide (KAR ba mide per OKS ide)

Synonyms urea peroxide

Brand Names Auro® Ear Drops [OTC]; Debrox® Otic [OTC]; E•R•O Ear [OTC]; Gly-Oxide® Oral [OTC]; Mollifene® Ear Wax Removing Formula [OTC]; Murine® Ear Drops [OTC]; Orajel® Perioseptic [OTC]; Proxigel® Oral [OTC]

Therapeutic Category Anti-infective Agent, Oral; Otic Agent, Cerumenolytic

Use
Oral: Relief of minor inflammation of gums, oral mucosal surfaces and lips including canker sores and dental irritation; adjunct in oral hygiene
Otic: Emulsify and disperse ear wax

Usual Dosage Children >12 years and Adults:
Oral: Apply several drops undiluted to affected area of the mouth 4 times/day and at bedtime for up to 7 days, expectorate after 2-3 minutes; as an adjunct to oral hygiene after brushing, swish 10 drops for 2-3 minutes, then expectorate; gel: massage on affected area 4 times/day
Otic: Instill 5-10 drops twice daily for up to 4 days; keep drops in ear for several minutes by keeping head tilted or placing cotton in ear

Dosage Forms
Gel, oral (Proxigel®): 10% (34 g)
Solution:
Oral:
Gly-Oxide®: 10% in glycerin (15 mL, 60 mL)
Orajel® Perioseptic: 15% in glycerin (13.3 mL)
Otic (Auro® Ear Drops, Debrox®, Mollifene® Ear Wax Removing, Murine® Ear Drops): 6.5% in glycerin (15 mL, 30 mL)

carbamylcholine chloride *see* carbachol *on previous page*

Carbastat® Ophthalmic *see* carbachol *on previous page*

carbenicillin (kar ben i SIL in)

Synonyms carbenicillin indanyl sodium; carindacillin

Brand Names Geocillin®

Therapeutic Category Penicillin

Use Treatment of urinary tract infections, asymptomatic bacteriuria, or prostatitis caused by susceptible strains of *Pseudomonas aeruginosa*, *E. coli*, indole-positive *Proteus*, and *Enterobacter*

Usual Dosage Oral:
Children: 30-50 mg/kg/day divided every 6 hours; maximum dose: 2-3 g/day
Adults: 1-2 tablets every 6 hours

Dosage Forms Tablet, film coated, as indanyl sodium ester: 382 mg [base]

carbenicillin indanyl sodium *see* carbenicillin *on this page*

carbidopa (kar bi DOE pa)

Brand Names Lodosyn®

Therapeutic Category Anti-Parkinson's Agent; Dopaminergic Agent (Antiparkinson's)

Use With levodopa in the treatment of parkinsonism to enable a lower dosage of the latter to be used and a more rapid response to be obtained, and to decrease side-effects; for details of administration and dosage

Usual Dosage Adults: Oral: 70-100 mg/day; maximum daily dose: 200 mg

Dosage Forms Tablet: 25 mg

carbidopa and levodopa *see* levodopa and carbidopa *on page 305*

carbinoxamine and pseudoephedrine
(kar bi NOKS a meen & soo doe e FED rin)

Brand Names Biohist-LA®; Carbiset® Tablet; Carbiset-TR® Tablet; Carbodec® Syrup; Carbodec® Tablet; Carbodec TR® Tablet; Cardec-S® Syrup; Rondec® Drops; Rondec® Filmtab®; Rondec® Syrup; Rondec-TR®

Therapeutic Category Antihistamine/Decongestant Combination

Use Temporary relief of nasal congestion, running nose, sneezing, itching of nose or throat, and itchy, watery eyes due to the common cold, hay fever, or other respiratory allergies

Usual Dosage Oral:

Children:

Drops: 1-18 months: 0.25-1 mL 4 times/day

Syrup:

18 months to 6 years: 2.5 mL 3-4 times/day

>6 years: 5 mL 2-4 times/day

Adults:

Liquid: 5 mL 4 times/day

Tablet: 1 tablet 4 times/day

Dosage Forms

Drops: Carbinoxamine maleate 2 mg and pseudoephedrine hydrochloride 25 mg per mL (30 mL with dropper)

Syrup: Carbinoxamine maleate 4 mg and pseudoephedrine hydrochloride 60 mg per 5 mL (120 mL, 480 mL)

Tablet:

Film-coated: Carbinoxamine maleate 4 mg and pseudoephedrine hydrochloride 60 mg

Sustained release: Carbinoxamine maleate 8 mg and pseudoephedrine hydrochloride 120 mg

carbinoxamine, pseudoephedrine, and dextromethorphan
(kar bi NOKS a meen, soo doe e FED rin, & deks troe meth OR fan)

Brand Names Carbodec DM®; Cardec DM®; Pseudo-Car® DM; Rondamine-DM® Drops; Rondec®-DM; Tussafed® Drops

Therapeutic Category Antihistamine/Decongestant/Antitussive

Use Relief of coughs and upper respiratory symptoms, including nasal congestion, associated with allergy or the common cold

Usual Dosage

Infants: Drops:

1-3 months: 1/4 mL 4 times/day

3-6 months: 1/2 mL 4 times/day

6-9 months: 3/4 mL 4 times/day

9-18 months: 1 mL 4 times/day

Children 1 1/2 to 6 years: Syrup: 2.5 mL 4 times/day

Children >6 years and Adults: Syrup: 5 mL 4 times/day

Dosage Forms

Drops: Carbinoxamine maleate 2 mg, pseudoephedrine hydrochloride 25 mg, and dextromethorphan hydrobromide 4 mg per mL (30 mL)

Syrup: Carbinoxamine maleate 4 mg, pseudoephedrine hydrochloride 60 mg, and dextromethorphan hydrobromide 15 mg per 5 mL (120 mL, 480 mL, 4000 mL)

Carbiset® Tablet *see* carbinoxamine and pseudoephedrine *on this page*

Carbiset-TR® Tablet *see* carbinoxamine and pseudoephedrine *on this page*

Carbocaine® *see* mepivacaine *on page 329*

Carbodec DM® *see* carbinoxamine, pseudoephedrine, and dextromethorphan *on this page*

Carbodec® Syrup *see* carbinoxamine and pseudoephedrine *on this page*

Carbodec® Tablet *see* carbinoxamine and pseudoephedrine *on this page*

Carbodec TR® Tablet *see* carbinoxamine and pseudoephedrine *on previous page*

carbol-fuchsin solution (kar bol-FOOK sin soe LOO shun)
Synonyms Castellani paint
Therapeutic Category Antifungal Agent
Use Treatment of superficial mycotic infections
Usual Dosage Topical: Apply to affected area 2-4 times/day
Dosage Forms Solution: Basic fuchsin 0.3%, boric acid 1%, phenol 4.5%, resorcinol 10%, acetone 5%, and alcohol 10%

carbolic acid *see* phenol *on page 410*

carboplatin (KAR boe pla tin)
Synonyms cbdca
Brand Names Paraplatin®
Therapeutic Category Antineoplastic Agent
Use Palliative treatment of ovarian carcinoma; also used in the treatment of small cell lung cancer, squamous cell carcinoma of the esophagus; solid tumors of the bladder, cervix and testes; pediatric brain tumor, neuroblastoma
Usual Dosage I.V. (refer to individual protocols):
Children:
Solid tumor: 560 mg/m^2 once every 4 weeks
Brain tumor: 175 mg/m^2 once weekly for 4 weeks with a 2-week recovery period between courses; dose is then adjusted on platelet count and neutrophil count values
Adults: Single agent: 360 mg/m^2 once every 4 weeks; dose is then adjusted on platelet count and neutrophil count values
Dosage Forms Powder for injection, lyophilized: 50 mg, 150 mg, 450 mg

carboprost tromethamine (KAR boe prost tro METH a meen)
Brand Names Hemabate™
Therapeutic Category Prostaglandin
Use Termination of pregnancy
Usual Dosage I.M.: Initial: 250 mcg, then 250 mcg at 1¹/₂-hour to 3¹/₂-hour intervals depending on uterine response; a 500 mcg dose may be administered if uterine response is not adequate after several 250 mcg doses
Dosage Forms Injection: Carboprost 250 mcg and tromethamine 83 mcg per mL (1 mL)

Carboptic® Ophthalmic *see* carbachol *on page 89*

carbose d *see* carboxymethylcellulose *on this page*

carboxymethylcellulose (kar boks ee meth il SEL yoo lose)
Synonyms carbose d; carboxymethylcellulose sodium
Brand Names Cellufresh® [OTC]; Celluvisc® [OTC]
Therapeutic Category Ophthalmic Agent, Miscellaneous
Use Preservative-free artificial tear substitute
Usual Dosage Adults: Ophthalmic: Instill 1-2 drops into eye(s) 3-4 times/day
Dosage Forms Solution, ophthalmic, as sodium, preservative free: 0.5% (0.3 mL); 1% (0.3 mL)

carboxymethylcellulose sodium *see* carboxymethylcellulose *on this page*

Cardec DM® *see* carbinoxamine, pseudoephedrine, and dextromethorphan *on previous page*

Cardec-S® Syrup *see* carbinoxamine and pseudoephedrine *on previous page*

Cardene® *see* nicardipine *on page 373*

Cardene® SR *see* nicardipine *on page 373*

Cardilate® *see* erythrityl tetranitrate *on page 199*

Cardio-Green® *see* indocyanine green *on page 282*

Cardioquin® *see* quinidine *on page 455*

Cardizem® **CD** *see* diltiazem *on page 170*

Cardizem® **Injectable** *see* diltiazem *on page 170*

Cardizem® **SR** *see* diltiazem *on page 170*

Cardizem® **Tablet** *see* diltiazem *on page 170*

Cardura® *see* doxazosin *on page 183*

carindacillin *see* carbenicillin *on page 90*

carisoprodate *see* carisoprodol *on this page*

Carisoprodate *see* carisoprodol, aspirin, and codeine *on this page*

carisoprodol (kar i soe PROE dole)
Synonyms carisoprodate; isobamate
Brand Names Soma®
Therapeutic Category Skeletal Muscle Relaxant
Use Skeletal muscle relaxant
Usual Dosage Adults: Oral: 350 mg 3-4 times/day; administer last dose at bedtime; compound: 1-2 tablets 4 times/day
Dosage Forms Tablet: 350 mg

carisoprodol and aspirin (kar i soe PROE dole & AS pir in)
Brand Names Soma® Compound
Therapeutic Category Skeletal Muscle Relaxant
Use Skeletal muscle relaxant
Usual Dosage Adults: Oral: 1-2 tablets 4 times/day
Dosage Forms Tablet: Carisoprodol 200 mg and aspirin 325 mg

carisoprodol, aspirin, and codeine
(kar i soe PROE dole, AS pir in, and KOE deen)
Synonyms Carisoprodate; Isobamate
Brand Names Soma® Compound w/Codeine
Therapeutic Category Skeletal Muscle Relaxant
Controlled Substance C-III
Use Skeletal muscle relaxant
Usual Dosage Adults: Oral: 1-2 tablets 4 times/day
Dosage Forms Tablet: Carisoprodol 200 mg, aspirin 325 mg, and codeine phosphate 16 mg

Carmol-HC® **Topical** *see* urea and hydrocortisone *on page 542*

Carmol® **Topical [OTC]** *see* urea *on page 542*

carmustine (kar MUS teen)
Synonyms bcnu
Brand Names BiCNU®; Gliadel®
Therapeutic Category Antineoplastic Agent
Use Brain tumors, multiple myeloma, Hodgkin's disease, and non-Hodgkin's lymphomas; some activity in malignant melanoma; glioblastoma multiforme (wafer)
Usual Dosage Children and Adults:
I.V. infusion (refer to individual protocols): 75-100 mg/m^2/day for 2 days or 150-200 mg/m^2 every 6 weeks as a single dose or divided into daily injections on 2 successive days; next dose is to be determined based on hematologic response to the previous dose
Wafer: Implant 8 wafer in resected brain cavity, if size and shape allow
(Continued)

carmustine *(Continued)*

Dosage Forms
Powder for injection: 100 mg/vial packaged with 3 mL of absolute alcohol for use as a sterile diluent
Wafer: 7.7 mg

Carnation Instant Breakfast® [OTC] *see* enteral nutritional products *on page 194*

Carnitor® Injection *see* levocarnitine *on page 304*

Carnitor® Oral *see* levocarnitine *on page 304*

carteolol (KAR tee oh lole)

Synonyms carteolol hydrochloride
Brand Names Cartrol® Oral; Ocupress® Ophthalmic
Therapeutic Category Beta-Adrenergic Blocker
Use Management of hypertension; treatment of increased intraocular pressure
Usual Dosage Adults:
Oral: 2.5 mg as a single daily dose, maintenance dose: 2.5-5 mg once daily
Ophthalmic: 1 drop in eye(s) twice daily
Dosage Forms
Solution, ophthalmic, as hydrochloride (Ocupress®): 1% (5 mL, 10 mL)
Tablet, as hydrochloride (Cartrol®): 2.5 mg, 5 mg

carteolol hydrochloride *see* carteolol *on this page*

Carter's Little Pills® [OTC] *see* bisacodyl *on page 67*

Cartrol® Oral *see* carteolol *on this page*

carvedilol (KAR ve dil ole)

Brand Names Coreg®
Therapeutic Category Beta-Adrenergic Blocker
Use Management of hypertension, congestive heart failure; can be used alone or in combination with other agents, especially thiazide-type diuretics
Usual Dosage Adults: Oral: 6.25 mg twice daily, if tolerated, should be maintained for 1-2 weeks, then increased to 12.5 mg twice daily; dosage may be increased to a maximum of 25 mg twice daily; if pulse rate drops <55 beats/minute, the dosage should be reduced
Dosage Forms Tablet: 3.125 mg, 6.25 mg, 12.5 mg, 25 mg

casanthranol and docusate *see* docusate and casanthranol *on page 180*

cascara sagrada (kas KAR a sah GRAH dah)

Therapeutic Category Laxative
Use Temporary relief of constipation; sometimes used with milk of magnesia ("black and white" mixture)
Usual Dosage Note: Cascara sagrada fluid extract is 5 times more potent than cascara sagrada aromatic fluid extract

Oral (aromatic fluid extract):
Infants: 1.25 mL/day (range: 0.5-1.5 mL) as needed
Children 2-11 years: 2.5 mL/day (range: 1-3 mL) as needed
Children ≥12 years and Adults: 5 mL/day (range: 2-6 mL) as needed at bedtime (1 tablet as needed at bedtime)
Dosage Forms
Aromatic fluid extract: 120 mL, 473 mL
Tablet: 325 mg

Casodex® *see* bicalutamide *on page 66*

Castellani paint *see* carbol-fuchsin solution *on page 92*

castor oil (KAS tor oyl)
Synonyms oleum ricini
Brand Names Alphamul® [OTC]; Emulsoil® [OTC]; Fleet® Flavored Castor Oil [OTC]; Neoloid® [OTC]; Purge® [OTC]
Therapeutic Category Laxative
Use Preparation for rectal or bowel examination or surgery; rarely used to relieve constipation; also applied to skin as emollient and protectant
Usual Dosage Oral:
Castor oil:
Infants <2 years: 1-5 mL or 15 mL/m^2/dose as a single dose
Children 2-11 years: 5-15 mL as a single dose
Children ≥12 years and Adults: 15-60 mL as a single dose
Emulsified castor oil:
Infants: 2.5-7.5 mL/dose
Children <2 years: 5-15 mL/dose
Children 2-11 years: 7.5-30 mL/dose
Children ≥12 years and Adults: 30-60 mL/dose
Dosage Forms
Emulsion, oral:
Alphamul®: 60% (90 mL, 3780 mL)
Emulsoil®: 95% (63 mL)
Fleet® Flavored Castor Oil: 67% (45 mL, 90 mL)
Neoloid®: 36.4% (118 mL)
Liquid, oral:
100% (60 mL, 120 mL, 480 mL)
Purge®: 95% (30 mL, 60 mL)

Cataflam® Oral *see* diclofenac *on page 164*

Catapres® Oral *see* clonidine *on page 130*

Catapres-TTS® Transdermal *see* clonidine *on page 130*

Caverject® Injection *see* alprostadil *on page 18*

cbdca *see* carboplatin *on page 92*

ccnu *see* lomustine *on page 312*

C-Crystals® [OTC] *see* ascorbic acid *on page 42*

2-cda *see* cladribine *on page 125*

cddp *see* cisplatin *on page 125*

Cebid® Timecelles® [OTC] *see* ascorbic acid *on page 42*

Ceclor® *see* cefaclor *on this page*

Ceclor® CD *see* cefaclor *on this page*

Cecon® [OTC] *see* ascorbic acid *on page 42*

Cedax® *see* ceftibuten *on page 100*

CeeNU® *see* lomustine *on page 312*

Ceepryn® [OTC] *see* cetylpyridinium *on page 105*

cefaclor (SEF a klor)
Brand Names Ceclor®; Ceclor® CD
Therapeutic Category Cephalosporin (Second Generation)
Use Infections caused by susceptible organisms including *Staph aureus*, *S. pneumoniae*, and *H. influenzae*; treatment of otitis media, sinusitis, and infections involving the respiratory tract, skin and skin structure, bone and joint, and urinary tract
(Continued)

cefaclor *(Continued)*

Usual Dosage Oral:
Children >1 month: 20-40 mg/kg/day divided every 8-12 hours; maximum dose: 2 g/day (twice daily option is for treatment of otitis media or pharyngitis)
Adults: 250-500 mg every 8 hours or daily dose can be administered in 2 divided doses

Dosage Forms
Capsule: 250 mg, 500 mg
Powder for oral suspension (strawberry flavor): 125 mg/5 mL (75 mL, 150 mL); 187 mg/ 5 mL (50 mL, 100 mL); 250 mg/5 mL (75 mL, 150 mL); 375 mg/5 mL (50 mL, 100 mL)
Tablet, extended release: 375 mg, 500 mg

cefadroxil (sef a DROKS il)

Synonyms cefadroxil monohydrate
Brand Names Duricef®
Therapeutic Category Cephalosporin (First Generation)
Use Treatment of susceptible bacterial infections including group A beta-hemolytic streptococcal pharyngitis or tonsillitis; skin and soft tissue infections caused by streptococci or staphylococci; urinary tract infections caused by *Klebsiella, E. coli,* and *Proteus mirabilis*

Usual Dosage Oral:
Children: 30 mg/kg/day divided twice daily up to a maximum of 2 g/day
Adults: 1-2 g/day in 2 divided doses

Dosage Forms
Capsule, as monohydrate: 500 mg
Suspension, oral, as monohydrate: 125 mg/5 mL, 250 mg/5 mL, 500 mg/5 mL (50 mL, 100 mL)
Tablet, as monohydrate: 1 g

cefadroxil monohydrate *see* cefadroxil *on this page*

Cefadyl® *see* cephapirin *on page 103*

cefamandole (sef a MAN dole)

Synonyms cefamandole nafate
Brand Names Mandol®
Therapeutic Category Cephalosporin (Second Generation)
Use Treatment of susceptible bacterial infection; mainly respiratory tract, skin and skin structure, bone and joint, urinary tract and gynecologic as well as septicemia, perioperative prophylaxis

Usual Dosage I.M., I.V.:
Children: 100-150 mg/kg/day in divided doses every 4-6 hours
Adults: 4-12 g/24 hours divided every 4-6 hours 500-1000 mg every 4-8 hours

Dosage Forms Powder for injection, as nafate: 500 mg (10 mL); 1 g (10 mL, 100 mL); 2 g (20 mL, 100 mL); 10 g (100 mL)

cefamandole nafate *see* cefamandole *on this page*

cefazolin (sef A zoe lin)

Synonyms cefazolin sodium
Brand Names Ancef®; Kefzol®; Zolicef®
Therapeutic Category Cephalosporin (First Generation)
Use Treatment of respiratory tract, skin and skin structure, urinary tract, biliary tract, bone and joint infections and septicemia due to susceptible gram-positive cocci (except enterococcus); some gram-negative bacilli including *E. coli, Proteus,* and *Klebsiella* may be susceptible; perioperative prophylaxis

Usual Dosage I.M., I.V.:
Infants and Children: 50-100 mg/kg/day in 3 divided doses; maximum dose: 6 g/day
Adults: 1-2 g every 8 hours

Dosage Forms
Infusion, premixed, as sodium, in D_5W (frozen) (Ancef®): 500 mg (50 mL); 1 g (50 mL)
Injection, as sodium (Kefzol®): 500 mg, 1 g
Powder for injection, as sodium (Ancef®, Zolicef®): 250 mg, 500 mg, 1 g, 5 g, 10 g, 20 g

cefazolin sodium *see cefazolin on previous page*

cefepime (SEF e pim)
Synonyms cefepime hydrochloride
Brand Names Maxipime®
Therapeutic Category Cephalosporin (Fourth Generation)
Use Treatment of respiratory tract infections (including bronchitis and pneumonia), cellu-litis and other skin and soft tissue infections, and urinary tract infections; considered a fourth generation cephalosporin because it has good gram-negative coverage similar to third generation cephalosporins, but better gram-positive coverage
Usual Dosage I.V.:
Children: Unlabeled: 50 mg/kg every 8 hours; maximum dose: 2 g
Adults:
Most infections: 1-2 g every 12 hours for 5-10 days; higher doses or more frequent administration may be required in pseudomonal infections
Urinary tract infections, uncomplicated: 500 mg every 12 hours
Dosage Forms Powder for Injection, as hydrochloride: 500 mg, 1 g, 2 g

cefepime hydrochloride *see cefepime on this page*

cefixime (sef IKS eem)
Brand Names Suprax®
Therapeutic Category Cephalosporin (Third Generation)
Use Treatment of urinary tract infections, otitis media, respiratory infections due to susceptible organisms including *S. pneumoniae* and *Pyogenes*, *H. influenzae*, *M. catar-rhalis*, and many *Enterobacteriaceae*; documented poor compliance with other oral antimicrobials; outpatient therapy of serious soft tissue or skeletal infections due to susceptible organisms; single-dose oral treatment of uncomplicated cervical/urethral gonorrhea due to *N. gonorrhoeae*; treatment of shigellosis in areas with a high rate of resistance to TMP-SMX
Usual Dosage Oral:
Children: 8 mg/kg/day in 1-2 divided doses; maximum dose: 400 mg/day
Children >50 kg or >12 years and Adults: 400 mg/day in 1-2 divided doses
Dosage Forms
Powder for oral suspension (strawberry flavor): 100 mg/5 mL (50 mL, 100 mL)
Tablet, film coated: 200 mg, 400 mg

Cefizox® *see ceftizoxime on page 100*

cefmetazole (sef MET a zole)
Synonyms cefmetazole sodium
Brand Names Zefazone®
Therapeutic Category Cephalosporin (Second Generation)
Use Second generation cephalosporin with an antibacterial spectrum similar to cefoxitin, useful on many aerobic and anaerobic gram-positive and gram-negative bacteria
Usual Dosage Adults: I.V.:
Infections: 2 g every 6-12 hours for 5-14 days
Prophylaxis: 2 g 30-90 minutes before surgery
Dosage Forms Powder for injection, as sodium: 1 g, 2 g

cefmetazole sodium *see cefmetazole on this page*

Cefobid® *see cefoperazone on next page*

Cefol® Filmtab® *see vitamins, multiple (oral, adult) on page 556*

cefonicid (se FON i sid)

Synonyms cefonicid sodium
Brand Names Monocid®
Therapeutic Category Cephalosporin (Second Generation)
Use Treatment of susceptible bacterial infection; mainly respiratory tract, skin and skin structure, bone and joint, urinary tract and gynecologic as well as septicemia; second generation cephalosporin
Usual Dosage Adults: I.M., I.V.: 1 g every 24 hours
Dosage Forms Powder for injection, as sodium: 500 mg, 1 g, 10 g

cefonicid sodium *see cefonicid on this page*

cefoperazone (sef oh PER a zone)

Synonyms cefoperazone sodium
Brand Names Cefobid®
Therapeutic Category Cephalosporin (Third Generation)
Use Treatment of susceptible bacterial infections, mainly respiratory tract, skin and skin structure, urinary tract and sepsis; as a third generation cephalosporin, cefoperazone has activity against gram-negative bacilli (eg, *E. coli*, *Klebsiella*, and *Haemophilus*) but variable activity against *Streptococcus* and *Staphylococcus* species; it has activity against *Pseudomonas aeruginosa*, but less than ceftazidime
Usual Dosage I.M., I.V.:
Children: 100-150 mg/kg/day divided every 8-12 hours
Adults: 2-4 g/day in divided doses every 12 hours (up to 12 g/day)
Dosage Forms
Injection, as sodium, premixed (frozen): 1 g (50 mL); 2 g (50 mL)
Powder for injection, as sodium: 1 g, 2 g

cefoperazone sodium *see cefoperazone on this page*

Cefotan® *see cefotetan on this page*

cefotaxime (sef oh TAKS eem)

Synonyms cefotaxime sodium
Brand Names Claforan®
Therapeutic Category Cephalosporin (Third Generation)
Use Treatment of susceptible lower respiratory tract, skin and skin structure, bone and joint, intra-abdominal and genitourinary tract infections; treatment of a documented or suspected meningitis due to susceptible organisms such as *H. influenzae* and *N. meningitidis*; nonpseudomonal gram-negative rod infection in a patient at risk of developing aminoglycoside-induced nephrotoxicity and/or ototoxicity; infection due to an organism whose susceptibilities clearly favor cefotaxime over cefuroxime or an aminoglycoside
Usual Dosage I.M., I.V.:
Infants and Children 1 month to 12 years:
<50 kg: 100-200 mg/kg/day in 3-4 divided doses
Meningitis: 200 mg/kg/day in 4 divided doses
>50 kg: Moderate to severe infection: 1-2 g every 6-8 hours; life-threatening infection: 2 g/dose every 4 hours; maximum dose: 12 g/day
Children >12 years and Adults: 1-2 g every 6-8 hours (up to 12 g/day)
Dosage Forms
Infusion, as sodium, premixed, in D_5W (frozen): 1 g (50 mL); 2 g (50 mL)
Powder for injection, as sodium: 500 mg, 1 g, 2 g, 10 g

cefotaxime sodium *see cefotaxime on this page*

cefotetan (SEF oh tee tan)

Synonyms cefotetan disodium
Brand Names Cefotan®

Therapeutic Category Cephalosporin (Second Generation)

Use Treatment of susceptible lower respiratory tract, skin and skin structure, bone and joint, genitourinary tract, sepsis, gynecologic, and intra-abdominal infections; active against anaerobes including *Bacteroides* species of gastrointestinal tract, gram-negative enteric bacilli including *E. coli*, *Klebsiella*, and *Proteus*; active against many strains of *N. gonorrhoeae*; perioperative prophylaxis

Usual Dosage I.M., I.V.:

Children: 40-80 mg/kg/day divided every 12 hours

Adults: 1-6 g/day in divided doses every 12 hours, 1-2 g may be administered every 24 hours for urinary tract infection

Dosage Forms Powder for injection, as disodium: 1 g (10 mL, 100 mL); 2 g (20 mL, 100 mL); 10 g (100 mL)

cefotetan disodium *see* cefotetan *on previous page*

cefoxitin (se FOKS i tin)

Synonyms cefoxitin sodium

Brand Names Mefoxin®

Therapeutic Category Cephalosporin (Second Generation)

Use Treatment of susceptible lower respiratory tract, skin and skin structure, bone and joint, genitourinary tract, sepsis, gynecologic, and intra-abdominal infections; active against anaerobes including *Bacteroides* species of the gastrointestinal tract, gram-negative enteric bacilli including *E. coli*, *Klebsiella*, and *Proteus*; active against many strains of *N. gonorrhoeae*; perioperative prophylaxis

Usual Dosage I.M., I.V.:

Infants >3 months and Children:

Mild-moderate infection: 80-100 mg/kg/day in divided doses every 4-6 hours

Severe infection: 100-160 mg/kg/day in divided doses every 4-6 hours

Maximum dose: 12 g/day

Adults: 1-2 g every 6-8 hours (I.M. injection is painful)

Dosage Forms

Infusion, as sodium, premixed, in D_5W (frozen): 1 g (50 mL); 2 g (50 mL)

Powder for injection, as sodium: 1 g, 2 g, 10 g

cefoxitin sodium *see* cefoxitin *on this page*

cefpodoxime (sef pode OKS eem)

Synonyms cefpodoxime proxetil

Brand Names Vantin®

Therapeutic Category Cephalosporin (Second Generation)

Use Treatment of susceptible acute, community-acquired pneumonia caused by *S. pneumoniae* or nonbeta-lactamase producing *H. influenzae*; alternative regimen for acute uncomplicated gonorrhea caused by *N. gonorrhoeae*; uncomplicated skin and skin structure infections caused by *S. aureus* or *S. pyogenes*; acute otitis media caused by *S. pneumoniae*, *H. influenzae*, or *M. catarrhalis*; pharyngitis or tonsillitis; and uncomplicated urinary tract infections caused by *E. coli*, *Klebsiella*, and *Proteus*

Usual Dosage Oral:

Children >6 months to 12 years: 10 mg/kg/day divided every 12 hours for 10 days

Adults: 100-400 mg every 12 hours for 7-14 days

Dosage Forms

Granules for oral suspension, as proxetil (lemon creme flavor): 50 mg/5 mL (100 mL); 100 mg/5 mL (100 mL)

Tablet, film coated, as proxetil: 100 mg, 200 mg

cefpodoxime proxetil *see* cefpodoxime *on this page*

cefprozil (sef PROE zil)
Brand Names Cefzil®
Therapeutic Category Cephalosporin (Second Generation)
Use Infections caused by susceptible organisms including *S. pneumoniae, H. influenzae, M. catarrhalis, S. aureus, S. pyogenes*; treatment of infections involving the respiratory tract, skin and skin structure, and otitis media
Usual Dosage Oral:
Infants and Children >6 months to 12 years: 15 mg/kg every 12 hours for 10 days
Children >13 years and Adults: 250-500 mg every 12-24 hours for 10 days
Dosage Forms
Powder for oral suspension, as anhydrous: 125 mg/5 mL (50 mL, 75 mL, 100 mL); 250 mg/5 mL (50 mL, 75 mL, 100 mL)
Tablet, as anhydrous: 250 mg, 500 mg

ceftazidime (SEF tay zi deem)
Brand Names Ceptaz™; Fortaz®; Tazicef®; Tazidime®
Therapeutic Category Cephalosporin (Third Generation)
Use Treatment of infections of the respiratory tract, urinary tract, skin and skin structure, intra-abdominal, osteomyelitis, sepsis, and meningitis caused by susceptible gram-negative aerobic organisms *Enterobacteriaceae pseudomonas*; pseudomonal infection in patient at risk of developing aminoglycoside-induced nephrotoxicity and/or ototoxicity; empiric therapy for febrile, granulocytopenic patients
Usual Dosage
Infants and Children 1 month to 12 years: 30-50 mg/kg/dose every 8 hours; maximum dose: 6 g/day
Adults: 1-2 g every 8-12 hours (250-500 mg every 12 hours for urinary tract infections)
Dosage Forms
Infusion, premixed (frozen) (Fortaz®): 1 g (50 mL); 2 g (50 mL)
Powder for injection: 500 mg, 1 g, 2 g, 6 g

ceftibuten (sef TYE byoo ten)
Brand Names Cedax®
Therapeutic Category Cephalosporin (Third Generation)
Use Oral cephalosporin for bronchitis, otitis media, and strep throat
Usual Dosage Oral:
Children: 9 mg/kg/day for 10 days; maximum daily dose: 400 mg
Children ≥12 years and Adults: 400 mg once daily for 10 days
Dosage Forms
Capsule: 400 mg
Powder for oral suspension (cherry flavor): 90 mg/5 mL (30 mL, 60 mL, 120 mL); 180 mg/5 mL (30 mL, 60 mL, 120 mL)

Ceftin® Oral *see* cefuroxime *on next page*

ceftizoxime (sef ti ZOKS eem)
Synonyms ceftizoxime sodium
Brand Names Cefizox®
Therapeutic Category Cephalosporin (Third Generation)
Use Treatment of susceptible bacterial infections, mainly respiratory tract, skin and skin structure, bone and joint, urinary tract and sepsis; as a third generation cephalosporin, ceftizoxime has activity against gram-negative enteric bacilli (eg, *E. coli, Klebsiella*), and cocci (eg, *Neisseria*), and variable activity against gram-positive cocci (*Staphylococcus* and *Streptococcus*); it has some anaerobic coverage but is less active against *B. fragilis* than cefoxitin; also indicated for *Neisseria gonorrhoeae* infections (including uncomplicated cervical and urethral gonorrhea and gonorrhea pelvic inflammatory disease), and *Haemophilus influenzae* meningitis

Usual Dosage I.M., I.V.:
Children ≥6 months: 50 mg/kg every 6-8 hours to 200 mg/kg/day to maximum of 12 g/24 hours
Adults: 1-2 g every 8-12 hours, up to 2 g every 4 hours or 4 g every 8 hours for life-threatening infections

Dosage Forms
Injection, as sodium, in D_5W (frozen): 1 g (50 mL); 2 g (50 mL)
Powder for injection, as sodium: 500 mg, 1 g, 2 g, 10 g

ceftizoxime sodium *see* ceftizoxime *on previous page*

ceftriaxone (sef trye AKS one)
Synonyms ceftriaxone sodium
Brand Names Rocephin®
Therapeutic Category Cephalosporin (Third Generation)
Use Treatment of sepsis, meningitis, infections of the lower respiratory tract, skin and skin structure, bone and joint, intra-abdominal and urinary tract due to susceptible organisms as a third generation cephalosporin, ceftriaxone has activity against gram-negative aerobic bacteria (ie, *H. influenzae*, Enterobacteriaceae, *Neisseria*) and variable activity against gram-positive cocci; documented or suspected infection due to susceptible organisms in home care patients and patients without I.V. line access; treatment of documented or suspected gonococcal infection or chancroid; emergency room management of patients at high risk for bacteremia, periorbital or buccal cellulitis, salmonellosis or shigellosis and pneumonia of unestablished etiology (<5 years of age)
Usual Dosage
Gonococcal ophthalmia: 25-50 mg/kg/day administered every 24 hours
Infants and Children: 50-100 mg/kg/day in 1-2 divided doses
Meningitis: 100 mg/kg/day divided every 12 hours; loading dose of 75 mg/kg may be administered at the start of therapy
Chancroid, uncomplicated gonorrhea: I.M.:
<45 kg: 125 mg as a single dose
>45 kg: 250 mg as a single dose
Adults: 1-2 g every 12-24 hours depending on the type and severity of the infection; maximum dose: 4 g/day
Dosage Forms
Infusion, as sodium, premixed (frozen): 1 g in $D_{3.8}W$ (50 mL); 2 g in $D_{2.4}W$ (50 mL)
Injection, as sodium: 350 mg/mL
Powder for injection, as sodium: 250 mg, 500 mg, 1 g, 2 g, 10 g

ceftriaxone sodium *see* ceftriaxone *on this page*

cefuroxime (se fyoor OKS eem)
Synonyms cefuroxime axetil; cefuroxime sodium
Brand Names Ceftin® Oral; Kefurox® Injection; Zinacef® Injection
Therapeutic Category Cephalosporin (Second Generation)
Use Second generation cephalosporin useful in infections caused by susceptible staphylococci, group B streptococci, pneumococci, *H. influenzae* (type A and B), *E. coli*, *Enterobacter*, and *Klebsiella*; treatment of susceptible infections of the upper and lower respiratory tract, otitis media, urinary tract, skin and soft tissue, bone and joint, and sepsis
Usual Dosage
Children:
Oral:
<12 years: 125 mg twice daily
>12 years: 250 mg twice daily
I.M., I.V.: 75-150 mg/kg/day divided every 8 hours; maximum dose: 9 g/day
Adults:
Oral: 125-500 mg twice daily, depending on severity of infection
(Continued)

cefuroxime *(Continued)*

I.M., I.V.: 100-150 mg/kg/day in divided doses every 6-8 hours; maximum: 6 g/24 hours
Dosage Forms
Infusion, as sodium, premixed (frozen) (Zinacef®): 750 mg (50 mL); 1.5 g (50 mL)
Powder:
For injection, as sodium: 750 mg, 1.5 g, 7.5 g
For injection, as sodium (Kefurox®, Zinacef®): 750 mg, 1.5 g, 7.5 g
For oral suspension, as axetil (tutti-frutti flavor) (Ceftin®): 125 mg/5 mL (50 mL, 100 mL, 200 mL)
Tablet, as axetil (Ceftin®): 125 mg, 250 mg, 500 mg

cefuroxime axetil *see* cefuroxime *on previous page*

cefuroxime sodium *see* cefuroxime *on previous page*

Cefzil® *see* cefprozil *on page 100*

Celestone® *see* betamethasone *on page 64*

Celestone® Soluspan® *see* betamethasone *on page 64*

CellCept® *see* mycophenolate *on page 359*

Cellufresh® [OTC] *see* carboxymethylcellulose *on page 92*

cellulose, oxidized (SEL yoo lose, OKS i dyzed)

Synonyms absorbable cotton
Brand Names Oxycel®; Surgicel®
Therapeutic Category Hemostatic Agent
Use Temporary packing for the control of capillary, venous, or small arterial hemorrhage
Usual Dosage Minimal amounts of an appropriate size are laid on the bleeding site
Dosage Forms
Pad (Oxycel®): 3" x 3", 8 ply
Pledget (Oxycel®): 2" x 1" x 1"
Strip:
Oxycel®:
18" x 2", 4 ply
5" x 1/2", 4 ply
36" x 1/2", 4 ply
Surgicel®:
2" x 14"
4" x 8"
2" x 3"
1/2" x 2"

cellulose sodium phosphate (sel yoo lose SOW dee um FOS fate)

Synonyms csp; sodium cellulose phosphate
Brand Names Calcibind®
Therapeutic Category Urinary Tract Product
Use Adjunct to dietary restriction to reduce renal calculi formation in absorptive hypercalciuria type I
Usual Dosage Adults: Oral: 5 g 3 times/day with meals; decrease dose to 5 g with main meal and 2.5 g with each of two other meals when urinary calcium declines to <150 mg/day
Dosage Forms Powder: 2.5 g packets (90s), 300 g bulk pack

Celluvisc® [OTC] *see* carboxymethylcellulose *on page 92*

Celontin® *see* methsuximide *on page 340*

Cel-U-Jec® *see* betamethasone *on page 64*

Cenafed® [OTC] *see* pseudoephedrine *on page 449*

Cenafed® Plus Tablet [OTC] *see* triprolidine and pseudoephedrine *on page 536*

Cena-K® *see* potassium chloride *on page 427*

Cenolate® *see* sodium ascorbate *on page 482*

Cēpacol® Anesthetic Troches [OTC] *see* cetylpyridinium and benzocaine *on page 105*

Cēpacol® Troches [OTC] *see* cetylpyridinium *on page 105*

Cēpastat® [OTC] *see* phenol *on page 410*

cephalexin (sef a LEKS in)
Synonyms cephalexin monohydrate
Brand Names Biocef; Keflex®; Keftab®
Therapeutic Category Cephalosporin (First Generation)
Use Treatment of susceptible bacterial infections, including those caused by group A beta-hemolytic *Streptococcus, Staphylococcus, Klebsiella pneumoniae, E. coli*, and *Proteus mirabilis*; not active against enterococci; used to treat susceptible infections of the respiratory tract, skin and skin structure, bone, genitourinary tract, and otitis media
Usual Dosage Oral:
Children: 25-50 mg/kg/day every 6 hours; severe infections: 50-100 mg/kg/day in divided doses every 6 hours; maximum: 3 g/24 hours
Adults: 250-1000 mg every 6 hours
Dosage Forms
Capsule, as monohydrate: 250 mg, 500 mg
Powder for oral suspension, as monohydrate: 125 mg/5 mL (5 mL unit dose, 60 mL, 100 mL, 200 mL); 250 mg/5 mL (5 mL unit dose, 100 mL, 200 mL)
Suspension, oral, as monohydrate, pediatric: 100 mg/mL [5 mg/drop] (10 mL)
Tablet:
As monohydrate: 250 mg, 500 mg, 1 g
As hydrochloride: 500 mg

cephalexin monohydrate *see* cephalexin *on this page*

cephalothin (sef A loe thin)
Synonyms cephalothin sodium
Therapeutic Category Cephalosporin (First Generation)
Use Treatment of respiratory tract, skin and skin structure, urinary tract, bone and joint infections, endocarditis, and septicemia due to susceptible gram-positive cocci (except enterococcus); some gram-negative bacilli including *E. coli, Proteus*, and *Klebsiella* may be susceptible; perioperative prophylaxis
Usual Dosage I.M., I.V.:
Children: 75-125 mg/kg/day divided every 4-6 hours; maximum dose: 10 g in a 24-hour period
Adults: 500 mg to 2 g every 4-6 hours
Dosage Forms
Infusion, as sodium, in D_5W (frozen): 1 g (50 mL); 2 g (50 mL)
Powder for injection, as sodium: 1 g, 2 g, 20 g

cephalothin sodium *see* cephalothin *on this page*

cephapirin (sef a PYE rin)
Synonyms cephapirin sodium
Brand Names Cefadyl®
Therapeutic Category Cephalosporin (First Generation)
Use Treatment of respiratory tract, skin and skin structure, urinary tract, bone and joint infections, endocarditis and septicemia due to susceptible gram-positive cocci (except enterococcus); some gram-negative bacilli including *E. coli, Proteus*, and *Klebsiella*, may be susceptible; perioperative prophylaxis
(Continued)

cephapirin *(Continued)*

Usual Dosage I.M., I.V.:
Children: 10-20 mg/kg every 6 hours up to 4 g/24 hours
Adults: 1 g every 6 hours up to 12 g/day
Dosage Forms Powder for injection, as sodium: 500 mg, 1 g, 2 g, 4 g, 20 g

cephapirin sodium *see cephapirin on previous page*

cephradine *(SEF ra deen)*

Brand Names Velosef®
Therapeutic Category Cephalosporin (First Generation)
Use Treatment of susceptible bacterial infections, including those caused by group A beta-hemolytic *Streptococcus*
Usual Dosage Oral:
Children ≥9 months: 25-100 mg/kg/day in equally divided doses every 6-12 hours up to 4 g/day
Adults: 2-4 g/day in 4 equally divided doses up to 8 g/day
Dosage Forms
Capsule: 250 mg, 500 mg
Powder for oral suspension: 125 mg/5 mL (5 mL, 100 mL, 200 mL); 250 mg/5 mL (5 mL, 100 mL, 200 mL)

Cephulac® *see lactulose on page 300*

Ceptaz™ *see ceftazidime on page 100*

Cerebyx® *see fosphenytoin on page 234*

Ceredase® *see alglucerase on page 16*

Cerezyme® *see imiglucerase on page 280*

cerivastatin *(se ree va STAT in)*

Synonyms cerivastatin sodium
Brand Names Baycol®
Therapeutic Category HMG-CoA Reductase Inhibitor
Use Adjunct to dietary therapy to for the reduction of elevated total and LDL cholesterol levels in patients with primary hypercholesterolemia and mixed dyslipidemia when the response to dietary restriction of saturated fat and cholesterol and other nonpharmacological measures alone has been inadequate
Usual Dosage Adults: Oral: 0.3 mg once daily in the evening; may be taken with or without food
Dosage Forms Tablet, as sodium: 0.2 mg, 0.3 mg

cerivastatin sodium *see cerivastatin on this page*

Cerose-DM® [OTC] *see chlorpheniramine, phenylephrine, and dextromethorphan on page 116*

Cerubidine® *see daunorubicin hydrochloride on page 150*

Cerumenex® Otic *see triethanolamine polypeptide oleate-condensate on page 531*

Cervidil® Vaginal Insert *see dinoprostone on page 172*

ces *see estrogens, conjugated on page 205*

Cetacaine® *see benzocaine, butyl aminobenzoate, tetracaine, and benzalkonium chloride on page 60*

Cetamide® Ophthalmic *see sulfacetamide sodium on page 496*

Cetapred® Ophthalmic *see sulfacetamide sodium and prednisolone on page 497*

cetirizine (se TI ra zeen)
Synonyms cetirizine hydrochloride; P-071; UCB-P071
Brand Names Zyrtec™
Therapeutic Category Antihistamine
Use Perennial and seasonal allergic rhinitis and other allergic symptoms including urticaria
Usual Dosage Children ≥12 years and Adults: Oral: 5-10 mg once daily, depending upon symptom severity
Dosage Forms
Syrup, as hydrochloride: 5 mg/5 mL (120 mL)
Tablet, as hydrochloride: 5 mg, 10 mg

cetirizine hydrochloride see cetirizine on this page

cetylpyridinium (SEE til peer i DI nee um)
Synonyms cetylpyridinium chloride
Brand Names Ceepryn® [OTC]; Cēpacol® Troches [OTC]
Therapeutic Category Local Anesthetic
Use Temporary relief of sore throat
Usual Dosage Children >6 years and Adults: Oral: Dissolve 1 lozenge in the mouth every 2 hours as needed
Dosage Forms
Mouthwash, as chloride: 0.05% and alcohol 14% (180 mL)
Troches, as chloride: 1:1500 (24s)

cetylpyridinium and benzocaine
(SEE til peer i DI nee um & BEN zoe kane)
Synonyms benzocaine and cetylpyridinium chloride; cetylpyridinium chloride and benzocaine
Brand Names Cēpacol® Anesthetic Troches [OTC]
Therapeutic Category Local Anesthetic
Use Symptomatic relief of sore throat
Usual Dosage Oral: Use as needed for sore throat
Dosage Forms Troche: Cetylpyridinium chloride 1:1500 and benzocaine 10 mg per troche (18s)

cetylpyridinium chloride see cetylpyridinium on this page

cetylpyridinium chloride and benzocaine see cetylpyridinium and benzocaine on this page

Cevalin® [OTC] see ascorbic acid on page 42

Cevi-Bid® [OTC] see ascorbic acid on page 42

Ce-Vi-Sol® [OTC] see ascorbic acid on page 42

cg see chorionic gonadotropin on page 122

CharcoAid® [OTC] see charcoal on this page

charcoal (CHAR kole)
Synonyms activated carbon; liquid antidote; medicinal carbon
Brand Names Actidose-Aqua® [OTC]; Actidose® With Sorbitol [OTC]; CharcoAid® [OTC]; Charcocaps® [OTC]; Insta-Char® [OTC]; Liqui-Char® [OTC]; SuperChar® [OTC]
Therapeutic Category Antidote
Use Emergency treatment in poisoning by drugs and chemicals; repetitive doses for gastrointestinal dialysis in drug overdose to enhance the elimination of certain drugs (eg, theophylline, phenobarbital, and aspirin) and in uremia to adsorb various waste products
(Continued)

charcoal *(Continued)*

Usual Dosage Oral:
Acute poisoning: Single dose: Charcoal with sorbitol:
Children 1-12 years: 1-2 g/kg/dose or 15-30 g or approximately 5-10 times the weight of the ingested poison; 1 g adsorbs 100-1000 mg of poison; the use of repeat oral charcoal with sorbitol doses is not recommended. In young children sorbitol should be repeated no more than 1-2 times/day.
Adults: 30-100 g

Charcoal in water:
Single dose:
Infants <1 year: 1 g/kg
Children 1-12 years: 15-30 g or 1-2 g/kg
Adults: 30-100 g or 1-2 g/kg
Multiple dose:
Infants <1 year: 1 g/kg every 4-6 hours
Children 1-12 years: 20-60 g or 1-2 g/kg every 2-6 hours until clinical observations and serum drug concentration have returned to a subtherapeutic range
Adults: 20-60 g or 1-2 g/kg every 2-6 hours
Gastric dialysis: Adults: 20-50 g every 6 hours for 1-2 days

Dosage Forms
Capsule (Charcocaps®): 260 mg
Granules (CharcoAid® 2000): 15 g (120 mL)
Liquid, activated:
Actidose-Aqua®: 12.5 g (60 mL); 25 g (120 mL)
CharcoAid® 2000: 15 g (120 mL); 50 g (240 mL)
Liqui-Char®: 12.5 g (60 mL); 15 g (75 mL); 25 g (120 mL); 30 g (120 mL); 50 g (240 mL)
SuperChar®: 30 g (240 mL)
Liquid, activated, with propylene glycol: 12.5 g (60 mL); 25 g (120 mL)
Liquid, activated, with sorbitol:
Actidose® With Sorbitol: 25 g (120 mL); 50 g (240 mL)
CharcoAid® 2000: 15 g (120 mL); 50 g (240 mL)
SuperChar®: 30 g (240 mL)
Powder for suspension, activated:
15 g, 30 g, 40 g, 120 g, 240 g
SuperChar®: 30 g
Suspension, activated, with sorbitol (CharcoAid®): 15 g (120 mL); 30 g (150 mL)

Charcocaps® [OTC] *see* charcoal *on previous page*

Chealamide® *see* edetate disodium *on page 190*

Chemet® *see* succimer *on page 494*

Chenix® *see* chenodiol *on this page*

chenodeoxycholic acid *see* chenodiol *on this page*

chenodiol *(kee noe DYE ole)*

Synonyms chenodeoxycholic acid
Brand Names Chenix®
Therapeutic Category Bile Acid
Use Oral dissolution of cholesterol gallstones in selected patients
Usual Dosage Adults: Oral: 13-16 mg/kg/day in 2 divided doses, starting with 250 mg twice daily the first 2 weeks and increasing by 250 mg/day each week thereafter until the recommended or maximum tolerated dose is achieved
Dosage Forms Tablet, film coated: 250 mg

Cheracol® *see* guaifenesin and codeine *on page 247*

Cheracol® D [OTC] *see* guaifenesin and dextromethorphan *on page 248*

Chibroxin™ Ophthalmic *see* norfloxacin *on page 379*

chicken pox vaccine *see* varicella virus vaccine *on page 546*

Chiggertox® **[OTC]** *see* benzocaine *on page 59*

Children's Advil® **Oral Suspension [OTC]** *see* ibuprofen *on page 278*

Children's Dynafed® **Jr [OTC]** *see* acetaminophen *on page 3*

Children's Hold® **[OTC]** *see* dextromethorphan *on page 160*

Children's Kaopectate® **[OTC]** *see* attapulgite *on page 48*

Children's Motrin® **Oral Suspension [OTC]** *see* ibuprofen *on page 278*

Children's Silapap® **[OTC]** *see* acetaminophen *on page 3*

Children's Silfedrine® **[OTC]** *see* pseudoephedrine *on page 449*

children's vitamins *see* vitamin, multiple (pediatric) *on page 554*

Chlo-Amine® **[OTC]** *see* chlorpheniramine *on page 113*

Chlorafed® **Liquid [OTC]** *see* chlorpheniramine and pseudoephedrine *on page 114*

chloral *see* chloral hydrate *on this page*

chloral hydrate (KLOR al HYE drate)

Synonyms chloral; hydrated chloral; trichloroacetaldehyde monohydrate
Brand Names Aquachloral® Supprettes®
Therapeutic Category Hypnotic, Nonbarbiturate
Controlled Substance C-IV
Use Short-term sedative and hypnotic (<2 weeks), sedative/hypnotic prior to nonpainful therapeutic or diagnostic procedures (eg, EEG, CT scan, MRI, ophthalmic exam, dental procedure)
Usual Dosage
Children:
Sedation, anxiety: Oral, rectal: 5-15 mg/kg/dose every 8 hours, maximum: 500 mg/dose
Prior to EEG: Oral, rectal: 20-25 mg/kg/dose, 30-60 minutes prior to EEG; may repeat in 30 minutes to maximum of 100 mg/kg or 2 g total
Hypnotic: Oral, rectal: 20-40 mg/kg/dose up to a maximum of 50 mg/kg/24 hours or 1 g/dose or 2 g/24 hours
Sedation, nonpainful procedure: Oral: 50-75 mg/kg/dose 30-60 minutes prior to procedure; may repeat 30 minutes after initial dose if needed, to a total maximum dose of 120 mg/kg or 1 g total
Adults: Oral, rectal:
Sedation, anxiety: 250 mg 3 times/day
Hypnotic: 500-1000 mg at bedtime or 30 minutes prior to procedure, not to exceed 2 g/24 hours
Dosage Forms
Capsule: 250 mg, 500 mg
Suppository, rectal: 324 mg, 500 mg, 648 mg
Syrup: 250 mg/5 mL (10 mL); 500 mg/5 mL (5 mL, 10 mL, 480 mL)

chlorambucil (klor AM byoo sil)

Brand Names Leukeran®
Therapeutic Category Antineoplastic Agent
Use Management of chronic lymphocytic leukemia (CLL), Hodgkin's and non-Hodgkin's lymphoma; breast and ovarian carcinoma, testicular carcinoma, choriocarcinoma; Waldenström's macroglobulinemia, and nephrotic syndrome unresponsive to conventional therapy
Usual Dosage Children and Adults: Oral (refer to individual protocols):
General short courses: 0.1-0.2 mg/kg/day or 4-8 mg/m^2/day for 2-3 weeks for remission induction, then adjust dose on basis of blood counts; maintenance therapy: 0.03-0.1 mg/kg/day
(Continued)

chlorambucil *(Continued)*

Nephrotic syndrome: 0.1-0.2 mg/kg/day every day for 5-15 weeks with low-dose prednisone
Chronic lymphocytic leukemia:
  Biweekly regimen: Initial: 0.4 mg/kg dose is increased by 0.1 mg/kg every 2 weeks until a response occurs and/or myelosuppression occurs
  Monthly regimen: Initial: 0.4 mg/kg, increase dose by 0.2 mg/kg every 4 weeks until a response occurs and/or myelosuppression occurs
Malignant lymphomas:
  Non-Hodgkins lymphoma: 0.1 mg/kg/day
  Hodgkins: 0.2 mg/kg/day
Dosage Forms Tablet, sugar coated: 2 mg

chloramphenicol (klor am FEN i kole)

Brand Names AK-Chlor® Ophthalmic; Chloromycetin®; Chloroptic® Ophthalmic
Therapeutic Category Antibiotic, Ophthalmic; Antibiotic, Otic; Antibiotic, Miscellaneous
Use Treatment of serious infections due to organisms resistant to other less toxic antibiotics or when its penetrability into the site of infection is clinically superior to other antibiotics to which the organism is sensitive; useful in infections caused by *Bacteroides, H. influenzae, Neisseria meningitidis, S. pneumoniae, Salmonella,* and *Rickettsia*
Usual Dosage
I.V.:
  Infants and Children: 50-75 mg/kg/day divided every 6 hours; maximum daily dose: 4 g/day
  Adults: 50 mg/kg/day in divided doses every 6 hours; maximum daily dose: 4 g/day
  Ophthalmic: Children and Adults: Instill 1-2 drops or small amount of ointment every 3-6 hours; increase interval between applications after 48 hours
Dosage Forms
  Capsule: 250 mg
  Ointment, ophthalmic: 1% [10 mg/g] (3.5 g)
  AK-Chlor®, Chloromycetin®, Chloroptic® S.O.P.: 1% [10 mg/g] (3.5 g)
  Powder for injection, as sodium succinate: 1 g
  Powder for ophthalmic solution (Chloromycetin®): 25 mg/vial (15 mL)
  Solution: 0.5% [5 mg/mL] (7.5 mL, 15 mL)
  Ophthalmic (AK-Chlor®, Chloroptic®): 0.5% [5 mg/mL] (2.5 mL, 7.5 mL, 15 mL)
  Otic (Chloromycetin®): 0.5% (15 mL)

chloramphenicol and prednisolone

(klor am FEN i kole & pred NIS oh lone)
Brand Names Chloroptic-P® Ophthalmic
Therapeutic Category Antibiotic/Corticosteroid, Ophthalmic
Use Topical anti-infective and corticosteroid for treatment of ocular infections
Usual Dosage Ophthalmic: Instill 1-2 drops in eye(s) 2-4 times/day
Dosage Forms Ointment, ophthalmic: Chloramphenicol 1% and prednisolone 0.5% (3.5 g)

chloramphenicol, polymyxin b, and hydrocortisone

(klor am FEN i kole, pol i MIKS in bee, & hye droe KOR ti sone)
Therapeutic Category Antibiotic/Corticosteroid, Ophthalmic
Use Topical anti-infective and corticosteroid for treatment of ocular infections
Usual Dosage Ophthalmic: Apply ½" ribbon every 3-4 hours until improvement occurs
Dosage Forms Solution, ophthalmic: Chloramphenicol 1%, polymyxin B sulfate 10,000 units, and hydrocortisone acetate 0.5% per g (3.75 g)

Chloraseptic® Oral [OTC] *see* phenol *on page 410*

Chlorate® **[OTC]** *see* chlorpheniramine *on page 113*

chlordiazepoxide (klor dye az e POKS ide)

Synonyms methaminodiazepoxide hydrochloride
Brand Names Libritabs®; Librium®; Mitran® Oral; Reposans-10® Oral
Therapeutic Category Benzodiazepine
Controlled Substance C-IV
Use Management of anxiety and as a preoperative sedative, symptoms of alcohol withdrawal
Usual Dosage
Children >6 years: Anxiety: Oral, I.M.: 0.5 mg/kg/24 hours divided every 6-8 hours
Adults:
Anxiety: Oral: 15-100 mg divided 3-4 times/day
Severe anxiety: 20-25 mg 3-4 times/day
Preoperative sedation:
Oral: 5-10 mg 3-4 times/day, 1-day preop
I.M.: 50-100 mg 1-hour preop
Alcohol withdrawal symptoms: Oral, I.V.: 50-100 mg to start, dose may be repeated in
2-4 hours as necessary to a maximum of 300 mg/24 hours
Dosage Forms
Capsule, as hydrochloride: 5 mg, 10 mg, 25 mg
Powder for injection, as hydrochloride: 100 mg
Tablet: 5 mg, 10 mg, 25 mg

chlordiazepoxide and amitriptyline *see* amitriptyline and chlordiazepoxide *on page 27*

chlordiazepoxide and clidinium *see* clidinium and chlordiazepoxide *on page 127*

Chloresium® **[OTC]** *see* chlorophyll *on next page*

chlorhexidine gluconate (klor HEKS i deen GLOO koe nate)

Brand Names BactoShield® Topical [OTC]; Betasept® [OTC]; Dyna-Hex® Topical [OTC];
Exidine® Scrub [OTC]; Hibiclens® Topical [OTC]; Hibistat® Topical [OTC]; Peridex® Oral
Rinse; PerioGard®
Therapeutic Category Antibiotic, Oral Rinse; Antibiotic, Topical
Use Skin cleanser for surgical scrub, cleanser for skin wounds, germicidal hand rinse,
and as antibacterial dental rinse
Usual Dosage Oral rinse (Peridex®)
Precede use of solution by flossing and brushing teeth, completely rinse toothpaste
from mouth; swish 15 mL undiluted oral rinse around in mouth for 30 seconds, then
expectorate. Caution patient not to swallow the medicine; avoid eating for 2-3 hours
after treatment. (The cap on bottle of oral rinse is a measure for 15 mL.)
When used as a treatment of gingivitis, the regimen begins with oral prophylaxis.
Patient treats mouth with 15 mL chlorhexidine; swish for 30 seconds, then expectorate;
this is repeated twice daily (morning and evening). Patient should have a re-evaluation
followed by a dental prophylaxis every 6 months.
Dosage Forms
Foam, topical, with isopropyl alcohol 4% (BactoShield®): 4% (180 mL)
Liquid, topical, with isopropyl alcohol 4%:
Dyna-Hex® Skin Cleanser: 2% (120 mL, 240 mL, 480 mL, 960 mL, 4000 mL); 4% (120
mL, 240 mL, 480 mL, 4000 mL)
BactoShield® 2: 2% (960 mL)
BactoShield®, Betasept®, Exidine® Skin Cleanser, Hibiclens® Skin Cleanser: 4% (15
mL, 120 mL, 240 mL, 480 mL, 960 mL, 4000 mL)
Rinse:
Oral (mint flavor) (Peridex®, PerioGard®): 0.12% with alcohol 11.6% (480 mL)
Topical (Hibistat® Hand Rinse): 0.5% with isopropyl alcohol 70% (120 mL, 240 mL)
Sponge/Brush (Hibiclens®): 4% with isopropyl alcohol 4% (22 mL)
(Continued)

chlorhexidine gluconate *(Continued)*
Wipes (Hibistat®): 0.5% (50s)

2-chlorodeoxyadenosine *see* cladribine *on page 125*
chloroethane *see* ethyl chloride *on page 211*
Chloromycetin® *see* chloramphenicol *on page 108*
chlorophylin *see* chlorophyll *on this page*

chlorophyll (KLOR oh fil)
Synonyms chlorophylin
Brand Names Chloresium® [OTC]; Derifil® [OTC]; Nullo® [OTC]; PALS® [OTC]
Therapeutic Category Gastrointestinal Agent, Miscellaneous
Use Topically promotes normal healing, relieves pain and inflammation, and reduces malodors in wounds, burns, surface ulcers, abrasions and skin irritations; used orally to control fecal and urinary odors in colostomy, ileostomy, or incontinence
Usual Dosage
Oral: 1-2 tablets/day
Topical: Apply generously and cover with gauze, linen, or other appropriate dressing; do not change dressings more often than every 48-72 hours
Dosage Forms
Ointment, topical (Chloresium®): Chlorophyllin copper complex 0.5% (30 g, 120 g)
Solution, topical, in isotonic saline (Chloresium®): Chlorophyllin copper complex 0.2% (240 mL, 946 mL)
Tablet:
Chloresium®: Chlorophyllin copper complex 14 mg
Derifil®: Water soluble chlorophyll: 100 mg
Nullo®: Chlorophyllin copper complex 33.3 mg
PALS®: Chlorophyllin copper complex 100 mg
Sodium free, sugar free: 20 mg

chloroprocaine (klor oh PROE kane)
Synonyms chloroprocaine hydrochloride
Brand Names Nesacaine®; Nesacaine®-MPF
Therapeutic Category Local Anesthetic
Use For infiltration anesthesia and for peripheral and epidural anesthesia
Usual Dosage Dosage varies with anesthetic procedure, the area to be anesthetized, the vascularity of the tissues, depth of anesthesia required, degree of muscle relaxation required, and duration of anesthesia
Dosage Forms Injection, as hydrochloride:
Preservative free (Nesacaine®-MPF): 2% (30 mL); 3% (30 mL)
With preservative (Nesacaine®): 1% (30 mL); 2% (30 mL)

chloroprocaine hydrochloride *see* chloroprocaine *on this page*
Chloroptic® Ophthalmic *see* chloramphenicol *on page 108*
Chloroptic-P® Ophthalmic *see* chloramphenicol and prednisolone *on page 108*

chloroquine and primaquine (KLOR oh kwin & PRIM a kween)
Synonyms primaquine and chloroquine
Brand Names Aralen® Phosphate With Primaquine Phosphate
Therapeutic Category Aminoquinoline (Antimalarial)
Use Prophylaxis of malaria, regardless of species, in all areas where the disease is endemic
Usual Dosage Adults: Start at least 1 day before entering the endemic area; administer 1 tablet/week on the same day each week; continue for 8 weeks after leaving the endemic area

Dosage Forms Tablet: Chloroquine phosphate 500 mg [base 300 mg] and primaquine phosphate 79 mg [base 45 mg]

chloroquine phosphate (KLOR oh kwin FOS fate)
Brand Names Aralen® Phosphate
Therapeutic Category Aminoquinoline (Antimalarial)
Use Suppression or chemoprophylaxis of malaria; treatment of uncomplicated or mild-moderate malaria; extraintestinal amebiasis; rheumatoid arthritis; discoid lupus erythematosus, scleroderma, pemphigus
Usual Dosage Oral:
Malaria (excluding resistant *P. falciparum*):
Suppression or prophylaxis in endemic areas (begin 1-2 weeks prior to, and continue for 6-8 weeks after the period of potential exposure):
Children: 5 mg base/kg/dose weekly, up to a maximum of 300 mg/dose
Adults: 300 mg/dose weekly
Treatment:
Children: 10 mg base/kg/dose, up to a maximum of 600 mg base/dose one time, followed by 5 mg base/kg/dose one time after 6 hours, and then daily for 2 days (total dose of 25 mg base/kg)
Adults: 600 mg base/dose one time, followed by 300 mg base/dose one time after 6 hours, and then daily for 2 days
Extraintestinal amebiasis: Dosage expressed in mg base:
Children: 10 mg/kg once daily for 2-3 weeks (up to 300 mg base/day)
Adults: 600 mg base/day for 2 days followed by 300 mg base/day for at least 2-3 weeks
Rheumatoid arthritis: Adults: 150 mg base once daily
Melanoma treatment: Children: 10 mg/kg base/dose (maximum: 600 mg) as a single dose followed by 5 mg/kg base one time after 6 hours, then daily for 2 days
Dosage Forms Tablet: 250 mg [150 mg base]; 500 mg [300 mg base]

chlorothiazide (klor oh THYE a zide)
Brand Names Diurigen®; Diuril®
Therapeutic Category Diuretic, Thiazide
Use Management of mild to moderate hypertension; edema associated with congestive heart failure, pregnancy, or nephrotic syndrome
Usual Dosage I.V. has been limited in infants and children and is generally not recommended

Infants <6 months and patients with pulmonary interstitial edema:
Oral: 20-40 mg/kg/day in 2 divided doses
I.V.: 2-8 mg/kg/day in 2 divided doses
Infants >6 months and Children:
Oral: 20 mg/kg/day in 2 divided doses
I.V.: 4 mg/kg/day
Adults:
Oral: 500 mg to 2 g/day divided in 1-2 doses
I.V.: 100-500 mg/day
Dosage Forms
Powder for injection, lyophilized, as sodium: 500 mg
Suspension, oral: 250 mg/5 mL (237 mL)
Tablet: 250 mg, 500 mg

chlorothiazide and methyldopa (klor oh THYE a zide & meth il DOE pa)
Synonyms methyldopa and chlorothiazide
Brand Names Aldoclor®
Therapeutic Category Antihypertensive, Combination
Use Treatment of hypertension
Usual Dosage Oral: 1 tablet 2-3 times/day for first 48 hours, then adjust
(Continued)

chlorothiazide and methyldopa *(Continued)*
Dosage Forms Tablet:
150: Chlorothiazide 150 mg and methyldopa 250 mg
250: Chlorothiazide 250 mg and methyldopa 250 mg

chlorothiazide and reserpine (klor oh THYE a zide & re SER peen)
Synonyms reserpine and chlorothiazide
Therapeutic Category Antihypertensive, Combination
Use Management of hypertension
Usual Dosage Oral: 1-2 tablets 1-2 times/day
Dosage Forms Tablet:
250: Chlorothiazide 250 mg and reserpine 0.125 mg
500: Chlorothiazide 500 mg and reserpine 0.125 mg

chlorotrianisene (klor oh trye AN i seen)
Brand Names TACE®
Therapeutic Category Estrogen Derivative
Use Treat inoperable prostatic cancer; management of atrophic vaginitis, female hypogo-
nadism, vasomotor symptoms of menopause; prevention of postpartum breast engorge-
ment (no longer recommended because increased risk of thrombophlebitis)
Usual Dosage Adults: Oral:
Prostatic cancer: 12-25 mg/day
Atrophic vaginitis: 12-25 mg/day in 28-day cycles (21 days on and 7 days off)
Female hypogonadism: 12-25 mg for 21 days followed by I.M. progesterone 100 mg or
5 days of oral progestin; next course may begin on days of induced uterine bleeding
Menopause: 12-25 mg for 30 days
Postpartum breast engorgement: 12 mg 4 times/day for 7 days or 72 mg twice daily for
2 days
Dosage Forms Capsule: 12 mg, 25 mg

chloroxine (klor OKS een)
Brand Names Capitrol®
Therapeutic Category Antiseborrheic Agent, Topical
Use Treatment of dandruff or seborrheic dermatitis of the scalp
Usual Dosage Topical: Use twice weekly, massage into wet scalp, lather should remain
on the scalp for approximately 3 minutes, then rinsed; application should be repeated
and scalp rinsed thoroughly
Dosage Forms Shampoo: 2% (120 mL)

Chlorphed® [OTC] *see* brompheniramine *on page 73*

Chlorphed®-LA Nasal Solution [OTC] *see* oxymetazoline *on page 390*

chlorphenesin (klor FEN e sin)
Synonyms chlorphenesin carbamate
Brand Names Maolate®
Therapeutic Category Skeletal Muscle Relaxant
Use Adjunctive treatment of discomfort in short-term, acute, painful musculoskeletal
conditions
Usual Dosage Adults: Oral: 800 mg 3 times/day, then adjusted to lowest effective
dosage, usually 400 mg 4 times/day for up to a maximum of 2 months
Dosage Forms Tablet, as carbamate: 400 mg

chlorphenesin carbamate *see* chlorphenesin *on this page*

chlorpheniramine (klor fen IR a meen)

Synonyms chlorpheniramine maleate

Brand Names Aller-Chlor® [OTC]; AL-R® [OTC]; Chlo-Amine® [OTC]; Chlorate® [OTC]; Chlor-Pro® [OTC]; Chlor-Trimeton® [OTC]; Telachlor®; Teldrin® [OTC]

Therapeutic Category Antihistamine

Use Perennial and seasonal allergic rhinitis and other allergic symptoms including urticaria

Usual Dosage

Children: Oral: 0.35 mg/kg/day in divided doses every 4-6 hours

2-6 years: 1 mg every 4-6 hours, not to exceed 6 mg in 24 hours

6-12 years: 2 mg every 4-6 hours, not to exceed 12 mg/day or sustained release 8 mg at bedtime

Children >12 years and Adults: Oral: 4 mg every 4-6 hours, not to exceed 24 mg/day or sustained release 8-12 mg every 8-12 hours, not to exceed 24 mg/day

Adults: Allergic reactions: I.M., I.V., S.C.: 10-20 mg as a single dose; maximum recommended dose: 40 mg/24 hours

Elderly: 4 mg once or twice daily. **Note:** Duration of action may be 36 hours or more when serum concentrations are low.

Dosage Forms

Capsule, as maleate: 12 mg

As maleate, timed release: 8 mg, 12 mg

Injection, as maleate: 10 mg/mL (1 mL, 30 mL); 100 mg/mL (2 mL)

Syrup, as maleate: 2 mg/5 mL (120 mL, 473 mL)

Tablet, as maleate: 4 mg, 8 mg, 12 mg

Chewable: 2 mg

Timed release: 8 mg, 12 mg

chlorpheniramine and acetaminophen

(klor fen IR a meen & a seet a MIN oh fen)

Brand Names Coricidin® [OTC]

Therapeutic Category Antihistamine/Analgesic

Use Symptomatic relief of congestion, headache, aches, and pains of colds and flu

Usual Dosage Adults: Oral: 2 tablets every 4 hours, up to 20 tablets/day

Dosage Forms Tablet: Chlorpheniramine maleate 2 mg and acetaminophen 325 mg

chlorpheniramine and phenylephrine (klor fen IR a meen & fen il EF rin)

Synonyms phenylephrine and chlorpheniramine

Brand Names Dallergy-D® Syrup; Ed A-Hist® Liquid; Histatab® Plus Tablet [OTC]; Histor-D® Syrup; Rolatuss® Plain Liquid; Ru-Tuss® Liquid

Therapeutic Category Antihistamine/Decongestant Combination

Use Temporary relief of nasal congestion and eustachian tube congestion as well as runny nose, sneezing, itching of nose or throat, itchy and watery eyes

Usual Dosage Oral:

Children:

2-5 years: 2.5 mL every 4 hours

6-12 years: 5 mL every 4 hours

Adults: 10 mL every 4 hours or 1-2 regular tablets 3-4 times daily or 1 sustained release capsule every 12 hours

Dosage Forms

Capsule, sustained release: Chlorpheniramine maleate 8 mg and phenylephrine hydrochloride 20 mg

Liquid:

Dallergy-D®, Histor-D®, Rolatuss® Plain, Ru-Tuss®: Chlorpheniramine maleate 2 mg and phenylephrine hydrochloride 5 mg per 5 mL

Ed A-Hist® Liquid: Chlorpheniramine maleate 4 mg and phenylephrine hydrochloride 10 mg per 5 mL

(Continued)

chlorpheniramine and phenylephrine *(Continued)*

Tablet (Histatab® Plus): Chlorpheniramine maleate 2 mg and phenylephrine hydrochloride 5 mg

chlorpheniramine and phenylpropanolamine

(klor fen IR a meen & fen il proe pa NOLE a meen)

Synonyms phenylpropanolamine and chlorpheniramine

Brand Names Allerest® 12 Hour Capsule [OTC]; A.R.M.® Caplet [OTC]; Chlor-Rest® Tablet [OTC]; Demazin® Syrup [OTC]; Genamin® Cold Syrup [OTC]; Ornade® Spansule®; Resaid®; Rescon Liquid [OTC]; Silaminic® Cold Syrup [OTC]; Temazin® Cold Syrup [OTC]; Thera-Hist® Syrup [OTC]; Triaminic® Allergy Tablet [OTC]; Triaminic® Cold Tablet [OTC]; Triaminic® Syrup [OTC]; Tri-Nefrin® Extra Strength Tablet [OTC]; Triphenyl® Syrup [OTC]

Therapeutic Category Antihistamine/Decongestant Combination

Use Symptomatic relief of nasal congestion, runny nose, sneezing, itchy nose or throat, and itchy or watery eyes due to the common cold or allergic rhinitis

Usual Dosage Oral:

Children <12 years: 5 mL every 3-4 hours

Children >12 years and Adults: 1 sustained release capsule or tablet every 12 hours or 5-10 mL every 3-4 hours or 1-2 regular tablets 3-4 times/day

Dosage Forms

Capsule, sustained release: Chlorpheniramine maleate 12 mg and phenylpropanolamine hydrochloride 75 mg

Liquid:

Triphenyl®, Genamin®: Chlorpheniramine maleate 1 mg and phenylpropanolamine hydrochloride 6.25 mg per 5 mL

Demazin®, Rescon®, Silaminic®, Temazin®, Thera-Hist®: Chlorpheniramine maleate 2 mg and phenylpropanolamine hydrochloride 12.5 mg per 5 mL

Syrup: Chlorpheniramine maleate 2 mg and phenylpropanolamine hydrochloride 12.5 mg per 5 mL

Tablet:

Triaminic® Cold: Chlorpheniramine maleate 2 mg and phenylpropanolamine hydrochloride 12.5 mg

Chlor-Rest®: Chlorpheniramine maleate 2 mg and phenylpropanolamine hydrochloride 18.7 mg

A.R.M.®, Triaminic® Allergy, Tri-Nefrin® Extra Strength: Chlorpheniramine maleate 4 mg and phenylpropanolamine hydrochloride 25 mg

Tablet, sustained release: Chlorpheniramine maleate 12 mg and phenylpropanolamine hydrochloride 75 mg

chlorpheniramine and pseudoephedrine

(klor fen IR a meen & soo doe e FED rin)

Synonyms pseudoephedrine and chlorpheniramine

Brand Names Allerest® Maximum Strength [OTC]; Anamine® Syrup [OTC]; Anaplex® Liquid [OTC]; Chlorafed® Liquid [OTC]; Chlor-Trimeton® 4 Hour Relief Tablet [OTC]; Co-Pyronil® 2 Pulvules® [OTC]; Deconamine® Syrup [OTC]; Deconamine® Tablet [OTC]; Deconamine® SR; Fedahist® Tablet [OTC]; Hayfebrol® Liquid [OTC]; Histalet® Syrup [OTC]; Klerist-D® Tablet [OTC]; Pseudo-Gest Plus® Tablet [OTC]; Rhinosyn-PD® Liquid [OTC]; Rhinosyn® Liquid [OTC]; Ryna® Liquid [OTC]; Sudafed Plus® Tablet [OTC]; Sudafed Plus® Liquid [OTC]

Therapeutic Category Antihistamine/Decongestant Combination

Use Relief of nasal congestion associated with the common cold, hay fever, and other allergies, sinusitis, eustachian tube blockage, and vasomotor and allergic rhinitis

Usual Dosage Oral:

Capsule: 1 capsule every 12 hours

Liquid: 5 mL 3-4 times/day

Tablet: 1 tablet 3-4 times/day

Dosage Forms
Capsule:

Co-Pyronil® 2 Pulvules®: Chlorpheniramine maleate 4 mg and pseudoephedrine hydrochloride 60 mg

Capsule, sustained release: Chlorpheniramine maleate 4 mg and pseudoephedrine hydrochloride 60 mg; chlorpheniramine maleate 8 mg and pseudoephedrine hydrochloride 120 mg

Liquid:

Anamine®, Anaplex®, Chlorafed®, Deconamine®, Hayfebrol®, Rhinosyn-PD®, Ryna®: Chlorpheniramine maleate 2 mg and pseudoephedrine sulfate 30 mg per 5 mL

Rhinosyn®: Chlorpheniramine maleate 2 mg and pseudoephedrine sulfate 60 mg per 5 mL

Histalet®: Chlorpheniramine maleate 3 mg and pseudoephedrine sulfate 45 mg per 5 mL

Tablet:

Allerest® Maximum Strength: Chlorpheniramine maleate 2 mg and pseudoephedrine hydrochloride 30 mg

Deconamine®, Fedahist®, Klerist-D®, Pseudo-Gest Plus®, Sudafed Plus®: Chlorpheniramine maleate 4 mg and pseudoephedrine hydrochloride 60 mg

Chlor-Trimeton® 4 Hour Relief: Chlorpheniramine maleate 4 mg and pseudoephedrine sulfate 60 mg

chlorpheniramine, ephedrine, phenylephrine, and carbetapentane

(klor fen IR a meen, e FED rin, fen il EF rin, & kar bay ta PEN tane)

Brand Names Rentamine®; Rynatuss® Pediatric Suspension; Tri-Tannate Plus®
Therapeutic Category Antihistamine/Decongestant/Antitussive
Use Symptomatic relief of cough
Usual Dosage Children: Oral:
<2 years: Titrate dose individually
2-6 years: 2.5-5 mL every 12 hours
>6 years: 5-10 mL every 12 hours
Dosage Forms Liquid: Carbetapentane tannate 30 mg, ephedrine tannate 5 mg, phenylephrine tannate 5 mg, and chlorpheniramine tannate 4 mg per 5 mL

chlorpheniramine maleate *see* chlorpheniramine *on page 113*

chlorpheniramine, phenindamine, and phenylpropanolamine

(klor fen IR a meen, fen IN dah meen, & fen il proe pa NOLE a meen)

Brand Names Nolamine®
Therapeutic Category Antihistamine/Decongestant Combination
Use Relief of upper respiratory and nasal congestion
Usual Dosage Adults: Oral: 1 tablet every 8-12 hours
Dosage Forms Tablet, timed release: Chlorpheniramine maleate 4 mg, phenindamine tartrate 24 mg, and phenylpropanolamine hydrochloride 50 mg

chlorpheniramine, phenylephrine, and codeine

(klor fen IR a meen, fen il EF rin, & KOE deen)

Brand Names Pediacof®; Pedituss®
Therapeutic Category Antihistamine/Decongestant/Antitussive
Controlled Substance C-IV
Use Symptomatic relief of rhinitis, nasal congestion, and cough due to colds or allergy
Usual Dosage Children 6 months to 12 years: Oral: 1.25-10 mL every 4-6 hours
Dosage Forms Liquid: Chlorpheniramine maleate 0.75 mg, phenylephrine hydrochloride 2.5 mg, and codeine phosphate 5 mg with potassium iodide 75 mg per 5 mL

chlorpheniramine, phenylephrine, and dextromethorphan
(klor fen IR a meen, fen il EF rin, & deks troe meth OR fan)
Brand Names Cerose-DM® [OTC]
Therapeutic Category Antihistamine/Decongestant/Antitussive
Use Temporary relief of cough due to minor throat and bronchial irritation; relief of nasal congestion, runny nose, and sneezing
Usual Dosage Adults: Oral: 5-10 mL 4 times/day
Dosage Forms Liquid: Chlorpheniramine maleate 4 mg, phenylephrine hydrochloride 10 mg, and dextromethorphan hydrobromide 15 mg per 5 mL

chlorpheniramine, phenylephrine, and methscopolamine
(klor fen IR a meen, fen il EF rin, & meth skoe POL a meen)
Brand Names D.A.II® Tablet; Dallergy®; Dura-Vent/DA®; Extendryl® SR; Histor-D® Timecelles®
Therapeutic Category Antihistamine/Decongestant/Anticholinergic
Use Relief of nasal congestion, runny nose, and sneezing
Usual Dosage Adults: Oral: 1 capsule or caplet every 12 hours or 5 mL every 4-6 hours
Dosage Forms
 Caplet, sustained release: Chlorpheniramine maleate 8 mg, phenylephrine hydrochloride 20 mg, and methscopolamine nitrate 2.5 mg
 Capsule, sustained release: Chlorpheniramine maleate 8 mg, phenylephrine hydrochloride 10 mg, and methscopolamine nitrate 2.5 mg
 Syrup: Chlorpheniramine maleate 2 mg, phenylephrine hydrochloride 10 mg, and methscopolamine nitrate 0.625 mg per 5 mL
 Tablet: Chlorpheniramine maleate 4 mg, phenylephrine hydrochloride 10 mg, and methscopolamine nitrate 1.25 mg

chlorpheniramine, phenylephrine, and phenylpropanolamine
(klor fen IR a meen, fen il EF rin, & fen il proe pa NOLE a meen)
Brand Names Hista-Vadrin® Tablet
Therapeutic Category Antihistamine/Decongestant Combination
Use Symptomatic relief of rhinitis and nasal congestion due to colds or allergy
Usual Dosage Adults: Oral: 1 tablet every 6 hours
Dosage Forms Tablet: Chlorpheniramine maleate 6 mg, phenylephrine hydrochloride 5 mg, and phenylpropanolamine hydrochloride 40 mg

chlorpheniramine, phenylephrine, and phenyltoloxamine
(klor fen IR a meen, fen il EF rin, & fen il tole LOKS a meen)
Brand Names Comhist®; Comhist® LA
Therapeutic Category Antihistamine/Decongestant Combination
Use Symptomatic relief of rhinitis and nasal congestion due to colds or allergy
Usual Dosage Oral: 1 capsule every 8-12 hours or 1-2 tablets 3 times/day
Dosage Forms
 Capsule, sustained release (Comhist® LA): Chlorpheniramine maleate 4 mg, phenylephrine hydrochloride 20 mg, and phenyltoloxamine citrate 50 mg
 Tablet (Comhist®): Chlorpheniramine maleate 2 mg, phenylephrine hydrochloride 10 mg, and phenyltoloxamine citrate 25 mg

chlorpheniramine, phenylephrine, phenylpropanolamine, and belladonna alkaloids
(klor fen IR a meen, fen il EF rin, fen il proe pa NOLE a meen, & bel a DON a AL ka loydz)
Synonyms phenylephrine, chlorpheniramine, phenylpropanolamine, and belladonna alkaloids; phenylpropanolamine, chlorpheniramine, phenylephrine, and belladonna alkaloids
Brand Names Atrohist® Plus; Phenahist-TR®; Phenchlor® S.H.A.; Ru-Tuss®; Stahist®

Therapeutic Category Cold Preparation

Use Relief of symptoms resulting from irritation of sinus, nasal, and upper respiratory tract tissues, including nasal congestion, watering eyes, and postnasal drip; this product contains anticholinergic agents and should be reserved for patients who do not respond to other antihistamine/decongestants

Usual Dosage Children ≥12 years and Adults: Oral: 1 tablet morning and evening, swallowed whole

Dosage Forms Tablet, sustained release: Chlorpheniramine 8 mg, phenylephrine 25 mg, phenylpropanolamine 50 mg, hyoscyamine 0.19 mg, atropine 0.04 mg, and scopolamine 0.01 mg

chlorpheniramine, phenylpropanolamine, and acetaminophen

(klor fen IR a meen, fen il proe pa NOLE a meen, & a seet a MIN oh fen)

Brand Names Congestant D® [OTC]; Coricidin ©D'® [OTC]; Dapacin® Cold Capsule [OTC]; Duadacin® Capsule [OTC]; Tylenol® Cold Effervescent Medication Tablet [OTC]

Therapeutic Category Antihistamine/Decongestant/Analgesic

Use Symptomatic relief of nasal congestion and headache from colds/sinus congestion

Usual Dosage Adults: Oral: 2 capsules/tablets every 4 hours, up to 12/day

Dosage Forms

Capsule: Chlorpheniramine maleate 2 mg, phenylpropanolamine hydrochloride 12.5 mg, and acetaminophen 325 mg

Tablet: Chlorpheniramine maleate 2 mg, phenylpropanolamine hydrochloride 12.5 mg, and acetaminophen 325 mg

chlorpheniramine, phenylpropanolamine, and dextromethorphan

(klor fen IR a meen, fen il proe pa NOLE a meen, & deks troe meth OR fan)

Brand Names Triaminicol® Multi-Symptom Cold Syrup [OTC]

Therapeutic Category Antihistamine/Decongestant/Antitussive

Use Relief of runny nose, sneezing; cough suppressant; promote nasal and sinus drainage

Usual Dosage

Children 6-12 years: 5 mL every 4 hours

Adults: 10 mL every 4 hours

Dosage Forms Liquid: Chlorpheniramine maleate 2 mg, phenylpropanolamine hydrochloride 12.5 mg, and dextromethorphan hydrobromide 10 mg per 5 mL

chlorpheniramine, phenyltoloxamine, phenylpropanolamine, and phenylephrine

(klor fen IR a meen, fen il tole LOKS a meen, fen il proe pa NOLE a meen & fen il EF rin)

Brand Names Naldecon®; Naldelate®; Nalgest®; Nalspan®; New Decongestant®; Par Decon®; Tri-Phen-Chlor®; Uni-Decon®

Therapeutic Category Antihistamine/Decongestant Combination

Use Symptomatic treatment of nasal and eustachian tube congestion associated with sinusitis and acute upper respiratory infection; symptomatic relief of perennial and allergic rhinitis

Usual Dosage Oral:

Children:

3-6 months: 0.25 mL (pediatric drops) every 3-4 hours

6-12 months: 2.5 mL (pediatric syrup) or 0.5 mL (pediatric drops) every 3-4 hours

1-6 years: 5 mL (pediatric syrup) or 1 mL (pediatric drops) every 3-4 hours

6-12 years: 2.5 mL (syrup) or 10 mL (pediatric syrup) or 1/2 tablet every 3-4 hours

Children >12 years and 5 mL (syrup) or 1 tablet every 3-4 hours

(Continued)

117

chlorpheniramine, phenyltoloxamine, phenylpropanolamine, and phenylephrine *(Continued)*

Dosage Forms
Drops, pediatric: Chlorpheniramine maleate 0.5 mg, phenyltoloxamine citrate 2 mg, phenylpropanolamine hydrochloride 5 mg, and phenylephrine hydrochloride 1.25 mg per mL
Syrup: Chlorpheniramine maleate 2.5 mg, phenyltoloxamine citrate 7.5 mg, phenylpropanolamine hydrochloride 20 mg, and phenylephrine hydrochloride 5 mg per 5 mL
Syrup, pediatric: Chlorpheniramine maleate 0.5 mg, phenyltoloxamine citrate 2 mg, phenylpropanolamine hydrochloride 5 mg, and phenylephrine hydrochloride 1.25 mg per 5 mL
Tablet, sustained release: Chlorpheniramine maleate 5 mg, phenyltoloxamine citrate 15 mg, phenylpropanolamine hydrochloride 40 mg, and phenylephrine hydrochloride 10 mg

chlorpheniramine, pseudoephedrine, and codeine
(klor fen IR a meen, soo doe e FED rin, & KOE deen)
Brand Names Codehist® DH; Decohistine® DH; Dihistine® DH; Ryna-C® Liquid
Therapeutic Category Antihistamine/Decongestant/Antitussive
Controlled Substance C-V
Use Temporary relief of cough associated with minor throat or bronchial irritation; relief of nasal congestion due to common cold, allergic rhinitis, or sinusitis
Usual Dosage Oral:
Children:
25-50 lb: 1.25-2.50 mL every 4-6 hours, up to 4 doses in a 24-hour period
50-90 lb: 2.5-5 mL every 4-6 hours, up to 4 doses in a 24-hour period
Adults: 10 mL every 4-6 hours, up to 4 doses in a 24-hour period
Dosage Forms Liquid: Chlorpheniramine maleate 2 mg, pseudoephedrine hydrochloride 30 mg, and codeine phosphate 10 mg (120 mL, 480 mL)

chlorpheniramine, pyrilamine, and phenylephrine
(klor fen IR a meen, pye RIL a meen, & fen il EF rin)
Brand Names Rhinatate® Tablet; R-Tannamine® Tablet; R-Tannate® Tablet; Rynatan® Pediatric Suspension; Rynatan® Tablet; Tanoral® Tablet; Triotann® Tablet; Tri-Tannate® Tablet
Therapeutic Category Antihistamine/Decongestant Combination
Use Symptomatic relief of nasal congestion associated with upper respiratory tract condition
Usual Dosage Oral:
Children:
<2 years: Titrate dose individually
2-6 years: 2.5-5 mL every 12 hours
Children >6 years and Adults: 5-10 mL every 12 hours
Dosage Forms
Liquid: Chlorpheniramine tannate 2 mg, pyrilamine tannate 12.5 mg, and phenylephrine tannate 5 mg per 5 mL
Tablet: Chlorpheniramine tannate 8 mg, pyrilamine maleate 12.5 mg, and phenylephrine tannate 25 mg

chlorpheniramine, pyrilamine, phenylephrine, and phenylpropanolamine
(klor fen IR a meen, pye RIL a meen, fen il EF rin, & fen il proe pa NOLE a meen)
Brand Names Histalet Forte® Tablet
Therapeutic Category Antihistamine/Decongestant Combination
Use Symptomatic relief of rhinitis and nasal congestion due to colds or allergy
Usual Dosage Adults: Oral: 1 tablet 2-3 times/day

Dosage Forms Tablet: Chlorpheniramine maleate 4 mg, pyrilamine maleate 25 mg, phenylephrine hydrochloride 10 mg, and phenylpropanolamine hydrochloride 50 mg

Chlor-Pro® [OTC] *see* chlorpheniramine *on page 113*

chlorpromazine (klor PROE ma zeen)

Synonyms chlorpromazine hydrochloride
Brand Names Ormazine; Thorazine®
Therapeutic Category Phenothiazine Derivative
Use Treatment of nausea and vomiting; psychoses; Tourette's syndrome; mania; intractable hiccups (adults); behavioral problems (children)
Usual Dosage
Children >6 months:
Psychosis:
Oral: 0.5-1 mg/kg/dose every 4-6 hours; older children may require 200 mg/day or higher
I.M., I.V.: 0.5-1 mg/kg/dose every 6-8 hours; maximum I.M./I.V. dose for <5 years (22.7 kg) = 40 mg/day; maximum I.M./I.V. for 5-12 years (22.7-45.5 kg) = 75 mg/day
Nausea and vomiting:
Oral: 0.5-1 mg/kg/dose every 4-6 hours as needed
I.M., I.V.: 0.5-1 mg/kg/dose every 6-8 hours; maximum dose: Same as psychosis
Rectal: 1 mg/kg/dose every 6-8 hours as needed
Adults:
Psychosis:
Oral: Range: 30-800 mg/day in 1-4 divided doses, initiate at lower doses and titrate as needed; usual dose is 200 mg/day; some patients may require 1-2 g/day
I.M., I.V.: 25 mg initially, may repeat (25-50 mg) in 1-4 hours, gradually increase to a maximum of 400 mg/dose every 4-6 hours until patient controlled; usual dose 300-800 mg/day
Nausea and vomiting:
Oral: 10-25 mg every 4-6 hours
I.M., I.V.: 25-50 mg every 4-6 hours
Rectal: 50-100 mg every 6-8 hours
Intractable hiccups: Oral, I.M.: 25-50 mg 3-4 times/day
Dosage Forms
Capsule, as hydrochloride, sustained action: 30 mg, 75 mg, 150 mg, 200 mg, 300 mg
Concentrate, oral, as hydrochloride: 30 mg/mL (120 mL); 100 mg/mL (60 mL, 240 mL)
Injection, as hydrochloride: 25 mg/mL (1 mL, 2 mL, 10 mL)
Suppository, rectal, as base: 25 mg, 100 mg
Syrup, as hydrochloride: 10 mg/5 mL (120 mL)
Tablet, as hydrochloride: 10 mg, 25 mg, 50 mg, 100 mg, 200 mg

chlorpromazine hydrochloride *see* chlorpromazine *on this page*

chlorpropamide (klor PROE pa mide)

Brand Names Diabinese®
Therapeutic Category Antidiabetic Agent (Oral)
Use Control blood sugar in adult onset, noninsulin-dependent diabetes (type II)
Usual Dosage The dosage of chlorpropamide is variable and should be individualized based upon the patient's response

Adults: Oral: 250 mg once daily; initial dose in elderly patients: 100 mg once daily; subsequent dosages may be increased or decreased by 50-125 mg/day at 3- to 5-day intervals; maximum daily dose: 750 mg
Dosage Forms Tablet: 100 mg, 250 mg

Chlor-Rest® Tablet [OTC] *see* chlorpheniramine and phenylpropanolamine *on page 114*

chlortetracyline (klor tet ra SYE kleen)
Synonyms chlortetracyline hydrochloride
Brand Names Aureomycin®
Therapeutic Category Antibiotic, Ophthalmic; Antibiotic, Topical
Use Treatment of superficial infections of the skin due to susceptible organisms, also infection prophylaxis in minor skin abrasions
Usual Dosage Topical: Apply 1-5 times/day, cover with sterile bandage if needed
Dosage Forms Ointment, as hydrochloride:
Ophthalmic: 1% [10 mg/g] (3.5 g)
Topical: 3% (14.2 g, 30 g)

chlortetracyline hydrochloride *see* chlortetracyline *on this page*

chlorthalidone (klor THAL i done)
Brand Names Hygroton®; Thalitone®
Therapeutic Category Diuretic, Miscellaneous
Use Management of mild to moderate hypertension, used alone or in combination with other agents; treatment of edema associated with congestive heart failure, nephrotic syndrome, or pregnancy
Usual Dosage Oral:
Children: 2 mg/kg 3 times/week
Adults: 25-100 mg/day or 100 mg 3 times/week
Dosage Forms
Tablet: 25 mg, 50 mg, 100 mg
Hygroton®: 25 mg, 50 mg, 100 mg
Thalitone®: 15 mg, 25 mg

Chlor-Trimeton® [OTC] *see* chlorpheniramine *on page 113*
Chlor-Trimeton® 4 Hour Relief Tablet [OTC] *see* chlorpheniramine and pseudoephedrine *on page 114*

chlorzoxazone (klor ZOKS a zone)
Brand Names Flexaphen®; Paraflex®; Parafon Forte™ DSC
Therapeutic Category Skeletal Muscle Relaxant
Use Symptomatic treatment of muscle spasm and pain associated with acute musculo-skeletal conditions
Usual Dosage Oral:
Children: 20 mg/kg/day or 600 mg/m^2/day in 3-4 divided doses
Adults: 250-500 mg 3-4 times/day up to 750 mg 3-4 times/day
Dosage Forms
Caplet (Parafon Forte™ DSC): 500 mg
Capsule (Flexaphen®, Mus-Lax®): 250 mg with acetaminophen 300 mg
Tablet: Paraflex®: 250 mg

Cholac® *see* lactulose *on page 300*
Cholan-HMB® *see* dehydrocholic acid *on page 152*
Cholebrine® *see* radiological/contrast media (ionic) *on page 457*

cholecalciferol (kole e kal SI fer ole)
Synonyms d$_3$
Brand Names Delta-D®
Therapeutic Category Vitamin D Analog
Use Dietary supplement, treatment of vitamin D deficiency or prophylaxis of deficiency
Usual Dosage Adults: Oral: 400-1000 units/day
Dosage Forms Tablet: 400 units, 1000 units

cholera vaccine (KOL er a vak SEEN)
Therapeutic Category Vaccine, Inactivated Bacteria
Use Primary immunization for cholera prophylaxis
Usual Dosage I.M., S.C.:
Children:
6 months to 4 years: 0.2 mL with same dosage schedule
5-10 years: 0.3 mL with same dosage schedule
Children >10 years and Adults: 0.5 mL in 2 doses 1 week to 1 month or more apart
Dosage Forms Injection: Suspension of killed *Vibrio cholerae* (Inaba and Ogawa types)
8 units of each serotype per mL (1.5 mL, 20 mL)

cholestyramine resin (koe LES tir a meen REZ in)
Brand Names Prevalite®; Questran®; Questran® Light
Therapeutic Category Bile Acid Sequestrant
Use Adjunct in the management of primary hypercholesterolemia; pruritus associated with elevated levels of bile acids; diarrhea associated with excess fecal bile acids; pseudomembraneous colitis
Usual Dosage Dosages are expressed in terms of anhydrous resin. Oral:
Children: 240 mg/kg/day in 3 divided doses; need to titrate dose depending on indication
Adults: 3-4 g 3-4 times/day to a maximum of 16-32 g/day in 2-4 divided doses
Dosage Forms
Powder: 4 g of resin/9 g of powder (9 g, 378 g)
For oral suspension:
With aspartame: 4 g of resin/5 g of powder (5 g, 210 g)
With phenylalanine: 4 g of resin/5.5 g of powder (60s)

choline magnesium trisalicylate
(KOE leen mag NEE zhum trye sa LIS i late)
Brand Names Trilisate®
Therapeutic Category Analgesic, Non-narcotic; Nonsteroidal Anti-Inflammatory Agent (NSAID)
Use Management of osteoarthritis, rheumatoid arthritis, and other arthritides
Usual Dosage Oral (based on total salicylate content):
Children: 30-60 mg/kg/day administered in 3-4 divided doses
Adults: 500 mg to 1.5 g 1-3 times/day
Dosage Forms
Liquid: 500 mg/5 mL [choline salicylate 293 mg and magnesium salicylate 362 mg per 5 mL] (237 mL)
Tablet:
500 mg: Choline salicylate 293 mg and magnesium salicylate 362 mg
750 mg: Choline salicylate 440 mg and magnesium salicylate 544 mg
1000 mg: Choline salicylate 587 mg and magnesium salicylate 725 mg

choline salicylate (KOE leen sa LIS i late)
Brand Names Arthropan® [OTC]
Therapeutic Category Analgesic, Non-narcotic; Nonsteroidal Anti-Inflammatory Agent (NSAID)
Use Temporary relief of pain of rheumatoid arthritis, rheumatic fever, osteoarthritis, and other conditions for which oral salicylates are recommended; useful in patients in which there is difficulty in administering doses in a tablet or capsule dosage form, because of the liquid dosage form
Usual Dosage Adults: Oral: 5 mL every 3-4 hours, if necessary, but not more than 6 doses in 24 hours
Dosage Forms Liquid (mint flavor): 870 mg/5 mL (240 mL, 480 mL)

choline theophyllinate *see* oxtriphylline *on page 388*

Cholografin® Meglumine *see* radiological/contrast media (ionic) *on page 457*

Choloxin® *see* dextrothyroxine *on page 161*

chondroitin sulfate-sodium hyaluronate
(kon DROY tin SUL fate-SOW de um hye a loo ROE nate)
Synonyms sodium hyaluronate-chrondroitin sulfate
Brand Names Viscoat®
Therapeutic Category Ophthalmic Agent, Viscoelastic
Use Surgical aid in anterior segment procedures, protects corneal endothelium and coats intraocular lens thus protecting it
Usual Dosage Ophthalmic: Carefully introduce into anterior chamber after thoroughly cleaning the chamber with a balanced salt solution
Dosage Forms Solution: Sodium chondroitin 40 mg and sodium hyaluronate 30 mg (0.25 mL, 0.5 mL)

Chooz® [OTC] *see* calcium carbonate *on page 82*

Chorex® *see* chorionic gonadotropin *on this page*

chorionic gonadotropin (kor ee ON ik goe NAD oh troe pin)
Synonyms cg; hcg
Brand Names A.P.L.®; Chorex®; Choron®; Gonic®; Pregnyl®; Profasi® HP
Therapeutic Category Gonadotropin
Use Treatment of hypogonadotropic hypogonadism, prepubertal cryptorchidism; induce ovulation
Usual Dosage Children: I.M.:
Prepubertal cryptorchidism: 1000-2000 units/m^2/dose 3 times/week for 3 weeks
Hypogonadotropic hypogonadism: 500-1000 USP units 3 times/week for 3 weeks, followed by the same dose twice weekly for 3 weeks
Dosage Forms Powder for injection: 200 units/mL (10 mL, 25 mL); 500 units/mL (10 mL); 1000 units/mL (10 mL); 2000 units/mL (10 mL)

Choron® *see* chorionic gonadotropin *on this page*

Chromagen® OB [OTC] *see* vitamin, multiple (prenatal) *on page 554*

Chroma-Pak® *see* trace metals *on page 525*

chromium injection *see* trace metals *on page 525*

Chronulac® *see* lactulose *on page 300*

Chymex® *see* bentiromide *on page 58*

Chymodiactin® *see* chymopapain *on this page*

chymopapain (KYE moe pa pane)
Brand Names Chymodiactin®
Therapeutic Category Enzyme
Use Alternative to surgery in patients with herniated lumbar intervertebral disks
Usual Dosage 2000-4000 units/disk with a maximum cumulative dose not to exceed 8000 units for patients with multiple disk herniations
Dosage Forms Injection: 4000 units [4 nKat]; 10,000 units [10 nKat]

Cibacalcin® Injection *see* calcitonin *on page 81*

ciclopirox (sye kloe PEER oks)
Synonyms ciclopirox olamine
Brand Names Loprox®
Therapeutic Category Antifungal Agent
Use Treatment of tinea pedis, tinea cruris, tinea corporis, cutaneous candidiasis, tinea versicolor

Usual Dosage Children >10 years and Adults: Topical: Apply twice daily, gently massage into affected areas; safety and efficacy in children <10 years have not been established

Dosage Forms
Cream, topical, as olamine: 1% (15 g, 30 g, 90 g)
Lotion, as olamine: 1% (30 mL)

ciclopirox olamine *see* ciclopirox *on previous page*

cidofovir (si DOF o veer)
Brand Names Vistide®
Therapeutic Category Antiviral Agent
Use Treatment of CMV retinitis in patients with acquired immunodeficiency syndrome (AIDS)
Usual Dosage
Induction treatment: 5 mg/kg once weekly for 2 consecutive weeks
Maintenance treatment: 5 mg/kg administered once every 2 weeks
Probenecid must be administered orally with each dose of cidofovir
Probenecid dose: 2 g 3 hours prior to cidofovir dose, 1 g 2 hours and 8 hours after completion of the infusion; patients should also receive 1 L of normal saline intravenously prior to each infusion of cidofovir; saline should be infused over 1-2 hours
Dosage Forms Injection: 75 mg/mL (5 mL)

Ciloxan™ Ophthalmic *see* ciprofloxacin *on next page*

cimetidine (sye MET i deen)
Brand Names Tagamet®; Tagamet® HB [OTC]
Therapeutic Category Histamine H_2 Antagonist
Use Short-term treatment of active duodenal ulcers and benign gastric ulcers; long-term prophylaxis of duodenal ulcer; gastric hypersecretory states; gastroesophageal reflux
Usual Dosage Oral, I.M., I.V.:
Infants: 10-20 mg/kg/day divided every 6-12 hours
Children: 20-30 mg/kg/day in divided doses every 6 hours

Patients with an active bleed: Administer cimetidine as a continuous infusion

Adults:
Short-term treatment of active ulcers:
Oral: 300 mg 4 times/day or 800 mg at bedtime or 400 mg twice daily for up to 8 weeks
I.M., I.V.: 300 mg every 6 hours or 37.5 mg/hour by continuous infusion; I.V. dosage should be adjusted to maintain an intragastric pH of 5 or greater
Duodenal ulcer prophylaxis: Oral: 400-800 mg at bedtime
Gastric hypersecretory conditions: Oral, I.M., I.V.: 300-600 mg every 6 hours; dosage not to exceed 2.4 g/day

Dosage Forms
Infusion, as hydrochloride, in NS: 300 mg (50 mL)
Injection, as hydrochloride: 150 mg/mL (2 mL, 8 mL)
Liquid, oral, as hydrochloride (mint-peach flavor): 300 mg/5 mL with alcohol 2.8% (5 mL, 240 mL)
Tablet: 200 mg, 300 mg, 400 mg, 800 mg

Cinobac® Pulvules® *see* cinoxacin *on this page*

cinoxacin (sin OKS a sin)
Brand Names Cinobac® Pulvules®
Therapeutic Category Quinolone
Use Urinary tract infections
Usual Dosage Children >12 years and Adults: Oral: 1 g/day in 2-4 doses
(Continued)

cinoxacin *(Continued)*
Dosage Forms Capsule: 250 mg, 500 mg

ciprofloxacin (sip roe FLOKS a sin)
Synonyms ciprofloxacin hydrochloride
Brand Names Ciloxan™ Ophthalmic; Cipro™ Injection; Cipro™ Oral
Therapeutic Category Antibiotic, Ophthalmic; Quinolone
Use Treatment of documented or suspected pseudomonal infection of the respiratory or urinary tract, acute sinusitis, skin and soft tissue, bone and joint, eye and ear; documented multidrug-resistant, aerobic gram-negative bacilli and some gram-positive staphylococci; documented infectious diarrhea due to *Campylobacter jejuni*, *Shigella*, or *Salmonella*; osteomyelitis caused by susceptible organisms in which parenteral therapy is not feasible; ocular infections caused by susceptible bacterial organisms in patients with corneal ulcers or conjunctivitis
Usual Dosage
  Children: Oral: 20-30 mg/kg/day in 2 divided doses; maximum dose: 1.5 g/day
  Adults:
    Oral: 250-750 mg every 12 hours, depending on severity of infection and susceptibility
    Ophthalmic: Instill 1-2 drops in eye(s) every 2 hours while awake for 2 days and 1-2 drops every 4 hours while awake for the next 5 days
    I.V.: 200-400 mg every 12 hours depending on severity of infection
Dosage Forms
  Infusion, as hydrochloride:
    In D_5W: 400 mg (200 mL)
    In NS or D_5W: 200 mg (100 mL)
  Injection, as hydrochloride: 200 mg (20 mL); 400 mg (40 mL)
  Solution, ophthalmic, as hydrochloride: 3.5 mg/mL (2.5 mL, 5 mL)
  Tablet, as hydrochloride: 100 mg, 250 mg, 500 mg, 750 mg

ciprofloxacin hydrochloride *see* ciprofloxacin *on this page*

Cipro™ Injection *see* ciprofloxacin *on this page*

Cipro™ Oral *see* ciprofloxacin *on this page*

cisapride (SIS a pride)
Brand Names Propulsid®
Therapeutic Category Gastrointestinal Agent, Prokinetic
Use Treatment of nocturnal symptoms of gastroesophageal reflux disease (GERD), also demonstrated effectiveness for gastroparesis, refractory constipation, and nonulcer dyspepsia
Usual Dosage Adults: Oral: 10 mg 4 times/day at least 15 minutes before meals and at bedtime; in some patients the dosage will need to be increased to 20 mg to obtain a satisfactory result
Dosage Forms
  Suspension, oral (cherry cream flavor): 1 mg/mL (450 mL)
  Tablet, scored: 10 mg, 20 mg

cisatracurium (sis a tra KYOO ree um)
Synonyms cisatracurium besylate
Brand Names Nimbex®
Therapeutic Category Skeletal Muscle Relaxant
Use Neuromuscular blockade in patients with renal and/or hepatic failure; eases endotracheal intubation as an adjunct to general anesthesia and relaxes skeletal muscle during surgery or mechanical ventilation; does not relieve pain
Usual Dosage I.V. (not to be used I.M.):
  Children 2 to 12 years: Initial: 0.10 mg/kg followed by maintenance doses of 1-5 mcg/kg/minute as needed to maintain neuromuscular blockade

Infusion (requires use of an infusion pump): 0.1 mg/mL or 0.4 mg/mL in D_5W or NS
Dosage Forms Injection, as besylate: 2 mg/mL (5 mL, 10 mL); 10 mg/mL (20 mL)

cisatracurium besylate *see* cisatracurium *on previous page*

cisplatin (SIS pla tin)
Synonyms cddp
Brand Names Platinol®; Platinol®-AQ
Therapeutic Category Antineoplastic Agent
Use Management of metastatic testicular or ovarian carcinoma, advanced bladder cancer, osteosarcoma, Hodgkin's and non-Hodgkin's lymphoma, head or neck cancer, cervical cancer, lung cancer, brain tumors, neuroblastoma; used alone or in combination with other agents
Usual Dosage Children and Adults (refer to individual protocols): I.V.:
Intermittent dosing schedule: 37-75 mg/m^2 once every 2-3 weeks or 50-120 mg/m^2 once every 3-4 weeks
Daily dosing schedule: 15-20 mg/m^2/day for 5 days every 3-4 weeks
Dosage Forms
Injection, aqueous: 1 mg/mL (50 mL, 100 mL)
Powder for injection: 10 mg, 50 mg

13-*cis*-retinoic acid *see* isotretinoin *on page 292*

Citanest® Forte *see* prilocaine *on page 437*

Citanest® Plain *see* prilocaine *on page 437*

Citracal® [OTC] *see* calcium citrate *on page 83*

citrate of magnesia *see* magnesium citrate *on page 318*

citric acid and d-gluconic acid irrigant *see* citric acid bladder mixture *on this page*

citric acid bladder mixture (SI trik AS id BLAD dur MIKS chur)
Synonyms citric acid and d-gluconic acid irrigant; hemiacidrin
Brand Names Renacidin®
Therapeutic Category Irrigating Solution
Use Preparing solutions for irrigating indwelling urethral catheters; to dissolve or prevent formation of calcifications
Usual Dosage 30-60 mL of 10% (sterile) solution 2-3 times/day by means of a rubber syringe
Dosage Forms
Powder for solution: Citric acid 156-171 g, magnesium hydroxycarbonate 75-87 g, d-gluconic acid 21-30 g, magnesium acid citrate 9-15 g, calcium carbonate 2-6 g (150 g, 300 g)
Solution, irrigation: Citric acid 6.602 g, magnesium hydroxycarbonate 3.177 g, glucono-delta-lactone 0.198 g and benzoic acid 0.023 g per 100 mL (500 mL)

Citrotein® [OTC] *see* enteral nutritional products *on page 194*

citrovorum factor *see* leucovorin *on page 302*

Citrucel® [OTC] *see* methylcellulose *on page 341*

CI-719 *see* gemfibrozil *on page 239*

cla *see* clarithromycin *on next page*

cladribine (KLA dri been)
Synonyms 2-cda; 2-chlorodeoxyadenosine
Brand Names Leustatin™
Therapeutic Category Antineoplastic Agent
Use Hairy cell and chronic lymphocytic leukemias
(Continued)

cladribine *(Continued)*
Usual Dosage Adults: I.V. continuous infusion: 0.09 mg/kg/day
Dosage Forms Injection, preservative free: 1 mg/mL (10 mL)

Claforan® *see* cefotaxime *on page 98*

clarithromycin (kla RITH roe mye sin)
Synonyms cla
Brand Names Biaxin™
Therapeutic Category Macrolide (Antibiotic)
Use Treatment of upper and lower respiratory tract infections, acute otitis media, and infections of the skin and skin structure due to susceptible strains of *S. aureus, S. pyogenes, S. pneumoniae, H. influenzae, M. catarrhalis, Mycoplasma pneumoniae, C. trachomatis, Legionella* sp, and *M. avium*; prophylaxis of disseminated *M. avium* Complex (MAC) infections in HIV-infected patients
Usual Dosage Oral: 250-500 mg every 12 hours for 7-14 days
Upper respiratory tract: 250-500 mg every 12 hours for 10-14 days
Pharyngitis/tonsillitis: 250 mg every 12 hours for 10 days
Acute maxillary sinusitis: 500 mg every 12 hours for 14 days
Lower respiratory tract: 250-500 mg every 12 hours for 7-14 days
Acute exacerbation of chronic bronchitis due to:
S. pneumoniae: 250 mg every 12 hours for 7-14 days
M. catarrhalis: 250 mg every 12 hours for 7-14 days
H. influenzae: 500 mg every 12 hours for 7-14 days
Pneumonia due to:
S. pneumoniae: 250 mg every 12 hours for 7-14 days
M. pneumoniae: 250 mg every 12 hours for 7-14 days
Uncomplicated skin and skin structure: 250 mg every 12 hours for 7-14 days
Dosage Forms
Granules for oral suspension: 125 mg/5 mL (50 mL, 100 mL); 250 mg/5 mL (50 mL, 100 mL)
Tablet, film coated: 250 mg, 500 mg

Claritin® *see* loratadine *on page 313*

Claritin-D® *see* loratadine and pseudoephedrine *on page 314*

Claritin-D® **24-Hour** *see* loratadine and pseudoephedrine *on page 314*

clavulanic acid and ticarcillin *see* ticarcillin and clavulanate potassium *on page 519*

Clear Away® **Disc [OTC]** *see* salicylic acid *on page 472*

Clear By Design® **Gel [OTC]** *see* benzoyl peroxide *on page 61*

Clear Eyes® **[OTC]** *see* naphazoline *on page 364*

Clearsil® **Maximum Strength [OTC]** *see* benzoyl peroxide *on page 61*

Clear Tussin® **30** *see* guaifenesin and dextromethorphan *on page 248*

clemastine (KLEM as teen)
Synonyms clemastine fumarate
Brand Names Antihist-1® [OTC]; Tavist®; Tavist®-1 [OTC]
Therapeutic Category Antihistamine
Use Perennial and seasonal allergic rhinitis and other allergic symptoms including urticaria
Usual Dosage Oral:
Children:
<12 years: 0.67-1.34 mg every 8-12 hours as needed
>12 years: 1.34 mg twice daily to 2.68 mg 3 times/day; do not exceed 8.04 mg/day
Adults: 1.34 mg twice daily to 2.68 mg 3 times/day; do not exceed 8.04 mg/day

Dosage Forms
Syrup, as fumarate (citrus flavor): 0.67 mg/5 mL with alcohol 5.5% (120 mL)
Tablet, as fumarate: 1.34 mg, 2.68 mg

clemastine and phenylpropanolamine
KLEM as teen & fen il proe pa NOLE a meen)
Brand Names Antihist-D®; Tavist-D®
Therapeutic Category Antihistamine/Decongestant Combination
Use Symptomatic relief of allergic rhinitis; pruritus of the eyes, nose or throat, lacrimation and nasal congestion
Usual Dosage Children >12 years and Adults: Oral: 1 tablet every 12 hours
Dosage Forms Tablet: Clemastine fumarate 1.34 mg and phenylpropanolamine hydrochloride 75 mg

clemastine fumarate *see* clemastine *on previous page*

Cleocin HCl® *see* clindamycin *on this page*

Cleocin Pediatric® *see* clindamycin *on this page*

Cleocin Phosphate® *see* clindamycin *on this page*

Cleocin T® *see* clindamycin *on this page*

clidinium and chlordiazepoxide (kli DI nee um & klor dye az e POKS ide)
Synonyms chlordiazepoxide and clidinium
Brand Names Clindex®; Librax®
Therapeutic Category Anticholinergic Agent
Use Adjunct treatment of peptic ulcer, treatment of irritable bowel syndrome
Usual Dosage Oral: 1-2 capsules 3-4 times/day, before meals or food and at bedtime
Dosage Forms Capsule: Clidinium bromide 2.5 mg and chlordiazepoxide hydrochloride 5 mg

Climara® **Transdermal** *see* estradiol *on page 202*

Clinda-Derm® **Topical Solution** *see* clindamycin *on this page*

clindamycin (klin da MYE sin)
Synonyms clindamycin hydrochloride; clindamycin phosphate
Brand Names Cleocin HCl®; Cleocin Pediatric®; Cleocin Phosphate®; Cleocin T®; Clinda-Derm® Topical Solution; Clindets® Pledgets; C/T/S® Topical Solution
Therapeutic Category Acne Products; Antibiotic, Miscellaneous
Use Useful agent against most aerobic gram-positive staphylococci and streptococci (except enterococci); also useful against *Fusobacterium*, *Bacteroides* sp. and *Actinomyces* for treatment of respiratory tract infections, skin and soft tissue infections, sepsis, intra-abdominal infections, and infections of the female pelvis and genital tract; used topically in treatment of severe acne
Usual Dosage Avoid in neonates (contains benzyl alcohol)
Infants and Children:
Oral: 10-30 mg/kg/day in 3-4 divided doses
I.M., I.V.: 25-40 mg/kg/day in 3-4 divided doses
Children and Adults: Topical: Apply twice daily
Adults:
Oral: 150-450 mg/dose every 6-8 hours; maximum dose: 1.8 g/day
I.M., I.V.: 1.2-1.8 g/day in 2-4 divided doses; maximum dose: 4.8 g/day
Vaginal: 1 full applicator (100 mg) inserted intravaginally once daily before bedtime for 7 consecutive days
Dosage Forms
Capsule, as hydrochloride: 75 mg, 150 mg, 300 mg
Cream, vaginal: 2% (40 g)
Gel, topical, as phosphate: 1% [10 mg/g] (7.5 g, 30 g)
(Continued)

clindamycin *(Continued)*

Granules for oral solution, as palmitate: 75 mg/5 mL (100 mL)
Infusion, as phosphate, in D$_5$W: 300 mg (50 mL); 600 mg (50 mL)
Injection, as phosphate: 150 mg/mL (2 mL, 4 mL, 6 mL, 50 mL, 60 mL)
Lotion: 1% [10 mg/mL] (60 mL)
Pledgets: 1%
Solution, topical, as phosphate: 1% [10 mg/mL] (30 mL, 60 mL, 480 mL)

clindamycin hydrochloride *see* clindamycin *on previous page*

clindamycin phosphate *see* clindamycin *on previous page*

Clindets® Pledgets *see* clindamycin *on previous page*

Clindex® *see* clidinium and chlordiazepoxide *on previous page*

Clinoril® *see* sulindac *on page 500*

clioquinol (klye oh KWIN ole)

Brand Names Vioform® [OTC]
Therapeutic Category Antifungal Agent
Use Treatment of tinea pedis, tinea cruris, and skin infections caused by dermatophytic fungi (ring worm)
Usual Dosage Children and Adults: Topical: Apply 2-4 times/day; do not use for >7 days
Dosage Forms
Cream: 3% (30 g)
Ointment, topical: 3% (30 g)

clioquinol and hydrocortisone (klye oh KWIN ole & hye droe KOR ti sone)

Synonyms hydrocortisone and clioquinol
Brand Names Corque® Topical; Pedi-Cort V® Creme
Therapeutic Category Antifungal/Corticosteroid
Use Contact or atopic dermatitis; eczema; neurodermatitis; anogenital pruritus; mycotic dermatoses; moniliasis
Usual Dosage Topical: Apply in a thin film 3-4 times/day
Dosage Forms Cream: Clioquinol 3% and hydrocortisone 1% (20 g)

clobetasol (kloe BAY ta sol)

Synonyms clobetasol propionate
Brand Names Temovate®
Therapeutic Category Corticosteroid, Topical
Use Short-term relief of inflammation of moderate to severe corticosteroid-responsive dermatosis
Usual Dosage Topical: Apply twice daily for up to 2 weeks with no more than 50 g/week
Dosage Forms
Cream, as propionate: 0.05% (15 g, 30 g, 45 g)
Cream, as propionate, in emollient base: 0.05% (15 g, 30 g, 60 g)
Gel, as propionate: 0.05% (15 g, 30 g, 45 g)
Ointment, topical, as propionate: 0.05% (15 g, 30 g, 45 g)
Scalp application, as propionate: 0.05% (25 mL, 50 mL)

clobetasol propionate *see* clobetasol *on this page*

Clocort® Maximum Strength *see* hydrocortisone *on page 268*

clocortolone (kloe KOR toe lone)

Synonyms clocortolone pivalate
Brand Names Cloderm® Topical
Therapeutic Category Corticosteroid, Topical
Use Inflammation of corticosteroid-responsive dermatoses

Usual Dosage Topical: Apply sparingly and gently rub into affected area 1-4 times/day
Dosage Forms Cream, as pivalate: 0.1% (15 g, 45 g)

clocortolone pivalate *see* clocortolone *on previous page*

Cloderm® Topical *see* clocortolone *on previous page*

clofazimine (kloe FA zi meen)
Synonyms clofazimine palmitate
Brand Names Lamprene®
Therapeutic Category Leprostatic Agent
Use Treatment of dapsone-resistant lepromatous leprosy (*Mycobacterium leprae*); multibacillary dapsone-sensitive leprosy; erythema nodosum leprosum; *Mycobacterium avium-intracellulare* (MAI) infections
Usual Dosage Oral:
  Children: Leprosy: 1 mg/kg/day every 24 hours in combination with dapsone and rifampin
  Adults:
    Dapsone-resistant leprosy: 50-100 mg/day in combination with one or more antileprosy drugs for 2 years; then alone 50-100 mg/day
    Dapsone-sensitive multibacillary leprosy: 50-100 mg/day in combination with two or more antileprosy drugs for at least 2 years and continue until negative skin smears are obtained, then institute single drug therapy with appropriate agent
    Erythema nodosum leprosum: 100-200 mg/day for up to 3 months or longer then taper dose to 100 mg/day when possible
    MAI: Combination therapy using clofazimine 100 mg 1 or 3 times/day in combination with other antimycobacterial agents
Dosage Forms Capsule, as palmatate: 50 mg

clofazimine palmitate *see* clofazimine *on this page*

clofibrate (kloe FYE brate)
Brand Names Atromid-S®
Therapeutic Category Antihyperlipidemic Agent, Miscellaneous
Use Adjunct to dietary therapy in the management of hyperlipidemias associated with high triglyceride levels
Usual Dosage Adults: Oral: 500 mg 4 times/day
Dosage Forms Capsule: 500 mg

Clomid® *see* clomiphene *on this page*

clomiphene (KLOE mi feen)
Synonyms clomiphene citrate
Brand Names Clomid®; Milophene®; Serophene®
Therapeutic Category Ovulation Stimulator
Use Treatment of ovulatory failure in patients desiring pregnancy
Usual Dosage Oral: 50 mg/day for 5 days (first course); start the regimen on or about the fifth day of cycle; if ovulation occurs do not increase dosage; if not, increase next course to 100 mg/day for 5 days
Dosage Forms Tablet, as citrate: 50 mg

clomiphene citrate *see* clomiphene *on this page*

clomipramine (kloe MI pra meen)
Synonyms clomipramine hydrochloride
Brand Names Anafranil®
Therapeutic Category Antidepressant, Tricyclic (Tertiary Amine)
Use Treatment of obsessive-compulsive disorder (OCD)
(Continued)

clomipramine *(Continued)*

Usual Dosage Oral:
Children: Initial: 25 mg/day and gradually increase, as tolerated to a maximum of 3 mg/kg or 100 mg, whichever is smaller
Adults: Initial: 25 mg/day and gradually increase, as tolerated to 100 mg/day the first 2 weeks, may then be increased to a total of 250 mg/day
Dosage Forms Capsule, as hydrochloride: 25 mg, 50 mg, 75 mg

clomipramine hydrochloride *see* clomipramine *on previous page*

Clomycin® [OTC] *see* bacitracin, neomycin, polymyxin B, and lidocaine *on page 54*

clonazepam (kloe NA ze pam)

Brand Names Klonopin™
Therapeutic Category Benzodiazepine
Controlled Substance C-IV
Use Prophylaxis of absence (petit mal), petit mal variant (Lennox-Gastaut), akinetic, and myoclonic seizures
Usual Dosage Oral:
Children <10 years or 30 kg:
Initial daily dose: 0.01-0.03 mg/kg/day (maximum: 0.05 mg/kg/day) administered in 2-3 divided doses; increase by no more than 0.5 mg every third day until seizures are controlled or adverse effects are seen
Maintenance dose: 0.1-0.2 mg/kg/day divided 3 times/day; not to exceed 0.2 mg/kg/day
Adults:
Initial daily dose not to exceed 1.5 mg administered in 3 divided doses; may increase by 0.5-1 mg every third day until seizures are controlled or adverse effects seen
Maintenance dose: 0.05-0.2 mg/kg; do not exceed 20 mg/day
Dosage Forms Tablet: 0.5 mg, 1 mg, 2 mg

clonidine (KLOE ni deen)

Synonyms clonidine hydrochloride
Brand Names Catapres® Oral; Catapres-TTS® Transdermal; Duraclon® Injection
Therapeutic Category Alpha-Adrenergic Agonist
Use Management of hypertension; aid in the diagnosis of pheochromocytoma and growth hormone deficiency; has orphan drug status for epidural use for pain control; used for heroin withdrawal and smoking cessation therapy in adults

Investigational use: Alternate agent for the treatment of attention deficit disorder with hyperactivity (ADDH)
Usual Dosage
Epidural infusion (continuous): 30 mcg/hour, titrated up or down depending on pain relief
Oral:
Children: Initial: 5-10 mcg/kg/day in divided doses every 8-12 hours; increase gradually at 5- to 7-day intervals to 25 mcg/kg/day in divided doses every 6 hours; maximum: 0.9 mg/day
Clonidine tolerance test (test of growth hormone release from pituitary): 0.15 mg/m^2 or 4 mcg/kg as single dose
Adults: Initial dose: 0.1 mg twice daily, usual maintenance dose: 0.2-1.2 mg/day in 2-4 divided doses; maximum recommended dose: 2.4 mg/day
Nicotine withdrawal symptoms: 0.1 mg twice daily to maximum of 0.4 mg/day for 3-4 weeks
Elderly: Initial: 0.1 mg once daily at bedtime, increase gradually as needed
Transdermal: Apply once every 7 days; for initial therapy start with 0.1 mg and increase by 0.1 mg at 1- to 2-week intervals; dosages >0.6 mg do not improve efficacy

Dosage Forms
Injection, preservative free, as hydrochloride: 100 mcg/mL (10 mL)
Patch, transdermal, as hydrochloride: 1, 2, and 3 (0.1, 0.2, 0.3 mg/day, 7-day duration)
Tablet, as hydrochloride: 0.1 mg, 0.2 mg, 0.3 mg

clonidine and chlorthalidone (KLOE ni deen & klor THAL i done)
Brand Names Combipres®
Therapeutic Category Antihypertensive, Combination
Use Management of mild to moderate hypertension
Usual Dosage Oral: 1 tablet 1-2 times/day
Dosage Forms Tablet:
0.1: Clonidine 0.1 mg and chlorthalidone 15 mg
0.2: Clonidine 0.2 mg and chlorthalidone 15 mg
0.3: Clonidine 0.3 mg and chlorthalidone 15 mg

clonidine hydrochloride *see* clonidine *on previous page*

Clopra® *see* metoclopramide *on page 344*

clorazepate (klor AZ e pate)
Synonyms clorazepate dipotassium
Brand Names Gen-XENE®; Tranxene®
Therapeutic Category Anticonvulsant; Benzodiazepine
Controlled Substance C-IV
Use Treatment of generalized anxiety and panic disorders; management of alcohol withdrawal; adjunct anticonvulsant in management of partial seizures
Usual Dosage Oral:
Anticonvulsant:
Children:
<9 years: Dose not established
9-12 years: Initial: 3.75-7.5 mg/dose twice daily; increase dose by 3.75 mg at weekly intervals, not to exceed 60 mg/day in 2-3 divided doses
Children >12 years and Adults: Initial: Up to 7.5 mg/dose 2-3 times/day; increase dose by 7.5 mg at weekly intervals; usual dose: 0.5-1 mg/kg/day; not to exceed 90 mg/day (up to 3 mg/kg/day has been used)
Anxiety: Adults: 7.5-15 mg 2-4 times/day, or administered as single dose of 15-22.5 mg at bedtime
Alcohol withdrawal: Adults: Initial: 30 mg, then 15 mg 2-4 times/day on first day; maximum daily dose: 90 mg; gradually decrease dose over subsequent days
Dosage Forms
Capsule, as dipotassium: 3.75 mg, 7.5 mg, 15 mg
Tablet, as dipotassium: 3.75 mg, 7.5 mg, 15 mg
Single dose: 11.25 mg, 22.5 mg

clorazepate dipotassium *see* clorazepate *on this page*

Clorpactin® WCS-90 *see* oxychlorosene *on page 389*

clotrimazole (kloe TRIM a zole)
Brand Names Femizole-7® [OTC]; Fungoid® Solution; Gyne-Lotrimin® [OTC]; Lotrimin®; Lotrimin® AF Cream [OTC]; Lotrimin® AF Lotion [OTC]; Lotrimin® AF Solution [OTC]; Mycelex®; Mycelex®-7; Mycelex®-G
Therapeutic Category Antifungal Agent
Use Treatment of susceptible fungal infections, including oropharyngeal candidiasis, dermatophytoses, superficial mycoses, cutaneous candidiasis, as well as vulvovaginal candidiasis; limited data suggests that the use of clotrimazole troches may be effective for prophylaxis against oropharyngeal candidiasis in neutropenic patients
(Continued)

clotrimazole *(Continued)*

Usual Dosage
Children >3 years and Adults:
Oral: 10 mg troche dissolved slowly 5 times/day
Topical: Apply twice daily
Adults: Vaginal: 100 mg/day for 7 days or 200 mg/day for 3 days or 500 mg single dose or 5 g (1 applicatorful) of 1% vaginal cream daily for 7-14 days
Dosage Forms
Combination pack (Mycelex-7®): Vaginal tablet 100 mg (7's) and vaginal cream 1% (7 g)
Cream:
Topical (Lotrimin®, Lotrimin® AF, Mycelex®, Mycelex® OTC) : 1% (15 g, 30 g, 45 g, 90 g)
Vaginal (Femizole-7®, Gyne-Lotrimin®, Mycelex®-G): 1% (45 g, 90 g)
Lotion (Lotrimin®): 1% (30 mL)
Solution, topical (Fungoid®, Lotrimin®, Lotrimin® AF, Mycelex®, Mycelex® OTC): 1% (10 mL, 30 mL)
Tablet, vaginal (Gyne-Lotrimin®, Mycelex®-G): 100 mg (7s); 500 mg (1s)
Troche (Mycelex®): 10 mg
Twin pack (Mycelex®): Vaginal tablet 500 mg (1's) and vaginal cream 1% (7 g)

cloxacillin (kloks a SIL in)

Synonyms cloxacillin sodium
Brand Names Cloxapen®; Tegopen®
Therapeutic Category Penicillin
Use Treatment of susceptible bacterial infections of the respiratory tract, skin and skin structure, bone and joint caused by penicillinase-producing staphylococci
Usual Dosage Oral:
Children >1 month: 50-100 mg/kg/day in divided doses every 6 hours; up to a maximum of 4 g/day
Adults: 250-500 mg every 6 hours
Dosage Forms
Capsule, as sodium: 250 mg, 500 mg
Powder for oral suspension, as sodium: 125 mg/5 mL (100 mL, 200 mL)

cloxacillin sodium *see cloxacillin on this page*

Cloxapen® *see cloxacillin on this page*

clozapine (KLOE za peen)

Brand Names Clozaril®
Therapeutic Category Antipsychotic Agent, Dibenzodiazepine
Use Management of schizophrenic patients
Usual Dosage Adults: Oral: Initial: 25 mg once or twice daily, increase as tolerated to a target dose of 300-450 mg/day, may require doses as high as 600-900 mg/day
Dosage Forms Tablet: 25 mg, 100 mg

Clozaril® *see clozapine on this page*

Clysodrast® *see bisacodyl on page 67*

cmv-igiv *see cytomegalovirus immune globulin (intravenous-human) on page 146*

coagulant complex inhibitor *see anti-inhibitor coagulant complex on page 37*

coal tar (KOLE tar)

Synonyms crude coal tar; lcd; pix carbonis
Brand Names AquaTar® [OTC]; Denorex® [OTC]; DHS® Tar [OTC]; Duplex® T [OTC]; Estar® [OTC]; Fototar® [OTC]; Neutrogena® T/Derm; Oxipor® VHC [OTC]; Pentrax® [OTC]; Polytar® [OTC]; psoriGel® [OTC]; T/Gel® [OTC]; Zetar® [OTC]
Therapeutic Category Antipsoriatic Agent; Antiseborrheic Agent, Topical

Use Topically for controlling dandruff, seborrheic dermatitis, or psoriasis

Usual Dosage

Bath: Add appropriate amount to bath water, for adults usually 60-90 mL of a 5% to 20% solution or 15-25 mL of 30% lotion; soak 5-20 minutes, then pat dry; use once daily for 3 days

Shampoo: Rub shampoo onto wet hair and scalp, rinse thoroughly; repeat; leave on 5 minutes; rinse thoroughly; apply twice weekly for the first 2 weeks then once weekly or more often if needed

Skin: Apply to the affected area 1-4 times/day; decrease frequency to 2-3 times/week once condition has been controlled

Scalp psoriasis: Tar oil bath or coal tar solution may be painted sparingly to the lesions 3-12 hours before each shampoo

Psoriasis of the body, arms, legs: Apply at bedtime; if thick scales are present, use product with salicylic acid and apply several times during the day

Dosage Forms

Cream: 1% to 5%

Gel: Coal tar 5%

Lotion: 2.5% to 30%

Lotion: 2%; 5%; 25%

Shampoo: Coal tar extract 2% with salicylic acid 2% (60 mL)

Shampoo, topical: Coal tar: 0.5% to 5%

Solution:

Coal tar: 2.5%, 5%, 20%

Coal tar extract: 5%

Suspension, coal tar: 30% to 33.3%

coal tar and salicylic acid (KOLE tar & sal i SIL ik AS id)

Brand Names X-seb® T [OTC]

Therapeutic Category Antipsoriatic Agent; Antiseborrheic Agent, Topical

Use Treatment of seborrheal dermatitis, dandruff

Usual Dosage Topical: Shampoo twice weekly

Dosage Forms Shampoo: Coal tar solution 10% and salicylic acid 4% (120 mL)

coal tar, lanolin, and mineral oil (KOLE tar, LAN oh lin, & MIN er al oyl)

Brand Names Balnetar® [OTC]

Therapeutic Category Antipsoriatic Agent; Antiseborrheic Agent, Topical

Use Treatment of psoriasis, seborrheal dermatitis, atopic dermatitis, eczematoid dermatitis

Usual Dosage Add to bath water, soak for 5-20 minutes then pat dry

Dosage Forms Oil, bath: Water-dispersible emollient tar 2.5%, lanolin fraction, and mineral oil (240 mL)

cocaine (koe KANE)

Synonyms cocaine hydrochloride

Therapeutic Category Local Anesthetic

Controlled Substance C-II

Use Topical anesthesia for mucous membranes

Usual Dosage Topical: Use lowest effective dose; do not exceed 1 mg/kg; patient tolerance, anesthetic technique, vascularity of tissue and area to be anesthetized will determine dose needed

Dosage Forms

Powder, as hydrochloride: 5 g, 25 g

Solution, topical:

As hydrochloride: 4% [40 mg/mL] (2 mL, 4 mL, 10 mL); 10% [100 mg/mL] (4 mL, 10 mL)

Viscous, as hydrochloride: 4% [40 mg/mL] (4 mL, 10 mL); 10% [100 mg/mL] (4 mL, 10 mL)

(Continued)

cocaine *(Continued)*

Tablet, soluble, for topical solution, as hydrochloride: 135 mg

cocaine hydrochloride *see cocaine on previous page*

coccidioidin skin test (koks i dee OH i din skin test)

Brand Names Spherulin®

Therapeutic Category Diagnostic Agent

Use Intradermal skin test in diagnosis of coccidioidomycosis; differential diagnosis of this disease from histoplasmosis, sarcoidosis and other mycotic and bacterial infections. The skin test may be negative in severe forms of disease (anergy) or when prolonged periods of time have passed since infection.

Usual Dosage Children and Adults: Intradermally: 0.1 mL of 1:100 or flexor surface of forearm

Positive reaction: Induration of 5 mm or more; erythema without induration is considered negative; read the test at 24 and 48 hours, since some reactions may not be noticeable after 36 hours. A positive reaction indicates present or past infection with *Coccidioides immitis.*

Negative reaction: A negative test means the individual has not been sensitized to coccidioidin or has lost sensitivity

Dosage Forms Injection: 1:10 (0.5 mL); 1:100 (1 mL)

Codafed® Expectorant *see guaifenesin, pseudoephedrine, and codeine on page 251*

Codamine® *see hydrocodone and phenylpropanolamine on page 267*

Codamine® Pediatric *see hydrocodone and phenylpropanolamine on page 267*

Codehist® DH *see chlorpheniramine, pseudoephedrine, and codeine on page 118*

codeine (KOE deen)

Synonyms codeine phosphate; codeine sulfate; methylmorphine

Therapeutic Category Analgesic, Narcotic; Antitussive

Controlled Substance C-II

Use Treatment of mild to moderate pain; antitussive in lower doses

Usual Dosage Doses should be titrated to appropriate analgesic effect; when changing routes of administration, note that oral dose is $2/3$ as effective as parenteral dose

Analgesic: Oral, I.M., S.C.:
Children: 0.5-1 mg/kg/dose every 4-6 hours as needed; maximum: 60 mg/dose
Adults: 30 mg/dose; range: 15-60 mg every 4-6 hours as needed
Antitussive: Oral (for nonproductive cough):
Children: 1-1.5 mg/kg/day in divided doses every 4-6 hours as needed: Alternatively dose according to age:
2-6 years: 2.5-5 mg every 4-6 hours as needed; maximum: 30 mg/day
6-12 years: 5-10 mg every 4-6 hours as needed; maximum: 60 mg/day
Adults: 10-20 mg/dose every 4-6 hours as needed; maximum: 120 mg/day

Dosage Forms
Injection, as phosphate: 30 mg (1 mL, 2 mL); 60 mg (1 mL, 2 mL)
Solution, oral: 15 mg/5 mL
Tablet, as sulfate: 15 mg, 30 mg, 60 mg
Tablet, as phosphate, soluble: 30 mg, 60 mg
Tablet, as sulfate, soluble: 15 mg, 30 mg, 60 mg

codeine and acetaminophen *see acetaminophen and codeine on page 3*

codeine and aspirin *see aspirin and codeine on page 44*

codeine and bromodiphenhydramine *see bromodiphenhydramine and codeine on page 72*

codeine and butalbital compound *see* butalbital compound and codeine *on page 78*

codeine and guaifenesin *see* guaifenesin and codeine *on page 247*

codeine phosphate *see* codeine *on previous page*

codeine sulfate *see* codeine *on previous page*

Codiclear® DH *see* hydrocodone and guaifenesin *on page 267*

cod liver oil *see* vitamin a and vitamin d *on page 552*

Codoxy® *see* oxycodone and aspirin *on page 390*

Cogentin® *see* benztropine *on page 62*

Co-Gesic® *see* hydrocodone and acetaminophen *on page 266*

Cognex® *see* tacrine *on page 502*

Co-Hist® [OTC] *see* acetaminophen, chlorpheniramine, and pseudoephedrine *on page 5*

Colace® [OTC] *see* docusate *on page 179*

colaspase *see* asparaginase *on page 43*

Colax® [OTC] *see* docusate and phenolphthalein *on page 180*

colchicine (KOL chi seen)

Therapeutic Category Antigout Agent
Use Treat acute gouty arthritis attacks and to prevent recurrences of such attacks; management of familial Mediterranean fever
Usual Dosage
Treatment for acute gouty arthritis:
Oral: Initial: 0.5-1.2 mg, then 0.5-0.6 mg every 1-2 hours or 1-1.2 mg every 2 hours until relief or GI side effects occur to a maximum total dose of 8 mg, wait 3 days before initiating a second course
I.V.: Initial: 1-3 mg, then 0.5 mg every 6 hours until response, not to exceed 4 mg/day; following a full course of colchicine (4 mg), wait 7 days before initiating another course of colchicine (by any route)
Prophylaxis of recurrent attacks: Oral:
<1 attack/year: 0.5 or 0.6 mg/day/dose for 3-4 days/week
>1 attack/year: 0.5 or 0.6 mg/day/dose
Severe cases: 1-1.8 mg/day
Dosage Forms
Injection: 0.5 mg/mL (2 mL)
Tablet: 0.5 mg, 0.6 mg

colchicine and probenecid (KOL chi seen & proe BEN e sid)

Synonyms probenecid and colchicine
Therapeutic Category Antigout Agent
Use Treatment of chronic gouty arthritis when complicated by frequent, recurrent acute attacks of gout
Usual Dosage Adults: Oral: 1 tablet daily for 1 week, then 1 tablet twice daily thereafter
Dosage Forms Tablet: Colchicine 0.5 mg and probenecid 0.5 g

Cold & Allergy® Elixir [OTC] *see* brompheniramine and phenylpropanolamine *on page 73*

Coldlac-LA® *see* guaifenesin and phenylpropanolamine *on page 249*

Coldloc® *see* guaifenesin, phenylpropanolamine, and phenylephrine *on page 251*

Coldrine® [OTC] *see* acetaminophen and pseudoephedrine *on page 5*

Colestid® *see* colestipol *on next page*

colestipol (koe LES ti pole)
Synonyms colestipol hydrochloride
Brand Names Colestid®
Therapeutic Category Antihyperlipidemic Agent, Miscellaneous
Use Adjunct in the management of primary hypercholesterolemia; to relieve pruritus associated with elevated levels of bile acids, possibly used to decrease plasma half-life of digoxin as an adjunct in the treatment of toxicity
Usual Dosage Oral: 15-30 g/day in divided doses 2-4 times/day
Dosage Forms
Granules, as hydrochloride: 5 g packet, 300 g, 500 g
Tablet, as hydrochloride: 1 g

colestipol hydrochloride *see* colestipol *on this page*

colfosceril palmitate (kole FOS er il PALM i tate)
Synonyms dipalmitoylphosphatidylcholine; dppc; synthetic lung surfactant
Brand Names Exosurf® Neonatal™
Therapeutic Category Lung Surfactant
Use Neonatal respiratory distress syndrome (RDS):
Prophylactic therapy: Infants at risk for developing RDS with body weight <1350 g; infants with evidence of pulmonary immaturity with body weight >1350 g
Rescue therapy: Treatment of infants with RDS based on respiratory distress not attributable to any other causes and chest radiographic findings consistent with RDS
Usual Dosage
Prophylactic treatment: Administer 5 mL/kg as soon as possible; the second and third doses should be administered at 12 and 24 hours later to those infants remaining on ventilators
Rescue treatment: Administer 5 mL/kg as soon as the diagnosis of RDS is made; the second 5 mL/kg dose should be administered 12 hours later
Dosage Forms Powder for injection, lyophilized: 108 mg (10 mL)

colistimethate (koe lis ti METH ate)
Synonyms colistimethate sodium
Brand Names Coly-Mycin® M Parenteral
Therapeutic Category Antibiotic, Miscellaneous
Use Treatment of infections due to sensitive strains of certain gram-negative bacilli
Usual Dosage Children and Adults: I.M., I.V.: 2.5-5 mg/kg/day in 2-4 divided doses
Dosage Forms Powder for injection, as sodium, lyophilized: 150 mg

colistimethate sodium *see* colistimethate *on this page*

colistin, neomycin, and hydrocortisone
(koe LIS tin, nee oh MYE sin & hye droe KOR ti sone)
Brand Names Coly-Mycin® S Otic Drops
Therapeutic Category Antibiotic/Corticosteroid, Otic
Use Treatment of superficial and susceptible bacterial infections of the external auditory canal; for treatment of susceptible bacterial infections of mastoidectomy and fenestration cavities
Usual Dosage Otic:
Children: 3 drops in affected ear 3-4 times/day
Adults: 4 drops in affected ear 3-4 times/day
Dosage Forms Suspension, otic: Colistin sulfate 0.3%, neomycin sulfate 0.47%, and hydrocortisone acetate 1% (5 mL, 10 mL)

collagenase (KOL la je nase)
Brand Names Biozyme-C®; Santyl®
Therapeutic Category Enzyme

Use Promote debridement of necrotic tissue in dermal ulcers and severe burns
Usual Dosage Topical: Apply daily or every other day
Dosage Forms Ointment, topical: 250 units/g (15 g, 30 g)

collagen implants (KOL a jen im PLANTS)
Therapeutic Category Ophthalmic Agent, Miscellaneous
Use Relief of dry eyes; enhance the effect of ocular medications
Usual Dosage Implants inserted by physician
Dosage Forms Implant: 0.2 mm, 0.3 mm, 0.4 mm, 0.5 mm, 0.6 mm

Collyrium Fresh® Ophthalmic [OTC] see tetrahydrozoline on page 510

Colovage® see polyethylene glycol-electrolyte solution on page 423

Coly-Mycin® M Parenteral see colistimethate on previous page

Coly-Mycin® S Otic Drops see colistin, neomycin, and hydrocortisone on previous page

CoLyte® see polyethylene glycol-electrolyte solution on page 423

Combipres® see clonidine and chlorthalidone on page 131

Combivent® see ipratropium and albuterol on page 288

Combivir® see zidovudine and lamivudine on page 560

Comfort® Ophthalmic [OTC] see naphazoline on page 364

Comfort® Tears Solution [OTC] see artificial tears on page 42

Comhist® see chlorpheniramine, phenylephrine, and phenyltoloxamine on page 116

Comhist® LA see chlorpheniramine, phenylephrine, and phenyltoloxamine on page 116

Compazine® see prochlorperazine on page 439

compound e see cortisone acetate on page 139

compound f see hydrocortisone on page 268

compound s see zidovudine on page 559

Compound W® [OTC] see salicylic acid on page 472

Compoz® Gel Caps [OTC] see diphenhydramine on page 173

Compoz® Nighttime Sleep Aid [OTC] see diphenhydramine on page 173

Comtrex® Maximum Strength Non-Drowsy [OTC] see acetaminophen, dextromethorphan, and pseudoephedrine on page 6

Condylox® see podofilox on page 422

Conex® [OTC] see guaifenesin and phenylpropanolamine on page 249

Congess® Jr see guaifenesin and pseudoephedrine on page 250

Congess® Sr see guaifenesin and pseudoephedrine on page 250

Congestac® see guaifenesin and pseudoephedrine on page 250

Congestant D® [OTC] see chlorpheniramine, phenylpropanolamine, and acetaminophen on page 117

conjugated estrogen and methyltestosterone see estrogens and methyltestosterone on page 204

conjugated estrogens see estrogens, conjugated on page 205

Conray® see radiological/contrast media (ionic) on page 457

Constilac® see lactulose on page 300

Constulose® see lactulose on page 300

Contac® Cough Formula Liquid [OTC] see guaifenesin and dextromethorphan on page 248

Control® **[OTC]** *see* phenylpropanolamine *on page 413*

Contuss® *see* guaifenesin, phenylpropanolamine, and phenylephrine *on page 251*

Contuss® **XT** *see* guaifenesin and phenylpropanolamine *on page 249*

Copaxone® *see* glatiramer acetate *on page 241*

Cophene-B® *see* brompheniramine *on page 73*

Cophene XP® *see* hydrocodone, pseudoephedrine, and guaifenesin *on page 268*

copolymer-1 *see* glatiramer acetate *on page 241*

copper injection *see* trace metals *on page 525*

Co-Pyronil® **2 Pulvules**® **[OTC]** *see* chlorpheniramine and pseudoephedrine *on page 114*

Cordarone® *see* amiodarone *on page 26*

Cordran® *see* flurandrenolide *on page 231*

Cordran® **SP** *see* flurandrenolide *on page 231*

Coreg® *see* carvedilol *on page 94*

Corgard® *see* nadolol *on page 361*

Coricidin® **[OTC]** *see* chlorpheniramine and acetaminophen *on page 113*

Coricidin ©D'® **[OTC]** *see* chlorpheniramine, phenylpropanolamine, and acetaminophen *on page 117*

Corque® **Topical** *see* clioquinol and hydrocortisone *on page 128*

CortaGel® **[OTC]** *see* hydrocortisone *on page 268*

Cortaid® **Maximum Strength [OTC]** *see* hydrocortisone *on page 268*

Cortaid® **with Aloe [OTC]** *see* hydrocortisone *on page 268*

Cortatrigen® **Otic** *see* neomycin, polymyxin b, and hydrocortisone *on page 369*

Cort-Dome® *see* hydrocortisone *on page 268*

Cortef® *see* hydrocortisone *on page 268*

Cortef® **Feminine Itch** *see* hydrocortisone *on page 268*

Cortenema® *see* hydrocortisone *on page 268*

Corticaine® **Topical** *see* dibucaine and hydrocortisone *on page 164*

corticotropin (kor ti koe TROE pin)

Synonyms acth; adrenocorticotropic hormone

Brand Names Acthar®; H.P. Acthar® Gel

Therapeutic Category Adrenal Corticosteroid

Use Infantile spasms; diagnostic aid in adrenocortical insufficiency; acute exacerbations of multiple sclerosis; severe muscle weakness in myasthenia gravis

Usual Dosage

Acute exacerbation of multiple sclerosis: I.M.: 80-120 units/day for 2-3 weeks

Diagnostic purposes:

I.M., S.C.: 20 units 4 times/day

I.V.: 10-25 units in 500 mL 5% dextrose in water over 8 hours

Dosage Forms

Injection, repository (H.P. Acthar® Gel): 40 units/mL (1 mL, 5 mL); 80 units/mL (1 mL, 5 mL)

Powder for injection (Acthar®): 25 units, 40 units

Cortifoam® *see* hydrocortisone *on page 268*

cortisol hydrocortisone acetate *see* hydrocortisone *on page 268*

cortisone acetate (KOR ti sone AS e tate)
Synonyms compound e
Brand Names Cortone® Acetate
Therapeutic Category Adrenal Corticosteroid
Use Management of adrenocortical insufficiency
Usual Dosage Depends upon the condition being treated and the response of the patient
Children:
Anti-inflammatory or immunosuppressive:
Oral: 2.5-10 mg/kg/day or 20-300 mg/m^2/day in divided doses every 6-8 hours
I.M.: 1-5 mg/kg/day or 14-375 mg/m^2/day in divided doses every 12-24 hours
Physiologic replacement:
Oral: 0.5-0.75 mg/kg/day in divided doses every 8 hours
I.M.: 0.25-0.35 mg/kg/day once daily
Stress coverage for surgery: I.M.: 1 and 2 days before preanesthesia, and 1-3 days after surgery: 50-62.5 mg/m^2/day; 4 days after surgery: 31-50 mg/m^2/day
Adults: Oral, I.M.: 20-300 mg/day
Dosage Forms
Injection: 50 mg/mL (10 mL)
Tablet: 5 mg, 10 mg, 25 mg

Cortisporin® Ophthalmic Ointment *see* bacitracin, neomycin, polymyxin b, and hydrocortisone *on page 53*

Cortisporin® Ophthalmic Suspension *see* neomycin, polymyxin b, and hydrocortisone *on page 369*

Cortisporin® Otic *see* neomycin, polymyxin b, and hydrocortisone *on page 369*

Cortisporin® Topical Cream *see* neomycin, polymyxin b, and hydrocortisone *on page 369*

Cortisporin® Topical Ointment *see* bacitracin, neomycin, polymyxin b, and hydrocortisone *on page 53*

Cortizone®-5 [OTC] *see* hydrocortisone *on page 268*

Cortizone®-10 [OTC] *see* hydrocortisone *on page 268*

Cortone® Acetate *see* cortisone acetate *on this page*

Cortrosyn® Injection *see* cosyntropin *on this page*

Corvert® *see* ibutilide *on page 278*

Cosmegen® *see* dactinomycin *on page 147*

cosyntropin (koe sin TROE pin)
Synonyms synacthen; tetracosactide
Brand Names Cortrosyn® Injection
Therapeutic Category Diagnostic Agent
Use Diagnostic test to differentiate primary adrenal from secondary (pituitary) adrenocortical insufficiency
Usual Dosage
Adrenocortical insufficiency: I.M., I.V.:
Children <2 years: 0.125 mg injected over 2 minutes
Children >2 years and Adults: 0.25 mg injected over 2 minutes
When greater cortisol stimulation is needed, an I.V. infusion may be used: I.V. infusion: 0.25 mg administered over 4-8 hours
Congenital adrenal hyperplasia evaluation: 1 mg/m^2/dose up to a maximum of 1 mg
Dosage Forms Powder for injection: 0.25 mg

Cotazym® *see* pancrelipase *on page 394*

Cotazym-S® *see* pancrelipase *on page 394*

Cotrim® *see* co-trimoxazole *on this page*

Cotrim® **DS** *see* co-trimoxazole *on this page*

co-trimoxazole (koe trye MOKS a zole)

Synonyms smx-tmp; sulfamethoxazole and trimethoprim; tmp-smx; trimethoprim and sulfamethoxazole

Brand Names Bactrim™; Bactrim™ DS; Cotrim®; Cotrim® DS; Septra®; Septra® DS; Sulfatrim®

Therapeutic Category Sulfonamide

Use Treatment of urinary tract infections caused by susceptible *E. coli, Klebsiella, Enterobacter, Proteus mirabilis, Proteus* (indole positive); acute otitis media due to amoxicillin-resistant *H. influenzae, S. pneumoniae,* and *M. catarrhalis;* acute exacerbations of chronic bronchitis; prophylaxis and treatment of *Pneumocystis carinii* pneumonitis (PCP); treatment of susceptible shigellosis, typhoid fever, *Nocardia asteroides* infection, and *Xanthomonas maltophilia* infection; the I.V. preparation is used for treatment of *Pneumocystis carinii* pneumonitis, *Shigella,* and severe urinary tract infections

Usual Dosage Oral, I.V. (dosage recommendations are based on the trimethoprim component):

Children >2 months:

Mild to moderate infections: 6-12 mg TMP/kg/day in divided doses every 12 hours

Serious infection/*Pneumocystis*: 15-20 mg TMP/kg/day in divided doses every 6 hours

Urinary tract infection prophylaxis: 2 mg TMP/kg/dose daily

Prophylaxis of *Pneumocystis*: 5-10 mg TMP/kg/day or 150 mg TMP/m^2/day in divided doses every 12 hours 3 days/week; dose should not exceed 320 mg trimethoprim and 1600 mg sulfamethoxazole 3 days/week; Mon, Tue, Wed

Adults: Urinary tract infection/chronic bronchitis: 1 double strength tablet every 12 hours for 10-14 days

Dosage Forms The 5:1 ratio (SMX to TMP) remains constant in all dosage forms:

Injection: Sulfamethoxazole 80 mg and trimethoprim 16 mg per mL (5 mL, 10 mL, 20 mL, 30 mL, 50 mL)

Suspension, oral: Sulfamethoxazole 200 mg and trimethoprim 40 mg per 5 mL (20 mL, 100 mL, 150 mL, 200 mL, 480 mL)

Tablet: Sulfamethoxazole 400 mg and trimethoprim 80 mg

Double strength: Sulfamethoxazole 800 mg and trimethoprim 160 mg

Coumadin® *see* warfarin *on page 557*

Covera-HS® *see* verapamil *on page 548*

Cozaar® *see* losartan *on page 314*

cpm *see* cyclophosphamide *on page 144*

Creon® *see* pancreatin *on page 394*

Creon® **10** *see* pancrelipase *on page 394*

Creon® **20** *see* pancrelipase *on page 394*

Creo-Terpin® **[OTC]** *see* dextromethorphan *on page 160*

Cresylate® *see* m-cresyl acetate *on page 323*

Crinone® *see* progesterone *on page 440*

Criticare HN® **[OTC]** *see* enteral nutritional products *on page 194*

Crixivan® *see* indinavir *on page 282*

Crolom® **Ophthalmic Solution** *see* cromolyn sodium *on next page*

cromoglicic acid *see* cromolyn sodium *on next page*

cromolyn sodium (KROE moe lin SOW dee um)

Synonyms cromoglicic acid; disodium cromoglycate; dscg

Brand Names Crolom® Ophthalmic Solution; Gastrocrom® Oral; Intal® Inhalation Capsule; Intal® Nebulizer Solution; Intal® Oral Inhaler; Nasalcrom® Nasal Solution [OTC]

Therapeutic Category Mast Cell Stabilizer

Use Adjunct in the prophylaxis of allergic disorders, including rhinitis, conjunctivitis, and asthma; inhalation product may be used for prevention of exercise-induced bronchospasm

Ophthalmologic: Vernal conjunctivitis, vernal keratoconjunctivitis, and vernal keratitis
Systemic: Mastocytosis, food allergy, and treatment of inflammatory bowel disease

Usual Dosage

Children:

Inhalation: >2 years: 20 mg 4 times/day

Nebulization solution: >5 years: 2 inhalations 4 times/day by metered spray, or 20 mg 4 times/day (Spinhaler®); taper frequency to the lowest effective level

For prevention of exercise-induced bronchospasm: Single dose of 2 inhalations (aerosol) just prior to exercise

Nasal: >6 years: 1 spray in each nostril 3-4 times/day

Adults: Nasal: 1 spray in each nostril 3-4 times/day

Systemic mastocytosis: Oral:

Infants ≤2 years of age: 20 mg/kg/day in 4 divided doses, not to exceed 30 mg/kg/day

Children 2-12 years: 100 mg 4 times/day; not to exceed 40 mg/kg/day

Adults: 200 mg 4 times/day

Food allergy and inflammatory bowel disease: Oral:

Children: 100 mg 4 times/day 15-20 minutes before meals, not to exceed 40 mg/kg/day

Adults: 200 mg 4 times/day 15-20 minutes before meal, up to 400 mg 4 times/day

Dosage Forms

Capsule:

Oral (Gastrocrom®): 100 mg

Inhalation, oral (Intal®): 800 mcg/spray (8.1 g)

Solution:

For nebulization: 10 mg/mL (2 mL)

Intal®: 10 mg/mL (2 mL)

Nasal (Nasalcrom®): 40 mg/mL (13 mL)

Ophthalmic (Crolom®): 4% (2.5 mL, 10 mL)

crotaline antivenin, polyvalent *see* antivenin (*Crotalidae*) polyvalent *on page 38*

crotamiton (kroe TAM i tonn)

Brand Names Eurax® Topical

Therapeutic Category Scabicides/Pediculicides

Use Treatment of scabies (*Sarcoptes scabiei*) in infants and children

Usual Dosage Scabicide: Children and Adults: Topical: Wash thoroughly and scrub away loose scales, then towel dry; apply a thin layer and massage drug onto skin of the entire body from the neck to the toes (with special attention to skin folds, creases, and interdigital spaces). Repeat application in 24 hours; take a cleansing bath 48 hours after the final application.

Dosage Forms

Cream: 10% (60 g)

Lotion: 10% (60 mL, 454 mL)

crude coal tar *see* coal tar *on page 132*

crystalline penicillin *see* penicillin g, parenteral, aqueous *on page 401*

Crystamine® *see* cyanocobalamin *on next page*

Crysti 1000® *see* cyanocobalamin *on next page*

Crysticillin® A.S. *see* penicillin g procaine *on page 401*

Crystodigin® *see* digitoxin *on page 168*

csp *see* cellulose sodium phosphate *on page 102*

C/T/S® Topical Solution *see* clindamycin *on page 127*

ctx *see* cyclophosphamide *on page 144*

Cuprimine® *see* penicillamine *on page 399*

Curretab® Oral *see* medroxyprogesterone acetate *on page 326*

Cutivate™ *see* fluticasone *on page 232*

cya *see* cyclosporine *on page 145*

cyanide antidote kit (SYE a nide AN tee dote kit)
Therapeutic Category Antidote
Use Treatment of cyanide poisoning
Usual Dosage Cyanide poisoning: 0.3 mL ampul of amyl nitrite is crushed every minute and vapor is inhaled for 15-30 seconds until an I.V. sodium nitrite infusion is available. Following administration of 300 mg I.V. sodium nitrite, inject 12.5 g sodium thiosulfate I.V. (over ~10 minutes), if needed; injection of both may be repeated at ½ the original dose.
Dosage Forms Kit: Sodium nitrite 300 mg/10 mL (#2); sodium thiosulfate 12.5 g/50 mL (#2); amyl nitrite 0.3 mL (#12); also disposable syringes, stomach tube, tourniquet and instructions

cyanocobalamin (sye an oh koe BAL a min)
Synonyms vitamin b_{12}
Brand Names Crystamine®; Crysti 1000®; Cyanoject®; Cyomin®
Therapeutic Category Vitamin, Water Soluble
Use Pernicious anemia; vitamin B_{12} deficiency; increased B_{12} requirements due to pregnancy, thyrotoxicosis, hemorrhage, malignancy, liver or kidney disease
Usual Dosage
  Congenital pernicious anemia (if evidence of neurologic involvement): I.M.: 1000 mcg/day for at least 2 weeks; maintenance: 50 mcg/month
  Vitamin B_{12} deficiency: I.M., S.C.: (oral is not recommended due to poor absorption)
  Children: 100 mcg/day for 10-15 days (total dose of 1-1.5 mg), then once or twice weekly for several months; may taper to 250-1000 mcg every month
  Adults: 100 mcg/day for 6-7 days
  Hematologic signs only:
    Children: 10-50 mcg/day for 5-10 days, then maintenance: 100-250 mcg/dose every 2-4 weeks
    Adults: 30 mcg/day for 5-10 days, followed by 100-200 mcg/month
  Methylmalonic aciduria: I.M.: 1 mg/day
Dosage Forms
  Gel, nasal (Ener-B®): 400 mcg/0.1 mL
  Injection: 30 mcg/mL (30 mL); 100 mcg/mL (1 mL, 10 mL, 30 mL); 1000 mcg/mL (1 mL, 10 mL, 30 mL)
  Tablet [OTC]: 25 mcg, 50 mcg, 100 mcg, 250 mcg, 500 mcg, 1000 mcg

Cyanoject® *see* cyanocobalamin *on this page*

Cyclan® *see* cyclandelate *on this page*

cyclandelate (sye KLAN de late)
Brand Names Cyclan®; Cyclospasmol®
Therapeutic Category Vasodilator
Use Adjunctive therapy in peripheral vascular disease and possibly senility
Usual Dosage Oral: 400-800 mg/day in 2-4 divided doses

Dosage Forms
Capsule: 200 mg, 400 mg
Tablet: 200 mg, 400 mg

cyclizine (SYE kli zeen)
Synonyms cyclizine hydrochloride; cyclizine lactate
Brand Names Marezine® [OTC]
Therapeutic Category Antihistamine
Use Prevention and treatment of nausea, vomiting and vertigo associated with motion sickness; control of postoperative nausea and vomiting
Usual Dosage Oral:
Children 6-12 years: 25 mg up to 3 times/day
Adults: 50 mg taken 30 minutes before departure, may repeat in 4-6 hours if needed, up to 200 mg/day
Dosage Forms
Injection, as lactate: 50 mg/mL (1 mL)
Tablet, as hydrochloride: 50 mg

cyclizine hydrochloride *see* cyclizine *on this page*

cyclizine lactate *see* cyclizine *on this page*

cyclobenzaprine (sye kloe BEN za preen)
Synonyms cyclobenzaprine hydrochloride
Brand Names Flexeril®
Therapeutic Category Skeletal Muscle Relaxant
Use Treatment of muscle spasm associated with acute painful musculoskeletal conditions; supportive therapy in tetanus
Usual Dosage Oral:
Children: Dosage has not been established
Adults: 20-40 mg/day in 2-4 divided doses; maximum dose: 60 mg/day
Dosage Forms Tablet, as hydrochloride: 10 mg

cyclobenzaprine hydrochloride *see* cyclobenzaprine *on this page*

Cyclocort® Topical *see* amcinonide *on page 23*

Cyclogyl® *see* cyclopentolate *on this page*

Cyclomydril® Ophthalmic *see* cyclopentolate and phenylephrine *on this page*

cyclopentolate (sye kloe PEN toe late)
Synonyms cyclopentolate hydrochloride
Brand Names AK-Pentolate®; Cyclogyl®; I-Pentolate®
Therapeutic Category Anticholinergic Agent
Use Diagnostic procedures requiring mydriasis and cycloplegia
Usual Dosage Ophthalmic:
Infants: Instill 1 drop of 0.5% into each eye 5-10 minutes before examination
Children: Instill 1 drop of 0.5%, 1%, or 2% in eye followed by 1 drop of 0.5% or 1% in 5 minutes, if necessary
Adults: Instill 1 drop of 1% followed by another drop in 5 minutes; 2% solution in heavily pigmented iris
Dosage Forms Solution, ophthalmic, as hydrochloride: 0.5% (2 mL, 5 mL, 15 mL); 1% (2 mL, 5 mL, 15 mL); 2% (2 mL, 5 mL, 15 mL)

cyclopentolate and phenylephrine (sye kloe PEN toe late & fen il EF rin)
Synonyms phenylephrine and cyclopentolate
Brand Names Cyclomydril® Ophthalmic
Therapeutic Category Anticholinergic/Adrenergic Agonist
Use Induce mydriasis greater than that produced with cyclopentolate HCl alone
(Continued)

cyclopentolate and phenylephrine (Continued)

Usual Dosage Ophthalmic: Instill 1 drop every 5-10 minutes, not to exceed 3 instillations
Dosage Forms Solution, ophthalmic: Cyclopentolate hydrochloride 0.2% and phenylephrine hydrochloride 1% (2 mL, 5 mL)

cyclopentolate hydrochloride see cyclopentolate on previous page

cyclophosphamide (sye kloe FOS fa mide)

Synonyms cpm; ctx; cyt
Brand Names Cytoxan® Injection; Cytoxan® Oral; Neosar® Injection
Therapeutic Category Antineoplastic Agent
Use Management of Hodgkin's disease, malignant lymphomas, multiple myeloma, leukemias, sarcomas, mycosis fungoides, neuroblastoma, ovarian carcinoma, breast carcinoma, a variety of other tumors; nephrotic syndrome, lupus erythematosus, severe rheumatoid arthritis, and rheumatoid vasculitis
Usual Dosage
Children with no hematologic problems:
  Induction:
   Oral: 2-8 mg/kg/day
   I.V.: 10-20 mg/kg/day divided once daily
  Maintenance: Oral: 2-5 mg/kg (50-150 mg/m^2) twice weekly
  Pediatric solid tumors: I.V.: 250-1800 mg/m^2 once daily for 1-5 days every 21-28 days
Adults with no hematologic problems:
  Induction:
   Oral: 1-5 mg/kg/day
   I.V.: 40-50 mg/kg (1.5-1.8 g/m^2) in divided doses over 2-5 days
  Maintenance:
   Oral: 1-5 mg/kg/day
   I.V.: 10-15 mg/kg (350-550 mg/m^2) every 7-10 days or 3-5 mg/kg (110-185 mg/m^2) twice weekly
Children and Adults: I.V.:
  SLE: 500-750 mg/m^2 every month; maximum: 1 g/m^2
  JRA/vasculitis: 10 mg/kg every 2 weeks
  BMT conditioning regimen: I.V.: 50 mg/kg/day once daily for 3-4 days
  Nephrotic syndrome: Oral: 2-3 mg/kg/day every day for up to 12 weeks when corticosteroids are unsuccessful
Dosage Forms
Powder for injection: 100 mg, 200 mg, 500 mg, 1 g, 2 g
Lyophilized: 100 mg, 200 mg, 500 mg, 1 g, 2 g
Tablet: 25 mg, 50 mg

cycloserine (sye kloe SER een)

Brand Names Seromycin® Pulvules®
Therapeutic Category Antibiotic, Miscellaneous
Use Adjunctive treatment in pulmonary or extrapulmonary tuberculosis; treatment of acute urinary tract infections caused by *E. coli* or *Enterobacter* sp when less toxic conventional therapy has failed or is contraindicated
Usual Dosage Oral:
Tuberculosis:
  Children: 10-20 mg/kg/day in 2 divided doses up to 1000 mg/day
  Adults: Initial: 250 mg every 12 hours for 14 days, then administer 500 mg to 1 g/day in 2 divided doses
Urinary tract infection: Adults: 250 mg every 12 hours for 14 days
Dosage Forms Capsule: 250 mg

Cyclospasmol® see cyclandelate on page 142

cyclosporin a see cyclosporine on next page

cyclosporine (SYE kloe spor een)
Synonyms cya; cyclosporin a
Brand Names Neoral® Oral; Sandimmune® Injection; Sandimmune® Oral
Therapeutic Category Immunosuppressant Agent
Use Immunosuppressant used with corticosteroids to prevent graft vs host disease in patients with kidney, liver, heart, and bone marrow transplants; has been used in the treatment of nephrotic syndrome in patients with documented focal glomerulosclerosis when corticosteroids and cyclophosphamide were unsuccessful
Usual Dosage Children and Adults:
Oral: Initial: 14-18 mg/kg/dose daily, beginning 4-12 hours prior to organ transplantation; maintenance: 5-10 mg/kg/day
I.V.: Initial: 5-6 mg/kg/day in divided doses every 12-24 hours; patients should be switched to oral cyclosporine as soon as possible
Dosage Forms
Capsule (Sandimmune®): 25 mg, 100 mg
Soft gel (Sandimmune®): 50 mg
Soft gel for microemulsion (Neoral®): 25 mg, 100 mg
Injection (Sandimmune®): 50 mg/mL (5 mL)
Solution:
Oral (Sandimmune®): 100 mg/mL (50 mL)
Oral for microemulsion (Neoral®): 100 mg/mL (50 mL)

Cycofed® Pediatric *see* guaifenesin, pseudoephedrine, and codeine *on page 251*

Cycrin® Oral *see* medroxyprogesterone acetate *on page 326*

Cyklokapron® *see* tranexamic acid *on page 526*

Cylert® *see* pemoline *on page 399*

Cylex® [OTC] *see* benzocaine *on page 59*

Cyomin® *see* cyanocobalamin *on page 142*

cyproheptadine (si proe HEP ta deen)
Synonyms cyproheptadine hydrochloride
Brand Names Periactin®
Therapeutic Category Antihistamine
Use Perennial and seasonal allergic rhinitis and other allergic symptoms including urticaria
Usual Dosage Oral:
Children: 0.25 mg/kg/day in 2-3 divided doses or
2-6 years: 2 mg every 8-12 hours (not to exceed 12 mg/day)
7-14 years: 4 mg every 8-12 hours (not to exceed 16 mg/day)
Adults: 12-16 mg/day every 8 hours (not to exceed 0.5 mg/kg/day)
Dosage Forms
Syrup, as hydrochloride: 2 mg/5 mL with alcohol 5% (473 mL)
Tablet, as hydrochloride: 4 mg

cyproheptadine hydrochloride *see* cyproheptadine *on this page*

Cystadane® *see* betaine anhydrous *on page 64*

Cystagon® *see* cysteamine *on this page*

cysteamine (sis TEE a meen)
Synonyms cysteamine bitartrate
Brand Names Cystagon®
Therapeutic Category Urinary Tract Product
Use Nephropathic cystinosis in children and adults
Usual Dosage Initiate therapy with 1/4 to 1/8 of maintenance dose; titrate slowly upward over 4-6 weeks
(Continued)

cysteamine *(Continued)*

Children <12 years: Oral: Maintenance: 1.3 g/m^2/day divided into 4 doses
Children >12 years and Adults (>110 lbs): Oral: 2 g/day in 4 divided doses; dosage may in increased to 1.95 g/m^2/day if cystine levels are <1 nmol/^{1}/$_2$ cystine/mg protein, although intolerance and incidence of adverse events may be increased
Dosage Forms Capsule, as bitartrate: 50 mg, 150 mg

cysteamine bitartrate *see* cysteamine *on previous page*

cysteine (SIS teen)

Synonyms cysteine hydrochloride
Therapeutic Category Nutritional Supplement
Use Total parenteral nutrition of infants as an additive to meet the I.V. amino acid requirements
Usual Dosage Combine 500 mg of cysteine with 12.5 g of amino acid, then dilute with 50% dextrose
Dosage Forms Injection, as hydrochloride: 50 mg/mL (10 mL)

cysteine hydrochloride *see* cysteine *on this page*

Cystografin® *see* radiological/contrast media (ionic) *on page 457*

Cystospaz® *see* hyoscyamine *on page 275*

Cystospaz-M® *see* hyoscyamine *on page 275*

cyt *see* cyclophosphamide *on page 144*

Cytadren® *see* aminoglutethimide *on page 25*

cytarabine (sye TARE a been)

Synonyms arabinosylcytosine; ara-c; cytarabine hydrochloride; cytosine arabinosine hydrochloride
Brand Names Cytosar-U®
Therapeutic Category Antineoplastic Agent
Use In combination regimens for the treatment of leukemias and non-Hodgkin's lymphomas
Usual Dosage Children and Adults (refer to individual protocols):
Induction remission:
I.T.: 5-75 mg/m^2 once daily for 4 days or 1 every 4 days until CNS
I.V.: 200 mg/m^2/day for 5 days at 2-week intervals; 100-200 mg/m^2/day for 5- to 10-day therapy course or every day until remission administered I.V. continuous drip, or in 2-3 divided doses findings normalize
Maintenance remission:
I.M., S.C.: 1-1.5 mg/kg single dose for maintenance at 1- to 4-week intervals
I.V.: 70-200 mg/m^2/day for 2-5 days at monthly intervals
High-dose therapies: Doses as high as 1-3 g/m^2 have been used for refractory or secondary leukemias or refractory non-Hodgkins lymphoma; dosages of 3 g/m^2 every 12 hours for up to 12 doses have been used
Dosage Forms
Powder for injection, as hydrochloride: 100 mg, 500 mg, 1 g, 2 g
Cytosar-U®: 100 mg, 500 mg, 1 g, 2 g

cytarabine hydrochloride *see* cytarabine *on this page*

CytoGam™ *see* cytomegalovirus immune globulin (intravenous-human) *on this page*

cytomegalovirus immune globulin (intravenous-human)

(sye toe meg a low VYE rus i MYUN GLOB yoo lin in tra VEE nus, HYU man)
Synonyms cmv-igiv
Brand Names CytoGam™

Therapeutic Category Immune Globulin

Use Attenuation of primary CMV disease associated with kidney transplantation

Usual Dosage I.V.: Initial: Administer at 15 mg/kg/hour, then increase to 30 mg/kg/hour after 30 minutes if no untoward reactions, then increase to 60 mg/kg/hour after another 30 minutes, volume not to exceed 75 mL/hour

Dosage Forms Powder for injection, lyophilized, detergent treated: 2500 mg ± 250 mg (50 mL)

Cytomel® Oral *see* liothyronine *on page 309*

Cytosar-U® *see* cytarabine *on previous page*

cytosine arabinosine hydrochloride *see* cytarabine *on previous page*

Cytotec® *see* misoprostol *on page 352*

Cytovene® *see* ganciclovir *on page 237*

Cytoxan® Injection *see* cyclophosphamide *on page 144*

Cytoxan® Oral *see* cyclophosphamide *on page 144*

d₃ *see* cholecalciferol *on page 120*

25-d₃ *see* calcifediol *on page 80*

d-3-mercaptovaline *see* penicillamine *on page 399*

d4T *see* stavudine *on page 492*

dacarbazine (da KAR ba zeen)

Synonyms dic; imidazole carboxamide

Brand Names DTIC-Dome®

Therapeutic Category Antineoplastic Agent

Use Singly or in various combination therapy to treat malignant melanoma, Hodgkin's disease, soft-tissue sarcomas (fibrosarcomas, rhabdomyosarcoma), islet cell carcinoma, medullary carcinoma of the thyroid, and neuroblastoma

Usual Dosage Refer to individual protocols. I.V.:

Children:

Solid tumors: 200-470 mg/m²/day over 5 days every 21-28 days

Neuroblastoma: 800-900 mg/m² as a single dose every 3-4 weeks in combination therapy

Adults:

Malignant melanoma: 2-4.5 mg/kg/day for 10 days, repeat in 4 weeks or may use 250 mg/m²/day for 5 days, repeat in 3 weeks

Hodgkin's disease: 150 mg/m²/day for 5 days, repeat every 4 weeks or 375 mg/m² on day 1, repeat in 15 days of each 28-day cycle in combination with other agents

Dosage Forms Injection: 100 mg (10 mL, 20 mL); 200 mg (20 mL, 30 mL); 500 mg (50 mL)

Dacodyl® [OTC] *see* bisacodyl *on page 67*

dactinomycin (dak ti noe MYE sin)

Synonyms act; actinomycin d

Brand Names Cosmegen®

Therapeutic Category Antineoplastic Agent

Use Management, either alone or in combination with other treatment modalities of Wilms' tumor, rhabdomyosarcoma, neuroblastoma, retinoblastoma, Ewing's sarcoma, trophoblastic neoplasms, testicular carcinoma, and other malignancies

Usual Dosage Refer to individual protocols; dosage should be based on body surface area in obese or edematous patients

Children >6 months and Adults: I.V.: 15 mcg/kg/day or 400-600 mcg/m²/day for 5 days, may repeat every 3-6 weeks; or 2.5 mg/m² administered in divided doses over 1 week; 0.75-2 mg/m² as a single dose administered at intervals of 1-4 weeks have been used

(Continued)

dactinomycin *(Continued)*
Dosage Forms Powder for injection, lyophilized: 0.5 mg

D.A.II® Tablet *see chlorpheniramine, phenylephrine, and methscopolamine on page 116*

Dairy Ease® [OTC] *see lactase on page 299*

Dakin's solution *see sodium hypochlorite solution on page 485*

Dakrina® Ophthalmic Solution [OTC] *see artificial tears on page 42*

Dalalone® *see dexamethasone on page 156*

Dalalone D.P.® *see dexamethasone on page 156*

Dalalone L.A.® *see dexamethasone on page 156*

Dalgan® *see dezocine on page 162*

Dallergy® *see chlorpheniramine, phenylephrine, and methscopolamine on page 116*

Dallergy-D® Syrup *see chlorpheniramine and phenylephrine on page 113*

Dalmane® *see flurazepam on page 231*

d-alpha tocopherol *see vitamin e on page 553*

dalteparin (dal TE pa rin)
Brand Names Fragmin®
Therapeutic Category Anticoagulant
Use Prevent deep vein thrombosis following abdominal surgery
Usual Dosage Adults: S.C.: 2500 units 1-2 hours prior to surgery, then once daily for 5-10 days postoperatively
Dosage Forms Injection: Prefilled syringe: 2500 units (16 mg) in 0.2 mL

Damason-P® *see hydrocodone and aspirin on page 266*

danaparoid (da NAP a roid)
Synonyms danaparoid sodium
Brand Names Orgaran®
Therapeutic Category Anticoagulant
Use Prophylaxis of postoperative deep vein thrombosis (DVT)
Usual Dosage Adults: S.C.: 750 anti-Xa units twice daily beginning 1-4 hours preoperatively, and then not sooner than 2 hours hours after surgery
Dosage Forms Injection, as sodium: 750 anti-Xa units/0.6 mL

danaparoid sodium *see danaparoid on this page*

danazol (DA na zole)
Brand Names Danocrine®
Therapeutic Category Androgen
Use Treatment of endometriosis, fibrocystic breast disease, and hereditary angioedema
Usual Dosage Adults: Oral:
  Endometriosis: 100-400 mg twice daily
  Fibrocystic breast disease: 50-200 mg twice daily for 2-6 months
  Hereditary angioedema: 400-600 mg/day in 2-3 divided doses
Dosage Forms Capsule: 50 mg, 100 mg, 200 mg

Danocrine® *see danazol on this page*

Dantrium® *see dantrolene on next page*

dantrolene (DAN troe leen)

Synonyms dantrolene sodium

Brand Names Dantrium®

Therapeutic Category Skeletal Muscle Relaxant

Use Treatment of spasticity associated with upper motor neuron disorders such as spinal cord injury, stroke, cerebral palsy, or multiple sclerosis; also used as treatment of malignant hyperthermia

Usual Dosage

Spasticity: Oral:

Children: Initial: 0.5 mg/kg/dose twice daily, increase frequency to 3-4 times/day at 4- to 7-day intervals, then increase dose by 0.5 mg/kg to a maximum of 3 mg/kg/dose 2-4 times/day up to 400 mg/day

Adults: 25 mg/day to start, increase frequency to 3-4 times/day, then increase dose by 25 mg every 4-7 days to a maximum of 100 mg 2-4 times/day or 400 mg/day

Hyperthermia: Children and Adults:

Oral: 4-8 mg/kg/day in 4 divided doses

I.V.: 1 mg/kg; may repeat dose up to cumulative dose of 10 mg/kg (mean effective dose: 2.5 mg/kg), then switch to oral dosage

Dosage Forms

Capsule, as sodium: 25 mg, 50 mg, 100 mg

Powder for injection, as sodium: 20 mg

dantrolene sodium *see* dantrolene *on this page*

Dapacin® Cold Capsule [OTC] *see* chlorpheniramine, phenylpropanolamine, and acetaminophen *on page 117*

dapiprazole (DA pi pray zole)

Synonyms dapiprazole hydrochloride

Brand Names Rēv-Eyes™

Therapeutic Category Alpha-Adrenergic Blocking Agent

Use Treatment of iatrogenically induced mydriasis produced by adrenergic or parasympatholytic agents

Usual Dosage Ophthalmic: Instill 2 drops followed 5 minutes later by an additional 2 drops applied to the conjunctiva

Dosage Forms Powder, lyophilized, as hydrochloride: 25 mg [0.5% solution when mixed with supplied diluent]

dapiprazole hydrochloride *see* dapiprazole *on this page*

dapsone (DAP sone)

Synonyms dds; diaminodiphenylsulfone

Brand Names Avlosulfon®

Therapeutic Category Sulfone

Use Treatment of leprosy due to susceptible strains of *M. leprae*; treatment of dermatitis herpetiformis; prophylaxis against *Pneumocystis carinii* in children who cannot tolerate sulfamethoxazole/trimethoprim or aerosolized pentamidine

Usual Dosage Oral:

Children: Leprosy: 1-2 mg/kg/24 hours; maximum: 100 mg/day

Adults:

Leprosy: 50-100 mg/day

Dermatitis herpetiformis: Start at 50 mg/day, increase to 300 mg/day, or higher to achieve full control, reduce dosage to minimum level as soon as possible

Dosage Forms Tablet: 25 mg, 100 mg

Daranide® *see* dichlorphenamide *on page 164*

Daraprim® *see* pyrimethamine *on page 453*

Darvocet-N® *see* propoxyphene and acetaminophen *on page 445*

Darvocet-N® 100 *see* propoxyphene and acetaminophen *on page 445*

Darvon® *see* propoxyphene *on page 445*

Darvon® Compound-65 Pulvules® *see* propoxyphene and aspirin *on page 446*

Darvon-N® *see* propoxyphene *on page 445*

daunomycin *see* daunorubicin hydrochloride *on this page*

daunorubicin citrate (liposomal)
(daw noe ROO bi sin SI trate lip po SOE mal)
Brand Names DaunoXome®
Therapeutic Category Antineoplastic Agent
Use Advanced HIV-associated Kaposi's sarcoma
Usual Dosage I.V. (**refer to individual protocols**):
  Children:
  ALL combination therapy: Remission induction: 25-45 mg/m^2 on day 1 every week for 4 cycles **or** 30-45 mg/m^2/day for 3 days
  In children <2 years or <0.5 m^2, daunorubicin should be based on weight - mg/kg: 1 mg/kg per protocol with frequency dependent on regimen employed
  Cumulative dose should not exceed 300 mg/m^2 in children >2 years or 10 mg/kg in children <2 years
  Adults: 30-60 mg/m^2/day for 3-5 days, repeat dose in 3-4 weeks
  Single agent induction for AML: 60 mg/m^2/day for 3 days; repeat every 3-4 weeks
  Combination therapy induction for AML: 45 mg/m^2/day for 3 days of the first course of induction therapy; subsequent courses: Every day for 2 days
  ALL combination therapy: 45 mg/m^2/day for 3 days
  Cumulative dose should not exceed 400-600 mg/m^2
Dosage Forms Injection: 2 mg/mL equivalent to 50 mg daunorubicin base

daunorubicin hydrochloride (daw noe ROO bi sin hye droe KLOR ide)
Synonyms daunomycin; dnr; rubidomycin hydrochloride
Brand Names Cerubidine®
Therapeutic Category Antineoplastic Agent
Use In combination with other agents in the treatment of leukemias (ALL, AML)
Usual Dosage I.V.:
  Children:
  Combination therapy: Remission induction for ALL: 25-45 mg/m^2 on day 1 every week for 4 cycles
  <2 years or <0.5 m^2: Manufacturer recommends that the dose is based on body weight rather than body surface area
  Adults: 30-60 mg/m^2/day for 3-5 days, repeat dose in 3-4 weeks; total cumulative dose should not exceed 400-600 mg/m^2
  Single agent induction for AML: 60 mg/m^2/day for 3 days; repeat every 3-4 weeks
  Combination therapy induction for AML: 45 mg/m^2/day for 3 days; Subsequent courses: Every day for 2 days
  Combination therapy: Remission induction for ALL: 45 mg/m^2 on days 1, 2, and 3
Dosage Forms Powder for injection, lyophilized: 20 mg

DaunoXome® *see* daunorubicin citrate (liposomal) *on this page*

Daypro™ *see* oxaprozin *on page 387*

Dayto Himbin® *see* yohimbine *on page 558*

DC 240® Softgels® [OTC] *see* docusate *on page 179*

dcf *see* pentostatin *on page 405*

DDAVP® *see* desmopressin acetate *on page 155*

ddc *see* zalcitabine *on page 559*

ddi *see* didanosine *on page 166*

dds *see* dapsone *on page 149*

1-deamino-8-d-arginine vasopressin *see* desmopressin acetate *on page 155*

Debrisan® **[OTC]** *see* dextranomer *on page 159*

Debrox® **Otic [OTC]** *see* carbamide peroxide *on page 90*

Decadron® *see* dexamethasone *on page 156*

Decadron®**-LA** *see* dexamethasone *on page 156*

Decadron® **Phosphate** *see* dexamethasone *on page 156*

Deca-Durabolin® **Injection** *see* nandrolone *on page 364*

Decaject® *see* dexamethasone *on page 156*

Decaject-LA® *see* dexamethasone *on page 156*

Decholin® *see* dehydrocholic acid *on next page*

Declomycin® *see* demeclocycline *on page 153*

Decofed® **Syrup [OTC]** *see* pseudoephedrine *on page 449*

Decohistine® **DH** *see* chlorpheniramine, pseudoephedrine, and codeine *on page 118*

Decohistine® **Expectorant** *see* guaifenesin, pseudoephedrine, and codeine *on page 251*

Deconamine® **SR** *see* chlorpheniramine and pseudoephedrine *on page 114*

Deconamine® **Syrup [OTC]** *see* chlorpheniramine and pseudoephedrine *on page 114*

Deconamine® **Tablet [OTC]** *see* chlorpheniramine and pseudoephedrine *on page 114*

Deconsal® **II** *see* guaifenesin and pseudoephedrine *on page 250*

Deconsal® **Sprinkle**® *see* guaifenesin and phenylephrine *on page 249*

Defen-LA® *see* guaifenesin and pseudoephedrine *on page 250*

deferoxamine (de fer OKS a meen)

Synonyms deferoxamine mesylate
Brand Names Desferal® Mesylate
Therapeutic Category Antidote
Use Acute iron intoxication; chronic iron overload secondary to multiple transfusions; diagnostic test for iron overload

Investigational use: Treatment of aluminum accumulation in renal failure
Usual Dosage
Children:
Acute iron intoxication:
I.M.: 90 mg/kg/dose every 8 hours; maximum: 6 g/day
I.V.: 15 mg/kg/hour; maximum: 6 g/day
Chronic iron overload:
I.V.: 15 mg/kg/hour
S.C.: 20-40 mg/kg/day over 8-12 hours
Aluminum-induced bone disease: 20-40 mg/kg every hemodialysis treatment, frequency dependent on clinical status of the patient
Adults:
Acute iron intoxication:
I.M.: 1 g stat, then 0.5 g every 4 hours for two doses, then 0.5 g every 4-12 hours up to 6 g/day
I.V.: 15 mg/kg/hour; maximum: 6 g/day
Chronic iron overload:
I.M.: 0.5-1 g every day
S.C.: 1-2 g every day over 8-24 hours
Dosage Forms Powder for injection, as mesylate: 500 mg

deferoxamine mesylate *see* deferoxamine *on previous page*

Deficol® **[OTC]** *see* bisacodyl *on page 67*

Degas® **[OTC]** *see* simethicone *on page 480*

Degest® **2 Ophthalmic [OTC]** *see* naphazoline *on page 364*

dehydrocholic acid (dee hye droe KOE lik AS id)
Brand Names Cholan-HMB®; Decholin®
Therapeutic Category Laxative
Use Relief of constipation; adjunct to various biliary tract conditions
Usual Dosage Children >12 years and Adults: Oral: 250-500 mg 2-3 times/day after meals up to 1.5 g/day
Dosage Forms Tablet: 250 mg

Deladumone® **Injection** *see* estradiol and testosterone *on page 203*

Del Aqua-5® **Gel** *see* benzoyl peroxide *on page 61*

Del Aqua-10® **Gel** *see* benzoyl peroxide *on page 61*

Delatest® **Injection** *see* testosterone *on page 507*

Delatestryl® **Injection** *see* testosterone *on page 507*

delavirdine (de la VIR deen)
Synonyms U-90152S
Brand Names Rescriptor™
Therapeutic Category Antiviral Agent
Use Treatment of HIV-1 infection in combination with appropriate antiretrovirals
Usual Dosage Adults: Oral: 400 mg 3 times/day
Dosage Forms Tablet: 100 mg

Delcort® *see* hydrocortisone *on page 268*

Delfen® **[OTC]** *see* nonoxynol 9 *on page 377*

Del-Mycin® **Topical** *see* erythromycin, topical *on page 201*

Delsym® **[OTC]** *see* dextromethorphan *on page 160*

Delta-Cortef® **Oral** *see* prednisolone *on page 434*

deltacortisone *see* prednisone *on page 436*

Delta-D® *see* cholecalciferol *on page 120*

deltadehydrocortisone *see* prednisone *on page 436*

deltahydrocortisone *see* prednisolone *on page 434*

Deltasone® *see* prednisone *on page 436*

Delta-Tritex® *see* triamcinolone *on page 528*

Del-Vi-A® *see* vitamin a *on page 552*

Demadex® *see* torsemide *on page 525*

Demazin® **Syrup [OTC]** *see* chlorpheniramine and phenylpropanolamine *on page 114*

demecarium (dem e KARE ee um)
Synonyms demecarium bromide
Brand Names Humorsol® Ophthalmic
Therapeutic Category Cholinesterase Inhibitor
Use Management of chronic simple glaucoma, chronic and acute angle-closure glaucoma; counter effects of cycloplegics

Usual Dosage Ophthalmic:
  Children: Instill 1 drop into eyes twice weekly to a maximum dosage of 1 or 2 drops twice daily for up to 4 months
  Adults: Instill 1-2 drops into eyes twice weekly to a maximum dosage of 1 or 2 drops twice daily for up to 4 months
Dosage Forms Solution, ophthalmic, as bromide: 0.125% (5 mL); 0.25% (5 mL)

demecarium bromide *see* demecarium *on previous page*

demeclocycline (dem e kloe SYE kleen)
Synonyms demeclocycline hydrochloride; demethylchlortetracycline
Brand Names Declomycin®
Therapeutic Category Tetracycline Derivative
Use Treatment of susceptible bacterial infections (acne, gonorrhea, pertussis, chronic bronchitis, and urinary tract infections) caused by both gram-negative and gram-positive organisms; treatment of chronic syndrome of inappropriate antidiuretic hormone (SIADH) secretion
Usual Dosage Oral:
  Children ≥8 years: 8-12 mg/kg/day divided every 6-12 hours
  Adults: 150 mg 4 times/day or 300 mg twice daily
    Uncomplicated gonorrhea: 600 mg stat, 300 mg every 12 hours for 4 days (3 g total)
    SIADH: Initial: 900-1200 mg/day or 13-15 mg/kg/day divided every 6-8 hours, then decrease to 0.6-0.9 g/day
Dosage Forms
  Capsule, as hydrochloride: 150 mg
  Tablet, as hydrochloride: 150 mg, 300 mg

demeclocycline hydrochloride *see* demeclocycline *on this page*

Demerol® *see* meperidine *on page 328*

4-demethoxydaunorubicin *see* idarubicin *on page 278*

demethylchlortetracycline *see* demeclocycline *on this page*

Demser® *see* metyrosine *on page 347*

Demulen® *see* ethinyl estradiol and ethynodiol diacetate *on page 208*

Denavir® *see* penciclovir *on page 399*

Denorex® **[OTC]** *see* coal tar *on page 132*

deodorized opium tincture *see* opium tincture *on page 384*

2'-deoxycoformycin *see* pentostatin *on page 405*

Depacon® *see* valproic acid and derivatives *on page 544*

Depakene® *see* valproic acid and derivatives *on page 544*

Depakote® *see* valproic acid and derivatives *on page 544*

depAndrogyn® **Injection** *see* estradiol and testosterone *on page 203*

depAndro® **Injection** *see* testosterone *on page 507*

Depen® *see* penicillamine *on page 399*

depGynogen® **Injection** *see* estradiol *on page 202*

depMedalone® **Injection** *see* methylprednisolone *on page 343*

Depo®**-Estradiol Injection** *see* estradiol *on page 202*

Depogen® **Injection** *see* estradiol *on page 202*

Depoject® **Injection** *see* methylprednisolone *on page 343*

Depo-Medrol® **Injection** *see* methylprednisolone *on page 343*

Deponit® **Patch** *see* nitroglycerin *on page 376*

Depopred® **Injection** *see* methylprednisolone *on page 343*

Depo-Provera® Injection *see* medroxyprogesterone acetate *on page 326*

Depo-Testadiol® Injection *see* estradiol and testosterone *on page 203*

Depotest® Injection *see* testosterone *on page 507*

Depotestogen® Injection *see* estradiol and testosterone *on page 203*

Depo®-Testosterone Injection *see* testosterone *on page 507*

deprenyl *see* selegiline *on page 476*

Deproist® Expectorant with Codeine *see* guaifenesin, pseudoephedrine, and codeine *on page 251*

Derifil® [OTC] *see* chlorophyll *on page 110*

Dermacort® *see* hydrocortisone *on page 268*

Dermaflex® Gel *see* lidocaine *on page 307*

Dermarest Dricort® *see* hydrocortisone *on page 268*

Derma-Smoothe/FS® *see* fluocinolone *on page 226*

Dermatop® *see* prednicarbate *on page 434*

Dermatophytin® *see* Trichophyton skin test *on page 531*

Dermatophytin-O *see* Candida albicans (Monilia) *on page 87*

DermiCort® *see* hydrocortisone *on page 268*

Dermolate® [OTC] *see* hydrocortisone *on page 268*

Dermoplast® [OTC] *see* benzocaine *on page 59*

Dermtex® HC with Aloe *see* hydrocortisone *on page 268*

des *see* diethylstilbestrol *on page 167*

Desferal® Mesylate *see* deferoxamine *on page 151*

desflurane (des FLOO rane)

Brand Names Suprane®
Therapeutic Category General Anesthetic
Use Induction or maintenance of anesthesia for adults in outpatient and inpatient surgery
Usual Dosage
  Children: Maintenance: Surgical levels of anesthesia may be maintained with concentrations of 5.2% to 10% desflurane, with or without nitrous oxide
  Adults: Titrate dose based on individual response; see table in the product packaging for specific details; minimum alveolar concentration (MAC) should be reduced in elderly patients
  Induction: Frequent starting concentration 3%; increased in 0.5% to 1% increments every 2-3 breaths; end tidal concentrations of 4% to 11% desflurane with and without nitrous oxide produce anesthesia within 2-4 minutes
  Maintenance: Surgical levels of anesthesia in adults may be maintained with concentrations of 2.5% to 8.5% desflurane, with or without nitrous oxide

  Note: Because of the higher vapor pressure and higher MAC of desflurane, special vaporizer canisters must be used. Equipment is **not** interchangeable with that for isoflurane.
Dosage Forms Liquid: 240 mL

desiccated thyroid *see* thyroid *on page 518*

desipramine (des IP ra meen)

Synonyms desipramine hydrochloride; desmethylimipramine hydrochloride
Brand Names Norpramin®; Pertofrane®
Therapeutic Category Antidepressant, Tricyclic (Secondary Amine)
Use Treatment of various forms of depression, often in conjunction with psychotherapy; analgesic in chronic pain, peripheral neuropathies

Usual Dosage Oral (not recommended for use in children <12 years):
Adolescents: Initial: 25-50 mg/day; gradually increase to 100 mg/day in single or divided doses; maximum: 150 mg/day
Adults: Initial: 75 mg/day in divided doses; increase gradually to 150-200 mg/day in divided or single dose; maximum: 300 mg/day

Dosage Forms
Capsule, as hydrochloride (Pertofrane®): 25 mg, 50 mg
Tablet, as hydrochloride (Norpramin®): 10 mg, 25 mg, 50 mg, 75 mg, 100 mg, 150 mg

desipramine hydrochloride *see* desipramine *on previous page*

Desitin® [OTC] *see* zinc oxide, cod liver oil, and talc *on page 561*

desmethylimipramine hydrochloride *see* desipramine *on previous page*

desmopressin acetate (des moe PRES in AS e tate)
Synonyms 1-deamino-8-d-arginine vasopressin
Brand Names DDAVP®; Stimate® Nasal
Therapeutic Category Vasopressin Analog, Synthetic
Use Treatment of diabetes insipidus and controlling bleeding in certain types of hemophilia
Usual Dosage
Children:
Diabetes insipidus: 3 months to 12 years: Intranasal: Initial: 5 mcg/day divided 1-2 times/day; range: 5-30 mcg/day divided 1-2 times/day
Hemophilia: >3 months: I.V.: 0.3 mcg/kg by slow infusion; may repeat dose if needed
Nocturnal enuresis: ≥6 years: Intranasal: Initial: 20 mcg at bedtime; range: 10-40 mcg
Adults:
Diabetes insipidus: I.V., S.C.: 2-4 mcg/day in 2 divided doses or $1/_{10}$ of the maintenance intranasal dose; intranasal: 5-40 mcg/day 1-3 times/day
Hemophilia: I.V.: 0.3 mcg/kg by slow infusion
Dosage Forms
Injection (DDAVP®): 4 mcg/mL (1 mL)
Solution, nasal:
DDAVP®: 100 mcg/mL (2.5 mL, 5 mL)
Stimate®: 1.5 mg/mL (2.5 mL)
Tablet (DDAVP®): 0.1 mg, 0.2 mg

Desogen® *see* ethinyl estradiol and desogestrel *on page 207*

desogestrel and ethinyl estradiol *see* ethinyl estradiol and desogestrel *on page 207*

desonide (DES oh nide)
Brand Names DesOwen® Topical; Tridesilon® Topical
Therapeutic Category Corticosteroid, Topical
Use Adjunctive therapy for inflammation in acute and chronic corticosteroid responsive dermatosis
Usual Dosage Topical: Apply 2-4 times/day
Dosage Forms
Cream, topical: 0.05% (15 g, 60 g)
Lotion: 0.05% (60 mL, 120 mL)
Ointment, topical: 0.05% (15 g, 60 g)

DesOwen® Topical *see* desonide *on this page*

desoximetasone (des oks i MET a sone)
Brand Names Topicort®; Topicort®-LP
Therapeutic Category Corticosteroid, Topical
Use Relief of inflammation and pruritic symptoms of corticosteroid-responsive dermatosis
(Continued)

desoximetasone *(Continued)*

Usual Dosage Topical:
Children: Apply sparingly in a very thin film to affected area 1-2 times/day
Adults: Apply sparingly in a thin film twice daily

Dosage Forms
Cream, topical:
Topicort®: 0.25% (15 g, 60 g, 120 g)
Topicort®-LP: 0.05% (15 g, 60 g)
Gel, topical: 0.05% (15 g, 60 g)
Ointment, topical (Topicort®): 0.25% (15 g, 60 g)

desoxyephedrine hydrochloride *see* methamphetamine *on page 335*

Desoxyn® *see* methamphetamine *on page 335*

desoxyphenobarbital *see* primidone *on page 437*

desoxyribonuclease and fibrinolysin *see* fibrinolysin and desoxyribonuclease *on page 222*

Desquam-E® **Gel** *see* benzoyl peroxide *on page 61*

Desquam-X® **Gel** *see* benzoyl peroxide *on page 61*

Desquam-X® **Wash** *see* benzoyl peroxide *on page 61*

Desyrel® *see* trazodone *on page 527*

Detussin® **Expectorant** *see* hydrocodone, pseudoephedrine, and guaifenesin *on page 268*

Devrom® **[OTC]** *see* bismuth subgallate *on page 68*

Dexacidin® *see* neomycin, polymyxin b, and dexamethasone *on page 369*

Dexacort® **Phosphate in Respihaler** *see* dexamethasone *on this page*

Dexacort® **Phosphate Turbinaire**® *see* dexamethasone *on this page*

dexamethasone *(deks a METH a sone)*

Synonyms dexamethasone acetate; dexamethasone sodium phosphate

Brand Names Aeroseb-Dex®; AK-Dex® Ophthalmic; Baldex®; Dalalone®; Dalalone D.P.®; Dalalone L.A.®; Decadron®; Decadron®-LA; Decadron® Phosphate; Decaject®; Decaject-LA®; Dexacort® Phosphate in Respihaler; Dexacort® Phosphate Turbinaire®; Dexasone®; Dexasone® L.A.; Dexone®; Dexone® LA; Dexotic®; Hexadrol®; Hexadrol® Phosphate; Maxidex®; Solurex®; Solurex L.A.®

Therapeutic Category Adrenal Corticosteroid

Use Systemically and locally for chronic inflammation, allergic, hematologic, neoplastic, and autoimmune diseases; may be used in management of cerebral edema, septic shock, and as a diagnostic agent

Usual Dosage
Children:
Antiemetic (prior to chemotherapy): 10 mg/m^2/dose for first dose then 5 mg/m^2/dose every 6 hours as needed
Physiologic replacement: Oral, I.M., I.V.: 0.03-0.15 mg/kg/day or 0.6-0.75 mg/m^2/day in divided doses every 6-12 hours
Extubation or airway edema: Oral, I.M., I.V.: 0.5-1 mg/kg/day in divided doses every 6 hours beginning 24 hours prior to extubation and continuing for 4-6 doses afterwards
Ophthalmic: Instill 3-4 times/day
Cerebral edema: Loading dose: 1-2 mg/kg/dose as a single dose; maintenance: 1 mg/kg/day (maximum: 16 mg/day) in divided doses every 4-6 hours
Bacterial meningitis in infants and children >2 months: I.V.: 0.6 mg/kg/day in 4 divided doses for the first 4 days of antibiotic treatment; start dexamethasone at the time of the first dose of antibiotic
Adults:
Anti-inflammatory: Oral, I.M., I.V.: 0.75-9 mg/day in divided doses every 6-12 hours

Cerebral edema: I.V. 10 mg stat, 4 mg I.M./I.V. every 6 hours until response is maximized, then switch to oral regimen, then taper off if appropriate

Diagnosis for Cushing's syndrome: Oral: 1 mg at 11 PM, draw blood at 8 AM

ANLL protocol: I.V.: 2 mg/m^2/dose every 8 hours for 12 doses

Dosage Forms

Acetate:

Injection:

Dalalone L.A.®, Decadron®-LA, Decaject-LA®, Dexasone® L.A., Dexone® LA, Solurex L.A.®: 8 mg/mL (1 mL, 5 mL)

Dalalone D.P.®: 16 mg/mL (1 mL, 5 mL)

Base:

Aerosol, topical:

Aeroseb-Dex®: 0.01% (58 g)

Elixir (Decadron®, Hexadrol®): 0.5 mg/5 mL (5 mL, 20 mL, 100 mL, 120 mL, 240 mL, 500 mL)

Solution:

Oral: 0.5 mg/5 mL (5 mL, 20 mL, 500 mL)

Oral concentrate: 0.5 mg/0.5 mL (30 mL)

Suspension, ophthalmic: 0.1% (5 mL)

Maxidex®: 0.1% (5 mL, 15 mL)

Tablet (Dexone®, Hexadrol®): 0.25 mg, 0.5 mg, 0.75 mg, 1 mg, 1.5 mg, 2 mg, 4 mg, 6 mg

Therapeutic pack: Six 1.5 mg tablets and eight 0.75 mg tablets

Sodium phosphate:

Aerosol, nasal (Dexacort®): 84 mcg/activation [170 metered doses] (12.6 g)

Aerosol, oral (Dexacort®): 84 mcg/activation [170 metered doses] (12.6 g)

Cream (Decadron® Phosphate): 0.1% (15 g, 30 g)

Injection:

Dalalone®, Decadron® Phosphate, Decaject®, Dexasone®, Hexadrol® Phosphate, Solurex®: 4 mg/mL (1 mL, 2 mL, 2.5 mL, 5 mL, 10 mL, 30 mL)

Hexadrol® Phosphate: 10 mg/mL (1 mL, 10 mL); 20 mg/mL (5 mL)

Decadron® Phosphate: 24 mg/mL (5 mL, 10 mL)

Ointment, ophthalmic: 0.05% (3.5 g)

AK-Dex®, Baldex®, Decadron® Phosphate, Maxidex®: 0.05% (3.5 g)

Solution, ophthalmic (AK-Dex®, Baldex®, Decadron® Phosphate, Dexotic®): 0.1% (5 mL)

dexamethasone acetate *see* dexamethasone *on previous page*

dexamethasone and neomycin *see* neomycin and dexamethasone *on page 368*

dexamethasone and tobramycin *see* tobramycin and dexamethasone *on page 522*

dexamethasone sodium phosphate *see* dexamethasone *on previous page*

Dexasone® *see* dexamethasone *on previous page*

Dexasone® L.A. *see* dexamethasone *on previous page*

Dexasporin® *see* neomycin, polymyxin b, and dexamethasone *on page 369*

Dexatrim® Pre-Meal [OTC] *see* phenylpropanolamine *on page 413*

dexbrompheniramine and pseudoephedrine

(deks brom fen EER a meen & soo doe e FED rin)

Synonyms pseudoephedrine and dexbrompheniramine

Brand Names Disobrom® [OTC]; Disophrol® Chronotabs® [OTC]; Disophrol® Tablet [OTC]; Drixomed®; Drixoral® [OTC]

Therapeutic Category Antihistamine/Decongestant Combination

Use Relief of symptoms of upper respiratory mucosal congestion in seasonal and perennial nasal allergies, acute rhinitis, rhinosinusitis and eustachian tube blockage

(Continued)

dexbrompheniramine and pseudoephedrine *(Continued)*

Usual Dosage Children >12 years and Adults: Oral: 1 tablet every 12 hours, may require 1 tablet every 8 hours

Dosage Forms
Tablet (Disophrol®): Dexbrompheniramine maleate 2 mg and pseudoephedrine sulfate 60 mg
Timed release (Disobrom®, Disophrol® Chrontabs®, Drixomed®, Drixoral®, Histrodrix®, Resporal®): Dexbrompheniramine maleate 6 mg and pseudoephedrine sulfate 120 mg

Dexchlor® *see* dexchlorpheniramine *on this page*

dexchlorpheniramine (deks klor fen EER a meen)

Synonyms dexchlorpheniramine maleate
Brand Names Dexchlor®; Poladex®; Polaramine®
Therapeutic Category Antihistamine
Use Perennial and seasonal allergic rhinitis and other allergic symptoms including urticaria

Usual Dosage Oral:
Children:
2-5 years: 0.5 mg every 4-6 hours
6-11 years: 1 mg every 4-6 hours or 4 mg timed release at bedtime
Adults: 2 mg every 4-6 hours or 4-6 mg timed release at bedtime or 8-10 hours

Dosage Forms
Syrup, as maleate (orange flavor): 2 mg/5 mL with alcohol 6% (480 mL)
Tablet, as maleate: 2 mg
Sustained action: 4 mg, 6 mg

dexchlorpheniramine maleate *see* dexchlorpheniramine *on this page*

Dexedrine® *see* dextroamphetamine *on next page*

Dexferrum® Injection *see* iron dextran complex *on page 289*

Dexone® *see* dexamethasone *on page 156*

Dexone® LA *see* dexamethasone *on page 156*

Dexotic® *see* dexamethasone *on page 156*

dexpanthenol (deks PAN the nole)

Synonyms pantothenyl alcohol
Brand Names Ilopan-Choline® Oral; Ilopan® Injection; Panthoderm® Cream [OTC]
Therapeutic Category Gastrointestinal Agent, Stimulant
Use Prophylactic use to minimize paralytic ileus, treatment of postoperative distention

Usual Dosage
Children and Adults: Relief of itching and aid in skin healing: Topical: Apply to affected area 1-2 times/day
Adults:
Relief of gas retention: Oral: 2-3 tablets 3 times/day
Prevention of postoperative ileus: I.M.: 250-500 mg stat, repeat in 2 hours, followed by doses every 6 hours until danger passes
Paralyzed ileus: I.M.: 500 mg stat, repeat in 2 hours, followed by doses every 6 hours, if needed

Dosage Forms
Cream: 2% (30 g, 60 g)
Injection (Ilopan®): 250 mg/mL (2 mL, 10 mL, 30 mL)
Tablet (Ilopan-Choline®): 50 mg with choline bitartrate 25 mg

dexrazoxane (deks ray ZOKS ane)

Synonyms ICRF-187
Brand Names Zinecard®

Therapeutic Category Cardiovascular Agent, Other

Use Prevention of cardiomyopathy associated with doxorubicin administration

Usual Dosage I.V.: 1000 mg/m^2 30 minutes before administration of doxorubicin; maximal doses in patients with and without prior treatment with nitrosoureas, respectively = 750 mg/m^2 and 120 mg/m^2; 3500 mg/m^2/day for 3 days has been maximally used in pediatric patients. The recommended dosage ratio of dexrazoxane:doxorubicin is 10:1.

Dosage Forms Powder for injection, lyophilized: 250 mg, 500 mg (10 mg/mL when reconstituted)

dextran (DEKS tran)

Synonyms dextran, high molecular weight; dextran, low molecular weight

Brand Names Gentran®; LMD®; Macrodex®; Rheomacrodex®

Therapeutic Category Plasma Volume Expander

Use Fluid replacement and blood volume expander used in the treatment of hypovolemia, shock, or near shock states

Usual Dosage I.V.:
Children: Total dose should not be >20 mL/kg during first 24 hours
Adults: 500-1000 mL at rate of 20-40 mL/minute

Dosage Forms Injection:
High molecular weight:
6% dextran 75 in dextrose 5% (500 mL)
Gentran®: 6% dextran 75 in sodium chloride 0.9% (500 mL)
Gentran®, Macrodex®: 6% dextran 70 in sodium chloride 0.9% (500 mL)
Macrodex®: 6% dextran 70 in dextrose 5% (500 mL)

Low molecular weight: Gentran®, LMD®, Rheomacrodex®:
10% dextran 40 in dextrose 5% (500 mL)
10% dextran 40 in sodium chloride 0.9% (500 mL)

dextran 1 (DEKS tran won)

Brand Names Promit®

Therapeutic Category Plasma Volume Expander

Use Prophylaxis of serious anaphylactic reactions to I.V. infusion of dextran

Usual Dosage I.V. (time between dextran 1 and dextran solution should not exceed 15 minutes):
Children: 0.3 mL/kg 1-2 minutes before I.V. infusion of dextran
Adults: 20 mL 1-2 minutes before I.V. infusion of dextran

Dosage Forms Injection: 150 mg/mL (20 mL)

dextran, high molecular weight *see dextran on this page*
dextran, low molecular weight *see dextran on this page*

dextranomer (deks TRAN oh mer)

Brand Names Debrisan® [OTC]

Therapeutic Category Topical Skin Product

Use Clean exudative wounds; no controlled studies have found dextranomer to be more effective than conventional therapy

Usual Dosage Topical: Apply to affected area once or twice daily

Dosage Forms
Beads: 4 g, 25 g, 60 g, 120 g
Paste: 10 g foil packets

dextroamphetamine (deks troe am FET a meen)

Synonyms dextroamphetamine sulfate

Brand Names Dexedrine®

Therapeutic Category Amphetamine
(Continued)

dextroamphetamine (Continued)

Controlled Substance C-II

Use Adjunct in treatment of attention deficit disorder with hyperactivity (ADDH) in children, narcolepsy, exogenous obesity

Usual Dosage Oral:

Children:

Narcolepsy: 6-12 years: Initial: 5 mg/day, may increase at 5 mg increments in weekly intervals until side effects appear; maximum dose: 60 mg/day

Attention deficit disorder:

3-5 years: Initial: 2.5 mg/day administered every morning; increase by 2.5 mg/day in weekly intervals until optimal response is obtained, usual range is 0.1-0.5 mg/kg/dose every morning with maximum of 40 mg/day

≥6 years: 5 mg once or twice daily; increase in increments of 5 mg/day at weekly intervals until optimal response is reached, usual range is 0.1-0.5 mg/kg/dose every morning (5-20 mg/day) with maximum of 40 mg/day

Adults:

Narcolepsy: Initial: 10 mg/day, may increase at 10 mg increments in weekly intervals until side effects appear; maximum: 60 mg/day

Exogenous obesity: 5-30 mg/day in divided doses of 5-10 mg 30-60 minutes before meals

Dosage Forms

Capsule, as sulfate, sustained release: 5 mg, 10 mg, 15 mg

Elixir, as sulfate: 5 mg/5 mL (480 mL)

Tablet, as sulfate: 5 mg, 10 mg (5 mg tablets contain tartrazine)

dextroamphetamine and amphetamine

(deks troe am FET a meen & am FET a meen)

Brand Names Adderall®

Therapeutic Category Amphetamine

Use Treatment of narcolepsy; exogenous obesity; abnormal behavioral syndrome in children (minimal brain dysfunction); attention deficit hyperactive disorder (ADHD)

Usual Dosage Oral:

Narcolepsy:

Children:

6-12 years: 5 mg/day, increase by 5 mg at weekly intervals

>12 years: 10 mg/day, increase by 10 mg at weekly intervals

Adults: 5-60 mg/day in 2-3 divided doses

Attention deficit disorder: Children:

3-5 years: 2.5 mg/day, increase by 2.5 mg at weekly intervals

>6 years: 5 mg/day, increase by 5 mg at weekly intervals not to exceed 40 mg/day

Short-term adjunct to exogenous obesity: Children >12 years and Adults: 5-30 mg/day in divided doses

Dosage Forms Tablet:

10 mg [dextroamphetamine sulfate 2.5 mg, dextroamphetamine saccharate 2.5 mg and amphetamine aspartate 2.5 mg, amphetamine sulfate 2.5 mg]

30 mg [dextroamphetamine sulfate 7.5 mg, dextroamphetamine saccharate 7.5 mg and amphetamine aspartate 7.55 mg, amphetamine sulfate 7.5 mg]

dextroamphetamine sulfate see dextroamphetamine on previous page

dextromethorphan (deks troe meth OR fan)

Brand Names Benylin DM® [OTC]; Benylin® Pediatric [OTC]; Children's Hold® [OTC]; Creo-Terpin® [OTC]; Delsym® [OTC]; Drixoral® Cough Liquid Caps [OTC]; Hold® DM [OTC]; Pertussin® CS [OTC]; Pertussin® ES [OTC]; Robitussin® Cough Calmers [OTC]; Robitussin® Pediatric [OTC]; Scot-Tussin DM® Cough Chasers [OTC]; Silphen DM® [OTC]; St. Joseph® Cough Suppressant [OTC]; Sucrets® Cough Calmers [OTC];

Suppress® [OTC]; Trocal® [OTC]; Vicks Formula 44® [OTC]; Vicks Formula 44® Pediatric Formula [OTC]

Therapeutic Category Antitussive

Use Symptomatic relief of coughs caused by minor viral upper respiratory tract infections or inhaled irritants; most effective for a chronic nonproductive cough

Usual Dosage Oral:

Children:

2-5 years: 2.5-5 mg every 4 hours or 7.5 mg every 6-8 hours; extended release is 50 mg twice daily

6-11 years: 5-10 mg every 4 hours or 15 mg every 6-8 hours; extended release is 30 mg twice daily

Adults: 10-20 mg every 4 hours or 30 mg every 6-8 hours; extended release is 60 mg twice daily

Dosage Forms

Capsule (Drixoral® Cough Liquid Caps): 30 mg

Liquid:

Creo-Terpin®: 10 mg/15 mL (120 mL)

Pertussin® CS: 3.5 mg/5 mL (120 mL)

Robitussin® Pediatric, St. Joseph® Cough Suppressant: 7.5 mg/5 mL (60 mL, 120 mL, 240 mL)

Pertussin® ES, Vicks Formula 44®: 15 mg/5 mL (120 mL, 240 mL)

Liquid, sustained release, as polistirex (Delsym®): 30 mg/5 mL (89 mL)

Lozenges:

Scot-Tussin DM® Cough Chasers: 2.5 mg

Children's Hold®, Hold® DM, Robitussin® Cough Calmers, Sucrets® Cough Calmers: 5 mg

Suppress®, Trocal®: 7.5 mg

Syrup:

Benylin® Pediatric: 7.5 mg/mL (118 mL)

Benylin DM®, Silphen DM®: 10 mg/5 mL (120 mL, 3780 mL)

Vicks Formula 44® Pediatric Formula: 15 mg/15 mL (120 mL)

dextromethorphan, acetaminophen, and pseudoephedrine *see* acetaminophen, dextromethorphan, and pseudoephedrine *on page 6*

dextromethorphan and guaifenesin *see* guaifenesin and dextromethorphan *on page 248*

dextromethorphan, guaifenesin, and pseudoephedrine *see* guaifenesin, pseudoephedrine, and dextromethorphan *on page 252*

dextropropoxyphene *see* propoxyphene *on page 445*

dextrose, levulose and phosphoric acid *see* phosphorated carbohydrate solution *on page 415*

dextrothyroxine (deks troe thye ROKS een)

Synonyms dextrothyroxine sodium

Brand Names Choloxin®

Therapeutic Category Antihyperlipidemic Agent, Miscellaneous

Use Reduction of elevated serum cholesterol

Usual Dosage Oral:

Children: 0.1 mg/kg/day

Adults: 1-2 mg/day, up to 8 mg/day

Dosage Forms Tablet, as sodium: 2 mg, 4 mg, 6 mg

dextrothyroxine sodium *see* dextrothyroxine *on this page*

Dey-Dose® Isoproterenol *see* isoproterenol *on page 291*

Dey-Dose® Metaproterenol *see* metaproterenol *on page 332*

Dey-Drop® Ophthalmic Solution *see* silver nitrate *on page 479*

Dey-Lute® Isoetharine *see* isoetharine *on page 289*

dezocine (DEZ oh seen)

Brand Names Dalgan®
Therapeutic Category Analgesic, Narcotic
Use Relief of moderate to severe postoperative, acute renal and ureteral colic, and cancer pain
Usual Dosage Adults:
  I.M.: Initial: 5-20 mg; may be repeated every 3-6 hours as needed; maximum: 120 mg/day
  I.V.: Initial: 2.5-10 mg; may be repeated every 2-4 hours as needed
Dosage Forms Injection, single-dose vial: 5 mg/mL (2 mL); 10 mg/mL (2 mL); 15 mg/mL (2 mL)

dfp *see* isoflurophate *on page 290*

dhad *see* mitoxantrone *on page 353*

DHC Plus® *see* dihydrocodeine compound *on page 169*

D.H.E. 45® Injection *see* dihydroergotamine *on page 169*

dhpg sodium *see* ganciclovir *on page 237*

DHS® Tar [OTC] *see* coal tar *on page 132*

DHS Zinc® [OTC] *see* pyrithione zinc *on page 454*

DHT™ *see* dihydrotachysterol *on page 169*

Diaβeta® *see* glyburide *on page 243*

Diabetic Tussin DM® [OTC] *see* guaifenesin and dextromethorphan *on page 248*

Diabetic Tussin® EX [OTC] *see* guaifenesin *on page 247*

Diabinese® *see* chlorpropamide *on page 119*

Dialose® [OTC] *see* docusate *on page 179*

Dialose® Plus Capsule [OTC] *see* docusate and casanthranol *on page 180*

Dialose® Plus Tablet [OTC] *see* docusate and phenolphthalein *on page 180*

Dialume® [OTC] *see* aluminum hydroxide *on page 21*

Diamine T.D.® [OTC] *see* brompheniramine *on page 73*

diaminodiphenylsulfone *see* dapsone *on page 149*

Diamox® *see* acetazolamide *on page 6*

Diamox Sequels® *see* acetazolamide *on page 6*

Diaparene® [OTC] *see* methylbenzethonium chloride *on page 341*

Diapid® Nasal Spray *see* lypressin *on page 317*

Diar-aid® [OTC] *see* loperamide *on page 313*

Diasorb® [OTC] *see* attapulgite *on page 48*

diazepam (dye AZ e pam)

Brand Names Dizac® Injection; Valium®
Therapeutic Category Benzodiazepine
Controlled Substance C-IV
Use Management of general anxiety disorders, panic disorders; to provide preoperative sedation, light anesthesia, and amnesia; treatment of status epilepticus, alcohol withdrawal symptoms; used as a skeletal muscle relaxant
Usual Dosage
  Children:
  Sedation or muscle relaxation or anxiety:
  Oral: 0.12-0.8 mg/kg/day in divided doses every 6-8 hours

I.M., I.V.: 0.04-0.3 mg/kg/dose every 2-4 hours to a maximum of 0.6 mg/kg within an 8-hour period if needed

Status epilepticus: I.V.:

Infants 30 days to 5 years: 0.05-0.3 mg/kg/dose administered over 2-3 minutes, every 15-30 minutes to a maximum total dose of 5 mg; repeat in 2-4 hours as needed or 0.2-0.5 mg/dose every 2-5 minutes to a maximum total dose of 5 mg

>5 years: 0.05-0.3 mg/kg/dose administered over 2-3 minutes, every 15-30 minutes to a maximum total dose of 10 mg; repeat in 2-4 hours as needed or 1 mg/dose every 2-5 minutes to a maximum of 10 mg;

Adults:

Anxiety:

Oral: 2-10 mg 2-4 times/day

I.M., I.V.: 2-10 mg, may repeat in 3-4 hours if needed

Skeletal muscle relaxation:

Oral: 2-10 mg 2-4 times/day

I.M., I.V.: 5-10 mg, may repeat in 2-4 hours

Status epilepticus: I.V.: 0.2-0.5 mg/kg/dose every 15-30 minutes for 2-3 doses; maximum dose: 30 mg

Dosage Forms

Injection: 5 mg/mL (1 mL, 2 mL, 5 mL, 10 mL)

Emulsified (Dizac®): 5 mg/mL (3 mL)

Solution:

Oral (wintergreen-spice flavor): 5 mg/5 mL (5 mL, 10 mL, 500 mL)

Oral concentrate: 5 mg/mL (30 mL)

Tablet: 2 mg, 5 mg, 10 mg

diazoxide (dye az OKS ide)

Brand Names Hyperstat® I.V.; Proglycem® Oral

Therapeutic Category Antihypoglycemic Agent; Vasodilator

Use I.V.: Emergency lowering of blood pressure; Oral: Hypoglycemia related to hyperinsulinism secondary to islet cell adenoma, carcinoma, or hyperplasia; adenomatosis; nesidioblastosis (persistent hyperinsulinemic hypoglycemia of infancy); leucine sensitivity, or extrapancreatic malignancy

Usual Dosage

Hyperinsulinemic hypoglycemia: Oral:

Newborns and Infants: 8-15 mg/kg/day in divided doses every 8-12 hours

Children and Adults: 3-8 mg/kg/day in divided doses every 8-12 hours

Hypertension: Children and Adults: I.V.: 1-3 mg/kg (maximum: 150 mg in a single injection); repeat dose in 5-15 minutes until blood pressure adequately reduced; repeat administration every 4-24 hours; monitor blood pressure closely

Dosage Forms

Capsule (Proglycem®): 50 mg

Injection (Hyperstat®): 15 mg/mL (1 mL, 20 mL)

Suspension, oral (chocolate-mint flavor) (Proglycem®): 50 mg/mL (30 mL)

Dibent® Injection see dicyclomine on page 165

Dibenzyline® see phenoxybenzamine on page 410

dibucaine (DYE byoo kane)

Brand Names Nupercainal® [OTC]

Therapeutic Category Local Anesthetic

Use Fast, temporary relief of pain and itching due to hemorrhoids, minor burns, other minor skin conditions

Usual Dosage Children and Adults:

Rectal: Hemorrhoids: Insert ointment into rectum using a rectal applicator; administer each morning,evening, and after each bowel movement

Topical: Apply gently to the affected areas; no more than 30 g for adults or 7.5 g for children should be used in any 24-hour period

(Continued)

163

dibucaine *(Continued)*

Dosage Forms
Cream: 0.5% (45 g)
Ointment, topical: 1% (30 g, 60 g)

dibucaine and hydrocortisone (DYE byoo kane & hye droe KOR ti sone)

Synonyms hydrocortisone and dibucaine
Brand Names Corticaine® Topical
Therapeutic Category Anesthetic/Corticosteroid
Use Relief of the inflammatory and pruritic manifestations of corticosteroid-responsive dermatoses and for external anal itching
Usual Dosage Topical: Apply to affected areas 2-4 times/day
Dosage Forms Cream: Dibucaine 5% and hydrocortisone 5%

dic *see* dacarbazine *on page 147*

dicalcium phosphate *see* calcium phosphate, dibasic *on page 86*

Dicarbosil® [OTC] *see* calcium carbonate *on page 82*

dichlorodifluoromethane and trichloromonofluoromethane

(dye klor oh dye flor oh METH ane & tri klor oh mon oh flor oh METH ane)
Brand Names Fluori-Methane® Topical Spray
Therapeutic Category Analgesic, Topical
Use Management of myofascial pain, restricted motion, muscle pain; control of pain associated with injections
Usual Dosage Topical: Apply to area from approximately 12" away
Dosage Forms Spray, topical: Dichlorodifluoromethane 15% and trichloromonofluoromethane 85%

dichlorotetrafluoroethane and ethyl chloride *see* ethyl chloride and dichlorotetrafluoroethane *on page 212*

dichlorphenamide (dye klor FEN a mide)

Synonyms diclofenamide
Brand Names Daranide®
Therapeutic Category Carbonic Anhydrase Inhibitor
Use Adjunct in treatment of open-angle glaucoma and perioperative treatment for angle-closure glaucoma
Usual Dosage Adults: Oral: 100-200 mg to start followed by 100 mg every 12 hours until desired response is obtained; maintenance dose: 25-50 mg 1-3 times/day
Dosage Forms Tablet: 50 mg

dichysterol *see* dihydrotachysterol *on page 169*

diclofenac (dye KLOE fen ak)

Synonyms diclofenac potassium; diclofenac sodium
Brand Names Cataflam® Oral; Voltaren® Ophthalmic; Voltaren® Oral; Voltaren-XR® Oral
Therapeutic Category Analgesic, Non-narcotic; Nonsteroidal Anti-Inflammatory Agent (NSAID)
Use Acute treatment of mild to moderate pain; acute and chronic treatment of rheumatoid arthritis, ankylosing spondylitis, and osteoarthritis; used for juvenile rheumatoid arthritis, gout, dysmenorrhea; ophthalmic solution for postoperative inflammation after cataract extraction
Usual Dosage Adults:
Oral:
Rheumatoid arthritis: 150-200 mg/day in 2-4 divided doses
Osteoarthritis: 100-150 mg/day in 2-3 divided doses

Ankylosing spondylitis: 100-125 mg/day in 4-5 divided doses

Ophthalmic: Instill 1 drop into affected eye 4 times/day beginning 24 hours after cataract surgery and continuing for 2 weeks

Dosage Forms

Solution, ophthalmic, as sodium (Voltaren®): 0.1% (2.5 mL, 5 mL)

Tablet:

Enteric coated, as sodium: 25 mg, 50 mg, 75 mg

Voltaren®: 25 mg, 50 mg, 75 mg

Extended release, as sodium (Voltaren-XR®): 100 mg

As potassium (Cataflam®): 50 mg

diclofenac potassium see diclofenac on previous page

diclofenac sodium see diclofenac on previous page

diclofenamide see dichlorphenamide on previous page

diclofenamide (dye kloks a SIL in)

Synonyms dicloxacillin sodium

Brand Names Dycill®; Dynapen®; Pathocil®

Therapeutic Category Penicillin

Use Treatment of skin and soft tissue infections, pneumonia and follow-up therapy of osteomyelitis caused by susceptible penicillinase-producing staphylococci

Usual Dosage Oral:

Children <40 kg: 12.5-50 mg/kg/day divided every 6 hours; doses of 50-100 mg/kg/day in divided doses every 6 hours have been used for follow-up therapy of osteomyelitis

Children >40 kg and Adults: 125-500 mg every 6 hours

Dosage Forms

Capsule, as sodium: 125 mg, 250 mg, 500 mg

Powder for oral suspension, as sodium: 62.5 mg/5 mL (80 mL, 100 mL, 200 mL)

dicloxacillin sodium see dicloxacillin on this page

dicumarol (dye KOO ma role)

Synonyms bishydroxycoumarin

Therapeutic Category Anticoagulant

Use Prophylaxis and treatment of thromboembolic disorders

Usual Dosage Adults: Oral: 25-200 mg/day based on prothrombin time (PT) determinations

Dosage Forms Tablet: 25 mg, 50 mg, 100 mg

dicyclomine (dye SYE kloe meen)

Synonyms dicyclomine hydrochloride; dicycloverine hydrochloride

Brand Names Antispas® Injection; Bentyl® Hydrochloride Injection; Bentyl® Hydrochloride Oral; Byclomine® Injection; Dibent® Injection; Di-Spaz® Injection; Di-Spaz® Oral; Or-Tyl® Injection

Therapeutic Category Anticholinergic Agent

Use Treatment of functional disturbances of GI motility such as irritable bowel syndrome

Usual Dosage

Oral:

Infants >6 months: 5 mg/dose 3-4 times/day

Children: 10 mg/dose 3-4 times/day

Adults: Begin with 80 mg/day in 4 equally divided doses, then increase up to 160 mg/day

I.M. **(should not be used I.V.)**: 80 mg/day in 4 divided doses (20 mg/dose)

Dosage Forms

Capsule, as hydrochloride: 10 mg, 20 mg

Injection, as hydrochloride: 10 mg/mL (2 mL, 10 mL)

Syrup, as hydrochloride: 10 mg/5 mL (118 mL, 473 mL, 946 mL)

(Continued)

dicyclomine *(Continued)*
Tablet, as hydrochloride: 20 mg

dicyclomine hydrochloride *see* dicyclomine *on previous page*

dicycloverine hydrochloride *see* dicyclomine *on previous page*

didanosine (dye DAN oh seen)
Synonyms ddi
Brand Names Videx®
Therapeutic Category Antiviral Agent
Use Treatment of patients with advanced HIV infection which is resistant to zidovudine therapy or in those patients with zidovudine intolerance; has been used in asymptomatic patients with very low CD4$^+$ lymphocyte counts (<200 cells/mm^3) with or without AIDS-related complex
Usual Dosage Administer on an empty stomach: Oral:
Children (dosing is based on body surface area (m^2)):
  <0.4: 25 mg tablets twice daily or 31 mg powder twice daily
  0.5-0.7: 50 mg tablets twice daily or 62 mg powder twice daily
  0.8-1: 75 mg tablets twice daily or 94 mg powder twice daily
  1.1-1.4: 100 mg tablets twice daily or 125 mg powder twice daily
Adults: Dosing is based on patient weight:
  35-49 kg: 125 mg tablets twice daily or 167 mg buffered powder twice daily
  50-74 kg: 200 mg tablets twice daily or 250 mg buffered powder twice daily
  ≥75 mg: 300 mg tablets twice daily or 375 mg buffered powder twice daily

Note: Children >1 year and Adults should receive 2 tablets per dose and children <1 year should receive 1 tablet per dose for adequate buffering and absorption; tablets should be chewed
Dosage Forms
Powder for oral solution:
  Buffered (single dose packet): 100 mg, 167 mg, 250 mg, 375 mg
  Pediatric: 2 g, 4 g
  Tablet, buffered, chewable (mint flavor): 25 mg, 50 mg, 100 mg, 150 mg

dideoxycytidine *see* zalcitabine *on page 559*

Didrex® *see* benzphetamine *on page 62*

Didronel® *see* etidronate disodium *on page 212*

dienestrol (dye en ES trole)
Brand Names DV® Vaginal Cream; Ortho-Dienestrol® Vaginal
Therapeutic Category Estrogen Derivative
Use Symptomatic management of atrophic vaginitis in postmenopausal women
Usual Dosage Adults: Vaginal: 1-2 applicatorfuls/day for 2 weeks and then ½ of that dose for 2 weeks; maintenance dose: 1 applicatorful 1-3 times/week for 3 weeks each month
Dosage Forms Cream, vaginal: 0.01% (30 g, 78 g)

dietary supplements *see* enteral nutritional products *on page 194*

diethylpropion (dye eth il PROE pee on)
Synonyms amfepramone; diethylpropion hydrochloride
Brand Names Tenuate®; Tenuate® Dospan®
Therapeutic Category Anorexiant
Controlled Substance C-IV
Use Short-term adjunct in exogenous obesity
Usual Dosage Adults: Oral: 25 mg 3 times/day before meals or food or 75 mg controlled release tablet at midmorning

Dosage Forms
Tablet, as hydrochloride: 25 mg
Tablet, as hydrochloride, controlled release: 75 mg

diethylpropion hydrochloride *see* diethylpropion *on previous page*

diethylstilbestrol (dye eth il stil BES trole)
Synonyms des; diethylstilbestrol diphosphate sodium; stilbestrol
Brand Names Stilphostrol®
Therapeutic Category Estrogen Derivative
Use Management of severe vasomotor symptoms of menopause, for estrogen replacement, and for palliative treatment of inoperable metastatic prostatic carcinoma
Usual Dosage Adults:
Hypogonadism and ovarian failure: Oral: 0.2-0.5 mg/day
Menopausal symptoms: Oral: 0.1-2 mg/day for 3 weeks and then off 1 week
Postmenopausal breast carcinoma: Oral: 15 mg/day
Prostate carcinoma: Oral: 1-3 mg/day
Prostatic cancer: I.V.: 0.5 g to start, then 1 g every 2-5 days followed by 0.25-0.5 g 1-2 times/week as maintenance
Diphosphate:
Oral: 50 mg 3 times/day; increase up to 200 mg or more 3 times/day
I.V.: Administer 0.5 g, dissolved in 250 mL of saline or D_5W, administer slowly the first 10-15 minutes then adjust rate so that the entire amount is administered in 1 hour
Dosage Forms
Injection, as diphosphate sodium (Stilphostrol®): 0.25 g (5 mL)
Tablet: 1 mg, 2.5 mg, 5 mg
Stilphostrol®: 50 mg

diethylstilbestrol diphosphate sodium *see* diethylstilbestrol *on this page*

difenoxin and atropine (dye fen OKS in & A troe peen)
Brand Names Motofen®
Therapeutic Category Antidiarrheal
Controlled Substance C-IV
Use Treatment of diarrhea
Usual Dosage Adults: Oral: Initial: 2 tablets, then 1 tablet after each loose stool; 1 tablet every 3-4 hours, up to 8 tablets in a 24-hour period; if no improvement after 48 hours, continued administration is not indicated
Dosage Forms Tablet: Difenoxin hydrochloride 1 mg and atropine sulfate 0.025 mg

Differin® *see* adapalene *on page 10*

diflorasone (dye FLOR a sone)
Synonyms diflorasone diacetate
Brand Names Florone®; Florone E®; Maxiflor®; Psorcon™
Therapeutic Category Corticosteroid, Topical
Use Relief of inflammation and pruritic symptoms of corticosteroid-responsive dermatosis
Usual Dosage Topical:
Cream: Apply 2-4 times/day
Ointment: Apply sparingly 1-3 times/day
Dosage Forms
Cream, as diacetate: 0.05% (15 g, 30 g, 60 g)
Ointment, topical, as diacetate: 0.05% (15 g, 30 g, 60 g)

diflorasone diacetate *see* diflorasone *on this page*

Diflucan® *see* fluconazole *on page 225*

diflunisal (dye FLOO ni sal)
Brand Names Dolobid®
Therapeutic Category Analgesic, Non-narcotic; Nonsteroidal Anti-Inflammatory Agent (NSAID)
Use Management of inflammatory disorders usually including rheumatoid arthritis and osteoarthritis; can be used as an analgesic for treatment of mild to moderate pain
Usual Dosage Adults: Oral:
  Pain: Initial: 500-1000 mg followed by 250-500 mg every 8-12 hours
  Inflammatory condition: 500-1000 mg/day in 2 divided doses
Dosage Forms Tablet: 250 mg, 500 mg

Di-Gel® [OTC] *see* aluminum hydroxide, magnesium hydroxide, and simethicone
on page 22

Digepepsin® *see* pancreatin on page 394

Digibind® *see* digoxin immune fab on next page

digitoxin (di ji TOKS in)
Brand Names Crystodigin®
Therapeutic Category Antiarrhythmic Agent, Miscellaneous; Cardiac Glycoside
Use Congestive heart failure; atrial fibrillation; atrial flutter; paroxysmal atrial tachycardia; and cardiogenic shock
Usual Dosage Oral:
  Children: Doses are very individualized; the maintenance range after neonatal period, the recommended digitalizing dose is as follows:
  <1 year: 0.045 mg/kg
  1-2 years: 0.04 mg/kg
  2 years: 0.03 mg/kg which is equivalent to 0.75 mg/m^2
  Maintenance: Approximately $1/10$ of the digitalizing dose
  Adults:
  Rapid loading dose: Initial: 0.6 mg followed by 0.4 mg and then 0.2 mg at intervals of 4-6 hours
  Slow loading dose: 0.2 mg twice daily for a period of 4 days followed by a maintenance dose
  Maintenance: 0.05-0.3 mg/day
  Most common dose: 0.15 mg/day
Dosage Forms Tablet: 0.1 mg, 0.2 mg

digoxin (di JOKS in)
Brand Names Lanoxicaps®; Lanoxin®
Therapeutic Category Antiarrhythmic Agent, Miscellaneous; Cardiac Glycoside
Use Treatment of congestive heart failure; slows the ventricular rate in tachyarrhythmias such as atrial fibrillation, atrial flutter, supraventricular tachycardia
Usual Dosage Adults (based on lean body weight and normal renal function for age. Decrease dose in patients with decreased renal function)

  Total digitalizing dose: Administer $1/2$ as initial dose, then administer $1/4$ of the total digitalizing dose (TDD) in each of 2 subsequent doses at 8- to 12-hour intervals; obtain EKG 6 hours after each dose to assess potential toxicity
  Oral: 0.75-1.5 mg
  I.M., I.V.: 0.5-1 mg
  Daily maintenance dose:
  Oral: 0.125-0.5 mg
  I.M., I.V.: 0.1-0.4 mg
Dosage Forms
  Capsule: 50 mcg, 100 mcg, 200 mcg
  Elixir, pediatric (lime flavor): 50 mcg/mL with alcohol 10% (60 mL)
  Injection: 250 mcg/mL (1 mL, 2 mL)
  Pediatric: 100 mcg/mL (1 mL)

Tablet: 125 mcg, 250 mcg, 500 mcg

digoxin immune fab (di JOKS in i MYUN fab)
Synonyms antidigoxin fab fragments
Brand Names Digibind®
Therapeutic Category Antidote
Use Treatment of potentially life-threatening digoxin or digitoxin intoxication in carefully selected patients
Usual Dosage To determine the dose of digoxin immune Fab, first determine the total body load of digoxin (TBL) as follows (using either an approximation of the amount ingested or a postdistribution serum digoxin concentration):

TBL of digoxin (in mg) = C (in ng/mL) x 5.6 x body weight (in kg)/1000 or TBL = mg of digoxin ingested (as tablets or elixir) x 0.8; C = postdistribution digoxin concentration

Dose of digoxin immune Fab (in mg) I.V. = TBL x 66.7 or dose of digoxin immune Fab (in number of 40 mg vials) = [C of digoxin (in ng/mL) x body weight (in kg)]/100
Dosage Forms Powder for injection, lyophilized: 40 mg

Dihistine® DH *see* chlorpheniramine, pseudoephedrine, and codeine *on page 118*

Dihistine® Expectorant *see* guaifenesin, pseudoephedrine, and codeine *on page 251*

dihydrocodeine compound (dye hye droe KOE deen KOM pound)
Brand Names DHC Plus®; Synalgos®-DC
Therapeutic Category Analgesic, Narcotic
Controlled Substance C-III
Use Management of mild to moderate pain that requires relaxation
Usual Dosage Adults: Oral: 1-2 capsules every 4-6 hours as needed for pain
Dosage Forms Capsule:
DHC Plus®: Dihydrocodeine bitartrate 16 mg, acetaminophen 356.4 mg, and caffeine 30 mg
Synalgos®-DC: Dihydrocodeine bitartrate 16 mg, aspirin 356.4 mg, and caffeine 30 mg

dihydroergotamine (dye hye droe er GOT a meen)
Synonyms dihydroergotamine mesylate
Brand Names D.H.E. 45® Injection
Therapeutic Category Ergot Alkaloid
Use Abort or prevent vascular headaches
Usual Dosage
I.M.: 1 mg at first sign of headache; 1 mg every 6 hours for 2 doses (not to exceed 6 mg in 24 hours)
I.V.: Up to 2 mg for faster effects
Dosage Forms Injection, as mesylate: 1 mg/mL (1 mL)

dihydroergotamine mesylate *see* dihydroergotamine *on this page*

dihydroergotoxine *see* ergoloid mesylates *on page 198*

dihydrohydroxycodeinone *see* oxycodone *on page 389*

dihydromorphinone *see* hydromorphone *on page 271*

dihydrotachysterol (dye hye droe tak IS ter ole)
Synonyms dichysterol
Brand Names DHT™; Hytakerol®
Therapeutic Category Vitamin D Analog
Use Treatment of hypocalcemia associated with hypoparathyroidism; prophylaxis of hypocalcemic tetany following thyroid surgery; suppress hyperparathyroidism and treat renal osteodystrophy in patients with chronic renal failure
(Continued)

dihydrotachysterol *(Continued)*

Usual Dosage Oral:
Hypoparathyroidism:
Infants and young Children: 0.1-0.5 mg/day
Older Children and Adults: 0.5-1 mg/day
Nutritional rickets: 0.5 mg as a single dose or 13-50 mcg/day until healing occurs
Renal osteodystrophy: 0.6-6 mg/24 hours; maintenance: 0.25-0.6 mg/24 hours adjusted
  as necessary to achieve normal serum calcium levels and promote bone healing
Dosage Forms
Capsule (Hytakerol®): 0.125 mg
Solution:
  Oral concentrate (DHT™): 0.2 mg/mL (30 mL)
  Oral, in oil (Hytakerol®): 0.25 mg/mL (15 mL)
Tablet (DHT™): 0.125 mg, 0.2 mg, 0.4 mg

dihydroxyaluminum sodium carbonate

(dye hye DROKS i a LOO mi num SOW dee um KAR bun ate)
Brand Names Rolaids® [OTC]
Therapeutic Category Antacid
Use Symptomatic relief of upset stomach associated with hyperacidity
Usual Dosage Oral: Chew 1-2 tablets as needed
Dosage Forms Tablet, chewable: 334 mg

1,25 dihydroxycholecalciferol *see* calcitriol *on page 81*

dihydroxypropyl theophylline *see* dyphylline *on page 188*

diiodohydroxyquin *see* iodoquinol *on page 287*

diisopropyl fluorophosphate *see* isoflurophate *on page 290*

Dilacor™ XR *see* diltiazem *on this page*

Dilantin® *see* phenytoin *on page 414*

Dilatrate®-SR *see* isosorbide dinitrate *on page 292*

Dilaudid® *see* hydromorphone *on page 271*

Dilaudid-5® *see* hydromorphone *on page 271*

Dilaudid-HP® *see* hydromorphone *on page 271*

Dilocaine® *see* lidocaine *on page 307*

Dilor® *see* dyphylline *on page 188*

diltiazem (dil TYE a zem)

Brand Names Cardizem® CD; Cardizem® Injectable; Cardizem® SR; Cardizem® Tablet;
Dilacor™ XR; Tiamate®; Tiazac®
Therapeutic Category Calcium Channel Blocker
Use
Oral: Hypertension; chronic stable angina or angina from coronary artery spasm
Injection: Atrial fibrillation or atrial flutter; paroxysmal supraventricular tachycardias
  (PSVT)
Usual Dosage Adults:
Oral: 30-120 mg 3-4 times/day; dosage should be increased gradually, at 1- to 2-day
  intervals until optimum response is obtained; usual maintenance dose: 240-360 mg/
  day
Sustained-release capsules (SR): Initial dose of 60-120 mg twice daily
Sustained-release capsules (CD, XR): 180-300 mg once daily
I.V.: Initial: 0.25 mg/kg as a bolus over 2 minutes, then continuous infusion of 5-15 mg/
  hour for up to 24 hours

Dosage Forms
Capsule, sustained release:
Cardizem® CD: 120 mg, 180 mg, 240 mg, 300 mg
Cardizem® SR: 60 mg, 90 mg, 120 mg
Dilacor™ XR: 180 mg, 240 mg
Tiazac®: 120 mg, 180 mg, 240 mg, 300 mg, 360 mg
Injection: 5 mg/mL (5 mL, 10 mL)
 Cardizem®: 5 mg/mL (5 mL, 10 mL)
Tablet (Cardizem®): 30 mg, 60 mg, 90 mg, 120 mg
Tablet, extended release (Tiamate®): 120 mg, 180 mg, 240 mg

Dimacol® Caplets [OTC] *see* guaifenesin, pseudoephedrine, and dextromethorphan *on page 252*

Dimaphen® Elixir [OTC] *see* brompheniramine and phenylpropanolamine *on page 73*

Dimaphen® Tablets [OTC] *see* brompheniramine and phenylpropanolamine *on page 73*

dimenhydrinate (dye men HYE dri nate)
Brand Names Calm-X® Oral [OTC]; Dimetabs® Oral; Dinate® Injection; Dramamine® Oral [OTC]; Dymenate® Injection; Hydrate® Injection; TripTone® Caplets® [OTC]
Therapeutic Category Antihistamine
Use Treatment and prevention of nausea, vertigo, and vomiting associated with motion sickness
Usual Dosage Oral:
Children:
2-5 years: 12.5-25 mg every 6-8 hours, maximum: 75 mg/day
6-12 years: 25-50 mg every 6-8 hours, maximum: 75 mg/day
 or
Alternately: 5 mg/kg/day in 4 divided doses, not to exceed 300 mg/day
Adults: 50-100 mg every 4-6 hours, not to exceed 400 mg/day
Dosage Forms
Capsule: 50 mg
Injection: 50 mg/mL (1 mL, 5 mL, 10 mL)
Liquid: 12.5 mg/4 mL (90 mL, 473 mL); 16.62 mg/5 mL (480 mL)
Tablet: 50 mg
Chewable: 50 mg

dimercaprol (dye mer KAP role)
Synonyms bal; British anti-lewisite; dithioglycerol
Brand Names BAL in Oil®
Therapeutic Category Chelating Agent
Use Antidote to gold, arsenic, and mercury poisoning; adjunct to edetate calcium disodium in lead poisoning
Usual Dosage Children and Adults: I.M.:
Mild arsenic and gold poisoning: 2.5 mg/kg/dose every 6 hours for 2 days, then every 12 hours on the third day, and once daily thereafter for 10 days
Severe arsenic and gold poisoning: 3 mg/kg/dose every 4 hours for 2 days then every 6 hours on the third day, then every 12 hours thereafter for 10 days
Mercury poisoning: Initial: 5 mg/kg followed by 2.5 mg/kg/dose 1-2 times/day for 10 days
Lead poisoning (use with edetate calcium disodium):
Mild: 3 mg/kg/dose every 4 hours for 5-7 days
Severe: 4 mg/kg/dose every 4 hours for 5-7 days
Acute encephalopathy: Initial: 4 mg/kg/dose, then every 4 hours
Dosage Forms Injection: 100 mg/mL (3 mL)

Dimetabs® Oral *see* dimenhydrinate *on this page*

Dimetane®-DC *see* brompheniramine, phenylpropanolamine, and codeine *on page 74*

Dimetane® Decongestant Elixir [OTC] *see* brompheniramine and phenylephrine *on page 73*

Dimetane® Extentabs® [OTC] *see* brompheniramine *on page 73*

Dimetapp® 4-Hour Liqui-Gel Capsule [OTC] *see* brompheniramine and phenylpropanolamine *on page 73*

Dimetapp® Elixir [OTC] *see* brompheniramine and phenylpropanolamine *on page 73*

Dimetapp® Extentabs® [OTC] *see* brompheniramine and phenylpropanolamine *on page 73*

Dimetapp® Sinus Caplets [OTC] *see* pseudoephedrine and ibuprofen *on page 450*

Dimetapp® Tablet [OTC] *see* brompheniramine and phenylpropanolamine *on page 73*

dimethoxyphenyl penicillin sodium *see* methicillin *on page 336*

β,β-dimethylcysteine *see* penicillamine *on page 399*

dimethyl sulfoxide (dye meth il sul FOKS ide)
Synonyms dmso
Brand Names Rimso®-50
Therapeutic Category Urinary Tract Product
Use Symptomatic relief of interstitial cystitis
Usual Dosage Instill 50 mL directly into bladder and allow to remain for 15 minutes; repeat every 2 weeks until maximum symptomatic relief is obtained
Dosage Forms Solution: 50% [500 mg/mL] (50 mL)

dimethyl tubocurarine iodide *see* metocurine iodide *on page 345*

Dinate® Injection *see* dimenhydrinate *on previous page*

dinoprostone (dye noe PROST one)
Synonyms pge_2; prostaglandin e_2
Brand Names Cervidil® Vaginal Insert; Prepidil® Vaginal Gel; Prostin E_2® Vaginal Suppository
Therapeutic Category Prostaglandin
Use Terminate pregnancy from 12th through 28th week of gestation; evacuate uterus in cases of missed abortion or intrauterine fetal death; manage benign hydatidiform mole
Usual Dosage Vaginal: Insert 1 suppository high in vagina, repeat at 3- to 5-hour intervals until abortion occurs up to 240 mg (maximum dose)
Dosage Forms
Insert, vaginal (Cervidil®): 10 mg
Gel, vaginal: 0.5 mg in 3 g syringes [each package contains a 10-mm and 20-mm shielded catheter]
Suppository, vaginal: 20 mg

dinoprost tromethamine (DYE noe prost tro METH a meen)
Synonyms $pgf_{2\alpha}$; prostaglandin f_2 alpha
Brand Names Prostin F_2 Alpha®
Therapeutic Category Prostaglandin
Use Abort 2nd trimester pregnancy
Usual Dosage 40 mg (8 mL) via transabdominal tap; if abortion not completed in 24 hours, another 10-40 mg may be administered
Dosage Forms Injection: 5 mg/mL (4 mL, 8 mL)

Diocto® [OTC] *see* docusate *on page 179*

Diocto C® **[OTC]** *see* docusate and casanthranol *on page 180*

Diocto-K® **[OTC]** *see* docusate *on page 179*

Diocto-K Plus® **[OTC]** *see* docusate and casanthranol *on page 180*

Dioctolose Plus® **[OTC]** *see* docusate and casanthranol *on page 180*

dioctyl calcium sulfosuccinate *see* docusate *on page 179*

dioctyl potassium sulfosuccinate *see* docusate *on page 179*

dioctyl sodium sulfosuccinate *see* docusate *on page 179*

Dioeze® **[OTC]** *see* docusate *on page 179*

Dionosil Oily® *see* radiological/contrast media (ionic) *on page 457*

Dioval® **Injection** *see* estradiol *on page 202*

Diovan® *see* valsartan *on page 545*

dipalmitoylphosphatidylcholine *see* colfosceril palmitate *on page 136*

Dipentum® *see* olsalazine *on page 383*

Diphen® **Cough [OTC]** *see* diphenhydramine *on this page*

Diphenhist® **[OTC]** *see* diphenhydramine *on this page*

diphenhydramine (dye fen HYE dra meen)

Synonyms diphenhydramine hydrochloride

Brand Names AllerMax® Oral [OTC]; Banophen® Oral [OTC]; Belix® Oral [OTC]; Benadryl® Injection; Benadryl® Oral [OTC]; Benadryl® Topical; Ben-Allergin-50® Injection; Benylin® Cough Syrup [OTC]; Bydramine® Cough Syrup [OTC]; Compoz® Gel Caps [OTC]; Compoz® Nighttime Sleep Aid [OTC]; Diphen® Cough [OTC]; Diphenhist® [OTC]; Dormarex® 2 Oral [OTC]; Dormin® Oral [OTC]; Genahist® Oral; Hydramyn® Syrup [OTC]; Hyrexin-50® Injection; Maximum Strength Nytol® [OTC]; Miles Nervine® Caplets [OTC]; Nytol® Oral [OTC]; Phendry® Oral [OTC]; Siladryl® Oral [OTC]; Silphen® Cough [OTC]; Sleep-eze 3® Oral [OTC]; Sleepinal® [OTC]; Sleepwell 2-nite® [OTC]; Snooze Fast® [OTC]; Sominex® Oral [OTC]; Tusstat® Syrup; Twilite® Oral [OTC]; Uni-Bent® Cough Syrup; 40 Winks® [OTC]

Therapeutic Category Antihistamine

Use Symptomatic relief of allergic symptoms caused by histamine release which include nasal allergies and allergic dermatosis; mild nighttime sedation, prevention of motion sickness, as an antitussive; treatment of phenothiazine-induced dystonic reactions

Usual Dosage

Children: Oral, I.M., I.V.: 5 mg/kg/day or 150 mg/m^2/day in divided doses every 6-8 hours, not to exceed 300 mg/day

Adults:

Oral: 25-50 mg every 4-6 hours

I.M., I.V.: 10-50 mg in a single dose every 2-4 hours, not to exceed 400 mg/day

Topical: For external application, not longer than 7 days

Dosage Forms

Capsule, as hydrochloride: 25 mg, 50 mg

Cream, as hydrochloride: 1%, 2%

Elixir, as hydrochloride: 12.5 mg/5 mL (5 mL, 10 mL, 20 mL, 120 mL, 480 mL, 3780 mL)

Injection, as hydrochloride: 10 mg/mL (10 mL, 30 mL); 50 mg/mL (1 mL, 10 mL)

Lotion, as hydrochloride: 1% (75 mL)

Solution, topical spray, as hydrochloride: 1% (60 mL)

Syrup, as hydrochloride: 12.5 mg/5 mL (5 mL, 120 mL, 240 mL, 480 mL, 3780 mL)

Tablet, as hydrochloride: 25 mg, 50 mg

diphenhydramine and pseudoephedrine

(dye fen HYE dra meen & soo doe e FED rin)

Brand Names Actifed® Allergy Tablet (Night) [OTC]; Banophen® Decongestant Capsule [OTC]; Benadryl® Decongestant Allergy Tablet [OTC]

(Continued)

diphenhydramine and pseudoephedrine *(Continued)*

Therapeutic Category Antihistamine/Decongestant Combination

Use Relief of symptoms of upper respiratory mucosal congestion in seasonal and perennial nasal allergies, acute rhinitis, rhinosinusitis, and eustachian tube blockage

Usual Dosage Adults: Oral: 1 capsule or tablet every 4-6 hours, up to 4/day

Dosage Forms

Capsule: Diphenhydramine hydrochloride 25 mg and pseudoephedrine hydrochloride 60 mg

Tablet:

Actifed® Allergy (Night): Diphenhydramine hydrochloride 25 mg and pseudoephedrine hydrochloride 30 mg

Benadryl® Decongestant Allergy: Diphenhydramine hydrochloride 25 mg and pseudoephedrine hydrochloride 60 mg

diphenhydramine hydrochloride *see* diphenhydramine *on previous page*

diphenidol *(dye FEN i dole)*

Synonyms diphenidol hydrochloride

Brand Names Vontrol®

Therapeutic Category Antiemetic

Use Control of nausea and vomiting; peripheral vertigo and associated nausea and vomiting, Ménière's disease, and middle and inner ear surgery

Usual Dosage Oral:

Children: Nausea, vomiting: 0.88 mg/kg (0.4 mg/lb); normal dosage for children weighing 50-100 lbs: 25 mg administered not more often than every 4 hours; total daily (24 hours) dose should not exceed 5.5 mg/kg (2.5 mg/lb)

Adults: Vertigo, nausea, vomiting: 25 mg every 4 hours; some patients may require 50 mg

Dosage Forms Tablet, as hydrochloride: 25 mg

diphenidol hydrochloride *see* diphenidol *on this page*

diphenoxylate and atropine *(dye fen OKS i late & A troe peen)*

Synonyms atropine and diphenoxylate

Brand Names Logen®; Lomanate®; Lomotil®; Lonox®

Therapeutic Category Antidiarrheal

Controlled Substance C-V

Use Treatment of diarrhea

Usual Dosage Oral (as diphenoxylate): Initial dose:

Children: 0.3-0.4 mg/kg/day in 2-4 divided doses

<2 years: Not recommended

2-5 years: 2 mg 3 times/day

5-8 years: 2 mg 4 times/day

8-12 years: 2 mg 5 times/day

Adults: 15-20 mg/day in 3-4 divided doses

Reduce dosage as soon as initial control of symptoms is achieved

Dosage Forms

Solution, oral: Diphenoxylate hydrochloride 2.5 mg and atropine sulfate 0.025 mg per 5 mL (4 mL, 10 mL, 60 mL)

Tablet: Diphenoxylate hydrochloride 2.5 mg and atropine sulfate 0.025 mg

diphenylhydantoin *see* phenytoin *on page 414*

diphtheria and tetanus toxoid *(dif THEER ee a & TET a nus TOKS oyd)*

Synonyms dt; td; tetanus and diphtheria toxoid

Therapeutic Category Toxoid

Use Active immunity against diphtheria and tetanus

Usual Dosage I.M.:

Infants and Children:

6 weeks to 1 year: Three 0.5 mL doses at least 4 weeks apart; administer a reinforcing dose 6-12 months after the third injection

1-6 years: Administer two 0.5 mL doses at least 4 weeks apart; reinforcing dose 6-12 months after second injection; if final dose is administered after seventh birthday, use adult preparation

4-6 years (booster immunization): 0.5 mL; not necessary if all 4 doses were administered after fourth birthday - routinely administer booster doses at 10-year intervals with the adult preparation

Children >7 years and Adults: 2 primary doses of 0.5 mL each, administered at an interval of 4-6 weeks; third (reinforcing) dose of 0.5 mL 6-12 months later; boosters every 10 years

Dosage Forms Injection:

Pediatric use:

Diphtheria 6.6 Lf units and tetanus 5 Lf units per 0.5 mL (5 mL)

Diphtheria 10 Lf units and tetanus 5 Lf units per 0.5 mL (0.5 mL, 5 mL)

Diphtheria 12.5 Lf units and tetanus 5 Lf units per 0.5 mL (5 mL)

Diphtheria 15 Lf units and tetanus 10 Lf units per 0.5 mL (5 mL)

Adult use:

Diphtheria 1.5 Lf units and tetanus 5 Lf units per 0.5 mL (0.5 mL, 5 mL)

Diphtheria 2 Lf units and tetanus 5 Lf units per 0.5 mL (5 mL)

Diphtheria 2 Lf units and tetanus 10 Lf units per 0.5 mL (5 mL)

diphtheria antitoxin (dif THEER ee a an tee TOKS in)

Therapeutic Category Antitoxin

Use Passive prevention and treatment of diphtheria

Usual Dosage I.M. or slow I.V. infusion: Dosage varies with a range from 20,000 units to 120,000 units

Dosage Forms Injection: 500 units/mL (20 mL, 40 mL)

diphtheria, tetanus toxoids, and acellular pertussis vaccine

(dif THEER ee a, TET a nus TOKS oyds & ay CEL yoo lar per TUS sis vak SEEN)

Synonyms dtap

Brand Names Acel-Imune®; Infanrix®; Tripedia®

Therapeutic Category Toxoid

Use Fourth or fifth immunization of children 15 months to 7 years of age (prior to seventh birthday) who have been previously immunized with 3 or 4 doses of whole-cell pertussis DTP vaccine

Usual Dosage I.M.: After at least 3 doses of whole-cell DTP, administer 0.5 mL at ~18 months (at least 6 months after third DTWP dose), then another dose at 4-5 years of age

Dosage Forms Injection:

Acel-Immune®: Diphtheria 7.5 Lf units, tetanus 5 Lf units, and acellular pertussis vaccine 40 mcg per 0.5 mL (7.5 mL)

Infanrix®: Diphtheria 25 Lf units, tetanus 10 Lf units, and acellular pertussis vaccine 25 mcg per 0.5 mL (7.5 mL)

Tripedia®: Diphtheria 6.7 Lf units, tetanus 5 Lf units, and acellular pertussis vaccine 46.8 mcg per 0.5 mL (7.5 mL)

diphtheria, tetanus toxoids, and whole-cell pertussis vaccine

(dif THEER ee a & TET a nus TOKS oyds & hole-sel per TUS sis vak SEEN)

Synonyms dpt

Brand Names Tri-Immunol®

Therapeutic Category Toxoid

(Continued)

diphtheria, tetanus toxoids, and whole-cell pertussis vaccine (Continued)

Use Active immunization of infants and children through 6 years of age (between 2 months and the seventh birthday) against diphtheria, tetanus, and pertussis; recommended for both primary immunization and routine recall; start immunization at once if whooping cough or diphtheria is present in the community

Usual Dosage The primary immunization for children 2 months to 6 years of age, ideally beginning at the age of 2-3 months or at 6-week check-up. Administer 0.5 mL I.M. on 3 occasions at 4- to 8-week intervals with a re-enforcing dose administered 1 year after the third injection. The booster doses (0.5 mL I.M.) are administered when the child is 4-6 years of age.

Dosage Forms Injection:
Diphtheria 6.7 Lf units, tetanus 5 Lf units, and pertussis 4 protective units per 0.5 mL (7.5 mL)
Tri-Immunol®: Diphtheria 12.5 Lf units, tetanus 5 Lf units, and pertussis 4 protective units per 0.5 mL (7.5 mL)

diphtheria, tetanus toxoids, whole-cell pertussis, and haemophilus b conjugate vaccine

(dif THEER ee a, TET a nus TOKS oyds, hole-sel per TUS sis, & hem OF fil us bee KON joo gate vak SEEN)

Synonyms DTwP-HIB

Brand Names Tetramune®

Therapeutic Category Toxoid

Use Active immunization of infants and children through 5 years of age (between 2 months and the sixth birthday) against diphtheria, tetanus, and pertussis and Haemophilus b disease when indications for immunization with DTP vaccine and HIB vaccine coincide

Usual Dosage The primary immunization for children 2 months to 5 years of age, ideally beginning at the age of 2-3 months or at 6-week check-up; administer 0.5 mL I.M. on 3 occasions at ~2 month intervals, followed by a fourth 0.5 mL dose at ~15 months of age

Dosage Forms Injection: Diphtheria toxoid 12.5 Lf units, tetanus toxoid 5 Lf units, and whole-cell pertussis vaccine 4 units, and Haemophilus influenzae type b oligosaccharide 10 mcg per 0.5 mL (5 mL)

dipivalyl epinephrine see dipivefrin on this page

dipivefrin (dye PI ve frin)

Synonyms dipivalyl epinephrine; dipivefrin hydrochloride; dpe

Brand Names AKPro® Ophthalmic; Propine® Ophthalmic

Therapeutic Category Adrenergic Agonist Agent

Use Reduces elevated intraocular pressure in chronic open-angle glaucoma; treatment of ocular hypertension

Usual Dosage Adults: Ophthalmic: Initial: 1 drop every 12 hours

Dosage Forms Solution, ophthalmic, as hydrochloride: 0.1% (5 mL, 10 mL, 15 mL)

dipivefrin hydrochloride see dipivefrin on this page

Diprivan® Injection see propofol on page 445

Diprolene® see betamethasone on page 64

Diprolene® AF see betamethasone on page 64

dipropylacetic acid see valproic acid and derivatives on page 544

Diprosone® see betamethasone on page 64

dipyridamole (dye peer ID a mole)
Brand Names Persantine®
Therapeutic Category Antiplatelet Agent; Vasodilator
Use Maintain patency after surgical grafting procedures including coronary artery bypass; with warfarin to decrease thrombosis in patients after artificial heart valve replacement; for chronic management of angina pectoris; with aspirin to prevent coronary artery thrombosis; in combination with aspirin or warfarin to prevent other thromboembolic disorders; dipyridamole may also be administered 2 days prior to open heart surgery to prevent platelet activation by extracorporeal bypass pump; diagnostic agent I.V. (dipyridamole stress test) for coronary artery disease
Usual Dosage
Children: Oral: 3-6 mg/kg/day in 3 divided doses
Dipyridamole stress test (for evaluation of myocardial perfusion): I.V.: 0.14 mg/kg/minute for a total of 4 minutes
Adults: Oral: 75-400 mg/day in 3-4 divided doses
Dosage Forms
Injection: 10 mg/2 mL
Tablet: 25 mg, 50 mg, 75 mg

dirithromycin (dye RITH roe mye sin)
Brand Names Dynabac®
Therapeutic Category Macrolide (Antibiotic)
Use Treatment of mild to moderate upper and lower respiratory tract infections, infections of the skin and skin structure, and sexually transmitted diseases due to susceptible strains
Usual Dosage Adults: Oral: 500 mg once daily for 7-14 days
Dosage Forms Tablet, enteric coated: 250 mg

Disalcid® *see* salsalate *on page 473*

disalicylic acid *see* salsalate *on page 473*

Disanthrol® [OTC] *see* docusate and casanthranol *on page 180*

Disobrom® [OTC] *see* dexbrompheniramine and pseudoephedrine *on page 157*

disodium cromoglycate *see* cromolyn sodium *on page 141*

d-isoephedrine hydrochloride *see* pseudoephedrine *on page 449*

Disolan® [OTC] *see* docusate and phenolphthalein *on page 180*

Disonate® [OTC] *see* docusate *on page 179*

Disophrol® Chronotabs® [OTC] *see* dexbrompheniramine and pseudoephedrine *on page 157*

Disophrol® Tablet [OTC] *see* dexbrompheniramine and pseudoephedrine *on page 157*

disopyramide (dye soe PEER a mide)
Synonyms disopyramide phosphate
Brand Names Norpace®
Therapeutic Category Antiarrhythmic Agent, Class I-A
Use Suppression and prevention of unifocal and multifocal ventricular premature complexes, coupled ventricular premature complexes, and/or paroxysmal ventricular tachycardia; also effective in the conversion and prevention of recurrence of atrial fibrillation, atrial flutter, and paroxysmal atrial tachycardia
Usual Dosage Oral:
Children:
<1 year: 10-30 mg/kg/24 hours in 4 divided doses
1-4 years: 10-20 mg/kg/24 hours in 4 divided doses
4-12 years: 10-15 mg/kg/24 hours in 4 divided doses
12-18 years: 6-15 mg/kg/24 hours in 4 divided doses
(Continued)

disopyramide *(Continued)*

Adults:
  <50 kg: 100 mg every 6 hours or 200 mg every 12 hours (controlled release)
  >50 kg: 150 mg every 6 hours or 300 mg every 12 hours (controlled release); if no response, may increase to 200 mg every 6 hours; maximum dose required for patients with severe refractory ventricular tachycardia is 400 mg every 6 hours
Dosage Forms Capsule:
  As phosphate: 100 mg, 150 mg
  Sustained action, as phosphate: 100 mg, 150 mg

disopyramide phosphate *see* disopyramide *on previous page*

Disotate® *see* edetate disodium *on page 190*

Di-Spaz® Injection *see* dicyclomine *on page 165*

Di-Spaz® Oral *see* dicyclomine *on page 165*

disulfiram *(dye SUL fi ram)*

Brand Names Antabuse®
Therapeutic Category Aldehyde Dehydrogenase Inhibitor Agent
Use Management of chronic alcoholics
Usual Dosage Oral:
  Maximum daily dose: 500 mg/day in a single dose for 1-2 weeks
  Average maintenance dose: 250 mg/day; range: 125-500 mg; duration of therapy is to continue until the patient is fully recovered socially and a basis for permanent self control has been established; maintenance therapy may be required for months or even years
Dosage Forms Tablet: 250 mg, 500 mg

dithioglycerol *see* dimercaprol *on page 171*

dithranol *see* anthralin *on page 36*

Ditropan® *see* oxybutynin *on page 389*

Diucardin® *see* hydroflumethiazide *on page 271*

Diurigen® *see* chlorothiazide *on page 111*

Diuril® *see* chlorothiazide *on page 111*

divalproex sodium *see* valproic acid and derivatives *on page 544*

Dizac® Injection *see* diazepam *on page 162*

Dizmiss® [OTC] *see* meclizine *on page 324*

dl-alpha tocopherol *see* vitamin e *on page 553*

dl-norephedrine hydrochloride *see* phenylpropanolamine *on page 413*

d-mannitol *see* mannitol *on page 321*

4-dmdr *see* idarubicin *on page 278*

D-Med® Injection *see* methylprednisolone *on page 343*

dmso *see* dimethyl sulfoxide *on page 172*

dnase *see* dornase alfa *on page 181*

dnr *see* daunorubicin hydrochloride *on page 150*

Doan's®, Original [OTC] *see* magnesium salicylate *on page 319*

dobutamine *(doe BYOO ta meen)*

Synonyms dobutamine hydrochloride
Brand Names Dobutrex® Injection
Therapeutic Category Adrenergic Agonist Agent
Use Short-term management of patients with cardiac decompensation

Usual Dosage I.V. infusion:
Children: 2.5-15 mcg/kg/minute, titrate to desired response
Adults: 2.5-15 mcg/kg/minute; maximum: 40 mcg/kg/minute, titrate to desired response
Dosage Forms Injection, as hydrochloride: 12.5 mg/mL (20 mL)

dobutamine hydrochloride *see* dobutamine *on previous page*

Dobutrex® Injection *see* dobutamine *on previous page*

docetaxel (doe se TAKS el)
Brand Names Taxotere®
Therapeutic Category Antineoplastic Agent
Use Treatment of breast cancer
Usual Dosage Adults: I.V.: 60-100 mg/m² administered over 1 hour every 3 weeks
Dosage Forms Injection: 10 mg/mL (2 mL, 8 mL)

Docucal-P® [OTC] *see* docusate and phenolphthalein *on next page*

docusate (DOK yoo sate)
Synonyms dioctyl calcium sulfosuccinate; dioctyl potassium sulfosuccinate; dioctyl sodium sulfosuccinate; docusate calcium; docusate potassium; docusate sodium; doss; dss
Brand Names Colace® [OTC]; DC 240® Softgels® [OTC]; Dialose® [OTC]; Diocto® [OTC]; Diocto-K® [OTC]; Dioeze® [OTC]; Disonate® [OTC]; DOK® [OTC]; DOS® Softgel® [OTC]; D-S-S® [OTC]; Kasof® [OTC]; Modane® Soft [OTC]; Pro-Cal-Sof® [OTC]; Regulax SS® [OTC]; Sulfalax® [OTC]; Surfak® [OTC]
Therapeutic Category Stool Softener
Use Stool softener in patients who should avoid straining during defecation and constipation associated with hard, dry stools
Usual Dosage Docusate salts are interchangeable; the amount of sodium, calcium, or potassium per dosage unit is clinically insignificant

Infants and Children <3 years: Oral: 10-40 mg/day in 1-4 divided doses
Children: Oral:
3-6 years: 20-60 mg/day in 1-4 divided doses
6-12 years: 40-150 mg/day in 1-4 divided doses
Adolescents and Adults: Oral: 50-500 mg/day in 1-4 divided doses
Older Children and Adults: Rectal: Add 50-100 mg of docusate liquid to enema fluid (saline or water); administer as retention or flushing enema
Dosage Forms
Capsule:
As calcium:
DC 240® Softgels®, Pro-Cal-Sof®, Sulfalax®: 240 mg
Surfak®: 50 mg, 240 mg
As potassium:
Diocto-K®: 100 mg
Kasof®: 240 mg
As sodium:
Colace®: 50 mg, 100 mg
Dioeze®: 250 mg
Disonate®: 100 mg, 240 mg
DOK®: 100 mg, 250 mg
DOS® Softgel®: 100 mg, 250 mg
D-S-S®: 100 mg
Modane® Soft: 100 mg
Regulax SS®: 100 mg, 250 mg
Liquid, as sodium (Diocto®, Colace®, Disonate®, DOK®): 150 mg/15 mL (30 mL, 60 mL, 480 mL)
Solution, oral, as sodium (Doxinate®): 50 mg/mL with alcohol 5% (60 mL, 3780 mL)
(Continued)

docusate *(Continued)*

Syrup, as sodium:
50 mg/15 mL (15 mL, 30 mL)
Colace®, Diocto®, Disonate®, DOK®: 60 mg/15 mL (240 mL, 480 mL, 3780 mL)
Tablet, as sodium (Dialose®): 100 mg

docusate and casanthranol (DOK yoo sate & ka SAN thra nole)

Synonyms casanthranol and docusate; dss with casanthranol
Brand Names Dialose® Plus Capsule [OTC]; Diocto C® [OTC]; Diocto-K Plus® [OTC]; Dioctolose Plus® [OTC]; Disanthrol® [OTC]; DSMC Plus® [OTC]; Genasoft® Plus [OTC]; Peri-Colace® [OTC]; Pro-Sof® Plus [OTC]; Regulace® [OTC]; Silace-C® [OTC]
Therapeutic Category Laxative/Stool Softner
Use Treatment of constipation generally associated with dry, hard stools and decreased intestinal motility
Usual Dosage Oral:
Children: 5-15 mL of syrup at bedtime or 1 capsule at bedtime
Adults: 1-2 capsules or 15-30 mL syrup at bedtime, may be increased to 2 capsules or 30 mL twice daily or 3 capsules at bedtime
Dosage Forms
Capsule:
Dialose® Plus, Diocto-K Plus®, Dioctolose Plus®, DSMC Plus®: Docusate potassium 100 mg and casanthranol 30 mg
Disanthrol®, Genasoft® Plus, Peri-Colace®, Pro-Sof® Plus, Regulace®: Docusate sodium 100 mg and casanthranol 30 mg
Syrup (Diocto C®, Peri-Colace®, Silace-C®): Docusate sodium 60 mg and casanthranol 30 mg per 15 mL with alcohol 10% (240 mL, 480 mL, 4000 mL)

docusate and phenolphthalein (DOK yoo sate & fee nole THAY leen)

Brand Names Colax® [OTC]; Dialose® Plus Tablet [OTC]; Disolan® [OTC]; Docucal-P® [OTC]; Doxidan® [OTC]; Ex-Lax®, Extra Gentle Pills [OTC]; Feen-a-Mint® Pills [OTC]; Femilax® [OTC]; Modane® Plus [OTC]; Phillips'® LaxCaps® [OTC]; Unilax® [OTC]
Therapeutic Category Laxative/Stool Softner
Use Management of chronic functional constipation
Usual Dosage Oral:
Children 6-12 years: 1 capsule daily administered at bedtime for 2-3 nights until bowel movements are normal
Children >12 years and Adults: 1-2 capsules daily administered at bedtime for 2-3 nights until bowel movements are normal
Dosage Forms
Capsule:
Disolan®: Docusate sodium 100 mg and phenolphthalein 65 mg
Docucal-P®, Doxidan®: Docusate calcium 60 mg and phenolphthalein 65 mg
Ex-Lax®, Extra Gentle Pills: Docusate sodium 60 mg and phenolphthalein 65 mg
Phillips'® LaxCaps®: Docusate sodium 83 mg and phenolphthalein 90 mg
Unilax®: Docusate sodium 230 mg and phenolphthalein 130 mg
Tablet: Colax®, Dialose® Plus, Feen-A-Mint® Pills, Femilax®, Modane® Plus: Docusate sodium 100 mg and phenolphthalein 65 mg

docusate calcium *see* docusate *on previous page*

docusate potassium *see* docusate *on previous page*

docusate sodium *see* docusate *on previous page*

DOK® [OTC] *see* docusate *on previous page*

Dolacet® *see* hydrocodone and acetaminophen *on page 266*

Dolene® *see* propoxyphene *on page 445*

Dolobid® *see* diflunisal *on page 168*

Dolophine® see methadone *on page 335*

Dolorac® **[OTC]** see capsaicin *on page 87*

Domeboro® **Topical [OTC]** see aluminum acetate and calcium acetate *on page 20*

donepezil (don EH pa zil)
Brand Names Aricept®
Therapeutic Category Acetylcholinesterase Inhibitor
Use Treatment of mild to moderate dementia of the Alzheimer's type
Usual Dosage Adults: Oral: Initial: 5 mg at bedtime; may be increased to 10 mg at bedtime after 4-6 weeks; a 10 mg dose may provide additional benefit for some patients
Dosage Forms Tablet: 5 mg, 10 mg

Donnamar® see hyoscyamine *on page 275*

Donnapectolin-PG® see hyoscyamine, atropine, scopolamine, kaolin, pectin, and opium *on page 276*

Donnatal® see hyoscyamine, atropine, scopolamine, and phenobarbital *on page 276*

Donnazyme® see pancreatin *on page 394*

dopamine (DOE pa meen)
Synonyms dopamine hydrochloride
Brand Names Intropin® Injection
Therapeutic Category Adrenergic Agonist Agent
Use Adjunct in the treatment of shock which persists after adequate fluid volume replacement
Usual Dosage I.V. infusion:
Children: 1-20 mcg/kg/minute, maximum: 50 mcg/kg/minute continuous infusion, titrate to desired response
Adults: 1 mcg/kg/minute up to 50 mcg/kg/minute, titrate to desired response
If dosages >20-30 mcg/kg/minute are needed, a more direct acting pressor may be more beneficial (ie, epinephrine, norepinephrine)

Hemodynamic effects of dopamine are dose-dependent:
Low-dose: 1-5 mcg/kg/minute, increased renal blood flow and urine output
Intermediate-dose: 5-15 mcg/kg/minute, increased renal blood flow, heart rate, cardiac contractility, and cardiac output
High-dose: >15 mcg/kg/minute, alpha-adrenergic effects begin to predominate, vasoconstriction, increased blood pressure
Dosage Forms
Infusion, as hydrochloride, in D_5W: 0.8 mg/mL (250 mL, 500 mL); 1.6 mg/mL (250 mL, 500 mL); 3.2 mg/mL (250 mL, 500 mL)
Injection, as hydrochloride: 40 mg/mL (5 mL, 10 mL, 20 mL); 80 mg/mL (5 mL, 20 mL); 160 mg/mL (5 mL)

dopamine hydrochloride see dopamine *on this page*

Dopar® see levodopa *on page 305*

Dopram® **Injection** see doxapram *on next page*

Doral® see quazepam *on page 454*

Dormarex® **2 Oral [OTC]** see diphenhydramine *on page 173*

Dormin® **Oral [OTC]** see diphenhydramine *on page 173*

dornase alfa (DOOR nase AL fa)
Synonyms dnase; recombinant human deoxyribonuclease
Brand Names Pulmozyme®
Therapeutic Category Enzyme
(Continued)

dornase alfa *(Continued)*

Use Management of cystic fibrosis patients to reduce the frequency of respiratory infections and to improve pulmonary function

Usual Dosage Children >5 years and Adults: Inhalation: 2.5 mg once daily through selected nebulizers in conjunction with a Pulmo-Aide® or a Pari-Proneb® compressor

Dosage Forms Solution, inhalation: 1 mg/mL (2.5 mL)

Doryx® Oral *see doxycycline on page 184*

dorzolamide *(dor ZOLE a mide)*

Synonyms dorzolamide hydrochloride

Brand Names Trusopt®

Therapeutic Category Carbonic Anhydrase Inhibitor

Use Lower intraocular pressure to treat glaucoma

Usual Dosage Adults: Ophthalmic: 1 drop in eye(s) 3 times/day

Dosage Forms Solution, ophthalmic, as hydrochloride: 2%

dorzolamide hydrochloride *see dorzolamide on this page*

doss *see docusate on page 179*

DOS® Softgel® [OTC] *see docusate on page 179*

Dostinex® *see cabergoline on page 79*

Dovonex® *see calcipotriene on page 81*

doxacurium *(doks a KYOO ri um)*

Synonyms doxacurium chloride

Brand Names Nuromax® Injection

Therapeutic Category Skeletal Muscle Relaxant

Use Doxacurium is indicated for use as an adjunct to general anesthesia. It provides skeletal muscle relaxation during surgery or endotracheal intubation; increases pulmonary compliance during mechanical ventilation

Usual Dosage I.V. (in obese patients, use ideal body weight to calculate dosage):
Children >2 years: Initial: 0.03-0.05 mg/kg followed by maintenance doses of 0.005-0.01 mg/kg after 30-45 minutes
Adults: Surgery: 0.05 mg/kg with thiopental/narcotic or 0.025 mg/kg with succinylcholine; maintenance dose: 0.005-0.01 mg/kg after 60-100 minutes

Dosage Forms Injection, as chloride: 1 mg/mL (5 mL)

doxacurium chloride *see doxacurium on this page*

doxapram *(DOKS a pram)*

Synonyms doxapram hydrochloride

Brand Names Dopram® Injection

Therapeutic Category Respiratory Stimulant

Use Respiratory and CNS stimulant; idiopathic apnea of prematurity refractory to xanthines

Usual Dosage I.V.:
Neonatal apnea (apnea of prematurity):
Initial: 0.5 mg/kg/hour
Maintenance: 0.5-2.5 mg/kg/hour, titrated to the lowest rate at which apnea is controlled
Adults: Respiratory depression following anesthesia:
Initial: 0.5-1 mg/kg; may repeat at 5-minute intervals; maximum total dose: 2 mg/kg; single doses should not exceed 1.5 mg/kg
I.V. infusion: Initial: 5 mg/minute until adequate response or adverse effects seen; decrease to 1-3 mg/minute; usual total dose: 0.5-4 mg/kg; maximum: 300 mg

Dosage Forms Injection, as hydrochloride: 20 mg/mL (20 mL)

doxapram hydrochloride *see* doxapram *on previous page*

doxazosin (doks AYE zoe sin)
Brand Names Cardura®
Therapeutic Category Alpha-Adrenergic Blocking Agent
Use Alpha-adrenergic blocking agent for treatment of hypertension
Usual Dosage Adults: Oral: 1 mg once daily, may be increased to 2 mg once daily thereafter up to 16 mg if needed
Dosage Forms Tablet: 1 mg, 2 mg, 4 mg, 8 mg

doxepin (DOKS e pin)
Synonyms doxepin hydrochloride
Brand Names Adapin® Oral; Sinequan® Oral; Zonalon® Topical Cream
Therapeutic Category Antidepressant, Tricyclic (Tertiary Amine); Topical Skin Product
Use
Oral: Treatment of various forms of depression, usually in conjunction with psychotherapy; treatment of anxiety disorders; analgesic for certain chronic and neuropathic pain
Topical: Adults: Short-term (<8 days) therapy of moderate pruritus due to atopic dermatitis or lichen simplex chronicus
Usual Dosage
Oral:
Adolescents: Initial: 25-50 mg/day in single or divided doses; gradually increase to 100 mg/day
Adults: Initial: 30-150 mg/day at bedtime or in 2-3 divided doses; may increase up to 300 mg/day; single dose should not exceed 150 mg; select patients may respond to 25-50 mg/day
Topical: Apply in a thin film 4 times/day
Dosage Forms
Capsule, as hydrochloride: 10 mg, 25 mg, 50 mg, 75 mg, 100 mg, 150 mg
Concentrate, oral, as hydrochloride: 10 mg/mL (120 mL)
Cream: 5% (30 g)

doxepin hydrochloride *see* doxepin *on this page*

Doxidan® [OTC] *see* docusate and phenolphthalein *on page 180*

Doxil™ *see* doxorubicin (liposomal) *on next page*

doxorubicin (doks oh ROO bi sin)
Synonyms adr; doxorubicin hydrochloride; hydroxydaunomycin hydrochloride
Brand Names Adriamycin PFS™; Adriamycin RDF™; Rubex®
Therapeutic Category Antineoplastic Agent
Use Treatment of various solid tumors including ovarian, breast, and bladder tumors; various lymphomas and leukemias (ANL, ALL), soft tissue sarcomas, neuroblastoma, osteosarcoma
Usual Dosage I.V. (refer to individual protocols; patient's ideal weight should be used to calculate body surface area):
Children: 35-75 mg/m^2 as a single dose, repeat every 21 days; or 20 mg/m^2 once weekly
Adults: 60-75 mg/m^2 as a single dose, repeat every 21 days or other dosage regimens like 20-30 mg/m^2/day for 2-3 days, repeat in 4 weeks or 20 mg/m^2 once weekly
The lower dose regimen should be administered to patients with decreased bone marrow reserve, prior therapy or marrow infiltration with malignant cells
Dosage Forms
Injection, as hydrochloride:
Aqueous, with NS: 2 mg/mL (5 mL, 10 mL, 25 mL)
Preservative free: 2 mg/mL (5 mL, 10 mL, 25 mL, 100 mL)
Powder for injection, as hydrochloride, lyophilized: 10 mg, 20 mg, 50 mg, 100 mg
(Continued)

doxorubicin *(Continued)*
Rapid dissolution formula: 10 mg, 20 mg, 50 mg, 150 mg

doxorubicin hydrochloride *see* doxorubicin *on previous page*

doxorubicin hydrochloride (liposomal) *see* doxorubicin (liposomal) *on this page*

doxorubicin (liposomal) (doks oh ROO bi sin lip pah SOW mal)
Synonyms doxorubicin hydrochloride (liposomal)
Brand Names Doxil™
Therapeutic Category Antineoplastic Agent
Use Treatment of AIDS-related Kaposi's sarcoma in patients with disease that has progressed on prior combination chemotherapy or in patients who are intolerant to such therapy
Usual Dosage I.V. (refer to individual protocols; patient's ideal weight should be used to calculate body surface area): I.V.: 20 mg/m^2 over 30 minutes, once every 3 weeks, for as long as patients respond satisfactorily and tolerate treatment
Dosage Forms Injection, as hydrochloride: 2 mg/mL (10 mL)

Doxychel® Injection *see* doxycycline *on this page*

Doxychel® Oral *see* doxycycline *on this page*

doxycycline (doks i SYE kleen)
Synonyms doxycycline hyclate; doxycycline monohydrate
Brand Names Bio-Tab® Oral; Doryx® Oral; Doxychel® Injection; Doxychel® Oral; Doxy® Oral; Monodox® Oral; Vibramycin® Injection; Vibramycin® Oral; Vibra-Tabs®
Therapeutic Category Tetracycline Derivative
Use
Children, Adolescents, and Adults: Treatment of Rocky Mountain spotted fever caused by susceptible *Rickettsia* or brucellosis
Older Children, Adolescents, and Adults: Treatment of Lyme disease, mycoplasmal disease, or *Legionella*; management of malignant pleural effusions when intrapleural therapy is indicated
Adolescents and Adults: Treatment of nongonococcal pelvic inflammatory disease and urethritis due to *Chlamydia*; treatment for victims of sexual assault
Usual Dosage Oral, I.V.:
Children ≥8 years: 2-4 mg/kg/day in 1-2 divided doses, not to exceed 200 mg/day
Adults: 100-200 mg/day in 1-2 divided doses
Dosage Forms
Capsule:
As hyclate:
Doxychel®, Vibramycin®: 50 mg
Doxy®, Doxychel®, Vibramycin®: 100 mg
As monohydrate (Monodox®): 50 mg, 100 mg
Coated pellets, as hyclate (Doryx®): 100 mg
Powder:
For injection, as hyclate (Doxy®, Doxychel®, Vibramycin® IV): 100 mg, 200 mg
For oral suspension, as monohydrate (raspberry flavor) (Vibramycin®): 25 mg/5 mL (60 mL)
Syrup, as calcium (raspberry-apple flavor) (Vibramycin®): 50 mg/5 mL (30 mL, 473 mL)
Tablet, as hyclate:
Doxychel®: 50 mg
Bio-Tab®, Doxychel®, Vibra-Tabs®: 100 mg

doxycycline hyclate *see* doxycycline *on this page*

doxycycline monohydrate *see* doxycycline *on this page*

Doxy® Oral *see* doxycycline *on this page*

dpa *see* valproic acid and derivatives *on page 544*

dpe *see* dipivefrin *on page 176*

d-penicillamine *see* penicillamine *on page 399*

DPH *see* phenytoin *on page 414*

dppc *see* colfosceril palmitate *on page 136*

dpt *see* diphtheria, tetanus toxoids, and whole-cell pertussis vaccine *on page 175*

Dramamine® II [OTC] *see* meclizine *on page 324*

Dramamine® Oral [OTC] *see* dimenhydrinate *on page 171*

Dri-Ear® Otic [OTC] *see* boric acid *on page 70*

Drisdol® Oral *see* ergocalciferol *on page 197*

Dristan® Cold Caplets [OTC] *see* acetaminophen and pseudoephedrine *on page 5*

Dristan® Long Lasting Nasal Solution [OTC] *see* oxymetazoline *on page 390*

Dristan® Saline Spray [OTC] *see* sodium chloride *on page 483*

Dristan® Sinus Caplets [OTC] *see* pseudoephedrine and ibuprofen *on page 450*

Drithocreme® *see* anthralin *on page 36*

Drithocreme® HP 1% *see* anthralin *on page 36*

Dritho-Scalp® *see* anthralin *on page 36*

Drixomed® *see* dexbrompheniramine and pseudoephedrine *on page 157*

Drixoral® [OTC] *see* dexbrompheniramine and pseudoephedrine *on page 157*

Drixoral® Cough & Congestion Liquid Caps [OTC] *see* pseudoephedrine and dextromethorphan *on page 450*

Drixoral® Cough Liquid Caps [OTC] *see* dextromethorphan *on page 160*

Drixoral® Cough & Sore Throat Liquid Caps [OTC] *see* acetaminophen and dextromethorphan *on page 4*

Drixoral® Non-Drowsy [OTC] *see* pseudoephedrine *on page 449*

Drixoral® Syrup [OTC] *see* brompheniramine and pseudoephedrine *on page 74*

dronabinol (droe NAB i nol)

Synonyms tetrahydrocannabinol; thc
Brand Names Marinol®
Therapeutic Category Antiemetic
Controlled Substance C-II
Use Treatment of nausea and vomiting secondary to cancer chemotherapy in patients who have not responded to conventional antiemetics; treatment of anorexia associated with weight loss in AIDS patients
Usual Dosage Oral:
Children: NCI protocol recommends 5 mg/m^2 starting 6-8 hours before chemotherapy and every 4-6 hours after to be continued for 12 hours after chemotherapy is discontinued
Adults: 5 mg/m^2 1-3 hours before chemotherapy, then administer 5 mg/m^2/dose every 2-4 hours after chemotherapy for a total of 4-6 doses/day; dose may be increased up to a maximum of 15 mg/m^2/dose if needed (dosage may be increased by 2.5 mg/m^2 increments)
Dosage Forms Capsule: 2.5 mg, 5 mg, 10 mg

droperidol (droe PER i dole)

Brand Names Inapsine®
Therapeutic Category Antiemetic; Antipsychotic Agent, Butyrophenone
(Continued)

droperidol *(Continued)*

Use Tranquilizer and antiemetic in surgical and diagnostic procedures; antiemetic for cancer chemotherapy; preoperative medication

Usual Dosage Titrate carefully to desired effect

Children 2-12 years:

Premedication: I.M.: 0.088-0.165 mg/kg; smaller doses may be sufficient for control of nausea or vomiting

Adjunct to general anesthesia: I.V. induction: 0.088-0.165 mg/kg

Nausea and vomiting: I.M., I.V.: 0.05-0.06 mg/kg/dose every 4-6 hours as needed

Adults:

Premedication: I.M., I.V.: 2.5-10 mg 30 minutes to 1 hour preoperatively

Adjunct to general anesthesia: I.V. induction: 0.22-0.275 mg/kg; maintenance: 1.25-2.5 mg/dose

Alone in diagnostic procedures: I.M.: Initial: 2.5-10 mg 30 minutes to 1 hour before; then 1.25-2.5 mg if needed

Nausea and vomiting: I.M., I.V.: 2.5-5 mg/dose every 3-4 hours as needed

Dosage Forms Injection: 2.5 mg/mL (1 mL, 2 mL, 5 mL, 10 mL)

droperidol and fentanyl (droe PER i dole & FEN ta nil)

Synonyms fentanyl and droperidol

Brand Names Innovar®

Therapeutic Category Analgesic, Narcotic

Use Produce and maintain analgesia and sedation during diagnostic or surgical procedures (neuroleptanalgesia and neuroleptanesthesia); adjunct to general anesthesia

Usual Dosage

Children:

Premedication: I.M.: 0.03 mL/kg 30-60 minutes prior to surgery

Adjunct to general anesthesia: I.V.: Total dose: 0.05 mL/kg as slow infusion (1 mL/1-2 minutes) until sleep occurs

Adults:

Premedication: I.M.: 0.5-2 mL 30-60 minutes prior to surgery

Adjunct to general anesthesia: I.V.: 0.09-0.11 mL/kg as slow infusion (1 mL/1-2 minutes) until sleep occurs

Dosage Forms Injection: Droperidol 2.5 mg and fentanyl 50 mcg per mL (2 mL, 5 mL)

Dr Scholl's Athlete's Foot [OTC] *see* tolnaftate *on page 523*

Dr Scholl's® Cracked Heel Relief Cream [OTC] *see* lidocaine *on page 307*

Dr Scholl's® Disk [OTC] *see* salicylic acid *on page 472*

Dr Scholl's Maximum Strength Tritin [OTC] *see* tolnaftate *on page 523*

Dr Scholl's® Wart Remover [OTC] *see* salicylic acid *on page 472*

Dry Eyes® Solution [OTC] *see* artificial tears *on page 42*

Dry Eye® Therapy Solution [OTC] *see* artificial tears *on page 42*

Dryox® Gel [OTC] *see* benzoyl peroxide *on page 61*

Dryox® Wash [OTC] *see* benzoyl peroxide *on page 61*

Drysol™ *see* aluminum chloride hexahydrate *on page 20*

dscg *see* cromolyn sodium *on page 141*

DSMC Plus® [OTC] *see* docusate and casanthranol *on page 180*

dss *see* docusate *on page 179*

D-S-S® [OTC] *see* docusate *on page 179*

dss with casanthranol *see* docusate and casanthranol *on page 180*

dt *see* diphtheria and tetanus toxoid *on page 174*

dtap *see* diphtheria, tetanus toxoids, and acellular pertussis vaccine *on page 175*

DTIC-Dome® *see* dacarbazine *on page 147*

dto *see* opium tincture *on page 384*

***d*-tubocurarine chloride** *see* tubocurarine *on page 539*

DTwP-HIB *see* diphtheria, tetanus toxoids, whole-cell pertussis, and *haemophilus* b conjugate vaccine *on page 176*

Duadacin® **Capsule [OTC]** *see* chlorpheniramine, phenylpropanolamine, and acetaminophen *on page 117*

Dulcolax® **[OTC]** *see* bisacodyl *on page 67*

Dull-C® **[OTC]** *see* ascorbic acid *on page 42*

DuoCet™ *see* hydrocodone and acetaminophen *on page 266*

Duo-Cyp® **Injection** *see* estradiol and testosterone *on page 203*

DuoFilm® **[OTC]** *see* salicylic acid *on page 472*

Duofilm® **Solution** *see* salicylic acid and lactic acid *on page 472*

Duo-Medihaler® **Aerosol** *see* isoproterenol and phenylephrine *on page 291*

DuoPlant® **Gel [OTC]** *see* salicylic acid *on page 472*

Duo-Trach® *see* lidocaine *on page 307*

Duotrate® *see* pentaerythritol tetranitrate *on page 402*

DuP 753 *see* losartan *on page 314*

Duphalac® *see* lactulose *on page 300*

Duplex® **T [OTC]** *see* coal tar *on page 132*

Duraclon® **Injection** *see* clonidine *on page 130*

Duract™ *see* bromfenac *on page 72*

Duragesic™ **Transdermal** *see* fentanyl *on page 219*

Dura-Gest® *see* guaifenesin, phenylpropanolamine, and phenylephrine *on page 251*

Duralone® **Injection** *see* methylprednisolone *on page 343*

Duramist® **Plus [OTC]** *see* oxymetazoline *on page 390*

Duramorph® **Injection** *see* morphine sulfate *on page 356*

Duranest® **Injection** *see* etidocaine *on page 212*

Duratest® **Injection** *see* testosterone *on page 507*

Duratestrin® **Injection** *see* estradiol and testosterone *on page 203*

Durathate® **Injection** *see* testosterone *on page 507*

Duration® **Nasal Solution [OTC]** *see* oxymetazoline *on page 390*

Duratuss-G® *see* guaifenesin *on page 247*

Dura-Vent® *see* guaifenesin and phenylpropanolamine *on page 249*

Dura-Vent/DA® *see* chlorpheniramine, phenylephrine, and methscopolamine *on page 116*

Duricef® *see* cefadroxil *on page 96*

Duvoid® *see* bethanechol *on page 66*

DV® **Vaginal Cream** *see* dienestrol *on page 166*

Dwelle® **Ophthalmic Solution [OTC]** *see* artificial tears *on page 42*

d-xylose (dee ZYE lose)
Synonyms wood sugar
Brand Names Xylo-Pfan® [OTC]
Therapeutic Category Diagnostic Agent
Use Evaluating intestinal absorption and diagnosing malabsorptive states
(Continued)

187

d-xylose *(Continued)*

Usual Dosage Oral:
Infants and young Children: 500 mg/kg as a 5% to 10% aqueous solution
Children: 5 g is dissolved in 250 mL water; additional fluids are permitted and are encouraged for children
Adults: 25 g dissolved in 200-300 mL water followed with an additional 200-400 mL water **or** 5 g dissolved in 200-300 mL water followed by an additional 200-400 mL water
Dosage Forms Powder for oral solution: 25 g

Dyazide® *see* hydrochlorothiazide and triamterene *on page 265*

Dycill® *see* dicloxacillin *on page 165*

Dyclone® *see* dyclonine *on this page*

dyclonine (DYE kloe neen)

Synonyms dyclonine hydrochloride
Brand Names Dyclone®; Sucrets® [OTC]
Therapeutic Category Local Anesthetic
Use Local anesthetic prior to laryngoscopy, bronchoscopy, or endotracheal intubation; used topically for temporary relief of pain associated with oral mucosa, skin, episiotomy, or anogenital lesions; the 0.5% topical solution may be used to block the gag reflex, and to relieve the pain of oral ulcers or stomatitis
Usual Dosage
Children and Adults: Topical solution:
Mouth sores: 5-10 mL of 0.5% or 1% to oral mucosa (swab or swish and then spit) 3-4 times/day as needed; maximum single dose: 200 mg (40 mL of 0.5% solution or 20 mL of 1% solution)
Bronchoscopy: Use 2 mL of the 1% solution or 4 mL of the 0.5% solution sprayed onto the larynx and trachea every 5 minutes until the reflex has been abolished
Children >3 years and Adults: Lozenge: Dissolve 1 in mouth slowly every 2 hours
Dosage Forms
Lozenges, as hydrochloride: 1.2 mg, 3 mg
Solution, topical, as hydrochloride: 0.5% (30 mL); 1% (30 mL)

dyclonine hydrochloride *see* dyclonine *on this page*

dyflos *see* isoflurophate *on page 290*

Dymelor® *see* acetohexamide *on page 7*

Dymenate® **Injection** *see* dimenhydrinate *on page 171*

Dynabac® *see* dirithromycin *on page 177*

Dynacin® **Oral** *see* minocycline *on page 351*

DynaCirc® *see* isradipine *on page 293*

Dynafed® **IB [OTC]** *see* ibuprofen *on page 278*

Dynafed®, **Maximum Strength [OTC]** *see* acetaminophen and pseudoephedrine *on page 5*

Dyna-Hex® **Topical [OTC]** *see* chlorhexidine gluconate *on page 109*

Dynapen® *see* dicloxacillin *on page 165*

dyphylline (DYE fi lin)

Synonyms dihydroxypropyl theophylline
Brand Names Dilor®; Lufyllin®
Therapeutic Category Theophylline Derivative
Use Bronchodilator in reversible airway obstruction due to asthma or COPD
Usual Dosage
Children: I.M.: 4.4-6.6 mg/kg/day in divided doses

Alphabetical Listing of Drugs

Adults:
Oral: Up to 15 mg/kg 4 times/day, individualize dosage
I.M.: 250-500 mg, do not exceed total dosage of 15 mg/kg every 6 hours
Dosage Forms
Elixir:
Lufyllin®: 100 mg/15 mL with alcohol 20% (473 mL, 3780 mL)
Dilor®: 160 mg/15 mL with alcohol 18% (473 mL)
Injection (Dilor®, Lufyllin®): 250 mg/mL (2 mL)
Tablet: 200 mg, 400 mg
Dilor®, Lufyllin®: 200 mg, 400 mg

Dyrenium® *see* triamterene *on page 530*

Easprin® *see* aspirin *on page 44*

echothiophate iodide (ek oh THYE oh fate EYE oh dide)
Synonyms ecostigmine iodide
Brand Names Phospholine Iodide® Ophthalmic
Therapeutic Category Cholinesterase Inhibitor
Use Reverse toxic CNS effects caused by anticholinergic drugs; used as miotic in treatment of glaucoma
Usual Dosage Adults: Ophthalmic: Glaucoma: Instill 1 drop twice daily into eyes with one dose just prior to bedtime; some patients have been treated with 1 dose/day or every other day. Use lowest concentration and frequency which gives satisfactory response, with a maximum dose of 0.125% once daily, although more intensive therapy may be used for short periods of time
Dosage Forms Powder for reconstitution, ophthalmic: 1.5 mg [0.03%] (5 mL); 3 mg [0.06%] (5 mL); 6.25 mg [0.125%] (5 mL); 12.5 mg [0.25%] (5 mL)

E-Complex-600® **[OTC]** *see* vitamin e *on page 553*

econazole (e KONE a zole)
Synonyms econazole nitrate
Brand Names Spectazole™
Therapeutic Category Antifungal Agent
Use Topical treatment of tinea pedis, tinea cruris, tinea corporis, tinea versicolor, and cutaneous candidiasis
Usual Dosage Children and Adults: Topical: Apply a sufficient amount to cover affected areas once daily; for cutaneous candidiasis: apply twice daily; candidal infections and tinea cruris, versicolor, and corporis should be treated for 2 weeks and tinea pedis for 1 month; occasionally, longer treatment periods may be required
Dosage Forms Cream, as nitrate: 1% (15 g, 30 g, 85 g)

econazole nitrate *see* econazole *on this page*

Econopred® **Ophthalmic** *see* prednisolone *on page 434*

Econopred® **Plus Ophthalmic** *see* prednisolone *on page 434*

ecostigmine iodide *see* echothiophate iodide *on this page*

Ecotrin® **[OTC]** *see* aspirin *on page 44*

Ecotrin® **Low Adult Strength [OTC]** *see* aspirin *on page 44*

Ed A-Hist® **Liquid** *see* chlorpheniramine and phenylephrine *on page 113*

edathamil disodium *see* edetate disodium *on next page*

Edecrin® *see* ethacrynic acid *on page 206*

edetate calcium disodium (ED e tate KAL see um dye SOW dee um)
Synonyms calcium edta
Brand Names Calcium Disodium Versenate®
(Continued)

edetate calcium disodium (Continued)

Therapeutic Category Chelating Agent

Use Treatment of acute and chronic lead poisoning; also used as an aid in the diagnosis of lead poisoning

Usual Dosage

Children:

Diagnosis of lead poisoning: Mobilization test: (Asymptomatic patients or lead levels <55 mcg/dL): (**Note:** Urine is collected for 24 hours after first EDTA dose and analyzed for lead content; if the ratio of mcg of lead in urine to mg calcium EDTA given is >1, then test is considered positive): Children: 500 mg/m^2 (maximum: 1 g/dose) I.M. or I.V. over 1 hour **or** 2 doses of 500 mg/m^2 at 12-hour intervals

Asymptomatic lead poisoning: (Blood lead concentration >55 mcg/dL or blood lead concentrations of 25-55 mcg/dL with blood erythrocyte protoporphyrin concentrations of ≥35 mcg/dL and positive mobilization test) or symptomatic lead poisoning without encephalopathy with lead level <100 mcg/dL: 1 g/m^2/day I.M./I.V. in divided doses every 8-12 hours for 3-5 days (usually 5 days); maximum: 1 g/24 hours or 50 mg/kg/day

Symptomatic lead poisoning with encephalopathy with lead level >100 mcg/dL (treatment with calcium EDTA and dimercaprol is preferred): 250 mg/m^2 I.M. or intermittent I.V. infusion 4 hours after dimercaprol, then at 4-hour intervals thereafter for 5 days (1.5 g/m^2/day); dose (1.5 g/m^2/day) can also be administered as a single I.V. continuous infusion over 12-24 hours/day for 5 days; maximum: 1 g/24 hours or 75 mg/kg/day

Note: Course of therapy may be repeated in 2-3 weeks until blood lead level is normal

Adults: I.M., I.V.:

Diagnosis of lead poisoning: 500 mg/m^2 (maximum: 1 g/dose) over 1 hour

Treatment: 2 g/day or 1.5 g/m^2/day in divided doses every 12-24 hours for 5 days; may repeat course one time after at least 2 days (usually after 2 weeks)

Dosage Forms Injection: 200 mg/mL (5 mL)

edetate disodium (ED e tate dye SOW dee um)

Synonyms edathamil disodium; edta; sodium edetate

Brand Names Chealamide®; Disotate®; Endrate®

Therapeutic Category Chelating Agent

Use Emergency treatment of hypercalcemia; control digitalis-induced cardiac dysrhythmias (ventricular arrhythmias)

Usual Dosage I.V.:

Hypercalcemia:

Children: 40-70 mg/kg slow infusion over 3-4 hours

Adults: 50 mg/kg/day over 3 or more hours

Dysrhythmias: Children and Adults: 15 mg/kg/hour up to 60 mg/kg/day

Dosage Forms Injection: 150 mg/mL (20 mL)

Edex® Injection *see* alprostadil *on page 18*

edrophonium (ed roe FOE nee um)

Synonyms edrophonium chloride

Brand Names Enlon® Injection; Reversol® Injection; Tensilon® Injection

Therapeutic Category Cholinergic Agent

Use Diagnosis of myasthenia gravis; differentiation of cholinergic crises from myasthenia crises; reversal of nondepolarizing neuromuscular blockers; treatment of paroxysmal atrial tachycardia

Usual Dosage

Infants: I.V.: Initial: 0.1 mg, followed by 0.4 mg if no response; total dose: 0.5 mg

Children:

Diagnosis: Initial: 0.04 mg/kg followed by 0.16 mg/kg if no response, to a maximum total dose of 5 mg for children ≤34 kg, or 10 mg for children >34 kg

Titration of oral anticholinesterase therapy: 0.04 mg/kg once; if strength improves, an increase in neostigmine or pyridostigmine dose is indicated

Adults:

Diagnosis: I.V.: 2 mg test dose administered over 15-30 seconds; 8 mg administered 45 seconds later if no response is seen. Test dose may be repeated after 30 minutes.

Titration of oral anticholinesterase therapy: 1-2 mg administered 1 hour after oral dose of anticholinesterase; if strength improves, an increase in neostigmine or pyridostigmine dose is indicated

Differentiation of cholinergic from myasthenic crisis: I.V.: 1 mg, may repeat after 1 minute (**Note:** Intubation and controlled ventilation may be required if patient has cholinergic crises.)

Reversal of nondepolarizing neuromuscular blocking agents (neostigmine with atropine usually preferred): I.V.: 10 mg, may repeat every 5-10 minutes up to 40 mg

Termination of paroxysmal atrial tachycardia: I.V.: 5-10 mg

Dosage Forms Injection, as chloride: 10 mg/mL (1 mL, 10 mL, 15 mL)

edrophonium chloride *see* edrophonium *on previous page*

ED-SPAZ® *see* hyoscyamine *on page 275*

edta *see* edetate disodium *on previous page*

E.E.S.® **Oral** *see* erythromycin *on page 199*

Effer-K™ *see* potassium bicarbonate and potassium citrate, effervescent *on page 427*

Effer-Syllium® **[OTC]** *see* psyllium *on page 451*

Effexor® *see* venlafaxine *on page 548*

Efidac/24® **[OTC]** *see* pseudoephedrine *on page 449*

eflornithine (ee FLOR ni theen)
Synonyms eflornithine hydrochloride
Brand Names Ornidyl® Injection
Therapeutic Category Antiprotozoal
Use Treatment of meningoencephalitic stage of *Trypanosoma brucei gambiense* infection (sleeping sickness)
Usual Dosage I.V. infusion: 100 mg/kg/dose administered every 6 hours (over 45 minutes) for 14 days
Dosage Forms Injection, as hydrochloride: 200 mg/mL (100 mL)

eflornithine hydrochloride *see* eflornithine *on this page*

Efodine® **[OTC]** *see* povidone-iodine *on page 431*

Efudex® **Topical** *see* fluorouracil *on page 229*

ehdp *see* etidronate disodium *on page 212*

Elase-Chloromycetin® **Topical** *see* fibrinolysin and desoxyribonuclease *on page 222*

Elase® **Topical** *see* fibrinolysin and desoxyribonuclease *on page 222*

Elavil® *see* amitriptyline *on page 27*

Eldecort® *see* hydrocortisone *on page 268*

Eldepryl® *see* selegiline *on page 476*

Eldercaps® **[OTC]** *see* vitamins, multiple (oral, adult) *on page 556*

Eldopaque® **[OTC]** *see* hydroquinone *on page 272*

Eldopaque Forte® *see* hydroquinone *on page 272*

Eldoquin® **[OTC]** *see* hydroquinone *on page 272*

Eldoquin® **Forte**® *see* hydroquinone *on page 272*

electrolyte lavage solution *see* polyethylene glycol-electrolyte solution *on page 423*

Elimite™ Cream *see* permethrin *on page 406*

Elixomin® *see* theophylline *on page 511*

Elixophyllin® *see* theophylline *on page 511*

Elmiron® *see* pentosan polysulfate sodium *on page 405*

Elocon® Topical *see* mometasone furoate *on page 355*

Elspar® *see* asparaginase *on page 43*

Eltroxin® *see* levothyroxine *on page 306*

Emcyt® *see* estramustine *on page 204*

Emecheck® [OTC] *see* phosphorated carbohydrate solution *on page 415*

Emetrol® [OTC] *see* phosphorated carbohydrate solution *on page 415*

Emgel™ Topical *see* erythromycin, topical *on page 201*

Eminase® *see* anistreplase *on page 36*

Emko® [OTC] *see* nonoxynol 9 *on page 377*

EMLA® *see* lidocaine and prilocaine *on page 308*

Empirin® [OTC] *see* aspirin *on page 44*

Empirin® With Codeine *see* aspirin and codeine *on page 44*

Emulsoil® [OTC] *see* castor oil *on page 95*

E-Mycin® Oral *see* erythromycin *on page 199*

enalapril (e NAL a pril)

Synonyms enalaprilat; enalapril maleate
Brand Names Vasotec®; Vasotec® I.V.
Therapeutic Category Angiotensin-Converting Enzyme (ACE) Inhibitors
Use Management of mild to severe hypertension, congestive heart failure, and asymptomatic left ventricular dysfunction
Usual Dosage Use lower listed initial dose in patients with hyponatremia, hypovolemia, severe congestive heart failure, decreased renal function, or in those receiving diuretics
  Children:
  Investigational initial oral doses of enalapril of 0.1 mg/kg/day increasing over 2 weeks to 0.12-0.43 mg/kg/day have been used to treat severe congestive heart failure in infants (n=8)
  Investigational I.V. doses of enalaprilat of 5-10 mcg/kg/dose administered every 8-24 hours (as determined by blood pressure readings) have been used for the treatment of neonatal hypertension (n=10); monitor patients carefully; select patients may require higher doses
  Adults:
  Oral: **Enalapril**: 2.5-5 mg/day then increase as required, usually 10-40 mg/day in 1-2 divided doses
  I.V.: **Enalaprilat**: 0.625-1.25 mg/dose, administered over 5 minutes every 6 hours
Dosage Forms
  Injection, as enalaprilat: 1.25 mg/mL (1 mL, 2 mL)
  Tablet, as maleate: 2.5 mg, 5 mg, 10 mg, 20 mg

enalapril and diltiazem (e NAL a pril & dil TYE a zem)

Brand Names Teczem®
Therapeutic Category Antihypertensive, Combination
Use Combination drug for treatment of hypertension
Dosage Forms Tablet, extended release: Enalapril maleate 5 mg and diltiazem maleate 180 mg

enalapril and felodipine (e NAL a pril & fe LOE di peen)
Brand Names Lexxel®
Therapeutic Category Antihypertensive Agent, Combination
Use Treatment of hypertension
Dosage Forms Tablet, extended release: Enalapril maleate 5 mg and felodipine 5 mg

enalapril and hydrochlorothiazide
(e NAL a pril & hye droe klor oh THYE a zide)
Brand Names Vaseretic® 10-25
Therapeutic Category Antihypertensive, Combination
Use Treatment of hypertension
Usual Dosage Oral: Dose is individualized
Dosage Forms Tablet: Enalapril maleate 10 mg and hydrochlorothiazide 25 mg

enalaprilat *see* enalapril *on previous page*

enalapril maleate *see* enalapril *on previous page*

encainide (en KAY nide)
Synonyms encainide hydrochloride
Brand Names Enkaid®
Therapeutic Category Antiarrhythmic Agent, Class I-C
Use Ventricular arrhythmias; supraventricular arrhythmias
Usual Dosage Adults: Oral: 25 mg every 8 hours; may increase to 35 mg every 8 hours after 3-5 days if needed; increase to 50 mg every 8 hours in another 3-5 days if response is not achieved
Dosage Forms Capsule, as hydrochloride: 25 mg, 35 mg, 50 mg

encainide hydrochloride *see* encainide *on this page*

Encare® [OTC] *see* nonoxynol 9 *on page 377*

Endal® *see* guaifenesin and phenylephrine *on page 249*

End Lice® Liquid [OTC] *see* pyrethrins *on page 452*

Endolor® *see* butalbital compound and acetaminophen *on page 78*

Endrate® *see* edetate disodium *on page 190*

Enduron® *see* methyclothiazide *on page 340*

Enduronyl® *see* methyclothiazide and deserpidine *on page 340*

Enduronyl® Forte *see* methyclothiazide and deserpidine *on page 340*

Enecat® *see* radiological/contrast media (ionic) *on page 457*

enflurane (EN floo rane)
Brand Names Ethrane®
Therapeutic Category General Anesthetic
Use General induction and maintenance of anesthesia (inhalation)
Usual Dosage Inhalation: 0.5% to 3%
Dosage Forms Liquid: 125 mL, 250 mL

Engerix-B® *see* hepatitis b vaccine *on page 259*

Enisyl® [OTC] *see* l-lysine *on page 311*

Enkaid® *see* encainide *on this page*

Enlon® Injection *see* edrophonium *on page 190*

Enomine® *see* guaifenesin, phenylpropanolamine, and phenylephrine *on page 251*

enoxacin (en OKS a sin)
Brand Names Penetrex™
Therapeutic Category Quinolone
Use Complicated and uncomplicated urinary tract infections caused by susceptible gram-negative and gram-positive bacteria
Usual Dosage Adults: Oral: 400 mg twice daily
Dosage Forms Tablet: 200 mg, 400 mg

enoxaparin (e noks ah PAIR in)
Synonyms enoxaparin sodium
Brand Names Lovenox® Injection
Therapeutic Category Anticoagulant
Use Prophylaxis and treatment of thromboembolic disorders (deep vein thrombosis)
Usual Dosage Adults: S.C.: 30 mg twice daily
Dosage Forms Injection, as sodium, preservative free: 30 mg/0.3 mL

enoxaparin sodium *see* enoxaparin *on this page*

Ensure® [OTC] *see* enteral nutritional products *on this page*

Ensure Plus® [OTC] *see* enteral nutritional products *on this page*

enteral nutritional products
Synonyms dietary supplements
Brand Names Amin-Aid® [OTC]; Carnation Instant Breakfast® [OTC]; Citrotein® [OTC]; Criticare HN® [OTC]; Ensure® [OTC]; Ensure Plus® [OTC]; Isocal® [OTC]; Magnacal® [OTC]; Microlipid™ [OTC]; Osmolite® HN [OTC]; Pedialyte® [OTC]; Polycose® [OTC]; Portagen® [OTC]; Pregestimil® [OTC]; Propac™ [OTC]; Soyalac® [OTC]; Vital HN® [OTC]; Vitaneed™ [OTC]; Vivonex® [OTC]; Vivonex® T.E.N. [OTC]
Therapeutic Category Nutritional Supplement
Dosage Forms
Liquid (Magnacal®): Calcium and sodium caseinate, maltodextrin, sucrose, partially hydrogenated soy oil, soy lecithin
Powder (Vivonex® T.E.N.): Amino acids, predigested carbohydrates, safflower oil

Entertainer's Secret® Spray [OTC] *see* saliva substitute *on page 473*

Entex® *see* guaifenesin, phenylpropanolamine, and phenylephrine *on page 251*

Entex® LA *see* guaifenesin and phenylpropanolamine *on page 249*

Entex® PSE *see* guaifenesin and pseudoephedrine *on page 250*

Entrobar® *see* radiological/contrast media (ionic) *on page 457*

Enulose® *see* lactulose *on page 300*

Enzone® *see* pramoxine and hydrocortisone *on page 433*

epeg *see* etoposide *on page 213*

ephedrine (e FED rin)
Synonyms ephedrine sulfate
Brand Names Kondon's Nasal® [OTC]; Pretz-D® [OTC]
Therapeutic Category Adrenergic Agonist Agent
Use Bronchial asthma; nasal congestion; acute bronchospasm; acute hypotensive states
Usual Dosage
Children:
Oral, S.C.: 3 mg/kg/day or 25-100 mg/m^2/day in 4-6 divided doses every 4-6 hours
I.M., slow I.V. push: 0.2-0.3 mg/kg/dose every 4-6 hours
Adults:
Oral: 25-50 mg every 3-4 hours as needed
I.M., S.C.: 25-50 mg, parenteral adult dose should not exceed 150 mg in 24 hours

I.V.: 5-25 mg/dose slow I.V. push repeated after 5-10 minutes as needed, then every 3-4 hours not to exceed 150 mg/24 hours

Dosage Forms
Capsule, as sulfate: 25 mg, 50 mg
Injection, as sulfate: 25 mg/mL (1 mL); 50 mg/mL (1 mL, 10 mL)
Jelly, as sulfate (Kondon's Nasal®): 1% (20 g)
Spray, as sulfate (Pretz-D®): 0.25% (15 mL)

ephedrine sulfate *see* ephedrine *on previous page*

Epi-C® *see* radiological/contrast media (ionic) *on page 457*

Epifrin® *see* epinephrine *on this page*

E-Pilo-x® Ophthalmic *see* pilocarpine and epinephrine *on page 417*

Epinal® *see* epinephryl borate *on next page*

epinephrine (ep i NEF rin)

Synonyms adrenaline; epinephrine bitartrate; epinephrine hydrochloride
Brand Names Adrenalin®; AsthmaHaler®; Bronitin®; Bronkaid® Mist [OTC]; Epifrin®; EpiPen® Auto-Injector; EpiPen® Jr Auto-Injector; Glaucon®; Primatene® Mist [OTC]; Sus-Phrine®
Therapeutic Category Adrenergic Agonist Agent
Use Treatment of bronchospasm, anaphylactic reactions, cardiac arrest, and management of open-angle (chronic simple) glaucoma
Usual Dosage
Bronchodilator:
Children: S.C.: 10 mcg/kg (0.01 mL/kg of 1:1000) (single doses not to exceed 0.5 mg); injection suspension (1:200): 0.005 mL/kg/dose (0.025 mg/kg/dose) to a maximum of 0.15 mL (0.75 mg for single dose) every 8-12 hours
Adults:
I.M., S.C. (1:1000): 0.1-0.5 mg every 10-15 minutes to 4 hours
Suspension (1:200) S.C.: 0.1-0.3 mL (0.5-1.5 mg)
I.V.: 0.1-0.25 mg (single dose maximum: 1 mg)

Cardiac arrest:
Neonates: I.V. or intratracheal: 0.01-0.03 mg/kg (0.1-0.3 mL/kg of 1:10,000 solution) every 3-5 minutes as needed; dilute intratracheal doses in 1-2 mL of normal saline
Infants and Children: Asystole or pulseless arrest:
I.V., intraosseous: First dose: 0.01 mg/kg (0.1 mL/kg of a 1:10,000 solution); subsequent doses: 0.1 mg/kg (0.1 mL/kg of a 1:1000 solution); doses as high as 0.2 mg/kg may be effective; repeat every 3-5 minutes
Intratracheal: 0.1 mg/kg (0.1 mL/kg of a 1:1000 solution); doses as high as 0.2 mg/kg may be effective
Adults: Asystole:
I.V.: 1 mg every 3-5 minutes; if this approach fails, alternative regimens include: Intermediate: 2-5 mg every 3-5 minutes; Escalating: 1 mg, 3 mg, 5 mg at 3-minute intervals; High: 0.1 mg/kg every 3-5 minutes
Intratracheal: Although optimal dose is unknown, doses of 2-2.5 times the I.V. dose may be needed

Bradycardia: Children:
I.V.: 0.01 mg/kg (0.1 mL/kg of 1:10,000 solution) every 3-5 minutes as needed (maximum: 1 mg/10 mL)
Intratracheal: 0.1 mg/kg (0.1 mL/kg of 1:1000 solution every 3-5 minutes); doses as high as 0.2 mg/kg may be effective
Refractory hypotension (refractory to dopamine/dobutamine): I.V. infusion administration requires the use of an infusion pump:
Children: Infusion rate 0.1-4 mcg/kg/minute
Adults: I.V. infusion: 1 mg in 250 mL NS/D$_5$W at 0.1-1 mcg/kg/minute; titrate to desired effect
(Continued)

epinephrine *(Continued)*

Hypersensitivity reaction:

Children: S.C.: 0.01 mg/kg every 15 minutes for 2 doses then every 4 hours as needed (single doses not to exceed 0.5 mg)

Adults: I.M., S.C.: 0.2-0.5 mg every 20 minutes to 4 hours (single dose maximum: 1 mg)

Nebulization:

Children <2 years: 0.25 mL of 1:1000 diluted in 3 mL NS with treatments ordered individually

Children >2 years and Adolescents: 0.5 mL of 1:1000 concentration diluted in 3 mL NS

Children >2 years and Adults (racemic epinephrine):

<10 kg: 2 mL of 1:8 dilution over 15 minutes every 1-4 hours

10-15 kg: 2 mL of 1:6 dilution over 15 minutes every 1-4 hours

15-20 kg: 2 mL of 1:4 dilution over 15 minutes every 1-4 hours

>20 kg: 2 mL of 1:3 dilution over 15 minutes every 1-4 hours

Adults: Instill 8-15 drops into nebulizer reservoirs; administer 1-3 inhalations 4-6 times/day

Ophthalmic: Instill 1-2 drops in eye(s) once or twice daily

Intranasal: Children ≥6 years and Adults: Apply locally as drops or spray or with sterile swab

Dosage Forms

Aerosol, oral:

Bitartrate (AsthmaHaler®, Bronitin®, Medihaler-Epi®, Primatene® Suspension): 0.3 mg/spray [epinephrine base 0.16 mg/spray] (10 mL, 15 mL, 22.5 mL)

Bronkaid®: 0.5% (10 mL, 15 mL, 22.5 mL)

Primatene®: 0.2 mg/spray (15 mL, 22.5 mL)

Auto-injector:

EpiPen®: Delivers 0.3 mg I.M. of epinephrine 1:1000 (2 mL)

EpiPen® Jr.: Delivers 0.15 mg I.M. of epinephrine 1:2000 (2 mL)

Solution:

Inhalation:

Adrenalin®: 1% [10 mg/mL, 1:100] (7.5 mL)

Injection:

Adrenalin®: 0.01 mg/mL [1:100,000] (5 mL); 0.1 mg/mL [1:10,000] (3 mL, 10 mL); 1 mg/mL [1:1000] (1 mL, 2 mL, 30 mL)

Suspension (Sus-Phrine®): 5 mg/mL [1:200] (0.3 mL, 5 mL)

Nasal (Adrenalin®): 0.1% [1 mg/mL, 1:1000] (30 mL)

Ophthalmic, as hydrochloride (Epifrin®, Glaucon®): 0.1% (1 mL, 30 mL); 0.5% (15 mL); 1% (1 mL, 10 mL, 15 mL); 2% (10 mL, 15 mL)

Topical (Adrenalin®): 0.1% [1 mg/mL, 1:1000] (10 mL, 30 mL)

epinephrine bitartrate *see* epinephrine *on previous page*

epinephrine hydrochloride *see* epinephrine *on previous page*

epinephryl borate *(ep i NEF ril BOR ate)*

Brand Names Epinal®

Therapeutic Category Adrenergic Agonist Agent

Use Reduces elevated intraocular pressure in chronic open-angle glaucoma

Usual Dosage Adults: Ophthalmic: Instill 1 drop into the eyes once or twice daily

Dosage Forms Solution, ophthalmic: 0.5% (7.5 mL); 1% (7.5 mL)

EpiPen® Auto-Injector *see* epinephrine *on previous page*

EpiPen® Jr Auto-Injector *see* epinephrine *on previous page*

Epitol® *see* carbamazepine *on page 89*

Epivir® *see* lamivudine *on page 301*

epo *see* epoetin alfa *on next page*

epoetin alfa (e POE e tin AL fa)
Synonyms epo; erythropoietin; rhuepo-α
Brand Names Epogen®; Procrit®
Therapeutic Category Colony Stimulating Factor
Use Anemia associated with end stage renal disease; anemia related to therapy with AZT-treated HIV-infected patients; anemia in cancer patients receiving chemotherapy; anemia of prematurity
Usual Dosage
In patients on dialysis epoetin alfa usually has been administered as an I.V. bolus 3 times/week. While the administration is independent of the dialysis procedure, it may be administered into the venous line at the end of the dialysis procedure to obviate the need for additional venous access; in patients with CRF not on dialysis, epoetin alfa may be administered either as an I.V. or S.C. injection.

AZT-treated HIV-infected patients: I.V., S.C.: Initial: 100 units/kg/dose 3 times/week for 8 weeks; after 8 weeks of therapy the dose can be adjusted by 50-100 units/kg increments 3 times/week to a maximum dose of 300 units/kg 3 times/week; if the hematocrit exceeds 40%, the dose should be discontinued until the hematocrit drops to 36%

Anemia of prematurity: S.C.: 25-100 units/kg/dose 3 times/week
Dosage Forms
1 mL single-dose vials: Preservative-free solution
  2000 units/mL
  3000 units/mL
  4000 units/mL
  10,000 units/mL
2 mL multidose vials: Preserved solution: 10,000 units/mL

Epogen® *see* epoetin alfa *on this page*

epoprostenol (e poe PROST en ole)
Synonyms epoprostenol sodium
Brand Names Flolan® Injection
Therapeutic Category Platelet Inhibitor
Use Long-term intravenous treatment of primary pulmonary hypertension (PPH)
Usual Dosage I.V. continuous infusion: 2 ng/kg/minute
Dosage Forms Injection, as sodium: 0.5 mg/vial and 1.5 mg/vial, each supplied with 50 mL of sterile diluent

epoprostenol sodium *see* epoprostenol *on this page*

epsom salts *see* magnesium sulfate *on page 320*

ept *see* teniposide *on page 504*

Equagesic® *see* aspirin and meprobamate *on page 45*

Equalactin® Chewable Tablet [OTC] *see* calcium polycarbophil *on page 86*

Equanil® *see* meprobamate *on page 330*

Equilet® [OTC] *see* calcium carbonate *on page 82*

Ercaf® *see* ergotamine *on next page*

Ergamisol® *see* levamisole *on page 303*

ergocalciferol (er goe kal SIF e role)
Synonyms activated ergosterol; viosterol; vitamin d$_2$
Brand Names Calciferol™ Injection; Calciferol™ Oral; Drisdol® Oral
Therapeutic Category Vitamin D Analog
Use Refractory rickets; hypophosphatemia; hypoparathyroidism
(Continued)

ergocalciferol *(Continued)*

Usual Dosage
Dietary supplementation: Oral:
Premature infants: 10-20 mcg/day (400-800 units), up to 750 mcg/day (30,000 units)
Infants and healthy Children: 10 mcg/day (400 units)
Renal failure: Oral:
Children: 0.1-1 mg/day (4000-40,000 units)
Adults: 0.5 mg/day (20,000 units)
Hypoparathyroidism: Oral:
Children: 1.25-5 mg/day (50,000-200,000 units) and calcium supplements
Adults: 625 mcg to 5 mg/day (25,000-200,000 units) and calcium supplements
Vitamin D-dependent rickets: Oral:
Children: 75-125 mcg/day (3000-5000 units)
Adults: 250 mcg to 1.5 mg/day (10,000-60,000 units)
Nutritional rickets and osteomalacia:
Oral:
Children and Adults (with normal absorption): 25 mcg/day (1000 units)
Children with malabsorption: 250-625 mcg/day (10,000-25,000 units)
I.M.: Adults: 250 mcg/day

Dosage Forms
Capsule (Drisdol®): 50,000 units [1.25 mg]
Injection (Calciferol™): 500,000 units/mL [12.5 mg/mL] (1 mL)
Liquid (Calciferol™, Drisdol®): 8000 units/mL [200 mcg/mL] (60 mL)
Tablet (Calciferol™): 50,000 units [1.25 mg]

ergoloid mesylates (ER goe loid MES i lates)
Synonyms dihydroergotoxine; hydrogenated ergot alkaloids
Brand Names Germinal®; Hydergine®; Hydergine® LC
Therapeutic Category Ergot Alkaloid
Use Treatment of cerebrovascular insufficiency in primary progressive dementia, Alzheimer's dementia, and senile onset
Usual Dosage Adults: Oral: 1 mg 3 times/day up to 4.5-12 mg/day; up to 6 months of therapy may be necessary
Dosage Forms
Capsule, liquid (Hydergine® LC): 1 mg
Liquid (Hydergine®): 1 mg/mL (100 mL)
Tablet:
Oral: 0.5 mg
Gerimal®, Hydergine®: 1 mg
Sublingual:
Gerimal®, Hydergine®: 0.5 mg, 1 mg

Ergomar® *see* ergotamine *on this page*

ergotamine (er GOT a meen)
Synonyms ergotamine tartrate; ergotamine tartrate and caffeine; ergotamine tartrate with belladonna alkaloids, and phenobarbital
Brand Names Cafatine®; Cafergot®; Cafetrate®; Ercaf®; Ergomar®; Wigraine®
Therapeutic Category Ergot Alkaloid
Use Prevent or abort vascular headaches, such as migraine or cluster
Usual Dosage
Older Children and Adolescents: Oral: 1 tablet at onset of attack; then 1 tablet every 30 minutes as needed, up to a maximum of 3 tablets per attack
Adults:
Oral (Cafergot®): 2 tablets at onset of attack; then 1 tablet every 30 minutes as needed; maximum: 6 tablets per attack; do not exceed 10 tablets/week
Oral (Ergostat®): 1 tablet under tongue at first sign, then 1 tablet every 30 minutes, 3 tablets/24 hours, 5 tablets/week

Rectal (Cafergot® suppositories, Wigraine® suppositories, Cafatine-PB® suppositories): 1 at first sign of an attack; follow with second dose after 1 hour, if needed; maximum dose: 2 per attack; do not exceed 5/week
Dosage Forms
Suppository, rectal (Cafatine®, Cafergot®, Cafetrate®, Wigraine®): Ergotamine tartrate 2 mg and caffeine 100 mg (12s)
Tablet (Ercaf®, Wigraine®): Ergotamine tartrate 1 mg and caffeine 100 mg
Sublingual (Ergomar®): Ergotamine tartrate 2 mg

ergotamine tartrate *see* ergotamine *on previous page*

ergotamine tartrate and caffeine *see* ergotamine *on previous page*

ergotamine tartrate with belladonna alkaloids, and phenobarbital *see* ergotamine *on previous page*

E•R•O Ear [OTC] *see* carbamide peroxide *on page 90*

erwinia asparaginase (ehr WIN ee ah a SPAIR a ji nase)
Synonyms NSC-106977; Porton Asparaginase
Therapeutic Category Antineoplastic Agent
Use Acute lymphocytic leukemia (ALL) in patients sensitive to *E. coli* L-asparaginase
Dosage Forms Injection: 10,000 units

Erwiniar® *see* asparaginase *on page 43*

Eryc® Oral *see* erythromycin *on this page*

Eryderm® Topical *see* erythromycin, topical *on page 201*

Erygel® Topical *see* erythromycin, topical *on page 201*

Erymax® Topical *see* erythromycin, topical *on page 201*

EryPed® Oral *see* erythromycin *on this page*

Ery-Tab® Oral *see* erythromycin *on this page*

erythrityl tetranitrate (e RI thri til te tra NYE trate)
Brand Names Cardilate®
Therapeutic Category Vasodilator
Use Prophylaxis and long-term treatment of frequent or recurrent anginal pain and reduced exercise tolerance associated with angina pectoris
Usual Dosage Adults: Oral: 5 mg under the tongue or in the buccal pouch 3 times/day or 10 mg before meals or food, chewed 3 times/day, increasing in 2-3 days if needed
Dosage Forms Tablet, oral or sublingual: 10 mg

Erythrocin® Oral *see* erythromycin *on this page*

erythromycin (er ith roe MYE sin)
Synonyms erythromycin estolate; erythromycin ethylsuccinate; erythromycin glucceptate; erythromycin lactobionate; erythromycin stearate
Brand Names E.E.S.® Oral; E-Mycin® Oral; Eryc® Oral; EryPed® Oral; Ery-Tab® Oral; Erythrocin® Oral; Ilosone® Oral; PCE® Oral
Therapeutic Category Macrolide (Antibiotic)
Use Treatment of mild to moderately severe infections of the upper and lower respiratory tract, pharyngitis and skin infections due to susceptible streptococci and staphylococci; other susceptible bacterial infections including mycoplasma pneumonia, *Legionella* pneumonia, diphtheria, pertussis, chancroid, *Chlamydia*, and *Campylobacter* gastroenteritis; used in conjunction with neomycin for decontaminating the bowel for surgery; dental procedure prophylaxis in penicillin allergic patients
Usual Dosage
Infants and Children:
Oral: Do not exceed 2 g/day
(Continued)

erythromycin *(Continued)*

Base and ethylsuccinate: 30-50 mg/kg/day divided every 6-8 hours
Estolate: 30-50 mg/kg/day divided every 8-12 hours
Stearate: 20-40 mg/kg/day divided every 6 hours
Pre-op bowel preparation: 20 mg/kg erythromycin base at 1, 2, and 11 PM on the day before surgery combined with mechanical cleansing of the large intestine and oral neomycin
I.V.: Lactobionate: 20-40 mg/kg/day divided every 6 hours, not to exceed 4 g/day
Adults:
Oral:
Base: 333 mg every 8 hours
Estolate, stearate or base: 250-500 mg every 6-12 hours
Ethylsuccinate: 400-800 mg every 6-12 hours
Pre-op bowel preparation: 1 g erythromycin base at 1, 2, and 11 PM on the day before surgery combined with mechanical cleansing of the large intestine and oral neomycin
I.V.: 15-20 mg/kg/day divided every 6 hours or administered as a continuous infusion over 24 hours

Dosage Forms
Erythromycin base:
Capsule:
Delayed release: 250 mg
Delayed release, enteric coated pellets (Eryc®): 250 mg
Tablet:
Delayed release: 333 mg
Enteric coated (E-Mycin®, Ery-Tab®, E-Base®): 250 mg, 333 mg, 500 mg
Film coated: 250 mg, 500 mg
Polymer coated particles (PCE®): 333 mg, 500 mg

Erythromycin estolate:
Capsule (Ilosone® Pulvules®): 250 mg
Suspension, oral (Ilosone®): 125 mg/5 mL (480 mL); 250 mg/5 mL (480 mL)
Tablet (Ilosone®): 500 mg

Erythromycin ethylsuccinate:
Granules for oral suspension (EryPed®): 400 mg/5 mL (60 mL, 100 mL, 200 mL)
Powder for oral suspension (E.E.S.®): 200 mg/5 mL (100 mL, 200 mL)
Suspension:
Oral (E.E.S.®, EryPed®): 200 mg/5 mL (5 mL, 100 mL, 200 mL, 480 mL); 400 mg/5 mL (5 mL, 60 mL, 100 mL, 200 mL, 480 mL)
Oral [drops] (EryPed®): 100 mg/2.5 mL (50 mL)
Tablet (E.E.S.®): 400 mg
Tablet, chewable (EryPed®): 200 mg

Erythromycin gluceptate: Injection: 1000 mg (30 mL)

Erythromycin lactobionate: Powder for injection: 500 mg, 1000 mg

Erythromycin stearate: Tablet, film coated (Eramycin®, Erythrocin®): 250 mg, 500 mg

erythromycin and benzoyl peroxide
(er ith roe MYE sin & BEN zoe il per OKS ide)
Brand Names Benzamycin®
Therapeutic Category Acne Products
Use Topical control of acne vulgaris
Usual Dosage Topical: Apply twice daily (morning and evening)
Dosage Forms Gel: Erythromycin 30 mg and benzoyl peroxide 50 mg per g

erythromycin and sulfisoxazole (er ith roe MYE sin & sul fi SOKS a zole)
Synonyms sulfisoxazole and erythromycin
Brand Names Eryzole®; Pediazole®
Therapeutic Category Macrolide (Antibiotic); Sulfonamide

Use Treatment of susceptible bacterial infections of the upper and lower respiratory tract; otitis media in children caused by susceptible strains of *Haemophilus influenzae*; other infections in patients allergic to penicillin

Usual Dosage Dosage recommendation is based on the product's erythromycin content; Oral:

Children ≥2 months: 40-50 mg/kg/day of erythromycin in divided doses every 6-8 hours; not to exceed 2 g erythromycin or 6 g sulfisoxazole/day or approximately 1.25 mL/kg/day divided every 6-8 hours
Adults: 400 mg erythromycin and 1200 mg sulfisoxazole every 6 hours

Dosage Forms Suspension, oral: Erythromycin ethylsuccinate 200 mg and sulfisoxazole acetyl 600 mg per 5 mL (100 mL, 150 mL, 200 mL, 250 mL)

erythromycin estolate *see* erythromycin *on page 199*
erythromycin ethylsuccinate *see* erythromycin *on page 199*
erythromycin gluceptate *see* erythromycin *on page 199*
erythromycin lactobionate *see* erythromycin *on page 199*
erythromycin stearate *see* erythromycin *on page 199*

erythromycin, topical (er ith roe MYE sin TOP i kal)

Brand Names Akne-Mycin® Topical; A/T/S® Topical; Del-Mycin® Topical; Emgel™ Topical; Eryderm® Topical; Erygel® Topical; Erymax® Topical; E-Solve-2® Topical; ETS-2%® Topical; Ilotycin® Ophthalmic; Staticin® Topical; T-Stat® Topical

Therapeutic Category Acne Products; Antibiotic, Ophthalmic; Antibiotic, Topical

Use Topical treatment of acne vulgaris

Usual Dosage Children and Adults:
Ophthalmic: Instill one or more times daily depending on the severity of the infection
Topical: Apply 2% solution over the affected area twice daily after the skin has been thoroughly washed and patted dry

Dosage Forms
Gel: 2% (30 g, 60 g)
Gel (A/T/S®, Emgel™, Erygel®): 2% (27 g, 30 g, 60 g)
Ointment:
Ophthalmic: 0.5% [5 mg/g] (3.5 g)
Ilotycin®: 0.5% [5 mg/g] (3.5 g)
Topical (Akne-mycin®): 2% (25 g)
Solution, topical:
Staticin®: 1.5% (60 mL)
Akne-mycin®, A/T/S®, Del-Mycin®, Eryderm®, ETS-2%®, Romycin®, Theramycin Z®, T-Stat®: 2% (60 mL, 66 mL, 120 mL)
Pad (T-Stat®): 2% (60s)
Pledgets: 2% (60s)
Swab: 2% (60s)

erythropoietin *see* epoetin alfa *on page 197*
Eryzole® *see* erythromycin and sulfisoxazole *on previous page*
eserine salicylate *see* physostigmine *on page 416*
Esgic® *see* butalbital compound and acetaminophen *on page 78*
Esgic-Plus® *see* butalbital compound and acetaminophen *on page 78*
Esidrix® *see* hydrochlorothiazide *on page 264*
Eskalith® *see* lithium *on page 311*

esmolol (ES moe lol)

Synonyms esmolol hydrochloride
Brand Names Brevibloc® Injection
Therapeutic Category Antiarrhythmic Agent, Class II; Beta-Adrenergic Blocker
(Continued)

esmolol *(Continued)*

Use Supraventricular tachycardia (primarily to control ventricular rate) and hypertension (especially perioperatively)

Usual Dosage Must be adjusted to individual response and tolerance

Children: An extremely limited amount of information regarding esmolol use in pediatric patients is currently available. Some centers have utilized doses of 100-500 mcg/kg administered over 1 minute for control of supraventricular tachycardias. Loading doses of 500 mcg/kg/minute over 1 minute with maximal doses of 50-250 mcg/kg/minute (mean 173) have been used in addition to nitroprusside in a small number of patients (7 patients; 7-19 years of age; median 13 years) to treat postoperative hypertension after coarctation of aorta repair.

Adults: I.V.: Loading dose: 500 mcg/kg over 1 minute; follow with a 50 mcg/kg/minute infusion for 4 minutes; if response is inadequate, rebolus with another 500 mcg/kg loading dose over 1 minute, and increase the maintenance infusion to 100 mcg/kg/minute. Repeat this process until a therapeutic effect has been achieved or to a maximum recommended maintenance dose of 200 mcg/kg/minute. Usual dosage range: 50-200 mcg/kg/minute with average dose = 100 mcg/kg/minute.

Dosage Forms Injection, as hydrochloride: 10 mg/mL (10 mL); 250 mg/mL (10 mL)

esmolol hydrochloride *see esmolol on previous page*

E-Solve-2® Topical *see erythromycin, topical on previous page*

Esoterica® Facial [OTC] *see hydroquinone on page 272*

Esoterica® Regular [OTC] *see hydroquinone on page 272*

Esoterica® Sensitive Skin Formula [OTC] *see hydroquinone on page 272*

Esoterica® Sunscreen [OTC] *see hydroquinone on page 272*

Estar® [OTC] *see coal tar on page 132*

estazolam (es TA zoe lam)

Brand Names ProSom™

Therapeutic Category Benzodiazepine

Controlled Substance C-IV

Use Short-term management of insomnia

Usual Dosage Adults: Oral: 1 mg at bedtime, some patients may require 2 mg

Dosage Forms Tablet: 1 mg, 2 mg

esterified estrogen and methyltestosterone *see estrogens and methyltestosterone on page 204*

esterified estrogens *see estrogens, esterified on page 205*

Estinyl® *see ethinyl estradiol on page 207*

Estivin® II Ophthalmic [OTC] *see naphazoline on page 364*

Estrace® Oral *see estradiol on this page*

Estraderm® Transdermal *see estradiol on this page*

estradiol (es tra DYE ole)

Synonyms estradiol cypionate; estradiol transdermal; estradiol valerate

Brand Names Alora® Transdermal; Climara® Transdermal; depGynogen® Injection; Depo®-Estradiol Injection; Depogen® Injection; Dioval® Injection; Estrace® Oral; Estraderm® Transdermal; Estra-L® Injection; Estring®; Estro-Cyp® Injection; Gynogen L.A.® Injection; Valergen® Injection; Vivelle™ Transdermal

Therapeutic Category Estrogen Derivative

Use Atrophic vaginitis, atrophic dystrophy of vulva, menopausal symptoms, female hypogonadism

Usual Dosage Adults (all dosage needs to be adjusted based upon the patient's response):

Male: Prostate cancer: Valerate:
I.M.: ≥30 mg or more every 1-2 weeks
Oral: 1-2 mg 3 times/day
Female:
Hypogonadism:
Oral: 1-2 mg/day in a cyclic regimen for 3 weeks on drug, then 1 week off drug
I.M.: Cypionate: 1.5-2 mg/month; valerate: 10-20 mg/month
Transdermal: 0.05 mg patch initially (titrate dosage to response) applied twice weekly in a cyclic regimen, for 3 weeks on drug and 1 week off drug
Atrophic vaginitis, kraurosis vulvae: Vaginal: Insert 2-4 g/day for 2 weeks then gradually reduce to ½ the initial dose for 2 weeks followed by a maintenance dose of 1 g 1-3 times/week
Moderate to severe vasomotor symptoms: I.M.:
Cypionate: 1-5 mg every 3-4 weeks
Valerate: 10-20 mg every 4 weeks
Postpartum breast engorgement: I.M.: Valerate: 10-25 mg at end of first stage of labor
Dosage Forms
Cream, vaginal (Estrace®): 0.1 mg/g (42.5 g)
Injection, as cypionate (depGynogen®, Depo®-Estradiol, Depogen®, Dura-Estrin®, Estra-D®, Estro-Cyp®, Estroject-L.A.®): 5 mg/mL (5 mL, 10 mL)
Injection, as valerate:
Valergen®: 10 mg/mL (5 mL, 10 mL); 20 mg/mL (1 mL, 5 mL, 10 mL); 40 mg/mL (5 mL, 10 mL)
Dioval®, Duragen®, Estra-L®, Gynogen L.A.®: 20 mg/mL (10 mL); 40 mg/mL (10 mL)
Tablet, micronized (Estrace®): 1 mg, 2 mg
Transdermal system:
Alora®:
0.05 mg/24 hours [18 cm^2], total estradiol 1.5 mg
0.075 mg/24 hours [27 cm^2], total estradiol 2.3 mg
0.1 mg/24 hours [36 cm^2], total estradiol 3 mg
Climara®:
0.05 mg/24 hours [12.5 cm^2], total estradiol 3.9 mg
0.1 mg/24 hours [25 cm^2], total estradiol 7.8 mg
Estraderm®:
0.05 mg/24 hours [10 cm^2], total estradiol 4 mg
0.1 mg/24 hours [20 cm^2], total estradiol 8 mg
Vivelle®:
0.0375 mg/day
0.05 mg/day
0.075 mg/day
Vaginal ring (Estring®): 2 mg gradually released over 90 days

estradiol and testosterone (es tra DYE ole & tes TOS ter one)
Synonyms estradiol cypionate and testosterone cypionate; estradiol valerate and testosterone enanthate; testosterone and estradiol
Brand Names Andro/Fem® Injection; Deladumone® Injection; depAndrogyn® Injection; Depo-Testadiol® Injection; Depotestogen® Injection; Duo-Cyp® Injection; Duratestrin® Injection; Valertest No.1® Injection
Therapeutic Category Estrogen and Androgen Combination
Use Vasomotor symptoms associated with menopause; postpartum breast engorgement
Usual Dosage Adults (all dosage needs to be adjusted based upon the patient's response)
Dosage Forms Injection:
Andro/Fem®, DepAndrogyn®, Depo-Testadiol®, Depotestogen®, Duo-Cyp®, Duratestrin®: Estradiol cypionate 2 mg and testosterone cypionate 50 mg per mL in cottonseed oil (1 mL, 10 mL)
Androgyn L.A.®, Deladumone®, Estra-Testrin®, Valertest No.1®: Estradiol valerate 4 mg and testosterone enanthate 90 mg per mL in sesame oil (5 mL, 10 mL)

estradiol cypionate *see* estradiol *on page 202*

estradiol cypionate and testosterone cypionate *see* estradiol and testosterone *on previous page*

estradiol transdermal *see* estradiol *on page 202*

estradiol valerate *see* estradiol *on page 202*

estradiol valerate and testosterone enanthate *see* estradiol and testosterone *on previous page*

Estra-L®️ Injection *see* estradiol *on page 202*

estramustine (es tra MUS teen)
Synonyms estramustine phosphate sodium
Brand Names Emcyt®️
Therapeutic Category Antineoplastic Agent
Use Palliative treatment of prostatic carcinoma
Usual Dosage Oral: 1 capsule for each 22 lb/day, in 3-4 divided doses
Dosage Forms Capsule, as phosphate sodium: 140 mg

estramustine phosphate sodium *see* estramustine *on this page*

Estratab®️ *see* estrogens, esterified *on next page*

Estratest®️ *see* estrogens and methyltestosterone *on this page*

Estratest®️ H.S. *see* estrogens and methyltestosterone *on this page*

Estring®️ *see* estradiol *on page 202*

Estro-Cyp®️ Injection *see* estradiol *on page 202*

estrogenic substance aqueous *see* estrone *on next page*

estrogens and medroxyprogesterone
(ES troe jenz & me DROKS ee proe JES te rone)
Brand Names Premphase™️; Prempro™️
Therapeutic Category Estrogen and Progestin Combination
Use Women with an intact uterus for the treatment of moderate to severe vasomotor symptoms associated with the menopause; treatment of atrophic vaginitis; primary ovarian failure; osteoporosis prophylactic
Usual Dosage Adults: Oral:
Premphase™️: Conjugated estrogen 0.625 mg [Premarin®️] and taken orally for 28 days and medroxyprogesterone acetate [Cycrin®️] 5 mg (14s) which are taken orally with a Premarin®️ tablet on days 15 through 28
Prempro™️: Conjugated estrogen 0.625 mg [Premarin®️] and medroxyprogesterone acetate [Cycrin®️] 2.5 mg are taken continuously one each day
Dosage Forms
Premphase™️: Two separate tablets in therapy pack: Conjugated estrogens 0.625 mg [Premarin®️] (28s) taken orally for 28 days and medroxyprogesterone acetate [Cycrin®️] 5 mg (14s) which are taken orally with a Premarin®️ tablet on days 15 through 28
Prempro™️: Conjugated estrogens 0.625 mg and medroxyprogesterone acetate 2.5 mg (14s)

estrogens and methyltestosterone
(ES troe jenz & meth il tes TOS te rone)
Synonyms conjugated estrogen and methyltestosterone; esterified estrogen and methyltestosterone
Brand Names Estratest®️; Estratest®️ H.S.; Premarin®️ With Methyltestosterone
Therapeutic Category Estrogen and Androgen Combination
Use Atrophic vaginitis; hypogonadism; primary ovarian failure; vasomotor symptoms of menopause; prostatic carcinoma; osteoporosis prophylactic

Usual Dosage Oral: Lowest dose that will control symptoms should be chosen, normally administered 3 weeks on and 1 week off

Dosage Forms Tablet:

Estratest®, Menogen®: Esterified estrogen 1.25 mg and methyltestosterone 2.5 mg

Estratest H.S.®, Menogen H.S.®: Esterified estrogen 0.625 mg and methyltestosterone 1.25 mg

Premarin® With Methyltestosterone: Conjugated estrogen 0.625 mg and methyltestosterone 5 mg; conjugated estrogen 1.25 mg and methyltestosterone 10 mg

estrogens, conjugated (ES troe jenz KON joo gate ed)

Synonyms ces; conjugated estrogens

Brand Names Premarin®

Therapeutic Category Estrogen Derivative

Use Dysfunctional uterine bleeding, atrophic vaginitis, hypogonadism, vasomotor symptoms of menopause

Usual Dosage Adults:

Male: Prostate cancer: Oral: 1.25-2.5 mg 3 times/day

Female:

Hypogonadism: Oral: 2.5-7.5 mg/day for 20 days, off 10 days and repeat until menses occur

Abnormal uterine bleeding:

Oral: 2.5-5 mg/day for 7-10 days; then decrease to 1.25 mg/day for 2 weeks

I.V.: 25 mg every 6-12 hours until bleeding stops

Moderate to severe vasomotor symptoms: Oral: 0.625-1.25 mg/day

Postpartum breast engorgement: Oral: 3.75 mg every 4 hours for 5 doses, then 1.25 mg every 4 hours for 5 days

Dosage Forms

Cream, vaginal: 0.625 mg/g (42.5 g)

Injection: 25 mg (5 mL)

Tablet: 0.3 mg, 0.625 mg, 0.9 mg, 1.25 mg, 2.5 mg

estrogens, esterified (ES troe jenz, es TER i fied)

Synonyms esterified estrogens

Brand Names Estratab®; Menest®

Therapeutic Category Estrogen Derivative

Use Atrophic vaginitis; hypogonadism; primary ovarian failure; vasomotor symptoms of menopause; prostatic carcinoma; osteoporosis prophylactic

Usual Dosage Adults: Oral:

Male: Prostate cancer: 1.25-2.5 mg 3 times/day

Female:

Hypogonadism: 2.5-7.5 mg/day for 20 days, off 10 days and repeat until menses occur

Moderate to severe vasomotor symptoms: 0.3-1.25 mg/day

Dosage Forms Tablet: 0.3 mg, 0.625 mg, 1.25 mg, 2.5 mg

estrone (ES trone)

Synonyms estrogenic substance aqueous

Brand Names Aquest®; Kestrone®

Therapeutic Category Estrogen Derivative

Use Atrophic vaginitis; hypogonadism; primary ovarian failure; vasomotor symptoms of menopause; prostatic carcinoma; osteoporosis prophylactic

Usual Dosage Adults: I.M.:

Vasomotor symptoms, atrophic vaginitis: 0.1-0.5 mg 2-3 times/week

Primary ovarian failure, hypogonadism: 0.1-1 mg/week, up to 2 mg/week

Prostatic carcinoma: 2-4 mg 2-3 times/week

Dosage Forms Injection: 2 mg/mL (10 mL, 30 mL); 5 mg/mL (10 mL)

estropipate (ES troe pih pate)
Synonyms piperazine estrone sulfate
Brand Names Ogen® Oral; Ogen® Vaginal; Ortho-Est® Oral
Therapeutic Category Estrogen Derivative
Use Atrophic vaginitis; hypogonadism; primary ovarian failure; vasomotor symptoms of menopause; prostatic carcinoma; osteoporosis prophylactic
Usual Dosage Adults: Female:
Moderate to severe vasomotor symptoms: Oral: 0.625-5 mg/day
Hypogonadism: Oral: 1.25-7.5 mg/day for 3 weeks followed by an 8- to 10-day rest period
Atrophic vaginitis or kraurosis vulvae: Vaginal: Instill 2-4 g/day 3 weeks on and 1 week off
Dosage Forms
Cream, vaginal: 0.15% [estropipate 1.5 mg/g] (42.5 g tube)
Tablet: 0.625 mg [estropipate 0.75 mg]; 1.25 mg [estropipate 1.5 mg]; 2.5 mg [estropipate 3 mg]; 5 mg [estropipate 6 mg]

Estrostep® 21 *see* ethinyl estradiol and norethindrone *on page 209*

Estrostep® Fe *see* ethinyl estradiol and norethindrone *on page 209*

ethacrynic acid (eth a KRIN ik AS id)
Synonyms sodium ethacrynate
Brand Names Edecrin®
Therapeutic Category Diuretic, Loop
Use Management of edema secondary to congestive heart failure; hepatic or renal disease, hypertension
Usual Dosage
Children:
Oral: 25 mg/day to start, increase by 25 mg/day at intervals of 2-3 days as needed, to a maximum of 3 mg/kg/day
I.V.: 1 mg/kg/dose, (maximum: 50 mg/dose); repeat doses not recommended
Adults:
Oral: 50-100 mg/day increased in increments of 25-50 mg at intervals of several days to a maximum of 400 mg/24 hours
I.V.: 0.5-1 mg/kg/dose (maximum: 50 mg/dose); repeat doses not recommended
Dosage Forms
Powder for injection, as ethacrynate sodium: 50 mg (50 mL)
Tablet: 25 mg, 50 mg

ethambutol (e THAM byoo tole)
Synonyms ethambutol hydrochloride
Brand Names Myambutol®
Therapeutic Category Antimycobacterial Agent
Use Treatment of tuberculosis and other mycobacterial diseases in conjunction with other antimycobacterial agents
Usual Dosage Oral (not recommended in children <12 years of age):
Children >12 years: 15 mg/kg/day once daily
Adolescents and Adults: 15-25 mg/kg/day once daily, not to exceed 2.5 g/day
Dosage Forms Tablet, as hydrochloride: 100 mg, 400 mg

ethambutol hydrochloride *see* ethambutol *on this page*

Ethamolin® *see* ethanolamine oleate *on next page*

eth and c *see* terpin hydrate and codeine *on page 506*

ethanoic acid *see* acetic acid *on page 7*

ethanol *see* alcohol, ethyl *on page 14*

ethanolamine oleate (ETH a nol a meen OH lee ate)
Brand Names Ethamolin®
Therapeutic Category Sclerosing Agent
Use Mild sclerosing agent used for bleeding esophageal varices
Usual Dosage Adults: 1.5-5 mL per varix, up to 20 mL total or 0.4 mL/kg; patients with severe hepatic dysfunction should receive less than recommended maximum dose
Dosage Forms Injection: 5% [50 mg/mL] (2 mL)

ethaverine (eth AV er een)
Synonyms ethaverine hydrochloride
Therapeutic Category Vasodilator
Use Peripheral and cerebral vascular insufficiency associated with arterial spasm
Usual Dosage Adults: Oral: 100 mg 3 times/day
Dosage Forms
Capsule, as hydrochloride: 100 mg
Tablet, as hydrochloride: 100 mg

ethaverine hydrochloride see ethaverine on this page

ethchlorvynol (eth klor VI nole)
Brand Names Placidyl®
Therapeutic Category Hypnotic, Nonbarbiturate
Controlled Substance C-IV
Use Short-term management of insomnia
Usual Dosage Oral: 500-1000 mg at bedtime
Dosage Forms Capsule: 200 mg, 500 mg, 750 mg

ethinyl estradiol (ETH in il es tra DYE ole)
Brand Names Estinyl®
Therapeutic Category Estrogen Derivative
Use Atrophic vaginitis; hypogonadism; primary ovarian failure; vasomotor symptoms of menopause; prostatic carcinoma; osteoporosis prophylactic
Usual Dosage Adults: Oral:
Hypogonadism: 0.05 mg 1-3 times/day for 2 weeks
Prostatic carcinoma: 0.15-2 mg/day
Vasomotor symptoms: 0.02-0.05 mg for 21 days, off 7 days and repeat
Dosage Forms Tablet: 0.02 mg, 0.05 mg, 0.5 mg

ethinyl estradiol and desogestrel
(ETH in il es tra DYE ole & des oh JES trel)
Synonyms desogestrel and ethinyl estradiol
Brand Names Desogen®; Ortho-Cept®
Therapeutic Category Contraceptive, Oral
Use Prevention of pregnancy
Usual Dosage Contraception: Oral: 1 tablet daily, beginning on day 5 of menstrual cycle (first day of menstrual flow is day 1). With 21-tablet packages, new dosing cycle begins 7 days after last tablet taken. With 28-tablet packages, dosage is 1 tablet daily without interruption; extra tablets are placebos, If next menstrual period does not begin on schedule, rule out pregnancy before starting new dosing cycle. If menstrual period begins, start new dosing cycle 7 days after last tablet was taken. if all doses have been taken on schedule and 1 menstrual period is missed, continue dosing cycle. If 2 consecutive menstrual periods are missed, pregnancy test is required before new dosing cycle is started.

One dose missed: Take as soon as remembered or take 2 tablets next day
Two doses missed: Take 2 tablets as soon as remembered or 2 tablets next 2 days
Three doses missed: Begin new compact of tablets starting on day 1 of next cycle
(Continued)

ethinyl estradiol and desogestrel *(Continued)*

Dosage Forms Tablet: Ethinyl estradiol 0.03 mg and desogestrel 0.15 mg (21s, 28s)

ethinyl estradiol and ethynodiol diacetate

(ETH in il es tra DYE ole & e thye noe DYE ole dye AS e tate)

Synonyms ethynodiol diacetate and ethinyl estradiol

Brand Names Demulen®; Zovia®

Therapeutic Category Contraceptive, Oral

Use Prevention of pregnancy; treatment of hypermenorrhea, endometriosis, female hypogonadism

Usual Dosage

For 21-tablet cycle packs, with 21 active tablets (28-day packs have 21 active tablets and 7 inert tablets): Administer 1 tablet daily starting on the fifth day of menstrual cycle, with day 1 being the first day of menstruation; begin taking a new cycle pack on the eighth day after taking the last tablet from the previous pack

With 28-tablet packages, dosage is 1 tablet daily without interruption; extra tablets are placebos or contain iron. If next menstrual period does not begin on schedule, rule out pregnancy before starting new dosing cycle. If menstrual period begins, start new dosing cycle 7 days after last tablet was administered. If all doses have been administered on schedule and 1 menstrual period is missed, continue dosing cycle. If 2 consecutive menstrual periods are missed, pregnancy test is required before new dosing cycle is started.

One dose missed: Administer as soon as remembered or administer 2 tablets next day

Two doses missed: Administer 2 tablets as soon as remembered or 2 tablets next 2 days

Three doses missed: Begin new compact of tablets starting on day 1 of next cycle

Dosage Forms Tablet:

1/35: Ethinyl estradiol 0.035 mg and ethynodiol diacetate 1 mg (21s, 28s)

1/50: Ethinyl estradiol 0.05 mg and ethynodiol diacetate 1 mg (21s, 28s)

ethinyl estradiol and levonorgestrel

(ETH in il es tra DYE ole & LEE voe nor jes trel)

Synonyms levonorgestrel and ethinyl estradiol

Brand Names Alesse®; Levlen®; Levora®; Nordette®; Tri-Levlen®; Triphasil®

Therapeutic Category Contraceptive, Oral

Use Prevention of pregnancy; treatment of hypermenorrhea, endometriosis, female hypogonadism

Usual Dosage

Contraception: Oral: 1 tablet daily, beginning on day 5 of menstrual cycle (first day of menstrual flow is day 1). With 20-tablet and 21-tablet packages, new dosing cycle begins 7 days after last tablet taken. With 28-tablet packages, dosage is 1 tablet daily without interruption; extra tablets are placebos or contain iron. If next menstrual period does not begin on schedule, rule out pregnancy before starting new dosing cycle. If menstrual period begins, start new dosing cycle 7 days after last tablet was taken. if all doses have been taken on schedule and 1 menstrual period is missed, continue dosing cycle. If 2 consecutive menstrual periods are missed, pregnancy test is required before new dosing cycle is started.

Triphasic oral contraceptive: 1 tablet/day in the sequence specified by the manufacturer

Dosage Forms Tablet:

Alesse®: Ethinyl estradiol 0.02 mg and levonorgestrel 0.1 mg (21s, 28s)

Levlen®, Levora®, Nordette®: Ethinyl estradiol 0.03 mg and levonorgestrel 0.15 mg (21s, 28s)

Tri-Levlen®, Triphasil®: Phase 1 (6 brown tablets): Ethinyl estradiol 0.03 mg and levonorgestrel 0.05 mg; Phase 2 (5 white tablets): Ethinyl estradiol 0.04 mg and levonorgestrel 0.075 mg; Phase 3 (10 yellow tablets): Ethinyl estradiol 0.03 mg and levonorgestrel 0.125 mg (21s, 28s)

ethinyl estradiol and norethindrone

(ETH in il es tra DYE ole & nor eth IN drone)

Synonyms norethindrone acetate and ethinyl estradiol

Brand Names Brevicon®; Estrostep® 21; Estrostep® Fe; Genora® 0.5/35; Genora® 1/35; Jenest-28™; Loestrin®; Modicon™; N.E.E.® 1/35; Nelova™ 0.5/35E; Nelova™ 10/11; Norethin™ 1/35E; Norinyl® 1+35; Ortho-Novum® 1/35; Ortho-Novum® 7/7/7; Ortho-Novum® 10/11; Ovcon® 35; Ovcon® 50; Tri-Norinyl®

Therapeutic Category Contraceptive, Oral

Use Prevention of pregnancy; treatment of hypermenorrhea, endometriosis, female hypogonadism

Usual Dosage

For 21-tablet cycle packs, with 21 active tablets (28-day packs have 21 active tablets and 7 inert tablets): Administer 1 tablet daily starting on the fifth day of menstrual cycle, with day 1 being the first day of menstruation; begin taking a new cycle pack on the eighth day after taking the last tablet from the previous pack

With 28-tablet packages, dosage is 1 tablet daily without interruption; extra tablets are placebos or contain iron. If next menstrual period does not begin on schedule, rule out pregnancy before starting new dosing cycle. If menstrual period begins, start new dosing cycle 7 days after last tablet was administered. If all doses have been administered on schedule and 1 menstrual period is missed, continue dosing cycle. If 2 consecutive menstrual periods are missed, pregnancy test is required before new dosing cycle is started.

One dose missed: Administer as soon as remembered or administer 2 tablets next day

Two doses missed: Administer 2 tablets as soon as remembered or 2 tablets next 2 days

Three doses missed: Begin new compact of tablets starting on day 1 of next cycle

Biphasic oral contraceptive (Ortho-Novum™ 10/11): 1 color tablet/day for 10 days, then next color tablet for 11 days

Triphasic oral contraceptive (Ortho-Novum™ 7/7/7, Tri-Norinyl®, Triphasil®): 1 tablet/day in the sequence specified by the manufacturer

Dosage Forms Tablet:

Brevicon®, Genora® 0.5/35, Modicon™, Nelova™ 0.5/35E: Ethinyl estradiol 0.035 mg and norethindrone 0.5 mg (21s, 28s)

Estrostep®:

Triangular tablet (white): Ethinyl estradiol 0.02 mg and norethindrone acetate 1 mg

Square tablet (white): Ethinyl estradiol 0.03 mg and norethindrone acetate 1 mg

Round tablet (white): Ethinyl estradiol 0.035 mg and norethindrone acetate 1 mg

Estrostep® Fe:

Triangular tablet (white): Ethinyl estradiol 0.02 mg and norethindrone acetate 1 mg

Square tablet (white): Ethinyl estradiol 0.03 mg and norethindrone acetate 1 mg

Round tablet (white): Ethinyl estradiol 0.035 mg and norethindrone acetate 1 mg

Brown tablet: Ferrous fumarate 75 mg

Loestrin® 1.5/30: Ethinyl estradiol 0.03 mg and norethindrone acetate 1.5 mg (21s)

Loestrin® Fe 1.5/30: Ethinyl estradiol 0.03 mg and norethindrone acetate 1.5 mg with ferrous fumarate 75 mg in 7 inert tablets (28s)

Loestrin® 1/20: Ethinyl estradiol 0.02 mg and norethindrone acetate 1 mg (21s)

Loestrin® Fe 1/20: Ethinyl estradiol 0.02 mg and norethindrone acetate 1 mg with ferrous fumarate 75 mg in 7 inert tablets (28s)

Genora® 1/35, N.E.E.® 1/35, Nelova® 1/35E, Norethin™ 1/35E, Norinyl® 1+35, Ortho-Novum® 1/35: Ethinyl estradiol 0.035 mg and norethindrone 1 mg (21s, 28s)

Jenest-28™: Phase 1 (7 white tablets): Ethinyl estradiol 0.035 mg and norethindrone 0.5 mg; Phase 2 (14 peach tablets): Ethinyl estradiol 0.035 mg and norethindrone 1 mg and 7 green inert tablets (28s)

Ortho-Novum® 7/7/7: Phase 1 (7 white tablets): Ethinyl estradiol 0.035 mg and norethindrone 0.5 mg; Phase 2 (7 light peach tablets): Ethinyl estradiol 0.035 mg and norethindrone 0.75 mg; Phase 3 (7 peach tablets): Ethinyl estradiol 0.035 mg and norethindrone 1 mg (21s, 28s)

(Continued)

ethinyl estradiol and norethindrone *(Continued)*

Ortho-Novum® 10/11: Phase 1 (10 white tablets): Ethinyl estradiol 0.035 mg and norethindrone 0.5 mg; Phase 2 (11 dark yellow tablets): Ethinyl estradiol 0.035 mg and norethindrone 1 mg (21s, 28s)

Ovcon® 35: Ethinyl estradiol 0.035 mg and norethindrone 0.4 mg (21s, 28s)

Ovcon® 50: Ethinyl estradiol 0.050 mg and norethindrone 1 mg (21s, 28s)

Tri-Norinyl®: Phase 1 (7 blue tablets): Ethinyl estradiol 0.035 mg and norethindrone 0.5 mg; Phase 2 (9 green tablets): Ethinyl estradiol 0.035 mg and norethindrone 1 mg; Phase 3 (5 blue tablets): Ethinyl estradiol 0.035 mg and norethindrone 0.5 mg (21s, 28s)

ethinyl estradiol and norgestimate

(ETH in il es tra DYE ole & nor JES ti mate)

Synonyms norgestimate and ethinyl estradiol

Brand Names Ortho-Cyclen®; Ortho Tri-Cyclen®

Therapeutic Category Contraceptive, Oral

Use Prevention of pregnancy

Usual Dosage

Contraception: Oral: 1 tablet daily, beginning on day 5 of menstrual cycle (first day of menstrual flow is day 1). With 21-tablet packages, new dosing cycle begins 7 days after last tablet administered. With 28-tablet packages, dosage is 1 tablet daily without interruption; extra tablets are placebos or contain iron. If next menstrual period does not begin on schedule, rule out pregnancy before starting new dosing cycle. If menstrual period begins, start new dosing cycle 7 days after last tablet was administered. If all doses have been administered on schedule and 1 menstrual period is missed, continue dosing cycle. If 2 consecutive menstrual periods are missed, pregnancy test is required before new dosing cycle is started.

One dose missed: Administer as soon as remembered or administer 2 tablets next day

Two doses missed: Administer 2 tablets as soon as remembered or 2 tablets next 2 days

Three doses missed: Begin new compact of tablets starting on day 1 of next cycle

Triphasic oral contraceptive: 1 tablet/day in the sequence specified by the manufacturer

Dosage Forms Tablet:

Ortho-Cyclen®: Ethinyl estradiol 0.035 mg and norgestimate 0.25 mg (21s, 28s)

Ortho Tri-Cyclen®: Phase 1 (7 white tablets): Ethinyl estradiol 0.035 mg and norgestimate 0.18 mg; Phase 2 (5 light blue tablets): Ethinyl estradiol 0.035 mg and norgestimate 0.215 mg; Phase 3 (10 blue tablets): Ethinyl estradiol 0.035 mg and norgestimate 0.25 mg (21s, 28s)

ethinyl estradiol and norgestrel (ETH in il es tra DYE ole & nor JES trel)

Synonyms norgestrel and ethinyl estradiol

Brand Names Lo/Ovral®; Ovral®

Therapeutic Category Contraceptive, Oral

Use Prevention of pregnancy; treatment of hypermenorrhea, endometriosis, female hypogonadism

Usual Dosage Contraception: Oral: 1 tablet daily, beginning on day 5 of menstrual cycle (first day of menstrual flow is day 1). With 20-tablet and 21-tablet packages, new dosing cycle begins 7 days after last tablet administered; with 28-tablet packages, dosage is 1 tablet daily without interruption; extra tablets are placebos or contain iron. If next menstrual period does not begin on schedule, rule out pregnancy before starting new dosing cycle; if menstrual period begins, start new dosing cycle 7 days after last tablet was administered; if all doses have been administered on schedule and 1 menstrual period is missed, continue dosing cycle; if two consecutive menstrual periods are missed, pregnancy test is required before new dosing cycle is started.

One dose missed: Administer as soon as remembered or administer 2 tablets next day

Two doses missed: Administer 2 tablets as soon as remembered or 2 tablets next 2 days

Three doses missed: Begin new compact of tablets starting on day 1 of next cycle
Dosage Forms Tablet:
Lo/Ovral®: Ethinyl estradiol 0.03 mg and norgestrel 0.3 mg (21s and 28s)
Ovral®: Ethinyl estradiol 0.05 mg and norgestrel 0.5 mg (21s and 28s)

Ethiodol® *see* radiological/contrast media (ionic) *on page 457*

ethiofos *see* amifostine *on page 24*

ethionamide (e thye on AM ide)

Brand Names Trecator®-SC
Therapeutic Category Antimycobacterial Agent
Use In conjunction with other antituberculosis agents in the treatment of tuberculosis and other mycobacterial diseases
Usual Dosage Oral:
Children: 15-20 mg/kg/day in 2 divided doses, not to exceed 1 g/day
Adults: 500-1000 mg/day in 1-3 divided doses
Dosage Forms Tablet, sugar coated: 250 mg

Ethmozine® *see* moricizine *on page 356*

ethosuximide (eth oh SUKS i mide)

Brand Names Zarontin®
Therapeutic Category Anticonvulsant
Use Management of absence (petit mal) seizures, myoclonic seizures, and akinetic epilepsy
Usual Dosage Oral:
Children 3-6 years: Initial: 250 mg; increment: 250 mg/day at 4- to 7-day intervals; maintenance: 20-40 mg/kg/day; maximum: 1500 mg/day in 2 divided doses
Children >6 years and Adults: Initial: 500 mg/day; maintenance: 20-40 mg/kg/day; increment: 250 mg/day at 4- to 7-day intervals; maximum: 1500 mg/day in 2 divided doses
Dosage Forms
Capsule: 250 mg
Syrup (raspberry flavor): 250 mg/5 mL (473 mL)

ethotoin (ETH oh toyn)

Synonyms ethylphenylhydantoin
Brand Names Peganone®
Therapeutic Category Hydantoin
Use Generalized tonic-clonic or complex-partial seizures
Usual Dosage Oral:
Children: 250 mg twice daily, up to 250 mg 4 times/day
Adults: 250 mg 4 times/day after meals, may be increased up to 3 g/day in divided doses 4 times/day
Dosage Forms Tablet: 250 mg, 500 mg

ethoxynaphthamido penicillin sodium *see* nafcillin *on page 361*

Ethrane® *see* enflurane *on page 193*

ethyl aminobenzoate *see* benzocaine *on page 59*

ethyl chloride (ETH il KLOR ide)

Synonyms chloroethane
Therapeutic Category Local Anesthetic
Use Local anesthetic in minor operative procedures and to relieve pain caused by insect stings and burns, and irritation caused by myofascial and visceral pain syndromes
Usual Dosage Topical: Dosage varies with use
Dosage Forms Spray: 100 mL, 120 mL

ethyl chloride and dichlorotetrafluoroethane
(ETH il KLOR ide & dye klor oh te tra floo or oh ETH ane)

Synonyms dichlorotetrafluoroethane and ethyl chloride

Brand Names Fluro-Ethyl® Aerosol

Therapeutic Category Local Anesthetic

Use Topical refrigerant anesthetic to control pain associated with minor surgical procedures, dermabrasion, injections, contusions, and minor strains

Usual Dosage Topical: Press gently on side of spray valve allowing the liquid to emerge as a fine mist approximately 2" to 4" from site of application

Dosage Forms Aerosol: Ethyl chloride 25% and dichlorotetrafluoroethane 75% (225 g)

ethylphenylhydantoin *see* ethotoin *on previous page*

ethynodiol diacetate and ethinyl estradiol *see* ethinyl estradiol and ethynodiol diacetate *on page 208*

Ethyol® *see* amifostine *on page 24*

etidocaine (e TI doe kane)

Synonyms etidocaine hydrochloride

Brand Names Duranest® Injection

Therapeutic Category Local Anesthetic

Use Infiltration anesthesia; peripheral nerve blocks; central neural blocks

Usual Dosage Varies with procedure; use 1% for peripheral nerve block, central nerve block, lumbar peridural caudal; use 1.5% for maxillary infiltration or inferior alveolar nerve block; use 1% or 1.5% for intra-abdominal or pelvic surgery, lower limb surgery, or caesarean section

Dosage Forms
Injection, as hydrochloride: 1% [10 mg/mL] (30 mL)
With epinephrine 1:200,000: 1% [10 mg/mL] (30 mL); 1.5% [15 mg/mL] (20 mL)

etidocaine hydrochloride *see* etidocaine *on this page*

etidronate disodium (e ti DROE nate dye SOW dee um)

Synonyms ehdp; sodium etidronate

Brand Names Didronel®

Therapeutic Category Bisphosphonate Derivative

Use Symptomatic treatment of Paget's disease and heterotopic ossification due to spinal cord injury; hypercalcemia associated with malignancy

Usual Dosage Adults: Oral:
Paget's disease: 5 mg/kg/day administered every day for no more than 6 months; may administer 10 mg/kg/day for up to 3 months. Daily dose may be divided if adverse GI effects occur.
Heterotopic ossification with spinal cord injury: 20 mg/kg/day for 2 weeks, then 10 mg/kg/day for 10 weeks (this dosage has been used in children, however, treatment greater than 1 year has been associated with a rachitic syndrome)
Hypercalcemia associated with malignancy: I.V.: 7.5 mg/kg/day for 3 days

Dosage Forms
Injection: 50 mg/mL (6 mL)
Tablet: 200 mg, 400 mg

etodolac (ee toe DOE lak)

Synonyms etodolic acid

Brand Names Lodine®; Lodine® XL

Therapeutic Category Analgesic, Non-narcotic; Nonsteroidal Anti-Inflammatory Agent (NSAID)

Use Acute and long-term use in the management of signs and symptoms of osteoarthritis and management of pain

Usual Dosage Adults: Oral:
Acute pain: 200-400 mg every 6-8 hours, as needed, not to exceed total daily doses of 1200 mg
Osteoarthritis: Initial: 800-1200 mg/day administered in divided doses: 400 mg 2 or 3 times/day; 300 mg 2, 3 or 4 times/day; 200 mg 3 or 4 times/day; total daily dose should not exceed 1200 mg; for patients weighing <60 kg, total daily dose should not exceed 20 mg/kg; extended release dose: one tablet daily

Dosage Forms
Capsule (Lodine®): 200 mg, 300 mg
Tablet: 400 mg
Lodine®: 400 mg
Tablet, extended release (Lodine® XL): 400 mg, 600 mg

etodolic acid *see* etodolac *on previous page*

etodolac (e TOM i date)
Brand Names Amidate® Injection
Therapeutic Category General Anesthetic
Use Induction of general anesthesia
Usual Dosage Children >10 years and Adults: I.V.: 0.2-0.6 mg/kg over period of 30-60 seconds
Dosage Forms Injection: 2 mg/mL (10 mL, 20 mL)

Etopophos® *see* etoposide phosphate *on this page*
Etopophos® Injection *see* etoposide *on this page*

etoposide (e toe POE side)
Synonyms epeg; vp-16
Brand Names Etopophos® Injection; Toposar® Injection; VePesid® Injection; VePesid® Oral
Therapeutic Category Antineoplastic Agent
Use Treatment of testicular and lung carcinomas, malignant lymphoma, Hodgkin's disease, leukemias (ALL, AML), neuroblastoma; also used in the treatment of Ewing's sarcoma, rhabdomyosarcoma, Wilms' tumor, brain tumors, and as a conditioning regimen for bone marrow transplantation in patients with advanced hematologic malignancies
Usual Dosage Refer to individual protocols
Pediatric solid tumors: I.V.: 60-120 mg/m²/day for 3-5 days every 3-6 weeks
Leukemia in children: I.V.: 100-200 mg/m²/day for 5 days
Testicular cancer: I.V.: 50-100 mg/m²/day on days 1-5 or 100 mg/m²/day on days 1, 3 and 5 every 3-4 weeks for 3-4 courses
Small cell lung cancer:
Oral: Twice the I.V. dose rounded to the nearest 50 mg administered once daily if total dose ≤400 mg or in divided doses if >400 mg
I.V.: 35 mg/m²/day for 4 days or 50 mg/m²/day for 5 days every 3-4 weeks
Dosage Forms
Capsule: 50 mg
Injection: 20 mg/mL (5 mL, 10 mL, 25 mL)
Powder for injection, lyophilized, as phosphate: 119.3 mg (100 mg base)

etoposide phosphate (e toe POE side FOS fate)
Brand Names Etopophos®
Therapeutic Category Antineoplastic Agent, Irritant; Antineoplastic Agent, Podophyllotoxin Derivative; Vesicant
Use Treatment of refractory testicular tumors and small cell lung cancer
Usual Dosage Refer to individual protocols
(Continued)

etoposide phosphate *(Continued)*

Adults:

Small cell lung cancer:

I.V. (in combination with other approved chemotherapeutic drugs): **Equivalent doses of etoposide phosphate to an etoposide dosage** range of 35 mg/m^2/day for 4 days to 50 mg/m^2/day for 5 days. Courses are repeated at 3- to 4-week intervals after adequate recovery from any toxicity.

Testicular cancer:

I.V. (in combination with other approved chemotherapeutic agents): **Equivalent dose of etoposide phosphate to etoposide dosage** range of 50-100 mg/m^2/day on days 1-5 to 100 mg/m^2/day on days 1, 3, and 5. Courses are repeated at 3- to 4-week intervals after adequate recovery from any toxicity.

Dosage adjustment in renal impairment:

Cl$_{cr}$ 15-50 mL/minute: Administer 75% of normal dose

Cl$_{cr}$ <15 mL minute: Data are not available and further dose reduction should be considered in these patients.

Hemodialysis: Supplemental dose is not necessary

Peritoneal dialysis: Supplemental dose is not necessary

CAPD effects: Unknown

CAVH effects: Unknown

Dosage adjustment in hepatic impairment:

Bilirubin 1.5-3 mg/dL or AST 60-180 units: Reduce dose by 50%

Bilirubin 3-5 mg/dL or AST >180 units: Reduce by 75%

Bilirubin >5 mg/dL: Do not administer

Dosage Forms Powder for injection, lyophilized: 119.3 mg (100 mg base)

Etrafon® *see* amitriptyline and perphenazine *on page 27*

etretinate (e TRET i nate)

Brand Names Tegison®

Therapeutic Category Antipsoriatic Agent

Use Treatment of severe recalcitrant psoriasis in patients intolerant of or unresponsive to standard therapies

Usual Dosage Adults: Oral: Individualized; Initial: 0.75-1 mg/kg/day in divided doses up to 1.5 mg/kg/day; maintenance dose established after 8-10 weeks of therapy 0.5-0.75 mg/kg/day

Dosage Forms Capsule: 10 mg, 25 mg

ETS-2%® **Topical** *see* erythromycin, topical *on page 201*

Eudal-SR® *see* guaifenesin and pseudoephedrine *on page 250*

Eulexin® *see* flutamide *on page 232*

Eurax® **Topical** *see* crotamiton *on page 141*

Eutron® *see* methyclothiazide and pargyline *on page 340*

Evac-Q-Mag® **[OTC]** *see* magnesium citrate *on page 318*

Evalose® *see* lactulose *on page 300*

Everone® **Injection** *see* testosterone *on page 507*

E-Vista® *see* hydroxyzine *on page 275*

E-Vitamin® **[OTC]** *see* vitamin e *on page 553*

Exact® **Cream [OTC]** *see* benzoyl peroxide *on page 61*

Excedrin®, **Extra Strength [OTC]** *see* acetaminophen, aspirin, and caffeine *on page 5*

Excedrin® **P.M. [OTC]** *see* acetaminophen and diphenhydramine *on page 4*

Exelderm® **Topical** *see* sulconazole *on page 495*

Exidine® **Scrub [OTC]** *see* chlorhexidine gluconate *on page 109*

Ex-Lax®, **Extra Gentle Pills [OTC]** *see* docusate and phenolphthalein *on page 180*

Exna® *see* benzthiazide *on page 62*

Exosurf® **Neonatal**™ *see* colfosceril palmitate *on page 136*

Exsel® *see* selenium sulfide *on page 476*

Extendryl® **SR** *see* chlorpheniramine, phenylephrine, and methscopolamine *on page 116*

Extra Action Cough Syrup [OTC] *see* guaifenesin and dextromethorphan *on page 248*

Extra Strength Adprin-B® **[OTC]** *see* aspirin *on page 44*

Extra Strength Bayer® **Enteric 500 Aspirin [OTC]** *see* aspirin *on page 44*

Extra Strength Bayer® **Plus [OTC]** *see* aspirin *on page 44*

Extra Strength Doan's® **[OTC]** *see* magnesium salicylate *on page 319*

Extra Strength Dynafed® **E.X. [OTC]** *see* acetaminophen *on page 3*

Eye-Lube-A® **Solution [OTC]** *see* artificial tears *on page 42*

Eye-Sed® **Ophthalmic [OTC]** *see* zinc sulfate *on page 561*

Eyesine® **Ophthalmic [OTC]** *see* tetrahydrozoline *on page 510*

Ezide® *see* hydrochlorothiazide *on page 264*

f₃t *see* trifluridine *on page 533*

factor ix complex (human) (FAK ter nyne KOM pleks HYU man)

Brand Names AlphaNine® SD; Konȳne® 80; Mononine®; Profilnine® Heat-Treated; Proplex® SX-T; Proplex® T

Therapeutic Category Blood Product Derivative

Use To control bleeding in patients with Factor IX deficiency (Hemophilia B or Christmas Disease); prevention/control of bleeding in hemophilia A patients with inhibitors to factor VIII; Proplex® T is indicated to prevent or control bleeding due to factor VII deficiency

Usual Dosage Factor IX deficiency (1 unit/kg raises IX levels 1%)

Children and Adults: I.V.:

Hospitalized patients: 20-50 units/kg/dose; may be higher in special cases; may be administered every 24 hours or more often in special cases

Inhibitor patients: 75-100 units/kg/dose; may be administered every 6-12 hours

Dosage Forms Injection:

AlphaNine® SD: Single dose vial

Konȳne® 80: 10 mL, 20 mL

Mononine®: 250 units, 500 units, 1000 units

Profilnine® Heat-Treated: Single dose vial

Proplex® SX-T: Vial

Proplex® T: Vial

factor viii *see* antihemophilic factor (human) *on page 37*

factor viii:c (porcine) (an tee hee moe FIL ik FAK ter POR seen)

Brand Names Hyate®:C

Therapeutic Category Blood Product Derivative

Use Treatment of congenital hemophiliacs with antibodies to human factor VIII:C and also for previously nonhemophiliac patients with spontaneously acquired inhibitors to human factor VIII:C; patients with inhibitors who are bleeding or who are to undergo surgery

Usual Dosage Clinical response should be used to assess efficacy rather than relying upon a particular laboratory value for recovery of factor VIII:C.

(Continued)

215

factor viii:c (porcine) *(Continued)*

Initial dose:
Antibody level to human factor VIII:C <50 Bethesda units/mL: 100-150 porcine units/kg (body weight) is recommended

Antibody level to human factor VIII:C >50 Bethesda units/mL: Activity of the antibody to porcine factor VIII:C should be determined; **an antiporcine antibody level** >20 Bethesda units/mL indicates that the patient is unlikely to benefit from treatment; for lower titers, a dose of 100-150 porcine units/kg is recommended

If a patient has previously been treated with Hyate®:C, this may provide a guide to his likely response and, therefore, assist in estimation of the preliminary dose

Subsequent doses: Following administration of the initial dose, if the recovery of factor VIII:C in the patient's plasma is not sufficient, a further higher dose should be administered; if recovery after the second dose is still insufficient, a third and higher dose may prove effective

Dosage Forms Powder for injection, lyophilized: 400-700 porcine units to be reconstituted with 20 mL sterile water

factor VIII recombinant *see* antihemophilic factor (recombinant) *on page 37*

Factrel® *see* gonadorelin *on page 245*

famciclovir (fam SYE kloe veer)

Brand Names Famvir™
Therapeutic Category Antiviral Agent
Use Management of acute herpes zoster (shingles)
Usual Dosage Adults: Oral: 500 mg every 8 hours for 7 days
Dosage Forms Tablet: 125 mg, 250 mg, 500 mg

famotidine (fa MOE ti deen)

Brand Names Pepcid®; Pepcid® AC Acid Controller [OTC]
Therapeutic Category Histamine H_2 Antagonist
Use Therapy and treatment of duodenal ulcer, gastric ulcer, control gastric pH in critically ill patients, symptomatic relief in gastritis, gastroesophageal reflux, active benign ulcer, and pathological hypersecretory conditions
Usual Dosage
Children: Oral, I.V.: Doses of 1-2 mg/kg/day have been used; maximum dose: 40 mg
Adults:
Oral:
Duodenal ulcer, gastric ulcer: 40 mg/day at bedtime for 4-8 weeks
Hypersecretory conditions: Initial: 20 mg every 6 hours, may increase up to 160 mg every 6 hours
GERD: 20 mg twice daily for 6 weeks
I.V.: 20 mg every 12 hours
Dosage Forms
Infusion, premixed in NS: 20 mg (50 mL)
Injection: 10 mg/mL (2 mL, 4 mL)
Powder for oral suspension (cherry-banana-mint flavor): 40 mg/5 mL (50 mL)
Tablet, film coated: 20 mg, 40 mg
Pepcid® AC Acid Controller: 10 mg

Famvir™ *see* famciclovir *on this page*

fat emulsion (fat e MUL shun)

Brand Names Intralipid®; Liposyn®; Nutrilipid®; Soyacal®
Therapeutic Category Intravenous Nutritional Therapy
Use Source of calories and essential fatty acids for patients requiring parenteral nutrition of extended duration
Usual Dosage Fat emulsion should not exceed 60% of the total daily calories

Initial dose:

Premature infants: 0.25-0.5 g/kg/day, increase by 0.25-0.5 g/kg/day to a maximum of 3-4 g/kg/day; maximum rate of infusion: 0.15 g/kg/hour (0.75 mL/kg/hour of 20% solution)

Infants and Children: 0.5-1 g/kg/day, increase by 0.5 g/kg/day to a maximum of 3-4 g/kg/day; maximum rate of infusion: 0.25 g/kg/hour (1.25 mL/kg/hour of 20% solution)

Adolescents and Adults: 1 g/kg/day, increase by 0.5-1 g/kg/day to a maximum of 2.5 g/kg/day; maximum rate of infusion: 0.25 g/kg/hour (1.25 mL/kg/hour of 20% solution); do not exceed 50 mL/hour (20%) or 100 mL/hour (10%)

Fatty acid deficiency: Children and Adults: 8% to 10% of total caloric intake; infuse once or twice weekly

Note: At the onset of therapy, the patient should be observed for any immediate allergic reactions such as dyspnea, cyanosis, and fever. Slower initial rates of infusion may be used for the first 10-15 minutes of the infusion (eg, 0.1 mL/minute of 10% or 0.05 mL/minute of 20% solution).

Dosage Forms Injection: 10% [100 mg/mL] (100 mL, 250 mL, 500 mL); 20% [200 mg/mL] (100 mL, 250 mL, 500 mL)

5-fc see flucytosine on page 225

Fedahist® Expectorant [OTC] see guaifenesin and pseudoephedrine on page 250

Fedahist® Expectorant Pediatric [OTC] see guaifenesin and pseudoephedrine on page 250

Fedahist® Tablet [OTC] see chlorpheniramine and pseudoephedrine on page 114

Feen-a-Mint® Pills [OTC] see docusate and phenolphthalein on page 180

Feiba VH Immuno® see anti-inhibitor coagulant complex on page 37

felbamate (FEL ba mate)

Brand Names Felbatol™

Therapeutic Category Anticonvulsant

Use Not a first-line agent; reserved for patients who do not adequately respond to alternative agents and whose epilepsy is so severe that benefit outweighs risk of liver failure or aplastic anemia; used as monotherapy and adjunctive therapy in patients ≥14 years of age with partial seizures with and without secondary generalization; adjunctive therapy in children ≥2 years of age who have partial and generalized seizures associated with Lennox-Gastaut syndrome

Usual Dosage Oral:

Monotherapy: 1200 mg/day in divided doses 3 or 4 times/day; titrate previously untreated patients under close clinical supervision, increasing the dosage in 600 mg increments every 2 weeks to 2400 mg/day based on clinical response and thereafter to 3600 mg/day in clinically indicated

Conversion to monotherapy: Initiate at 1200 mg/day in divided doses 3 or 4 times/day, reduce the dosage of the concomitant anticonvulsant(s) by 33% at the initiation of felbamate therapy; at week 2, increase the felbamate dosage to 2400 mg/day while reducing the dosage of the other anticonvulsant(s) up to an additional 33% of their original dosage; at week 3, increase the felbamate dosage up to 3600 mg/day and continue to reduce the dosage of the other anticonvulsant(s) as clinically indicated

Adjunctive therapy:
Week 1:
Felbamate: 1200 mg/day initial dose
Concomitant anticonvulsant(s): Reduce original dosage by 20% to 33%
Week 2:
Felbamate: 2400 mg/day (Therapeutic range)
Concomitant anticonvulsant(s): Reduce original dosage by up to an additional 33%
Week 3:
Felbamate: 3600 mg/day (Therapeutic range)
(Continued)

felbamate *(Continued)*

Concomitant anticonvulsant(s): Reduce original dosage as clinically indicated
Dosage Forms
Suspension, oral: 600 mg/5 mL (240 mL, 960 mL)
Tablet: 400 mg, 600 mg

Felbatol™ *see* felbamate *on previous page*

Feldene® *see* piroxicam *on page 420*

felodipine (fe LOE di peen)

Brand Names Plendil®
Therapeutic Category Calcium Channel Blocker
Use Management of angina pectoris due to coronary insufficiency, hypertension
Usual Dosage Oral:
Adults: Initial: 5 mg once daily; dosage range: 2.5-10 mg once daily; may increase dose up to a maximum of 10 mg
Elderly: Initial: 2.5 mg/day
Dosage Forms Tablet, extended release: 2.5 mg, 5 mg, 10 mg

Femcet® *see* butalbital compound and acetaminophen *on page 78*

Femguard® *see* sulfabenzamide, sulfacetamide, and sulfathiazole *on page 496*

Femilax® [OTC] *see* docusate and phenolphthalein *on page 180*

Femiron® [OTC] *see* ferrous fumarate *on page 220*

Femizole-7® [OTC] *see* clotrimazole *on page 131*

Femizol-M® [OTC] *see* miconazole *on page 348*

Fenesin™ *see* guaifenesin *on page 247*

Fenesin DM® *see* guaifenesin and dextromethorphan *on page 248*

fenofibrate (fen oh FYE brate)

Synonyms procetofene; proctofene
Brand Names Lipidil®
Therapeutic Category Antihyperlipidemic Agent, Miscellaneous
Use Adjunct to dietary therapy for the treatment of adults with very high elevations of serum triglyceride levels (types IV and V hyperlipidemia) who are at risk of pancreatitis and who do not respond adequately to a determined dietary effort; its efficacy can be enhanced by combination with other hypolipidemic agents that have a different mechanism of action; safety and efficacy may be greater than that of clofibrate
Usual Dosage Oral:
Children >10 years: 5 mg/kg/day
Adults: 100 mg 3 times/day with meals or 200 mg in the morning and 100 mg in the evening
Dosage Forms Capsule: 100 mg

fenoprofen (fen oh PROE fen)

Synonyms fenoprofen calcium
Brand Names Nalfon®
Therapeutic Category Analgesic, Non-narcotic; Nonsteroidal Anti-Inflammatory Agent (NSAID)
Use Symptomatic treatment of acute and chronic rheumatoid arthritis and osteoarthritis; relief of mild to moderate pain
Usual Dosage Oral:
Children: Juvenile arthritis: 900 mg/m^2/day, then increase over 4 weeks to 1.8 g/m^2/day
Adults:
Arthritis: 300-600 mg 3-4 times/day up to 3.2 g/day
Pain: 200 mg every 4-6 hours as needed

Dosage Forms
Capsule, as calcium: 200 mg, 300 mg
Tablet, as calcium: 600 mg

fenoprofen calcium *see* fenoprofen *on previous page*

fentanyl (FEN ta nil)

Synonyms fentanyl citrate
Brand Names Duragesic™ Transdermal; Fentanyl Oralet®; Sublimaze® Injection
Therapeutic Category Analgesic, Narcotic; General Anesthetic
Controlled Substance C-II
Use Sedation; relief of pain; preoperative medication; adjunct to general or regional anesthesia; management of chronic pain (transdermal product)
Oral transmucosal: Hospital setting use only as preoperative anesthetic agent or to induce conscious sedation before procedures
Usual Dosage Doses should be titrated to appropriate effects; wide range of doses, dependent upon desired degree of analgesia/anesthesia
Children:
Sedation for minor procedures/analgesia: I.M., I.V.:
1-3 years: 2-3 mcg/kg/dose; may repeat after 30-60 minutes as required
3-12 years: 1-2 mcg/kg/dose; may repeat at 30- to 60-minute intervals as required.
Note: Children 18-36 months of age may require 2-3 mcg/kg/dose
Continuous sedation/analgesia: Initial I.V. bolus: 1-2 mcg/kg then 1 mcg/kg/hour; titrate upward; usual: 1-3 mcg/kg/hour
Transdermal: Not recommended
Children <12 years and Adults:
Sedation for minor procedures/analgesia: 0.5-1 mcg/kg/dose; higher doses are used for major procedures
Preoperative sedation, adjunct to regional anesthesia, postoperative pain: I.M., I.V.: 50-100 mcg/dose
Adjunct to general anesthesia: I.M., I.V.: 2-50 mcg/kg
General anesthesia without additional anesthetic agents: I.V. 50-100 mcg/kg with O_2 and skeletal muscle relaxant
Transdermal: Initial: 25 mcg/hour system; if currently receiving opiates, convert to fentanyl equivalent and administer equianalgesic dosage (see package insert for further information)
Dosage Forms
Injection, as citrate: 0.05 mg/mL (2 mL, 5 mL, 10 mL, 20 mL, 50 mL)
Lozenge, oral transmucosal (raspberry flavored): 200 mcg, 300 mcg, 400 mcg
Transdermal system: 25 mcg/hour [10 cm^2]; 50 mcg/hour [20 cm^2]; 75 mcg/hour [30 cm^2]; 100 mcg/hour [40 cm^2] (all available in 5s)

fentanyl and droperidol *see* droperidol and fentanyl *on page 186*

fentanyl citrate *see* fentanyl *on this page*

Fentanyl Oralet® *see* fentanyl *on this page*

Feosol® [OTC] *see* ferrous sulfate *on page 221*

Feostat® [OTC] *see* ferrous fumarate *on next page*

Ferancee® [OTC] *see* ferrous salt and ascorbic acid *on next page*

Feratab® [OTC] *see* ferrous sulfate *on page 221*

Fergon® [OTC] *see* ferrous gluconate *on next page*

Fer-In-Sol® [OTC] *see* ferrous sulfate *on page 221*

Fer-Iron® [OTC] *see* ferrous sulfate *on page 221*

Fero-Grad 500® [OTC] *see* ferrous salt and ascorbic acid *on next page*

Fero-Gradumet® [OTC] *see* ferrous sulfate *on page 221*

Ferospace® **[OTC]** *see ferrous sulfate on next page*

Ferralet® **[OTC]** *see ferrous gluconate on this page*

Ferralyn® Lanacaps® **[OTC]** *see ferrous sulfate on next page*

Ferra-TD® **[OTC]** *see ferrous sulfate on next page*

Ferro-Sequels® **[OTC]** *see ferrous fumarate on this page*

ferrous fumarate (FER us FYOO ma rate)
Brand Names Femiron® [OTC]; Feostat® [OTC]; Ferro-Sequels® [OTC]; Fumasorb® [OTC]; Fumerin® [OTC]; Hemocyte® [OTC]; Ircon® [OTC]; Nephro-Fer™ [OTC]; Span-FF® [OTC]
Therapeutic Category Electrolyte Supplement
Use Prevention and treatment of iron deficiency anemias
Usual Dosage Oral:
  Children: 3 mg/kg 3 times/day
  Adults: 200 mg 3-4 times/day
Dosage Forms Amount of elemental iron is listed in brackets
  Capsule, controlled release (Span-FF®): 325 mg [106 mg]
  Drops (Feostat®): 45 mg/0.6 mL [15 mg/0.6 mL] (60 mL)
  Suspension, oral (Feostat®): 100 mg/5 mL [33 mg/5 mL] (240 mL)
  Tablet: 325 mg [106 mg]
   Chewable (chocolate flavor) (Feostat®): 100 mg [33 mg]
   Femiron®: 63 mg [20 mg]
   Fumerin®: 195 mg [64 mg]
   Fumasorb®, Ircon®: 200 mg [66 mg]
   Hemocyte®: 324 mg [106 mg]
   Nephro-Fer™: 350 mg [115 mg]
   Timed release (Ferro-Sequels®): Ferrous fumarate 150 mg [50 mg] and docusate sodium 100 mg

ferrous gluconate (FER us GLOO koe nate)
Brand Names Fergon® [OTC]; Ferralet® [OTC]; Simron® [OTC]
Therapeutic Category Electrolyte Supplement
Use Prevention and treatment of iron deficiency anemias
Usual Dosage Oral (dose expressed in terms of elemental iron):
  Iron deficiency anemia: 3-6 Fe mg/kg/day in 3 divided doses
  Maintenance:
   Preterm infants:
    Birthweight <1000 g: 4 Fe mg/kg/day
    Birthweight 1000-1500 g: 3 Fe mg/kg/day
    Birthweight 1500-2500 g: 2 Fe mg/kg/day
   Term Infants and Children: 1-2 Fe mg/kg/day in 3 divided doses, up to a maximum of 18 Fe mg/day
   Adults: 60-100 Fe mg/day in 3 divided doses
Dosage Forms Amount of elemental iron is listed in brackets
  Capsule, soft gelatin (Simron®): 86 mg [10 mg]
  Elixir (Fergon®): 300 mg/5 mL [34 mg/5 mL] with alcohol 7% (480 mL)
  Tablet: 300 mg [34 mg]; 325 mg [38 mg]
  Fergon®, Ferralet®: 320 mg [37 mg]
  Sustained release (Ferralet® Slow Release): 320 mg [37 mg]

ferrous salt and ascorbic acid (FER us SUL fate & a SKOR bik AS id)
Synonyms ascorbic acid and ferrous sulfate
Brand Names Ferancee® [OTC]; Fero-Grad 500® [OTC]
Therapeutic Category Vitamin
Use Treatment of iron deficiency in nonpregnant adults; treatment and prevention of iron deficiency in pregnant adults

Usual Dosage Adults: Oral: 1 tablet daily

Dosage Forms Amount of elemental iron is listed in brackets

Caplet, sustained release (Ferromar®): Ferrous fumarate 201.5 mg [65 mg] and ascorbic acid 200 mg

Tablet (Fero-Grad 500®): Ferrous sulfate 525 mg [105 mg] and ascorbic acid 500 mg

Chewable (Ferancee®): Ferrous fumarate 205 mg [67 mg] and ascorbic acid 150 mg

ferrous sulfate (FER us SUL fate)

Synonyms $FeSO_4$

Brand Names Feosol® [OTC]; Feratab® [OTC]; Fer-In-Sol® [OTC]; Fer-Iron® [OTC]; Fero-Gradumet® [OTC]; Ferospace® [OTC]; Ferralyn® Lanacaps® [OTC]; Ferra-TD® [OTC]; Mol-Iron® [OTC]; Slow FE® [OTC]

Therapeutic Category Electrolyte Supplement

Use Prevention and treatment of iron deficiency anemias

Usual Dosage Oral (dose expressed in terms of elemental iron):

Children:

Severe iron deficiency anemia: 4-6 mg Fe/kg/day in 3 divided doses

Mild to moderate iron deficiency anemia: 3 mg Fe/kg/day in 1-2 divided doses

Prophylaxis: 1-2 mg Fe/kg/day up to a maximum of 15 mg/day

Adults: Iron deficiency: 60-100 Fe/kg/day in divided doses

Dosage Forms Amount of elemental iron is listed in brackets

Capsule:

Exsiccated, timed release (Feosol®): 159 mg [50 mg]

Exsiccated, timed release (Ferralyn® Lanacaps®, Ferra-TD®): 250 mg [50 mg]

Ferospace®: 250 mg [50 mg]

Drops, oral:

Fer-In-Sol®: 75 mg/0.6 mL [15 mg/0.6 mL] (50 mL)

Fer-Iron®: 125 mg/mL [25 mg/mL] (50 mL)

Elixir (Feosol®): 220 mg/5 mL [44 mg/5 mL] with alcohol 5% (473 mL, 4000 mL)

Syrup (Fer-In-Sol®): 90 mg/5 mL [18 mg/5 mL] with alcohol 5% (480 mL)

Tablet: 324 mg [65 mg]

Exsiccated (Feosol®) 200 mg [65 mg]

Exsiccated, timed release (Slow FE®): 160 mg [50 mg]

Feratab®: 300 mg [60 mg]

Mol-Iron®: 195 mg [39 mg]

Timed release (Fero-Gradumet®): 525 mg [105 mg]

ferrous sulfate, ascorbic acid, and vitamin b-complex

(FER us SUL fate, a SKOR bik AS id, & VYE ta min bee KOM pleks)

Brand Names Iberet®-Liquid [OTC]

Therapeutic Category Vitamin

Use Treatment of conditions of iron deficiency with an increased need for B-complex vitamins and vitamin C

Usual Dosage Oral:

Children 1-3 years: 5 mL twice daily after meals

Children >4 years and Adults: 10 mL 3 times/day after meals

Dosage Forms Liquid:

Ferrous sulfate: 78.75 mg

Ascorbic acid: 375 mg

B_1: 4.5 mg

B_2: 4.5 mg

B_3: 22.5 mg

B_5: 7.5 mg

B_6: 3.75 mg

B_{12}: 18.75 mg all per 15 mL

ferrous sulfate, ascorbic acid, vitamin b-complex, and folic acid
(FER us SUL fate, a SKOR bik AS id, VYE ta min bee KOM pleks, & FOE lik AS id)
Brand Names Iberet-Folic-500®
Therapeutic Category Vitamin
Use Treatment of iron deficiency and prevention of concomitant folic acid deficiency where there is an associated deficient intake or increased need for B-complex vitamins
Usual Dosage Adults: Oral: 1 tablet daily
Dosage Forms Tablet, controlled release:
Ferrous sulfate: 105 mg
Ascorbic acid: 500 mg
B_1: 6 mg
B_2: 6 mg
B_3: 30 mg
B_5: 10 mg
B_6: 5 mg
B_{12}: 25 mcg
Folic acid: 800 mcg

Fertinex® Injection *see* urofollitropin *on page 543*

FeSO$_4$ *see* ferrous sulfate *on previous page*

Feverall™ [OTC] *see* acetaminophen *on page 3*

Feverall™ Sprinkle Caps [OTC] *see* acetaminophen *on page 3*

fexofenadine (feks oh FEN a deen)
Synonyms fexofenadine hydrochloride
Brand Names Allegra®
Therapeutic Category Antihistamine
Use Nonsedating antihistamine indicated for the relief of seasonal allergic rhinitis
Usual Dosage Children ≥12 years and Adults: Oral: 1 capsule (60 mg) twice daily
Dosage Forms Capsule, as hydrochloride: 60 mg

fexofenadine hydrochloride *see* fexofenadine *on this page*

Fiberall® Chewable Tablet [OTC] *see* calcium polycarbophil *on page 86*

Fiberall® Powder [OTC] *see* psyllium *on page 451*

Fiberall® Wafer [OTC] *see* psyllium *on page 451*

FiberCon® Tablet [OTC] *see* calcium polycarbophil *on page 86*

Fiber-Lax® Tablet [OTC] *see* calcium polycarbophil *on page 86*

fibrinolysin and desoxyribonuclease
(fye brin oh LYE sin & des oks i rye boe NOO klee ase)
Synonyms desoxyribonuclease and fibrinolysin
Brand Names Elase-Chloromycetin® Topical; Elase® Topical
Therapeutic Category Enzyme
Use Debriding agent; cervicitis; and irrigating agent in infected wounds
Usual Dosage Topical:
Ointment: 2-3 times/day
Wet dressing: 3-4 times/day
Dosage Forms
Ointment, topical:
Elase®: Fibrinolysin 1 unit and desoxyribonuclease 666.6 units per g (10 g, 30 g)
Elase-Chloromycetin®: Fibrinolysin 1 unit and desoxyribonuclease 666.6 units per g with chloramphenicol 10 mg per g (10 g, 30 g)
Powder, dry: Fibrinolysin 25 units and desoxyribonuclease 15,000 units per 30 g

filgrastim (fil GRA stim)

Synonyms g-csf; granulocyte colony stimulating factor
Brand Names Neupogen®
Therapeutic Category Colony Stimulating Factor
Use To reduce the duration of neutropenia and the associated risk of infection in patients with nonmyeloid malignancies receiving myelosuppressive chemotherapeutic regimens associated with a significant incidence of severe neutropenia with fever; it has also been used in AIDS patients on zidovudine and in patients with noncancer chemotherapy-induced neutropenia
Usual Dosage Children and Adults (refer to individual protocols): I.V., S.C.: 5-10 mcg/kg/day (~150-300 mcg/m²/day) once daily for up to 14 days until ANC = 10,000/mm³; dose escalations at 5 mcg/kg/day may be required in some individuals when response at 5 mcg/kg/day is not adequate; dosages of 0.6-120 mcg/kg/day have been used in children ranging in age from 3 months to 18 years
Dosage Forms Injection, preservative free: 300 mcg/mL (1 mL, 1.6 mL)

Filibon® [OTC] *see* vitamin, multiple (prenatal) *on page 554*

finasteride (fi NAS teer ide)

Brand Names Proscar®
Therapeutic Category Antiandrogen
Use Early data indicate that finasteride is useful in the treatment of benign prostatic hyperplasia
Usual Dosage Adults: Benign prostatic hyperplasia: Oral: 5 mg/day as a single dose; clinical responses occur within 12 weeks to 6 months of initiation of therapy; long-term administration is recommended for maximal response
Dosage Forms Tablet, film coated: 5 mg

Fiorgen PF® *see* butalbital compound and aspirin *on page 78*

Fioricet® *see* butalbital compound and acetaminophen *on page 78*

Fiorinal® *see* butalbital compound and aspirin *on page 78*

Fiorinal® With Codeine *see* butalbital compound and codeine *on page 78*

fisalamine *see* mesalamine *on page 331*

FK506 *see* tacrolimus *on page 502*

Flagyl® *see* metronidazole *on page 346*

Flarex® *see* fluorometholone *on page 229*

Flatulex® [OTC] *see* simethicone *on page 480*

Flavorcee® [OTC] *see* ascorbic acid *on page 42*

flavoxate (fla VOKS ate)

Synonyms flavoxate hydrochloride
Brand Names Urispas®
Therapeutic Category Antispasmodic Agent, Urinary
Use Antispasmodic to provide symptomatic relief of dysuria, nocturia, suprapubic pain, urgency, and incontinence
Usual Dosage Children >12 years and Adults: Oral: 100-200 mg 3-4 times/day
Dosage Forms Tablet, film coated, as hydrochloride: 100 mg

flavoxate hydrochloride *see* flavoxate *on this page*

Flaxedil® *see* gallamine triethiodide *on page 236*

flecainide (fle KAY nide)

Synonyms flecainide acetate
Brand Names Tambocor™
(Continued)

flecainide (Continued)

Therapeutic Category Antiarrhythmic Agent, Class I-C

Use Prevention and suppression of documented life-threatening ventricular arrhythmias (ie, sustained ventricular tachycardia); prevention of symptomatic, disabling supraventricular tachycardias in patients without structural heart disease

Usual Dosage Oral:

Children: Initial: 3 mg/kg/day in 3 divided doses; usual 3-6 mg/kg/day in 3 divided doses; up to 11 mg/kg/day for uncontrolled patients with subtherapeutic levels

Adults: Initial: 100 mg every 12 hours, increase by 100 mg/day (administer in 2 doses/ day) every 4 days to maximum of 400 mg/day; for patients receiving 400 mg/day who are not controlled and have trough concentrations <0.6 mcg/mL, dosage may be increased to 600 mg/day

Dosage Forms Tablet, as acetate: 50 mg, 100 mg, 150 mg

flecainide acetate see flecainide on previous page

Fleet® Babylax® Rectal [OTC] see glycerin on page 243

Fleet® Enema [OTC] see sodium phosphate on page 486

Fleet® Flavored Castor Oil [OTC] see castor oil on page 95

Fleet® Laxative [OTC] see bisacodyl on page 67

Fleet® Pain Relief [OTC] see pramoxine on page 432

Fleet® Phospho®-Soda [OTC] see sodium phosphate on page 486

Flexaphen® see chlorzoxazone on page 120

Flexeril® see cyclobenzaprine on page 143

Flo-Coat® see radiological/contrast media (ionic) on page 457

Flolan® Injection see epoprostenol on page 197

Flomax™ see tamsulosin on page 502

Flonase™ see fluticasone on page 232

Florical® [OTC] see calcium carbonate on page 82

Florinef® Acetate see fludrocortisone acetate on next page

Florone® see diflorasone on page 167

Florone E® see diflorasone on page 167

Floropryl® Ophthalmic see isoflurophate on page 290

Florvite® see vitamin, multiple (pediatric) on page 554

Flovent® see fluticasone on page 232

Floxin® see ofloxacin on page 382

floxuridine (floks YOOR i deen)

Synonyms fluorodeoxyuridine

Brand Names FUDR®

Therapeutic Category Antineoplastic Agent

Use Palliative management of carcinomas of head, neck, and brain as well as liver, gallbladder, and bile ducts

Usual Dosage Adults:

Intra-arterial infusion: 0.1-0.6 mg/kg/day for 14 days followed by heparinized saline for 14 days

Investigational: I.V.: 0.5-1 mg/kg/day for 6-15 days

Dosage Forms

Injection, preservative free: 100 mg/mL (5 mL)

Powder for injection: 500 mg (5 mL, 10 mL)

flubenisolone see betamethasone on page 64

fluconazole (floo KOE na zole)

Brand Names Diflucan®

Therapeutic Category Antifungal Agent

Use Treatment of susceptible fungal infections including oropharyngeal, esophageal, and vaginal candidiasis; treatment of systemic candidal infections including urinary tract infection, peritonitis, cystitis, and pneumonia; treatment and suppression of cryptococcal meningitis; prophylaxis of candidiasis in patients undergoing bone marrow transplantation; alternative to amphotericin B in patients with pre-existing renal impairment or when requiring concomitant therapy with other potentially nephrotoxic drugs

Usual Dosage Daily dose of fluconazole is the same for oral and I.V. administration

Infants & Children: Oral, I.V.: Safety profile of fluconazole has been studied in 577 children ages 1 day to 17 years. Doses as high as 12 mg/kg/day once daily (equivalent to adult doses of 400 mg/day) have been used to treat candidiasis in immunocompromised children; 10-12 mg/kg/day doses once daily have been used prophylactically against fungal infections in pediatric bone marrow transplantation patients. Do not exceed 600 mg/day.

Adults:

Vaginal candidiasis: Oral: 150 mg single dose

Prophylaxis against fungal infections in bone marrow transplantation patients: Oral, I.V.: 400 mg/day once daily

Dosage Forms

Injection: 2 mg/mL (100 mL, 200 mL)

Powder for oral suspension: 10 mg/mL (35 mL); 40 mg/mL (35 mL)

Tablet: 50 mg, 100 mg, 150 mg, 200 mg

flucytosine (floo SYE toe seen)

Synonyms 5-fc; 5-flurocytosine

Brand Names Ancobon®

Therapeutic Category Antifungal Agent

Use In combination with amphotericin B in the treatment of serious *Candida, Aspergillus, Cryptococcus*, and *Torulopsis* infections

Usual Dosage Children and Adults: Oral: 50-150 mg/kg/day in divided doses every 6 hours

Dosage Forms Capsule: 250 mg, 500 mg

Fludara® *see* fludarabine *on this page*

fludarabine (floo DARE a been)

Synonyms fludarabine phosphate

Brand Names Fludara®

Therapeutic Category Antineoplastic Agent

Use Treatment of B-cell chronic lymphocytic leukemia unresponsive to previous therapy with an alkylating agent containing regimen. Fludarabine has been tested in patients with refractory acute lymphocytic leukemia and acute nonlymphocytic leukemia, but required a highly toxic dose to achieve response.

Usual Dosage Adults: I.V.:

Chronic lymphocytic leukemia: 25 mg/m²/day over a 30-minute period for 5 days

Non-Hodgkin's lymphoma: Loading dose: 20 mg/m² followed by 30 mg/m²/day for 48 hours

Dosage Forms Powder for injection, as phosphate, lyophilized: 50 mg (6 mL)

fludarabine phosphate *see* fludarabine *on this page*

fludrocortisone acetate (floo droe KOR ti sone AS e tate)

Synonyms fluohydrocortisone acetate; 9α-fluorohydrocortisone acetate

Brand Names Florinef® Acetate

Therapeutic Category Adrenal Corticosteroid (Mineralocorticoid)

(Continued)

fludrocortisone acetate *(Continued)*

Use Addison's disease; partial replacement therapy for adrenal insufficiency; treatment of salt-losing forms of congenital adrenogenital syndrome; has been used with increased sodium intake for the treatment of idiopathic orthostatic hypotension
Usual Dosage Oral:
Infants and Children: 0.05-0.1 mg/day
Adults: 0.05-0.2 mg/day
Dosage Forms Tablet: 0.1 mg

Flumadine® *see* rimantadine *on page 466*

flumazenil (FLO may ze nil)
Brand Names Romazicon™
Therapeutic Category Antidote
Use Benzodiazepine antagonist; reverses sedative effects of benzodiazepines used in general anesthesia or conscious sedation; management of benzodiazepine overdose; not indicated for ethanol, barbiturate, general anesthetic or narcotic overdose
Usual Dosage Reversal of conscious sedation or general anesthesia: 0.2 mg (2 mL) administered I.V. over 15 seconds; if desired effect is not achieved after 60 seconds, repeat in 0.2 mg (2 mL) increments every 60 seconds up to a total of 1 mg (10 mL); in event of resedation, repeat doses may be administered at 20-minute intervals with no more than 1 mg (10 mL) administered at any one time, with a maximum of 3 mg in any 1 hour
Dosage Forms Injection: 0.1 mg/mL (5 mL, 10 mL)

flunisolide (floo NIS oh lide)
Brand Names AeroBid®-M Oral Aerosol Inhaler; AeroBid® Oral Aerosol Inhaler; Nasalide® Nasal Aerosol; Nasarel® Nasal Spray
Therapeutic Category Adrenal Corticosteroid
Use Steroid-dependent asthma; nasal solution is used for seasonal or perennial rhinitis
Usual Dosage
Children:
Oral inhalation: >6 years: 2 inhalations twice daily up to 4 inhalations/day
Nasal: 6-14 years: 1 spray each nostril 2-3 times/day, not to exceed 4 sprays/day each nostril
Adults:
Oral inhalation: 2 inhalations twice daily up to 8 inhalations/day
Nasal: 2 sprays each nostril twice daily; maximum dose: 8 sprays/day in each nostril
Dosage Forms
Inhalant:
Nasal (Nasalide®): 25 mcg/actuation [200 sprays] (25 mL)
Oral:
AeroBid®: 250 mcg/actuation [100 metered doses] (7 g)
AeroBid-M® (menthol flavor): 250 mcg/actuation [100 metered doses] (7 g)
Solution, spray: 0.025% [200 actuations] (25 mL)

fluocinolone (floo oh SIN oh lone)
Synonyms fluocinolone acetonide
Brand Names Derma-Smoothe/FS®; Fluonid®; Flurosyn®; FS Shampoo®; Synalar®; Synalar-HP®; Synemol®
Therapeutic Category Corticosteroid, Topical
Use Relief of susceptible inflammatory dermatosis
Usual Dosage Children and Adults: Topical: Apply 2-4 times/day
Dosage Forms
Cream, as acetonide: 0.01% (15 g, 60 g); 0.025% (15 g, 60 g)
Flurosyn®, Synalar®: 0.01% (15 g, 30 g, 60 g, 425 g)
Flurosyn®, Synalar®, Synemol®: 0.025% (15 g, 60 g, 425 g)

Synalar-HP®: 0.2% (12 g)
Ointment, topical, as acetonide: 0.025% (15 g, 60 g)
Flurosyn®, Synalar®: 0.025% (15 g, 30 g, 60 g, 425 g)
Oil, as acetonide (Derma-Smoothe/FS®): 0.01% (120 mL)
Shampoo, as acetonide (FS Shampoo®): 0.01% (180 mL)
Solution, topical, as acetonide: 0.01% (20 mL, 60 mL)
Fluonid®, Synalar®: 0.01% (20 mL, 60 mL)

fluocinolone acetonide *see* fluocinolone *on previous page*

fluocinonide (floo oh SIN oh nide)
Brand Names Lidex®; Lidex-E®
Therapeutic Category Corticosteroid, Topical
Use Inflammation of corticosteroid-responsive dermatoses
Usual Dosage Children and Adults: Topical: Apply thin layer to affected area 2-4 times/ day depending on the severity of the condition
Dosage Forms
Cream: 0.05% (15 g, 30 g, 60 g, 120 g)
Anhydrous, emollient (Lidex®): 0.05% (15 g, 30 g, 60 g, 120 g)
Aqueous, emollient (Lidex-E®): 0.05% (15 g, 30 g, 60 g, 120 g)
Gel, topical: 0.05% (15 g, 60 g)
Lidex®: 0.05% (15 g, 30 g, 60 g, 120 g)
Ointment, topical: 0.05% (15 g, 30 g, 60 g)
Lidex®: 0.05% (15 g, 30 g, 60 g, 120 g)
Solution, topical: 0.05% (20 mL, 60 mL)
Lidex®: 0.05% (20 mL, 60 mL)

Fluogen® *see* influenza virus vaccine *on page 283*

fluohydrocortisone acetate *see* fludrocortisone acetate *on page 225*

Fluonid® *see* fluocinolone *on previous page*

Fluoracaine® Ophthalmic *see* proparacaine and fluorescein *on page 444*

fluorescein sodium (FLURE e seen SOW dee um)
Synonyms soluble fluorescein
Brand Names AK-Fluor® Injection; Fluorescite® Injection; Fluorets® Ophthalmic Strips; Fluor-I-Strip®; Fluor-I-Strip-AT®; Flurate® Ophthalmic Solution; Fluress® Ophthalmic Solution; Ful-Glo® Ophthalmic Strips; Funduscein® Injection
Therapeutic Category Diagnostic Agent
Use Demonstrates defects of corneal epithelium; diagnostic aid in ophthalmic angiography
Usual Dosage
Injection: Perform intradermal skin test before use to avoid possible allergic reaction
Children: 3.5 mg/lb (7.5 mg/kg) injected rapidly into antecubital vein
Adults: 500-750 mg injected rapidly into antecubital vein
Strips: Moisten with sterile water or irrigating solution, touch conjunctiva with moistened tip, blink several times after application
Topical solution: Instill 1-2 drops, allow a few seconds for staining, then wash out excess with sterile irrigation solution
Dosage Forms
Injection (AK-Fluor®, Fluorescite®, Funduscein®, Ophthifluor®): 10% [100 mg/mL] (5 mL); 25% [250 mg/mL] (2 mL, 3 mL)
Ophthalmic:
Solution: 2% [20 mg/mL] (1 mL, 2 mL, 15 mL)
Flurate®, Fluress®: 0.25% [2.5 mg/mL] with benoxinate 0.4% (5 mL)
Strip:
Ful-Glo®: 0.6 mg
Fluorets®, Fluor-I-Strip-AT®: 1 mg
(Continued)

fluorescein sodium *(Continued)*
Fluor-I-Strip®: 9 mg

Fluorescite® Injection *see* fluorescein sodium *on previous page*

Fluorets® Ophthalmic Strips *see* fluorescein sodium *on previous page*

fluoride (FLOR ide)
Synonyms acidulated phosphate fluoride; sodium fluoride; stannous fluoride

Brand Names ACT® [OTC]; Fluorigard® [OTC]; Fluorinse®; Fluoritab®; Flura-Drops®; Flura-Loz®; Gel-Kam®; Gel-Tin® [OTC]; Karidium®; Karigel®; Karigel®-N; Listermint® with Fluoride [OTC]; Luride®; Luride® Lozi-Tab®; Luride®-SF Lozi-Tab®; Minute-Gel®; Pediaflor®; Pharmaflur®; Phos-Flur®; Point-Two®; PreviDent®; Stop® [OTC]; Thera-Flur®; Thera-Flur-N®

Therapeutic Category Mineral, Oral

Use Prevention of dental caries

Usual Dosage Oral: Dental rinse or gel:

Children 6-12 years: 5-10 mL rinse or apply to teeth and spit daily after brushing

Adults: 10 mL rinse or apply to teeth and spit daily after brushing

Dosage Forms Fluoride ion content listed in brackets

Drops, oral, as sodium:

Fluoritab®, Flura-Drops®: 0.55 mg/drop [0.25 mg/drop] (22.8 mL, 24 mL)

Karidium®, Luride®: 0.275 mg/drop [0.125 mg/drop] (30 mL, 60 mL)

Pediaflor®: 1.1 mg/mL [0.5 mg/mL] (50 mL)

Gel, topical:

Acidulated phosphate fluoride (Minute-Gel®): 1.23% (480 mL)

Sodium fluoride (Karigel®, Karigel®-N, PreviDent®): 1.1% [0.5%] (24 g, 30 g, 60 g, 120 g, 130 g, 250 g)

Stannous fluoride (Gel-Kam®, Gel-Tin®, Stop®): 0.4% [0.1%] (60 g, 65 g, 105 g, 120 g)

Lozenge, as sodium (Flura-Loz®) (raspberry flavor): 2.2 mg [1 mg]

Rinse, topical, as sodium:

ACT®, Fluorigard®: 0.05% [0.02%] (90 mL, 180 mL, 300 mL, 360 mL, 480 mL)

Fluorinse®, Point-Two®: 0.2% [0.09%] (240 mL, 480 mL, 3780 mL)

Listermint® with Fluoride: 0.02% [0.01%] (180 mL, 300 mL, 360 mL, 480 mL, 540 mL, 720 mL, 960 mL, 1740 mL)

Solution, oral, as sodium (Phos-Flur®): 0.44 mg/mL [0.2 mg/mL] (250 mL, 500 mL, 3780 mL)

Tablet, as sodium:

Chewable:

Fluoritab®, Luride Lozi-Tab®, Pharmaflur®: 1.1 mg [0.5 mg]

Fluoritab®, Karidium®, Luride® Lozi-Tab®, Luride®-SF Lozi-Tab®, Pharmaflur®: 2.2 mg [1 mg]

Oral: Flura®, Karidium®: 2.2 mg [1 mg]

Fluorigard® [OTC] *see* fluoride *on this page*

Fluori-Methane® Topical Spray *see* dichlorodifluoromethane and trichloromonofluoromethane *on page 164*

Fluorinse® *see* fluoride *on this page*

Fluor-I-Strip® *see* fluorescein sodium *on previous page*

Fluor-I-Strip-AT® *see* fluorescein sodium *on previous page*

Fluoritab® *see* fluoride *on this page*

fluorodeoxyuridine *see* floxuridine *on page 224*

9α-fluorohydrocortisone acetate *see* fludrocortisone acetate *on page 225*

fluorometholone (flure oh METH oh lone)
Brand Names Flarex®; Fluor-Op®; FML®; FML® Forte
Therapeutic Category Adrenal Corticosteroid
Use Inflammatory conditions of the eye, including keratitis, iritis, cyclitis, and conjunctivitis
Usual Dosage Children >2 years and Adults: Ophthalmic: 1-2 drops into conjunctival sac every hour during day, every 2 hours at night until favorable response is obtained, then use 1 drop every 4 hours; in mild or moderate inflammation: 1-2 drops into conjunctival sac 2-4 times/day. Ointment may be applied every 4 hours in severe cases or 1-3 times/day in mild to moderate cases.
Dosage Forms Ophthalmic:
Ointment (FML®): 0.1% (3.5 g)
Suspension:
Flarex®, Fluor-Op®, FML®: 0.1% (2.5 mL, 5 mL, 10 mL)
FML® Forte: 0.25% (2 mL, 5 mL, 10 mL, 15 mL)

Fluor-Op® *see* fluorometholone *on this page*

Fluoroplex® Topical *see* fluorouracil *on this page*

fluorouracil (flure oh YOOR a sil)
Synonyms 5-fluorouracil; 5-fu
Brand Names Adrucil® Injection; Efudex® Topical; Fluoroplex® Topical
Therapeutic Category Antineoplastic Agent
Use Treatment of carcinoma of stomach, colon, rectum, breast, and pancreas; also used topically for management of multiple actinic keratoses and superficial basal cell carcinomas
Usual Dosage Children and Adults (refer to individual protocol):
I.V.: Initial: 12 mg/kg/day (maximum: 800 mg/day) for 4-5 days; maintenance: 6 mg/kg every other day for 4 doses
Single weekly bolus dose of 15 mg/kg can be administered depending on the patient's reaction to the previous course of treatment; maintenance dose of 5-15 mg/kg/week as a single dose not to exceed 1 g/week
I.V. infusion: 15 mg/kg/day (maximum daily dose: 1 g) has been administered by I.V. infusion over 4 hours for 5 days
Oral: 20 mg/kg/day for 5 days every 5 weeks for colorectal carcinoma; 15 mg/kg/week for hepatoma
Topical: 5% cream twice daily
Dosage Forms
Cream, topical:
Efudex®: 5% (25 g)
Fluoroplex®: 1% (30 g)
Injection (Adrucil®): 50 mg/mL (10 mL, 20 mL, 50 mL, 100 mL)
Solution, topical:
Efudex®: 2% (10 mL); 5% (10 mL)
Fluoroplex®: 1% (30 mL)

5-fluorouracil *see* fluorouracil *on this page*

fluostigmin *see* isoflurophate *on page 290*

Fluothane® *see* halothane *on page 256*

fluoxetine (floo OKS e teen)
Synonyms fluoxetine hydrochloride
Brand Names Prozac®
Therapeutic Category Antidepressant, Selective Serotonin Reuptake Inhibitor
Use Treatment of major depression; preliminary studies report use for obsessive-compulsive disorders in children and adolescents
Usual Dosage Oral:
Children <18 years: Dose not established
(Continued)

fluoxetine *(Continued)*

Adults: 20 mg/day in the morning; may increase after several weeks by 20 mg/day increments; maximum: 80 mg/day; doses >20 mg should be divided into 2 daily doses
Note: Lower doses of 5 mg/day have been used for initial treatment
Dosage Forms
Capsule, as hydrochloride: 10 mg, 20 mg
Liquid, as hydrochloride (mint flavor): 20 mg/5 mL (120 mL)

fluoxetine hydrochloride *see* fluoxetine *on previous page*

fluoxymesterone (floo oks i MES te rone)
Brand Names Halotestin®
Therapeutic Category Androgen
Use Replacement of endogenous testicular hormone; in female used as palliative treatment of breast cancer, postpartum breast engorgement
Usual Dosage Adults: Oral:
Male:
Hypogonadism: 5-20 mg/day
Delayed puberty: 2.5-20 mg/day for 4-6 months
Female:
Breast carcinoma: 10-40 mg/day in divided doses for 1-3 months
Breast engorgement: 2.5 mg after delivery, 5-10 mg/day in divided doses for 4-5 days
Dosage Forms Tablet: 2 mg, 5 mg, 10 mg

fluphenazine (floo FEN a zeen)
Synonyms fluphenazine decanoate; fluphenazine enanthate; fluphenazine hydrochloride
Brand Names Permitil® Oral; Prolixin Decanoate® Injection; Prolixin Enanthate® Injection; Prolixin® Injection; Prolixin® Oral
Therapeutic Category Phenothiazine Derivative
Use Management of manifestations of psychotic disorders
Usual Dosage Adults:
Oral: 0.5-10 mg/day in divided doses every 6-8 hours; usual maximum dose 20 mg/day
I.M.: 2.5-10 mg/day in divided doses every 6-8 hours; usual maximum dose 10 mg/day
I.M., S.C. (Decanoate®): Oral to I.M., S.C. conversion ratio = 12.5 mg, I.M., S.C. every 3 weeks for every 10 mg of oral fluphenazine
Dosage Forms
Concentrate, as hydrochloride:
Permitil®: 5 mg/mL with alcohol 1% (118 mL)
Prolixin®: 5 mg/mL with alcohol 14% (120 mL)
Elixir, as hydrochloride (Prolixin®): 2.5 mg/5 mL with alcohol 14% (60 mL, 473 mL)
Injection:
As decanoate (Prolixin Decanoate®): 25 mg/mL (1 mL, 5 mL)
As enanthate (Prolixin Enanthate®): 25 mg/mL (5 mL)
As hydrochloride (Prolixin®): 2.5 mg/mL (10 mL)
Tablet, as hydrochloride:
Permitil®: 2.5 mg, 5 mg, 10 mg
Prolixin®: 1 mg, 2.5 mg, 5 mg, 10 mg

fluphenazine decanoate *see* fluphenazine *on this page*

fluphenazine enanthate *see* fluphenazine *on this page*

fluphenazine hydrochloride *see* fluphenazine *on this page*

Flura-Drops® *see* fluoride *on page 228*

Flura-Loz® *see* fluoride *on page 228*

flurandrenolide (flure an DREN oh lide)
Synonyms flurandrenolone
Brand Names Cordran®; Cordran® SP
Therapeutic Category Corticosteroid, Topical
Use Inflammation of corticosteroid-responsive dermatoses
Usual Dosage Topical:
  Children:
   Ointment or cream: Apply 1-2 times/day
   Tape: Apply once daily
  Adults: Cream, lotion, ointment: Apply 2-3 times/day
Dosage Forms
  Cream, emulsified base (Cordran® SP): 0.025% (30 g, 60 g); 0.05% (15 g, 30 g, 60 g)
  Lotion (Cordran®): 0.05% (15 mL, 60 mL)
  Ointment, topical (Cordran®): 0.025% (30 g, 60 g); 0.05% (15 g, 30 g, 60 g)
  Tape, topical (Cordran®): 4 mcg/cm^2 (7.5 cm x 60 cm, 7.5 cm x 200 cm rolls)

flurandrenolone *see* flurandrenolide *on this page*

Flurate® Ophthalmic Solution *see* fluorescein sodium *on page 227*

flurazepam (flure AZ e pam)
Synonyms flurazepam hydrochloride
Brand Names Dalmane®
Therapeutic Category Benzodiazepine
Controlled Substance C-IV
Use Short-term treatment of insomnia
Usual Dosage Oral:
  Children:
   <15 years: Dose not established
   >15 years: 15 mg at bedtime
  Adults: 15-30 mg at bedtime
Dosage Forms Capsule, as hydrochloride: 15 mg, 30 mg

flurazepam hydrochloride *see* flurazepam *on this page*

flurbiprofen (flure BI proe fen)
Synonyms flurbiprofen sodium
Brand Names Ansaid® Oral; Ocufen® Ophthalmic
Therapeutic Category Analgesic, Non-narcotic; Nonsteroidal Anti-Inflammatory Agent (NSAID)
Use
  Ophthalmic: For inhibition of intraoperative trauma-induced miosis; the value of flurbiprofen for the prevention and management of postoperative ocular inflammation and postoperative cystoid macular edema remains to be determined
  Systemic: Management of inflammatory disease and rheumatoid disorders; dysmenorrhea; pain
Usual Dosage
  Oral: Rheumatoid arthritis and osteoarthritis: 200-300 mg/day in 2, 3, or 4 divided doses
  Ophthalmic: Instill 1 drop every 30 minutes, 2 hours prior to surgery (total of 4 drops to each affected eye)
Dosage Forms
  Solution, ophthalmic, as sodium (Ocufen®): 0.03% (2.5 mL, 5 mL, 10 mL)
  Tablet, as sodium (Ansaid®): 50 mg, 100 mg

flurbiprofen sodium *see* flurbiprofen *on this page*

Fluress® Ophthalmic Solution *see* fluorescein sodium *on page 227*

5-flurocytosine *see* flucytosine *on page 225*

Fluro-Ethyl® **Aerosol** *see* ethyl chloride and dichlorotetrafluoroethane *on page 212*

Flurosyn® *see* fluocinolone *on page 226*

flutamide (FLOO ta mide)
Brand Names Eulexin®
Therapeutic Category Antiandrogen
Use In combination with LHRH agonistic analogs for the treatment of metastatic prostatic carcinoma
Usual Dosage Oral: 2 capsules every 8 hours
Dosage Forms Capsule: 125 mg

Flutex® *see* triamcinolone *on page 528*

fluticasone (floo TIK a sone)
Synonyms fluticasone propionate
Brand Names Cutivate™; Flonase™; Flovent®
Therapeutic Category Adrenal Corticosteroid; Corticosteroid, Topical
Use
Inhalation: Maintenance treatment of asthma as prophylactic therapy. It is also indicated for patients requiring oral corticosteroid therapy for asthma to assist in total discontinuation or reduction of total oral dose. NOT indicated for the relief of acute bronchospasm.
Intranasal: Management of seasonal and perennial allergic rhinitis in patients ≥12 years of age
Topical: Relief of inflammation and pruritus associated with corticosteroid-responsive dermatoses [medium potency topical corticosteroid]
Usual Dosage
Adolescents:
Topical: Apply sparingly in a thin film twice daily
Intranasal: Initially 1 spray (50 mcg/spray) per nostril once daily. Patients not adequately responding or patients with more severe symptoms may use 2 sprays (200 mcg) per nostril. Depending on response, dosage may be reduced to 100 mcg daily. Total daily dosage should not exceed 4 sprays (200 mcg)/day.
Adults:
Topical: Apply sparingly in a thin film twice daily
Inhalation, Oral:

Recommended Oral Inhalation Doses

Previous Therapy	Recommended Starting Dose	Recommended Highest Dose
Bronchodilator alone	88 mcg twice daily	440 mcg twice daily
Inhaled corticosteroids	88–220 mcg twice daily	440 mcg twice daily
Oral corticosteroids	880 mcg twice daily	880 mcg twice daily

Intranasal: Initially 2 sprays (50 mcg/spray) per nostril once daily. After the first few days, dosage may be reduced to 1 spray per nostril once daily for maintenance therapy. Maximum total daily dose should not exceed 4 sprays (200 mcg)/day.
Dosage Forms
Spray:
Aerosol, oral inhalation (Flovent®): 44 mcg/actuation (7.9 g = 60 actuations or 13 g = 120 actuations), 110 mcg/actuation (13 g = 120 actuations); 220 mcg/actuation (13 g = 120 actuations)
Intranasal (Flonase™): 50 mcg/actuation (9 g = 60 actuations, 16 g = 120 actuations)
Topical (Cutivate™):
Cream: 0.05% (15 g, 30 g, 60 g)
Ointment: 0.005% (15 g, 60 g)

fluticasone propionate *see* fluticasone *on previous page*

fluvastatin (FLOO va sta tin)
  Brand Names Lescol®
  Therapeutic Category HMG-CoA Reductase Inhibitor
  Use Adjunct to dietary therapy to decrease elevated serum total and LDL cholesterol concentrations in primary hypercholesterolemia
  Usual Dosage Adults: Oral: 20 mg at bedtime
  Dosage Forms Capsule: 20 mg, 40 mg

fluvoxamine (floo VOKS ah meen)
  Brand Names Luvox®
  Therapeutic Category Antidepressant, Selective Serotonin Reuptake Inhibitor
  Use Treatment of major depression and obsessive-compulsive disorder (OCD)
  Usual Dosage Adults: Initial: 50 mg at bedtime; adjust in 50 mg increments at 4- to 7-day intervals; usual dose range: 100-300 mg/day; divide total daily dose into 2 doses; administer larger portion at bedtime
  Dosage Forms Tablet: 50 mg, 100 mg

Fluzone® *see* influenza virus vaccine *on page 283*

FML® *see* fluorometholone *on page 229*

FML® Forte *see* fluorometholone *on page 229*

FML-S® Ophthalmic Suspension *see* sulfacetamide sodium and fluorometholone *on page 496*

Foille® [OTC] *see* benzocaine *on page 59*

Foille® Medicated First Aid [OTC] *see* benzocaine *on page 59*

folacin *see* folic acid *on this page*

folate *see* folic acid *on this page*

Folex® PFS *see* methotrexate *on page 338*

folic acid (FOE lik AS id)
  Synonyms folacin; folate; pteroylglutamic acid
  Brand Names Folvite®
  Therapeutic Category Vitamin, Water Soluble
  Use Treatment of megaloblastic and macrocytic anemias due to folate deficiency
  Usual Dosage Folic acid deficiency:
    Infants: 15 mcg/kg/dose daily or 50 mcg/day
    Children: Oral, I.M., I.V., S.C.: 1 mg/day initial dosage; maintenance dose: 1-10 years: 0.1-0.3 mg/day
    Children >11 years and Adults: Oral, I.M., I.V., S.C.: 1 mg/day initial dosage; maintenance dose: 0.5 mg/day
  Dosage Forms
    Injection, as sodium folate: 5 mg/mL (10 mL); 10 mg/mL (10 mL)
      Folvite®: 5 mg/mL (10 mL)
    Tablet: 0.1 mg, 0.4 mg, 0.8 mg, 1 mg
      Folvite®: 1 mg

folinic acid *see* leucovorin *on page 302*

Folvite® *see* folic acid *on this page*

Forane® *see* isoflurane *on page 290*

Formula Q® *see* quinine *on page 456*

5-formyl tetrahydrofolate *see* leucovorin *on page 302*

Fortaz® *see* ceftazidime *on page 100*

Fosamax® *see* alendronate *on page 15*

foscarnet (fos KAR net)
Synonyms pfa; phosphonoformic acid
Brand Names Foscavir® Injection
Therapeutic Category Antiviral Agent
Use Alternative to ganciclovir for treatment of CMV infections and is possibly the preferred initial agent for the treatment of CMV retinitis except for those patients with decreased renal function; treatment of acyclovir-resistant mucocutaneous herpes simplex virus infections in immunocompromised patients; and acyclovir-resistant herpes zoster infections
Usual Dosage
Induction treatment: 60 mg/kg 3 times/day for 14-21 days
Maintenance therapy: 90-120 mg/kg/day
Dosage Forms Injection: 24 mg/mL (250 mL, 500 mL)

Foscavir® **Injection** *see* foscarnet *on this page*

fosfomycin (fos foe MYE sin)
Synonyms fosfomycin tromethamine
Brand Names Monurol™
Therapeutic Category Antibiotic, Miscellaneous
Use Treatment of uncomplicated urinary tract infections
Usual Dosage Adults: Oral: Single dose of 3 g in 4 oz of water
Dosage Forms Powder, as tromethamine: 3 g, to be mixed in 4 oz of water

fosfomycin tromethamine *see* fosfomycin *on this page*

fosinopril (foe SIN oh pril)
Brand Names Monopril®
Therapeutic Category Angiotensin-Converting Enzyme (ACE) Inhibitors
Use Treatment of hypertension, either alone or in combination with other antihypertensive agents
Usual Dosage Adults: Oral: 20-40 mg/day
Dosage Forms Tablet: 10 mg, 20 mg, 40 mg

fosphenytoin (FOS fen i toyn)
Synonyms fosphenytoin sodium
Brand Names Cerebyx®
Therapeutic Category Hydantoin
Use Indicated for short-term parenteral administration when other means of phenytoin administration are unavailable, inappropriate or deemed less advantageous; the safety and effectiveness of fosphenytoin in this use has not been systematically evaluated for more than 5 days; may be used for the control of generalized convulsive status epilepticus and prevention and treatment of seizures occurring during neurosurgery
Usual Dosage The dose, concentration in solutions, and infusion rates for fosphenytoin are expressed as phenytoin sodium equivalents; fosphenytoin should always be prescribed and dispensed in phenytoin sodium equivalents

Status epilepticus: I.V.: Adults: Loading dose: Phenytoin equivalent 15-20 mg/kg I.V. administered at 100-150 mg/minute
Nonemergent loading and maintenance dosing: I.V. or I.M.: Adults:
Loading dose: Phenytoin equivalent 10-20 mg/kg I.V. or I.M. (max I.V. rate 150 mg/minute)
Initial daily maintenance dose: Phenytoin equivalent 4-6 mg/kg/day I.V. or I.M.
I.M. or I.V. substitution for oral phenytoin therapy: May be substituted for oral phenytoin sodium at the same total daily dose, however, Dilantin® capsules are ~90% bioavailable by the oral route; phenytoin, supplied as fosphenytoin, is 100% bioavailable by

both the I.M. and I.V. routes; for this reason, plasma phenytoin concentrations may increase when I.M. or I.V. fosphenytoin is substituted for oral phenytoin sodium therapy; in clinical trials I.M. fosphenytoin was administered as a single daily dose utilizing either 1 or 2 injection sites; some patients may require more frequent dosing

Dosage Forms Injection, as sodium: 150 mg [equivalent to phenytoin sodium 100 mg]; 750 mg, [equivalent to phenytoin sodium 500 mg]

fosphenytoin sodium *see* fosphenytoin *on previous page*

Fostex® [OTC] *see* sulfur and salicylic acid *on page 499*

Fostex® 10% BPO Gel [OTC] *see* benzoyl peroxide *on page 61*

Fostex® 10% Wash [OTC] *see* benzoyl peroxide *on page 61*

Fostex® Bar [OTC] *see* benzoyl peroxide *on page 61*

Fototar® [OTC] *see* coal tar *on page 132*

Fragmin® *see* dalteparin *on page 148*

Freezone® Solution [OTC] *see* salicylic acid *on page 472*

frusemide *see* furosemide *on next page*

FS Shampoo® *see* fluocinolone *on page 226*

5-fu *see* fluorouracil *on page 229*

FUDR® *see* floxuridine *on page 224*

Ful-Glo® Ophthalmic Strips *see* fluorescein sodium *on page 227*

Fulvicin® P/G *see* griseofulvin *on page 246*

Fulvicin-U/F® *see* griseofulvin *on page 246*

Fumasorb® [OTC] *see* ferrous fumarate *on page 220*

Fumerin® [OTC] *see* ferrous fumarate *on page 220*

Funduscein® Injection *see* fluorescein sodium *on page 227*

Fungizone® *see* amphotericin B *on page 31*

Fungoid® AF Topical Solution [OTC] *see* undecylenic acid and derivatives *on page 541*

Fungoid® Creme *see* miconazole *on page 348*

Fungoid® Solution *see* clotrimazole *on page 131*

Fungoid® Tincture *see* miconazole *on page 348*

Furacin® Topical *see* nitrofurazone *on page 375*

Furadantin® *see* nitrofurantoin *on page 375*

furazolidone (fyoor a ZOE li done)

Brand Names Furoxone®

Therapeutic Category Antiprotozoal

Use Treatment of bacterial or protozoal diarrhea and enteritis caused by susceptible organisms: *Giardia lamblia* and *Vibrio cholerae*

Usual Dosage Oral:

Children >1 month: 5-8.8 mg/kg/day in 3-4 divided doses for 7-10 days, not to exceed 400 mg/day

Adults: 100 mg 4 times/day for 7-10 days

Dosage Forms

Liquid: 50 mg/15 mL (60 mL, 473 mL)

Tablet: 100 mg

furazosin *see* prazosin *on page 433*

furosemide (fyoor OH se mide)

Synonyms frusemide
Brand Names Lasix®
Therapeutic Category Diuretic, Loop
Use Management of edema associated with congestive heart failure and hepatic or renal disease; used alone or in combination with antihypertensives in treatment of hypertension
Usual Dosage
Infants and Children:
  Oral: 2 mg/kg/dose increased in increments of 1 mg/kg/dose with each succeeding dose until a satisfactory effect is achieved to a maximum of 6 mg/kg/dose no more frequently than 6 hours
  I.M., I.V.: 1 mg/kg/dose, increasing by each succeeding dose at 1 mg/kg/dose at intervals of 6-12 hours until a satisfactory response up to 6 mg/kg/dose
Adults:
  Oral: Initial: 20-80 mg/dose, increase in increments of 20-40 mg/dose at intervals of 6-8 hours; usual maintenance dose interval is twice daily or every day
  I.M., I.V.: 20-40 mg/dose, may be repeated in 1-2 hours as needed and increased by 20 mg/dose with each succeeding dose up to 600 mg/day; usual dosing interval: 6-12 hours
Dosage Forms
Injection: 10 mg/mL (2 mL, 4 mL, 5 mL, 6 mL, 8 mL, 10 mL, 12 mL)
Solution, oral: 10 mg/mL (60 mL, 120 mL); 40 mg/5 mL (5 mL, 10 mL, 500 mL)
Tablet: 20 mg, 40 mg, 80 mg

Furoxone® *see* furazolidone *on previous page*

G-1® *see* butalbital compound and acetaminophen *on page 78*

gabapentin (GA ba pen tin)

Brand Names Neurontin®
Therapeutic Category Anticonvulsant
Use Adjunct for treatment of drug-refractory partial and secondarily generalized seizures
Usual Dosage Adults: Oral: 900-1800 mg/day administered in 3 divided doses; therapy is initiated with a rapid titration, beginning with 300 mg on day 1, 300 mg twice daily on day 2, and 300 mg 3 times/day on day 3

Discontinuing therapy or replacing with an alternative agent should be done gradually over a minimum of 7 days
Dosage Forms Capsule: 100 mg, 300 mg, 400 mg

gallamine triethiodide (GAL a meen trye eth EYE oh dide)

Brand Names Flaxedil®
Therapeutic Category Skeletal Muscle Relaxant
Use Produce skeletal muscle relaxation during surgery after general anesthesia has been induced
Usual Dosage I.V.: 1 mg/kg then repeat dose of 0.5-1 mg/kg in 30-40 minutes for prolonged procedures
Dosage Forms Injection: 20 mg/mL (10 mL)

gallium nitrate (GAL ee um NYE trate)

Brand Names Ganite™
Therapeutic Category Antidote
Use Treatment of clearly symptomatic cancer-related hypercalcemia that has not responded to adequate hydration
Usual Dosage Adults: I.V. infusion: 200 mg/m^2 for 5 consecutive days
Dosage Forms Injection: 25 mg/mL (20 mL)

Gamimune® N *see* immune globulin, intravenous *on page 281*

gamma benzene hexachloride *see* lindane *on page 309*

Gammagard® *see* immune globulin, intravenous *on page 281*

Gammagard® **S/D** *see* immune globulin, intravenous *on page 281*

gamma globulin *see* immune globulin, intramuscular *on page 281*

gammaphos *see* amifostine *on page 24*

Gammar-P® **I.V.** *see* immune globulin, intravenous *on page 281*

Gamulin® **Rh** *see* $Rh_o(D)$ immune globulin *on page 463*

ganciclovir (gan SYE kloe veer)
  Synonyms dhpg sodium; gcv sodium; nordeoxyguanosine
  Brand Names Cytovene®; Vitrasert®
  Therapeutic Category Antiviral Agent
  Use Treatment of cytomegalovirus (CMV) retinitis in immunocompromised patients, as
    well as CMV GI infections and pneumonitis; prevention of CMV disease in transplant
    patients who have been diagnosed with latent or active CMV; ganciclovir also has
    antiviral activity against herpes simplex virus types 1 and 2
  Usual Dosage Slow I.V. infusion
    Retinitis: Children >3 months and Adults: Induction therapy: 5 mg/kg/dose every 12
      hours for 14-21 days followed by maintenance therapy; maintenance therapy: 5 mg/kg/
      day as a single daily dose for 7 days/week or 6 mg/kg/day for 5 days/week
    Other CMV infections: 5 mg/kg/dose every 12 hours for 14-21 days or 2.5 mg/kg/dose
      every 8 hours; maintenance therapy: 5 mg/kg/day as a single daily dose for 7 days/
      week or 6 mg/kg/day for 5 days/week
  Dosage Forms
    Capsule: 250 mg
    Implant, intravitreal: 4.5 mg released gradually over 5-8 months
    Powder for injection, lyophilized: 500 mg (10 mL)

Ganite™ *see* gallium nitrate *on previous page*

Gantanol® *see* sulfamethoxazole *on page 498*

Gantrisin® *see* sulfisoxazole *on page 499*

Garamycin® **Injection** *see* gentamicin *on page 240*

Garamycin® **Ophthalmic** *see* gentamicin *on page 240*

Garamycin® **Topical** *see* gentamicin *on page 240*

Gas-Ban DS® **[OTC]** *see* aluminum hydroxide, magnesium hydroxide, and simethicone *on page 22*

Gas Relief® *see* simethicone *on page 480*

Gastrocrom® **Oral** *see* cromolyn sodium *on page 141*

Gastrografin® *see* radiological/contrast media (ionic) *on page 457*

Gastrosed™ *see* hyoscyamine *on page 275*

Gas-X® **[OTC]** *see* simethicone *on page 480*

Gaviscon®**-2 Tablet [OTC]** *see* aluminum hydroxide and magnesium trisilicate *on
page 22*

Gaviscon® **Liquid [OTC]** *see* aluminum hydroxide and magnesium carbonate *on
page 21*

Gaviscon® **Tablet [OTC]** *see* aluminum hydroxide and magnesium trisilicate *on
page 22*

g-csf *see* filgrastim *on page 223*

gcv sodium *see* ganciclovir *on this page*

Gee Gee® **[OTC]** *see* guaifenesin *on page 247*

gelatin, absorbable (JEL a tin, ab SORB a ble)

Synonyms absorbable gelatin sponge
Brand Names Gelfilm® Ophthalmic; Gelfoam® Topical
Therapeutic Category Hemostatic Agent
Use Adjunct to provide hemostasis in surgery; also used in oral and dental surgery; in open prostatic surgery
Usual Dosage Topical: Hemostasis: Apply packs or sponges dry or saturated with sodium chloride. When applied dry, hold in place with moderate pressure. When applied wet, squeeze to remove air bubbles. Prostatectomy cones are designed for use with the Foley bag catheter. The powder is applied as a paste prepared by adding approximately 4 mL of sterile saline solution to the powder.
Dosage Forms
Gelfilm® (sterile)
Film: 100 mm x 125 mm (1s)
Ophthalmic: 25 mm x 50 mm (6s)

Gelfoam®
Cones, prostatectomy:
Size 13 cm (13 cm in diameter) (6s)
Size 18 cm (18 cm in diameter) (6s)
Packs:
Size 2 cm (40 cm x 2 cm) (1s)
Size 6 cm (40 cm x 6 cm) (6s)
Packs, dental:
Size 2 (10 mm x 20 mm x 7 mm) (15s)
Size 4 (20 mm x 20 mm x 7 mm) (15s)
Sponges:
Size 12-3 mm (20 mm x 60 mm x 3 mm) (4s)
Size 12-7 mm (20 mm x 60 mm x 7 mm) (4s)
Size 50 (80 mm x 62.5 mm x 10 mm) (4s)
Size 100 (80 mm x 125 mm x 10 mm) (6s)
Size 100, compressed (80 mm x 125 mm) (6s)
Size 200 (80 mm x 250 mm x 10 mm) (6s)

gelatin, pectin, and methylcellulose

(JEL a tin, PEK tin, & meth il SEL yoo lose)
Brand Names Orabase® Plain [OTC]
Therapeutic Category Protectant, Topical
Use Temporary relief from minor oral irritations
Usual Dosage Oral: Press small dabs into place until the involved area is coated with a thin film; do not try to spread onto area; may be used as often as needed
Dosage Forms Paste, oral: 5 g, 15 g

Gelfilm® Ophthalmic *see* gelatin, absorbable *on this page*

Gelfoam® Topical *see* gelatin, absorbable *on this page*

Gel-Kam® *see* fluoride *on page 228*

Gelpirin® [OTC] *see* acetaminophen, aspirin, and caffeine *on page 5*

Gel-Tin® [OTC] *see* fluoride *on page 228*

Gelucast® *see* zinc gelatin *on page 561*

Gelusil® [OTC] *see* aluminum hydroxide, magnesium hydroxide, and simethicone *on page 22*

gemcitabine (jem SIT a been)

Synonyms gemcitabine hydrochloride
Brand Names Gemzar®
Therapeutic Category Antineoplastic Agent

Use Treatment of patients with inoperable pancreatic cancer
Usual Dosage Adults: I.V.: 1000 mg/^{2} over 30 minutes once weekly for up to 7 weeks
Dosage Forms Powder for injection, as hydrochloride, lyophilized: 20 mg/mL (10 mL, 50 mL)

gemcitabine hydrochloride *see* gemcitabine *on previous page*

gemfibrozil (jem FI broe zil)
Synonyms CI-719
Brand Names Lopid®
Therapeutic Category Antihyperlipidemic Agent, Miscellaneous
Use Hypertriglyceridemia in types IV and V hyperlipidemia; increases HDL cholesterol
Usual Dosage Oral: 1200 mg/day in 2 divided doses, 30 minutes before breakfast and supper
Dosage Forms
Capsule: 300 mg
Tablet, film coated: 600 mg

Gemzar® *see* gemcitabine *on previous page*

Genabid® *see* papaverine *on page 395*

Genac® **Tablet [OTC]** *see* triprolidine and pseudoephedrine *on page 536*

Genagesic® *see* guaifenesin and phenylpropanolamine *on page 249*

Genahist® **Oral** *see* diphenhydramine *on page 173*

Genamin® **Cold Syrup [OTC]** *see* chlorpheniramine and phenylpropanolamine *on page 114*

Genamin® **Expectorant [OTC]** *see* guaifenesin and phenylpropanolamine *on page 249*

Genapap® **[OTC]** *see* acetaminophen *on page 3*

Genasoft® **Plus [OTC]** *see* docusate and casanthranol *on page 180*

Genaspor® **[OTC]** *see* tolnaftate *on page 523*

Genatap® **Elixir [OTC]** *see* brompheniramine and phenylpropanolamine *on page 73*

Genatuss® **[OTC]** *see* guaifenesin *on page 247*

Genatuss DM® **[OTC]** *see* guaifenesin and dextromethorphan *on page 248*

Gencalc® **600 [OTC]** *see* calcium carbonate *on page 82*

Geneye® **Ophthalmic [OTC]** *see* tetrahydrozoline *on page 510*

Gen-K® *see* potassium chloride *on page 427*

Genoptic® **Ophthalmic** *see* gentamicin *on next page*

Genoptic® **S.O.P. Ophthalmic** *see* gentamicin *on next page*

Genora® **0.5/35** *see* ethinyl estradiol and norethindrone *on page 209*

Genora® **1/35** *see* ethinyl estradiol and norethindrone *on page 209*

Genora® **1/50** *see* mestranol and norethindrone *on page 332*

Genotropin® **Injection** *see* human growth hormone *on page 262*

Genpril® **[OTC]** *see* ibuprofen *on page 278*

Gentacidin® **Ophthalmic** *see* gentamicin *on next page*

Gentak® **Ophthalmic** *see* gentamicin *on next page*

gentamicin (jen ta MYE sin)

Synonyms gentamicin sulfate

Brand Names Garamycin® Injection; Garamycin® Ophthalmic; Garamycin® Topical; Genoptic® Ophthalmic; Genoptic® S.O.P. Ophthalmic; Gentacidin® Ophthalmic; Gentak® Ophthalmic; G-myticin® Topical; Jenamicin® Injection

Therapeutic Category Aminoglycoside (Antibiotic); Antibiotic, Ophthalmic; Antibiotic, Topical

Use Treatment of susceptible bacterial infections, normally due to gram-negative organisms including *Pseudomonas, Proteus, Serratia*, and gram-positive *Staphylococcus*; treatment of bone infections, CNS infections, respiratory tract infections, skin and soft tissue infections, as well as abdominal and urinary tract infections, endocarditis, and septicemia; used in combination with ampicillin as empiric therapy for sepsis in newborns; used topically to treat superficial infections of the skin or ophthalmic infections caused by susceptible bacteria

Usual Dosage Dosage should be based on an estimate of ideal body weight

Infants and Children >3 months: Intrathecal: 1-2 mg/day

Infants and Children <5 years: 2.5 mg/kg/dose every 8 hours

Children >5 years: 1.5-2.5 mg/kg/dose every 8 hours

Ophthalmic: Solution: 1-2 drops every 2-4 hours, up to 2 drops every hour for severe infections; ointment: 2-3 times/day

Topical: Apply 3-4 times/day

Adults:

Intrathecal: 4-8 mg/day

I.M., I.V.: 3-5 mg/kg/day in divided doses every 8 hours

Topical: Apply 3-4 times/day

Ophthalmic: Solution: 1-2 drops every 2-4 hours; ointment: 2-3 times/day

Dosage Forms

Cream, topical, as sulfate (Garamycin®, G-myticin®): 0.1% (15 g)

Infusion:

In D₅W, as sulfate: 60 mg, 80 mg, 100 mg

In NS, as sulfate: 40 mg, 60 mg, 80 mg, 90 mg, 100 mg, 120 mg

Injection, as sulfate: 40 mg/mL (1 mL, 1.5 mL, 2 mL)

Pediatric, as sulfate: 10 mg/mL (2 mL)

Intrathecal, preservative free, as sulfate (Garamycin®): 2 mg/mL (2 mL)

Ointment, as sulfate:

Ophthalmic: 0.3% [3 mg/g] (3.5 g)

Garamycin®, Genoptic® S.O.P., Gentacidin®, Gentak®: 0.3% [3 mg/g] (3.5 g)

Topical, as sulfate (Garamycin®, G-myticin®): 0.1% (15 g)

Solution, ophthalmic, as sulfate: 0.3% (5 mL, 15 mL)

Garamycin®, Genoptic®, Gentacidin®, Gentak®: 0.3% (1 mL, 5 mL, 15 mL)

gentamicin and prednisolone *see* prednisolone and gentamicin *on page 435*

gentamicin sulfate *see* gentamicin *on this page*

Gentran® *see* dextran *on page 159*

Gen-XENE® *see* clorazepate *on page 131*

Geocillin® *see* carbenicillin *on page 90*

Geref® Injection *see* sermorelin acetate *on page 478*

german measles vaccine *see* rubella virus vaccine, live *on page 471*

Germinal® *see* ergoloid mesylates *on page 198*

Gevrabon® [OTC] *see* vitamin b complex *on page 553*

gg *see* guaifenesin *on page 247*

GG-Cen® [OTC] *see* guaifenesin *on page 247*

glatiramer acetate (gla TIR a mer AS e tate)
Synonyms copolymer-1
Brand Names Copaxone®
Therapeutic Category Biological, Miscellaneous
Use Reduce the frequency of relapses in relapsing-remitting multiple sclerosis (MS)
Usual Dosage Adults: S.C.: 20 mg daily
Dosage Forms Injection: 20 mg (2 mL)

Glaucon® *see* epinephrine *on page 195*

GlaucTabs® *see* methazolamide *on page 336*

Gliadel® *see* carmustine *on page 93*

glibenclamide *see* glyburide *on page 243*

glimepiride (GLYE me pye ride)
Brand Names Amaryl®
Therapeutic Category Antidiabetic Agent (Oral)
Use
Management of noninsulin-dependent diabetes mellitus (type II) as an adjunct to diet and exercise to lower blood glucose
Use in combination with insulin to lower blood glucose in patients whose hyperglycemia cannot be controlled by diet and exercise in conjunction with an oral hypoglycemic agent
Usual Dosage Oral (allow several days between dose titrations):
Adults: Initial: 1-2 mg once daily, administered with breakfast or the first main meal; usual maintenance dose: 1-4 mg once daily; after a dose of 2 mg once daily, increase in increments of 2 mg at 1- to 2-week intervals based upon the patient's blood glucose response to a maximum of 8 mg once daily
Elderly: Initial: 1 mg/day

Combination with insulin therapy (fasting glucose level for instituting combination therapy is in the range of >150 mg/dL in plasma or serum depending on the patient): 8 mg once daily with the first main meal

After starting with low-dose insulin, upward adjustments of insulin can be done approximately weekly as guided by frequent measurements of fasting blood glucose. Once stable, combination-therapy patients should monitor their capillary blood glucose on an ongoing basis, preferably daily.
Dosage Forms Tablet: 1 mg, 2 mg, 4 mg

glipizide (GLIP i zide)
Synonyms glydiazinamide
Brand Names Glucotrol®; Glucotrol® XL
Therapeutic Category Antidiabetic Agent (Oral)
Use Management of noninsulin-dependent diabetes mellitus (type II)
Usual Dosage Adults: Oral: 2.5-40 mg/day; doses larger than 15-20 mg/day should be divided and administered twice daily
Dosage Forms
Tablet: 5 mg, 10 mg
Extended release: 5 mg, 10 mg

glucagon (GLOO ka gon)
Therapeutic Category Antihypoglycemic Agent
Use Hypoglycemia; diagnostic aid in the radiologic examination of GI tract when a hypotonic state is needed; used with some success as a cardiac stimulant in management of severe cases of beta-adrenergic blocking agent overdosage
(Continued)

241

glucagon (Continued)

Usual Dosage
Hypoglycemia or insulin shock therapy: I.M., I.V., S.C.:
Children: 0.025-0.1 mg/kg/dose, not to exceed 1 mg/dose, repeated in 20 minutes as needed
Adults: 0.5-1 mg, may repeat in 20 minutes as needed
Diagnostic aid: Adults: I.M., I.V.: 0.25-2 mg 10 minutes prior to procedure
Dosage Forms Powder for injection, lyophilized: 1 mg [1 unit]; 10 mg [10 units]

glucocerebrosidase see alglucerase on page 16

Glucophage® see metformin on page 333

glucose, instant (GLOO kose, IN stant)

Brand Names B-D Glucose® [OTC]; Glutose® [OTC]; Insta-Glucose® [OTC]
Therapeutic Category Antihypoglycemic Agent
Use Management of hypoglycemia
Usual Dosage Oral: 10-20 g
Dosage Forms
Gel, oral (Glutose®, Insta-Glucose®): Dextrose 40% (25 g, 30.8 g, 80 g)
Tablet, chewable (B-D Glucose®): 5 g

glucose polymers (GLOO kose POL i merz)

Brand Names Moducal® [OTC]; Polycose® [OTC]; Sumacal® [OTC]
Therapeutic Category Nutritional Supplement
Use Supplies calories for those persons not able to meet the caloric requirement with usual food intake
Usual Dosage Adults: Oral: Add to foods or beverages or mix in water
Dosage Forms
Liquid (Polycose®): 126 mL
Powder (Moducal®, Polycose®, Sumacal®): 350 g, 368 g, 400 g

Glucotrol® see glipizide on previous page

Glucotrol® XL see glipizide on previous page

glutamic acid (gloo TAM ik AS id)

Synonyms glutamic acid hydrochloride
Therapeutic Category Gastrointestinal Agent, Miscellaneous
Use Treatment of hypochlorhydria and achlorhydria
Usual Dosage Adults: Oral: 340 mg to 1.02 g 3 times/day before meals or food
Dosage Forms
Capsule, as hydrochloride: 340 mg
Powder: 100 g
Tablet: 500 mg

glutamic acid hydrochloride see glutamic acid on this page

glutethimide (gloo TETH i mide)

Therapeutic Category Hypnotic, Nonbarbiturate
Controlled Substance C-II
Use Short-term treatment of insomnia
Usual Dosage Oral:
Adults: 250-500 mg at bedtime, dose may be repeated but not less than 4 hours before intended awakening; maximum: 1 g/day
Elderly/debilitated patients: Total daily dose should not exceed 500 mg
Dosage Forms Tablet: 250 mg

Glutose® [OTC] see glucose, instant on this page

Glyate® **[OTC]** *see* guaifenesin *on page 247*

glyburide (GLYE byoor ide)
Synonyms glibenclamide
Brand Names Diaβeta®; Glynase™ PresTab™; Micronase®
Therapeutic Category Antidiabetic Agent (Oral)
Use Management of noninsulin-dependent diabetes mellitus (type II)
Usual Dosage Adults:
  Oral: 1.25-5 mg to start then 1.25-20 mg maintenance dose/day divided in 1-2 doses
  PresTab™: Initial: 0.75-3 mg/day, increase by 1.5 mg/day in weekly intervals; maximum:
  12 mg/day
Dosage Forms
  Tablet (Diaβeta®, Micronase®): 1.25 mg, 2.5 mg, 5 mg
  Tablet, micronized (Glynase™ PresTab™): 1.5 mg, 3 mg, 6 mg

glycerin (GLIS er in)
Synonyms glycerol
Brand Names Fleet® Babylax® Rectal [OTC]; Ophthalgan® Ophthalmic; Osmoglyn®
  Ophthalmic; Sani-Supp® Suppository [OTC]
Therapeutic Category Laxative; Ophthalmic Agent, Miscellaneous
Use Constipation; reduction of intraocular pressure; reduction of corneal edema; glycerin
  has been administered orally to reduce intracranial pressure
Usual Dosage
  Constipation: Rectal:
    Children <6 years: 1 infant suppository 1-2 times/day as needed or 2-5 mL as an
    enema
    Children >6 years and Adults: 1 adult suppository 1-2 times/day as needed or 5-15 mL
    as an enema

  Children and Adults:
    Reduction of intraocular pressure: Oral: 1-1.8 g/kg 1-1½ hours preoperatively; addi-
    tional doses may be administered at 5-hour intervals
    Reduction of corneal edema: Instill 1-2 drops in eye(s) every 3-4 hours
    Reduction of intracranial pressure: Oral: 1.5 g/kg/day divided every 4 hours; dose of 1
    g/kg/dose every 6 hours has also been used
Dosage Forms
  Solution:
    Ophthalmic, sterile (Ophthalgan®): Glycerin with chlorobutanol 0.55% (7.5 mL)
    Oral (lime flavor)(Osmoglyn®): 50% (220 mL)
    Rectal (Fleet Babylax®): 4 mL/applicator (6s)
    Suppository, rectal (Sani-Supp®): Glycerin with sodium stearate (infant and adult sizes)

glycerin, lanolin, and peanut oil (GLIS er in, LAN oh lin, & PEE nut oyl)
Brand Names Massé® Breast Cream [OTC]
Therapeutic Category Topical Skin Product
Use Nipple care of pregnant and nursing women
Usual Dosage Topical: Apply as often as needed
Dosage Forms Cream: 2 oz

glycerol *see* glycerin *on this page*

glycerol guaiacolate *see* guaifenesin *on page 247*

Glycerol-T® *see* theophylline and guaifenesin *on page 512*

glycerol triacetate *see* triacetin *on page 528*

glyceryl trinitrate *see* nitroglycerin *on page 376*

Glycofed® *see* guaifenesin and pseudoephedrine *on page 250*

glycopyrrolate (glye koe PYE roe late)
Synonyms glycopyrronium bromide
Brand Names Robinul®; Robinul® Forte
Therapeutic Category Anticholinergic Agent
Use Adjunct in treatment of peptic ulcer disease; inhibit salivation and excessive secretions of the respiratory tract; reversal of cholinergic agents such as neostigmine and pyridostigmine; control of upper airway secretions
Usual Dosage
Children: Control of secretions:
Oral: 40-100 mcg/kg/dose 3-4 times/day
I.M., I.V.: 4-10 mcg/kg/dose every 3-4 hours; maximum: 0.2 mg/dose or 0.8 mg/24 hours
Children:
Intraoperative: I.V.: 4 mcg/kg not to exceed 0.1 mg; repeat at 2- to 3-minute intervals as needed
Preoperative: I.M.:
<2 years: 4.4-8.8 mcg/kg 30-60 minutes before procedure
>2 years: 4.4 mcg/kg 30-60 minutes before procedure
Children and Adults: Reverse neuromuscular blockade: I.V.: 0.2 mg for each 1 mg of neostigmine or 5 mg of pyridostigmine administered
Adults:
Intraoperative: I.V.: 0.1 mg repeated as needed at 2- to 3-minute intervals
Peptic ulcer:
Oral: 1-2 mg 2-3 times/day
I.M., I.V.: 0.1-0.2 mg 3-4 times/day
Preoperative: I.M.: 4.4 mcg/kg 30-60 minutes before procedure
Dosage Forms
Injection, as bromide: 0.2 mg/mL (1 mL, 2 mL, 5 mL, 20 mL)
Robinul®: 0.2 mg/mL (1 mL, 2 mL, 5 mL, 20 mL)
Tablet, as bromide:
Robinul®: 1 mg
Robinul® Forte: 2 mg

glycopyrronium bromide *see* glycopyrrolate *on this page*

Glycotuss® [OTC] *see* guaifenesin *on page 247*

Glycotuss-dM® [OTC] *see* guaifenesin and dextromethorphan *on page 248*

glydiazinamide *see* glipizide *on page 241*

Glynase™ PresTab™ *see* glyburide *on previous page*

Gly-Oxide® Oral [OTC] *see* carbamide peroxide *on page 90*

Glyset® *see* miglitol *on page 351*

Glytuss® [OTC] *see* guaifenesin *on page 247*

gm-csf *see* sargramostim *on page 474*

G-myticin® Topical *see* gentamicin *on page 240*

GnRH *see* gonadorelin *on next page*

gold sodium thiomalate (gold SOW dee um thye oh MAL ate)
Brand Names Aurolate®
Therapeutic Category Gold Compound
Use Treatment of progressive rheumatoid arthritis
Usual Dosage I.M.:
Children: Initial: Test dose of 10 mg I.M. is recommended, followed by 1 mg/kg I.M. weekly for 20 weeks; not to exceed 50 mg in a single injection; maintenance: 1 mg/kg/dose at 2- to 4-week intervals thereafter for as long as therapy is clinically beneficial and toxicity does not develop. Administration for 2-4 months is usually required before clinical improvement is observed

Adults: 10 mg first week; 25 mg second week; then 25-50 mg/week until 1 g cumulative dose has been administered. If improvement occurs without adverse reactions, administer 25-50 mg every 2-3 weeks, then every 3-4 weeks.

Dosage Forms Injection: 25 mg/mL (1 mL); 50 mg/mL (1 mL, 2 mL, 10 mL)

GoLYTELY® *see* polyethylene glycol-electrolyte solution *on page 423*

gonadorelin (goe nad oh REL in)

Synonyms GnRH; gonadorelin acetate; gonadorelin hydrochloride; gonadotropin releasing hormone; LH-RH; LRH; luteinizing hormone releasing hormone

Brand Names Factrel®; Lutrepulse®

Therapeutic Category Diagnostic Agent; Gonadotropin

Use Evaluation of hypothalamic-pituitary gonadotropic function; used to evaluate abnormal gonadotropin regulation as in precocious puberty and delayed puberty; treatment of primary hypothalamic amenorrhea

Usual Dosage Female:

Diagnostic test: Children >12 years and Adults: I.V., S.C. hydrochloride salt: 100 mcg administered in women during early phase of menstrual cycle (day 1-7)

Primary hypothalamic amenorrhea: Adults: Acetate: I.V.: 5 mcg every 90 minutes via Lutrepulse® pump kit at treatment intervals of 21 days (pump will pulsate every 90 minutes for 7 days)

Dosage Forms

Injection, as acetate (Lutrepulse®): 0.8 mg, 3.2 mg

Injection, as hydrochloride (Factrel®): 100 mcg, 500 mcg

gonadorelin acetate *see* gonadorelin *on this page*

gonadorelin hydrochloride *see* gonadorelin *on this page*

gonadotropin releasing hormone *see* gonadorelin *on this page*

Gonak™ [OTC] *see* hydroxypropyl methylcellulose *on page 274*

Gonic® *see* chorionic gonadotropin *on page 122*

gonioscopic ophthalmic solution *see* hydroxypropyl methylcellulose *on page 274*

Goniosol® **[OTC]** *see* hydroxypropyl methylcellulose *on page 274*

Goody's® **Headache Powders** *see* acetaminophen, aspirin, and caffeine *on page 5*

Gordofilm® **Liquid** *see* salicylic acid *on page 472*

Gormel® **Creme [OTC]** *see* urea *on page 542*

goserelin (GOE se rel in)

Synonyms goserelin acetate

Brand Names Zoladex® Implant

Therapeutic Category Gonadotropin Releasing Hormone Analog

Use Palliative treatment of advanced prostate cancer and breast cancer

Usual Dosage Adults: S.C.:

Breast/prostatic cancer: 3.6 mg as a depot injection every 28 days into upper abdominal wall using sterile technique under the supervision of a physician. At the physician's option, local anesthesia may be used prior to injection. The injection should be repeated every 28 days as long as the patient can tolerate the side effects and there is satisfactory disease regression. While a delay of a few days is permissible, every effort should be made to adhere to the 28-day schedule.

Prostatic cancer: 10.8 mg as a depot injection every 12 weeks into upper abdominal wall using sterile technique under the supervision of a physician. At the physician's option, local anesthesia may be used prior to injection. The injection should be repeated every 12 weeks as long as the patient can tolerate the side effects and there is satisfactory disease regression. While a delay of a few days is permissible, every effort should be made to adhere to the 12 week schedule.

(Continued)

goserelin *(Continued)*

Dosage Forms Injection, implant, as acetate: 3.6 mg, 10.8 mg

goserelin acetate *see* goserelin *on previous page*

granisetron (gra NI se tron)
Brand Names Kytril™ Injection
Therapeutic Category Selective 5-HT$_3$ Receptor Antagonist
Use Prophylaxis and treatment of chemotherapy-related emesis
Usual Dosage
Oral: 1 tablet (1 mg) twice daily
I.V.:
10-40 mcg/kg for 1-3 doses. Doses should be administered as a single IVPB over 5 minutes to 1 hour, administer just prior to chemotherapy (15-60 minutes before). As intervention therapy for breakthrough nausea and vomiting, during the first 24 hours following chemotherapy, 2 or 3 repeat infusions (same dose) have been administered, separated by at least 10 minutes
Dosage Forms
Injection: 1 mg/mL
Tablet: 1 mg (2s), (20s)

Granulex *see* trypsin, balsam peru, and castor oil *on page 538*

granulocyte colony stimulating factor *see* filgrastim *on page 223*

granulocyte-macrophage colony stimulating factor *see* sargramostim *on page 474*

Grifulvin® V *see* griseofulvin *on this page*

Grisactin® Ultra *see* griseofulvin *on this page*

griseofulvin (gri see oh FUL vin)
Synonyms griseofulvin microsize; griseofulvin ultramicrosize
Brand Names Fulvicin® P/G; Fulvicin-U/F®; Grifulvin® V; Grisactin® Ultra; Gris-PEG®
Therapeutic Category Antifungal Agent
Use Treatment of tinea infections of the skin, hair, and nails caused by susceptible species of *Microsporum*, *Epidermophyton*, or *Trichophyton*
Usual Dosage Oral:
Children:
Microsize: 10-15 mg/kg/day in single or divided doses;
Ultramicrosize: >2 months: 5.5-7.3 mg/kg/day in single or divided doses
Adults:
Microsize: 500-1000 mg/day in single or divided doses
Ultramicrosize: 330-375 mg/day in single or divided doses; doses up to 750 mg/day have been used for infections more difficult to eradicate such as tinea unguium

Duration of therapy depends on the site of infection:
Tinea corporis: 2-4 weeks
Tinea capitis: 4-6 weeks or longer
Tinea pedis: 4-8 weeks
Tinea unguium: 3-6 months
Dosage Forms
Microsize:
Suspension, oral (Grifulvin® V): 125 mg/5 mL with alcohol 0.2% (120 mL)
Tablet: Fulvicin-U/F®, Grifulvin® V: 250 mg, 500 mg
Ultramicrosize:
Tablet:
Fulvicin® P/G: 165 mg, 330 mg
Fulvicin® P/G, Grisactin® Ultra, Gris-PEG®: 125 mg, 250 mg
Grisactin® Ultra: 330 mg

griseofulvin microsize *see* griseofulvin *on previous page*

griseofulvin ultramicrosize *see* griseofulvin *on previous page*

Gris-PEG® *see* griseofulvin *on previous page*

Guaifed® **[OTC]** *see* guaifenesin and pseudoephedrine *on page 250*

Guaifed®**-PD** *see* guaifenesin and pseudoephedrine *on page 250*

guaifenesin (gwye FEN e sin)

Synonyms gg; glycerol guaiacolate

Brand Names Anti-Tuss® Expectorant [OTC]; Breonesin® [OTC]; Diabetic Tussin® EX [OTC]; Duratuss-G®; Fenesin™; Gee Gee® [OTC]; Genatuss® [OTC]; GG-Cen® [OTC]; Glyate® [OTC]; Glycotuss® [OTC]; Glytuss® [OTC]; Guaifenex® LA; GuiaCough® Expectorant [OTC]; Guiatuss® [OTC]; Halotussin® [OTC]; Humibid® L.A.; Humibid® Sprinkle; Hytuss® [OTC]; Hytuss-2X® [OTC]; Liquibid®; Medi-Tuss® [OTC]; Monafed®; Muco-Fen-LA®; Mytussin® [OTC]; Naldecon® Senior EX [OTC]; Organidin® NR; Pneumomist®; Respa-GF®; Robitussin® [OTC]; Scot-Tussin® [OTC]; Siltussin® [OTC]; Sinumist®-SR Capsulets®; Touro Ex®; Tusibron® [OTC]; Uni-tussin® [OTC]

Therapeutic Category Expectorant

Use Temporary control of cough due to minor throat and bronchial irritation

Usual Dosage Oral:

Children:

<2 years: 12 mg/kg/day in 6 divided doses

2-5 years: 50-100 mg (2.5-5 mL) every 4 hours, not to exceed 600 mg/day

6-11 years: 100-200 mg (5-10 mL) every 4 hours, not to exceed 1.2 g/day

Children >12 years and Adults: 200-400 mg (10-20 mL) every 4 hours to a maximum of 2.4 g/day (60 mL/day)

Dosage Forms

Caplet, sustained release (Touro Ex®): 600 mg

Capsule (Breonesin®, GG-Cen®, Hytuss-2X®): 200 mg

Sustained release (Humibid® Sprinkle): 300 mg

Liquid:

Diabetic Tussin® EX, Organidin® NR, Tusibron®: 100 mg/5 mL (118 mL)

Naldecon® Senior EX: 200 mg/5 mL (118 mL, 480 mL)

Syrup (Anti-Tuss® Expectorant, Genatuss®, Glyate®, GuiaCough® Expectorant, Guiatuss®, Halotussin®, Malotuss®, Medi-Tuss®, Mytussin®, Robitussin®, Scot-tussin®, Siltussin®, Tusibron®, Uni-Tussin®): 100 mg/5 mL with alcohol 3.5% (30 mL, 120 mL, 240 mL, 473 mL, 946 mL)

Tablet:

Duratuss-G®: 1200 mg

Gee Gee®, Glytuss®, Organidin® NR: 200 mg

Glycotuss®, Hytuss®: 100 mg

Sustained release:

Fenesin™, Guaifenex® LA, Humibid® L.A., Liquibid®, Monafed®, Muco-Fen-LA®, Pneumomist®, Respa-GF®, Sinumist®-SR Capsulets®: 600 mg

guaifenesin and codeine (gwye FEN e sin & KOE deen)

Synonyms codeine and guaifenesin

Brand Names Brontex® Liquid; Brontex® Tablet; Cheracol®; Guaituss AC®; Guiatussin® with Codeine; Mytussin® AC; Robafen® AC; Robitussin® A-C; Tussi-Organidin® NR

Therapeutic Category Antitussive/Expectorant

Controlled Substance C-V

Use Temporary control of cough due to minor throat and bronchial irritation

Usual Dosage Oral:

Children:

2-6 years: 1-1.5 mg/kg codeine/day divided into 4 doses administered every 4-6 hours

6-12 years: 5 mL every 4 hours, not to exceed 30 mL/24 hours

>12 years: 10 mL every 4 hours, up to 60 mL/24 hours

(Continued)

guaifenesin and codeine *(Continued)*

Adults: 10 mL or one tablet every 6-8 hours

Dosage Forms

Liquid [C-V] (Brontex®): Guaifenesin 75 mg and codeine phosphate 2.5 mg per 5 mL
Syrup [C-V] (Cheracol®, Guaituss AC®, Guiatussin® with Codeine, Mytussin® AC, Robafen® AC, Robitussin® A-C, Tussi-Organidin® NR): Guaifenesin 100 mg and codeine phosphate 10 mg per 5 mL (60 mL, 120 mL, 480 mL)
Tablet [C-III] (Brontex®): Guaifenesin 300 mg and codeine phosphate 10 mg

guaifenesin and dextromethorphan

(gwye FEN e sin & deks troe meth OR fan)

Synonyms dextromethorphan and guaifenesin

Brand Names Benylin® Expectorant [OTC]; Cheracol® D [OTC]; Clear Tussin® 30; Contac® Cough Formula Liquid [OTC]; Diabetic Tussin DM® [OTC]; Extra Action Cough Syrup [OTC]; Fenesin DM®; Genatuss DM® [OTC]; Glycotuss-dM® [OTC]; Guaifenex® DM; GuiaCough® [OTC]; Guiatuss-DM® [OTC]; Halotussin® DM [OTC]; Humibid® DM [OTC]; Iobid DM®; Kolephrin® GG/DM [OTC]; Monafed® DM; Muco-Fen-DM®; Mytussin® DM [OTC]; Naldecon® Senior DX [OTC]; Phanatuss® Cough Syrup [OTC]; Phenadex® Senior [OTC]; Respa-DM®; Rhinosyn-DMX® [OTC]; Robafen DM® [OTC]; Robitussin®-DM [OTC]; Safe Tussin® 30 [OTC]; Scot-Tussin® Senior Clear [OTC]; Siltussin DM® [OTC]; Synacol® CF [OTC]; Syracol-CF® [OTC]; Tolu-Sed® DM [OTC]; Tusibron-DM® [OTC]; Tuss-DM® [OTC]; Tussi-Organidin® DM NR; Uni-tussin® DM [OTC]; Vicks® 44E [OTC]; Vicks® Pediatric Formula 44E [OTC]

Therapeutic Category Antitussive/Expectorant

Use Temporary control of cough due to minor throat and bronchial irritation

Usual Dosage Oral:

Children:

2-5 years: 2.5 mL every 6-8 hours; maximum: 10 mL/day
6-12 years: 5 mL every 6-8 hours; maximum: 20 mL/24 hours
>12 years: 10 mL every 6-8 hours; maximum: 40 mL/24 hours
Alternatively: 0.1-0.15 mL/kg/dose every 6-8 hours as needed
Adults: 10 mL every 6-8 hours

Dosage Forms

Syrup:

Benylin® Expectorant: Guaifenesin 100 mg and dextromethorphan hydrobromide 5 mg per 5 mL (118 mL, 236 mL)
Cheracol® D, Clear Tussin® 30, Genatuss DM®, Mytussin® DM, Robitussin®-DM, Siltussin DM®, Tolu-Sed® DM, Tussi-Organidin® DM NR: Guaifenesin 100 mg and dextromethorphan hydrobromide 10 mg per 5 mL (5 mL, 10 mL, 120 mL, 240 mL, 360 mL, 480 mL, 3780 mL)
Contac® Cough Formula Liquid: Guaifenesin 67 mg and dextromethorphan hydrobromide 10 mg per 5 mL (120 mL)
Extra Action Cough Syrup, GuiaCough®, Guiatuss DM®, Halotussin® DM, Rhinosyn-DMX®, Tusibron-DM®, Uni-tussin® DM: Guaifenesin 100 mg and dextromethorphan hydrobromide 15 mg per 5 mL (120 mL, 240 mL, 480 mL)
Kolephrin® GG/DM: Guaifenesin 150 mg and dextromethorphan hydrobromide 10 mg per 5 mL (120 mL)
Naldecon® Senior DX: Guaifenesin 200 mg and dextromethorphan hydrobromide 15 mg per 5 mL (118 mL, 480 mL)
Phanatuss®: Guaifenesin 85 mg and dextromethorphan hydrobromide 10 mg per 5 mL
Vicks® 44E: Guaifenesin 66.7 mg and dextromethorphan hydrobromide 6.7 mg per 5 mL
Tablet:
Extended release
Guaifenex DM®, Iobid DM®, Fenesin DM®, Humibid® DM, Monafed® DM, Respa-DM®: Guaifenesin 600 mg and dextromethorphan hydrobromide 30 mg
Glycotuss-dM®: Guaifenesin 100 mg and dextromethorphan hydrobromide 10 mg
Queltuss®: Guaifenesin 100 mg and dextromethorphan hydrobromide 15 mg

Syracol-CF®: Guaifenesin 200 mg and dextromethorphan hydrobromide 15 mg
Tuss-DM®: Guaifenesin 200 mg and dextromethorphan hydrobromide 10 mg

guaifenesin and hydrocodone see hydrocodone and guaifenesin on page 267

guaifenesin and phenylephrine (gwye FEN e sin & fen il EF rin)
Synonyms phenylephrine and guaifenesin
Brand Names Deconsal® Sprinkle®; Endal®; Sinupan®
Therapeutic Category Cold Preparation
Usual Dosage Adults: Oral: 1-2 tablets/capsules every 12 hours
Dosage Forms
Capsule, sustained release:
Deconsal® Sprinkle®: Guaifenesin 300 mg and phenylephrine hydrochloride 10 mg
Sinupan®: Guaifenesin 200 mg and phenylephrine hydrochloride 40 mg
Tablet, timed release (Endal®): Guaifenesin 300 mg and phenylephrine hydrochloride 20 mg

guaifenesin and phenylpropanolamine
(gwye FEN e sin & fen il proe pa NOLE a meen)
Synonyms phenylpropanolamine and guaifenesin
Brand Names Ami-Tex LA®; Coldlac-LA®; Conex® [OTC]; Contuss® XT; Dura-Vent®; Entex® LA; Genagesic®; Genamin® Expectorant [OTC]; Guaifenex® PPA 75; Guaipax®; Myminic® Expectorant [OTC]; Naldecon-EX® Children's Syrup [OTC]; Nolex® LA; Partuss® LA; Phenylfenesin® L.A.; Profen II®; Profen LA®; Rymed-TR®; Silaminic® Expectorant [OTC]; Sildicon-E® [OTC]; Snaplets-EX® [OTC]; Theramin® Expectorant [OTC]; Triaminic® Expectorant [OTC]; Tri-Clear® Expectorant [OTC]; Triphenyl® Expectorant [OTC]; ULR-LA®; Vicks® DayQuil® Sinus Pressure & Congestion Relief [OTC]
Therapeutic Category Expectorant/Decongestant
Use Symptomatic relief of those respiratory conditions where tenacious mucous plugs and congestion complicate the problem such as sinusitis, pharyngitis, bronchitis, asthma, and as an adjunctive therapy in serous otitis media
Usual Dosage Oral:
Children:
2-6 years: 2.5 mL every 4 hours
6-12 years: 1/2 tablet every 12 hours or 5 mL every 4 hours
Children >12 years and Adults: 1 tablet every 12 hours or 10 mL every 4 hours
Dosage Forms
Caplet:
Vicks® DayQuil® Sinus Pressure & Congestion Relief: Guaifenesin 200 mg and phenylpropanolamine hydrochloride 25 mg
Rymed-TR®: Guaifenesin 400 mg and phenylpropanolamine hydrochloride 75 mg
Drops:
Sildicon-E®: Guaifenesin 30 mg and phenylpropanolamine hydrochloride 6.25 mg per mL (30 mL)
Granules (Snaplets-EX®): Guaifenesin 50 mg and phenylpropanolamine hydrochloride 6.25 mg (pack)
Liquid:
Conex®, Genamin® Expectorant, Myminic® Expectorant, Silaminic® Expectorant, Theramine® Expectorant, Triaminic® Expectorant, Tri-Clear® Expectorant, Triphenyl® Expectorant: Guaifenesin 100 mg and phenylpropanolamine hydrochloride 12.5 mg per 5 mL (120 mL, 240 mL, 480 mL, 3780 mL)
Naldecon-EX® Children's Syrup: Guaifenesin 100 mg and phenylpropanolamine hydrochloride 6.25 mg per 5 mL (120 mL)
Tablet, extended release:
Ami-Tex LA®, Contuss® XT, Entex® LA, Guaipax®, Nolex® LA, Partuss® LA, Phenylfenesin® L.A., ULR-LA®: Guaifenesin 400 mg and phenylpropanolamine hydrochloride 75 mg
(Continued)

guaifenesin and phenylpropanolamine (Continued)

Dura-Vent®, Profen LA®: Guaifenesin 600 mg and phenylpropanolamine hydrochloride 75 mg

Coldlac-LA®, Guaifenex® PPA 75, Profen II®: Guaifenesin 600 mg and phenylpropanolamine hydrochloride 37.5 mg

guaifenesin and pseudoephedrine (gwye FEN e sin & soo doe e FED rin)

Synonyms pseudoephedrine and guaifenesin

Brand Names Congess® Jr; Congess® Sr; Congestac®; Deconsal® II; Defen-LA®; Entex® PSE; Eudal-SR®; Fedahist® Expectorant [OTC]; Fedahist® Expectorant Pediatric [OTC]; Glycofed®; Guaifed® [OTC]; Guaifed®-PD; Guaifenex® PSE; GuaiMAX-D®; Guaitab®; Guaivent®; Guai-Vent/PSE®; Guiatuss PE® [OTC]; Halotussin® PE [OTC]; Histalet® X; Nasabid™; Respa-1st®; Respaire®-60 SR; Respaire®-120 SR; Robitussin-PE® [OTC]; Robitussin® Severe Congestion Liqui-Gels [OTC]; Ru-Tuss® DE; Rymed®; Sinufed® Timecelles®; Touro LA®; Tuss-LA®; V-Dec-M®; Versacaps®; Zephrex®; Zephrex LA®

Therapeutic Category Expectorant/Decongestant

Use Enhance the output of respiratory tract fluid and reduce mucosal congestion and edema in the nasal passage

Usual Dosage Oral:

Children:

2-6 years: 2.5 mL every 4 hours not to exceed 15 mL/24 hours

6-12 years: 5 mL every 4 hours not to exceed 30 mL/24 hours

Children >12 years and Adults: 10 mL every 4 hours not to exceed 60 mL/24 hours

Dosage Forms

Capsule:

Guaivent®: Guaifenesin 250 mg and pseudoephedrine hydrochloride 120 mg

Robitussin® Severe Congestion Liqui-Gels: Guaifenesin 200 mg and pseudoephedrine hydrochloride 30 mg

Rymed®: Guaifenesin 250 mg and pseudoephedrine hydrochloride 30 mg

Capsule, extended release:

Congess® Jr: Guaifenesin 125 mg and pseudoephedrine hydrochloride 60 mg

Nasabid®: Guaifenesin 250 mg and pseudoephedrine hydrochloride 90 mg

Congess® Sr, Guaifed®, Respaire®-120 SR,: Guaifenesin 250 mg and pseudoephedrine hydrochloride 120 mg

Guaifed®-PD, Sinufed® Timecelles®, Versacaps®: Guaifenesin 300 mg and pseudoephedrine hydrochloride 60 mg

Respaire®-60 SR: Guaifenesin 200 mg and pseudoephedrine hydrochloride 60 mg

Tuss-LA® Capsule: Guaifenesin 500 mg and pseudoephedrine hydrochloride 120 mg

Drops, oral (Fedahist® Expectorant Pediatric): Guaifenesin 40 mg and pseudoephedrine hydrochloride 7.5 mg per mL (30 mL)

Syrup:

Fedahist® Expectorant, Guaifed®: Guaifenesin 200 mg and pseudoephedrine hydrochloride 30 mg per 5 mL (120 mL, 240 mL)

Guiatuss® PE, Halotussin® PE, Robitussin-PE®, Rymed®: Guaifenesin 100 mg and pseudoephedrine hydrochloride 30 mg per 5 mL (120 mL, 240 mL, 480 mL)

Histalet® X: Guaifenesin 200 mg and pseudoephedrine hydrochloride 45 mg per 5 mL (473 mL)

Tablet:

Congestac®, Guaitab®, Zephrex®: Guaifenesin 400 mg and pseudoephedrine hydrochloride 60 mg

Glycofed®: Guaifenesin 100 mg and pseudoephedrine hydrochloride 30 mg

Tablet, extended release:

Deconsal® II, Defen-LA®, Respa-1st®: Guaifenesin 600 mg and pseudoephedrine hydrochloride 60 mg

Entex® PSE, Guaifenex® PSE, GuaiMAX-D®, Guai-Vent/PSE®, Ru-Tuss® DE, Sudex®, Zephrex LA®: Guaifenesin 600 mg and pseudoephedrine hydrochloride 120 mg

Eudal-SR®, Histalet® X, Touro LA®: Guaifenesin 400 mg and pseudoephedrine hydro-chloride 120 mg

Tuss-LA® Tablet, V-Dec-M®: Guaifenesin 5mg and pseudoephedrine hydrochloride 120 mg

guaifenesin, phenylpropanolamine, and dextromethorphan
(gwye FEN e sin, fen il proe pa NOLE a meen, & deks troe meth OR fan)

Brand Names Anatuss® [OTC]; Guiatuss CF® [OTC]; Naldecon® DX Adult Liquid [OTC]; Profen II DM®; Robafen® CF [OTC]; Robitussin-CF® [OTC]; Siltussin-CF® [OTC]

Therapeutic Category Antitussive/Decongestant/Expectorant

Use Temporarily relieves nasal congestion and controls cough due to minor throat and bronchial irritation; helps loosen phlegm and thin bronchial secretions to make coughs more productive

Usual Dosage Oral:

Children:

2-6 years: 2.5 mL every 4 hours not to exceed 15 mL/24 hours

6-12 years: 5 mL every 4 hours not to exceed 30 mL/24 hours

Children >12 years and Adults: 10 mL every 4 hours not to exceed 60 mL/24 hours

Dosage Forms

Syrup:

Anatuss®: Guaifenesin 100 mg, phenylpropanolamine hydrochloride 25 mg, and dextromethorphan hydrobromide 15 mg per 5 mL (120 mL, 473 mL)

Guiatuss® CF, Robafen® CF, Robitussin-CF®: Guaifenesin 100 mg, phenylpropanola-mine hydrochloride 12.5 mg, and dextromethorphan hydrobromide 10 mg per 5 mL (120 mL, 240 mL, 360 mL, 480 mL)

Naldecon® DX Adult: Guaifenesin 200 mg, phenylpropanolamine hydrochloride 12.5 mg, and dextromethorphan hydrobromide 10 mg per 5 mL (120 mL, 473 mL)

Siltussin-CF®: Guaifenesin 100 mg, phenylpropanolamine hydrochloride 12.5 mg, and dextromethorphan hydrobromide 10 mg per 5 mL

Tablet: Anatuss®: Guaifenesin 100 mg, phenylpropanolamine hydrochloride 25 mg, and dextromethorphan hydrobromide 15 mg

Timed release (Profen II DM®): Guaifenesin 600 mg, phenylpropanolamine hydrochlo-ride 37.5 mg, and dextromethorphan hydrobromide 30 mg

guaifenesin, phenylpropanolamine, and phenylephrine
(gwye FEN e sin, fen il proe pa NOLE a meen, & fen il EF rin)

Brand Names Coldloc®; Contuss®; Dura-Gest®; Enomine®; Entex®; Guaifenex®; Guiatex®

Therapeutic Category Expectorant/Decongestant

Use Temporary relief of nasal congestion, running nose, sneezing, itching of nose and throat, and itchy, watery eyes due to common cold, hay fever, or other upper respiratory allergies

Usual Dosage Children >12 years and Adults: Oral: 1 capsule 4 times/day (every 6 hours) with food or fluid

Dosage Forms

Capsule (Contuss®, Dura-Gest®, Enomine®, Entex®, Guiatex®): Guaifenesin 200 mg, phenylpropanolamine hydrochloride 45 mg, and phenylephrine hydrochloride 5 mg

Liquid (Coldloc®, Contuss®, Entex®, Guaifenex®): Guaifenesin 100 mg, phenylpropanol-amine hydrochloride 20 mg, and phenylephrine hydrochloride 5 mg per 5 mL (118 mL, 480 mL)

Tablet (Respinol-G®): Guaifenesin 200 mg, phenylpropanolamine hydrochloride 45 mg, and phenylephrine hydrochloride 5 mg

guaifenesin, pseudoephedrine, and codeine
(gwye FEN e sin, soo doe e FED rin, & KOE deen)

Brand Names Codafed® Expectorant; Cycofed® Pediatric; Decohistine® Expectorant; Deproist® Expectorant with Codeine; Dihistine® Expectorant; Guiatuss DAC®; Guiatussin® DAC; Halotussin® DAC; Isoclor® Expectorant; Mytussin® DAC; Nucofed®; (Continued)

guaifenesin, pseudoephedrine, and codeine *(Continued)*

Nucofed® Pediatric Expectorant; Nucotuss®; Phenhist® Expectorant; Robitussin®-DAC; Ryna-CX®; Tussar® SF Syrup

Therapeutic Category Antitussive/Decongestant/Expectorant

Controlled Substance C-III; C-V

Use Temporarily relieves nasal congestion and controls cough due to minor throat and bronchial irritation; helps loosen phlegm and thin bronchial secretions to make coughs more productive

Usual Dosage Oral:

Children 6-12 years: 5 mL every 4 hours, not to exceed 40 mL/24 hours

Children >12 years and Adults: 10 mL every 4 hours, not to exceed 40 mL/24 hours

Dosage Forms Liquid:

C-III: Nucofed®, Nucotuss®: Guaifenesin 200 mg, pseudoephedrine hydrochloride 60 mg, and codeine phosphate 20 mg per 5 mL (480 mL)

C-V: Codafed® Expectorant, Cycofed® Pediatric, Decohistine® Expectorant, Deproist® Expectorant with Codeine, Dihistine® Expectorant, Guiatuss DAC®, Guiatussin® DAC, Halotussin® DAC, Isoclor® Expectorant, Mytussin® DAC, Nucofed® Pediatric Expectorant, Phenhist® Expectorant, Robitussin®-DAC, Ryna-CX®, Tussar® SF: Guaifenesin 100 mg, pseudoephedrine hydrochloride 30 mg, and codeine phosphate 10 mg per 5 mL (120 mL, 480 mL, 4000 mL)

guaifenesin, pseudoephedrine, and dextromethorphan

(gwye FEN e sin, soo doe e FED rin, & deks troe meth OR fan)

Synonyms dextromethorphan, guaifenesin, and pseudoephedrine; pseudoephedrine, dextromethorphan, and guaifenesin

Brand Names Anatuss® DM [OTC]; Dimacol® Caplets [OTC]; Rhinosyn-X® Liquid [OTC]; Ru-Tuss® Expectorant [OTC]; Sudafed® Cold & Cough Liquid Caps [OTC]

Therapeutic Category Cold Preparation

Usual Dosage Adults: Oral: 2 capsules (caplets) or 10 mL every 4 hours

Dosage Forms

Caplets (Dimacol®): Guaifenesin 100 mg, pseudoephedrine hydrochloride 30 mg, and dextromethorphan hydrobromide 10 mg

Capsule (Sudafed® Cold & Cough Liquid Caps): Guaifenesin 100 mg, pseudoephedrine hydrochloride 30 mg, and dextromethorphan hydrobromide 10 mg

Liquid (Anatuss® DM, Rhinosyn-X® Liquid, Ru-Tuss® Expectorant): Guaifenesin 100 mg, pseudoephedrine hydrochloride 30 mg, and dextromethorphan hydrobromide 10 mg per 5 mL

Guaifenex® *see* guaifenesin, phenylpropanolamine, and phenylephrine *on previous page*

Guaifenex® DM *see* guaifenesin and dextromethorphan *on page 248*

Guaifenex® LA *see* guaifenesin *on page 247*

Guaifenex® PPA 75 *see* guaifenesin and phenylpropanolamine *on page 249*

Guaifenex® PSE *see* guaifenesin and pseudoephedrine *on page 250*

GuaiMAX-D® *see* guaifenesin and pseudoephedrine *on page 250*

Guaipax® *see* guaifenesin and phenylpropanolamine *on page 249*

Guaitab® *see* guaifenesin and pseudoephedrine *on page 250*

Guaituss AC® *see* guaifenesin and codeine *on page 247*

Guaivent® *see* guaifenesin and pseudoephedrine *on page 250*

Guai-Vent/PSE® *see* guaifenesin and pseudoephedrine *on page 250*

guanabenz (GWAHN a benz)

Synonyms guanabenz acetate

Brand Names Wytensin®

Therapeutic Category Alpha-Adrenergic Agonist
Use Management of hypertension
Usual Dosage Adults: Oral: Initial: 4 mg twice daily, increase in increments of 4-8 mg/day every 1-2 weeks to a maximum of 32 mg twice daily
Dosage Forms Tablet, as acetate: 4 mg, 8 mg

guanabenz acetate *see* guanabenz *on previous page*

guanadrel (GWAHN a drel)

Synonyms guanadrel sulfate
Brand Names Hylorel®
Therapeutic Category Alpha-Adrenergic Agonist
Use Step 2 agent in stepped-care treatment of hypertension, usually with a diuretic
Usual Dosage Oral: Initial: 10 mg/day (5 mg twice daily); adjust dosage until blood pressure is controlled, usual dosage: 20-75 mg/day, administered twice daily
Dosage Forms Tablet, as sulfate: 10 mg, 25 mg

guanadrel sulfate *see* guanadrel *on this page*

guanethidine (gwahn ETH i deen)

Synonyms guanethidine monosulfate
Brand Names Ismelin®
Therapeutic Category Alpha-Adrenergic Agonist
Use Treatment of moderate to severe hypertension
Usual Dosage Oral:
Children: Initial: 0.2 mg/kg/day administered daily; maximum dose: up to 3 mg/kg/24 hours
Adults: Initial: 10-12.5 mg/day, then 25-50 mg/day in 3 divided doses
Dosage Forms Tablet, as monosulfate: 10 mg, 25 mg

guanethidine monosulfate *see* guanethidine *on this page*

guanfacine (GWAHN fa seen)

Synonyms guanfacine hydrochloride
Brand Names Tenex®
Therapeutic Category Alpha-Adrenergic Agonist
Use Management of hypertension
Usual Dosage Adults: Oral: 1 mg (usually at bedtime), may increase if needed at 3- to 4-week intervals to a maximum of 3 mg/day; 1 mg/day is most common dose
Dosage Forms Tablet, as hydrochloride: 1 mg

guanfacine hydrochloride *see* guanfacine *on this page*

guanidine (GWAHN i deen)

Synonyms guanidine hydrochloride
Therapeutic Category Cholinergic Agent
Use Reduction of the symptoms of muscle weakness associated with the myasthenic syndrome of Eaton-Lambert, not for myasthenia gravis
Usual Dosage Adults: Oral: Initial: 10-15 mg/kg/day in 3-4 divided doses, gradually increase to 35 mg/kg/day
Dosage Forms Tablet, as hydrochloride: 125 mg

guanidine hydrochloride *see* guanidine *on this page*
GuiaCough® [OTC] *see* guaifenesin and dextromethorphan *on page 248*
GuiaCough® Expectorant [OTC] *see* guaifenesin *on page 247*
Guiatex® *see* guaifenesin, phenylpropanolamine, and phenylephrine *on page 251*
Guiatuss® [OTC] *see* guaifenesin *on page 247*

Guiatuss CF® **[OTC]** *see* guaifenesin, phenylpropanolamine, and dextromethorphan *on page 251*

Guiatuss DAC® *see* guaifenesin, pseudoephedrine, and codeine *on page 251*

Guiatuss-DM® **[OTC]** *see* guaifenesin and dextromethorphan *on page 248*

Guiatussin® DAC *see* guaifenesin, pseudoephedrine, and codeine *on page 251*

Guiatussin® with Codeine *see* guaifenesin and codeine *on page 247*

Guiatuss PE® **[OTC]** *see* guaifenesin and pseudoephedrine *on page 250*

gum benjamin *see* benzoin *on page 61*

G-well® *see* lindane *on page 309*

Gynecort® **[OTC]** *see* hydrocortisone *on page 268*

Gyne-Lotrimin® **[OTC]** *see* clotrimazole *on page 131*

Gyne-Sulf® *see* sulfabenzamide, sulfacetamide, and sulfathiazole *on page 496*

Gynogen L.A.® Injection *see* estradiol *on page 202*

Gynol II® **[OTC]** *see* nonoxynol 9 *on page 377*

Habitrol™ Patch *see* nicotine *on page 373*

haemophilus b conjugate vaccine
(hem OF fi lus bee KON joo gate vak SEEN)
Synonyms Hib polysaccharide conjugate; prp-d
Brand Names HibTITER®; OmniHIB®; PedvaxHIB™; ProHIBiT®
Therapeutic Category Vaccine, Inactivated Bacteria
Use Immunization of children 24 months to 6 years of age against diseases caused by *H. influenzae* type b
Usual Dosage Children: I.M.: 0.5 mL as a single dose should be administered
Dosage Forms Injection:
HibTITER®, OmniHIB®: Capsular oligosaccharide 10 mcg and diphtheria CRM$_{197}$ protein ~25 mcg per 0.5 mL (0.5 mL, 2.5 mL, 5 mL)
PedvaxHIB™: Purified capsular polysaccharide 15 mcg and *Neisseria meningitidis* OMPC 250 mcg per dose (0.5 mL)
ProHIBiT®: Purified capsular polysaccharide 25 mcg and conjugated diphtheria toxoid protein 18 mcg per dose (0.5 mL, 2.5 mL, 5 mL)

halazepam (hal AZ e pam)
Brand Names Paxipam®
Therapeutic Category Benzodiazepine
Controlled Substance C-IV
Use Management of anxiety disorders; short-term relief of the symptoms of anxiety
Usual Dosage Adults: Oral: 20-40 mg 3 or 4 times/day
Dosage Forms Tablet: 20 mg, 40 mg

halcinonide (hal SIN oh nide)
Brand Names Halog®; Halog®-E
Therapeutic Category Corticosteroid, Topical
Use Inflammation of corticosteroid-responsive dermatoses
Usual Dosage Children and Adults: Topical: Apply sparingly 1-3 times/day, occlusive dressing may be used for severe or resistant dermatoses
Dosage Forms
Cream (Halog®): 0.025% (15 g, 60 g, 240 g); 0.1% (15 g, 30 g, 60 g, 240 g)
Emollient base (Halog®-E) : 0.1% (15 g, 30 g, 60 g)
Ointment, topical (Halog®): 0.1% (15 g, 30 g, 60 g, 240 g)
Solution (Halog®): 0.1% (20 mL, 60 mL)

Halcion® *see* triazolam *on page 530*

Haldol® *see* haloperidol *on this page*

Haldol® **Decanoate** *see* haloperidol *on this page*

Haldrone® *see* paramethasone acetate *on page 396*

Halenol® **Childrens [OTC]** *see* acetaminophen *on page 3*

Haley's M-O® **[OTC]** *see* magnesium hydroxide and mineral oil emulsion *on page 319*

Halfan® *see* halofantrine *on this page*

Halfprin® **81**® **[OTC]** *see* aspirin *on page 44*

halobetasol (hal oh BAY ta sol)
Synonyms halobetasol propionate
Brand Names Ultravate™
Therapeutic Category Corticosteroid, Topical
Use Relief of inflammatory and pruritic manifestations of corticosteroid-response dermatoses
Usual Dosage Children and Adults: Topical: Apply sparingly to skin twice daily, rub in gently and completely
Dosage Forms
Cream, as propionate: 0.05% (15 g, 45 g)
Ointment, topical, as propionate: 0.05% (15 g, 45 g)

halobetasol propionate *see* halobetasol *on this page*

halofantrine (ha loe FAN trin)
Synonyms halofantrine hydrochloride
Brand Names Halfan®
Therapeutic Category Antimalarial Agent
Use Treatment of mild to moderate acute malaria caused by susceptible strains of *Plasmodium falciparum* and *Plasmodium vivax*
Usual Dosage Oral:
Children <40 kg: 8 mg/kg every 6 hours for 3 doses
Adults: 500 mg every 6 hours for 3 doses
Dosage Forms
Suspension, as hydrochloride: 100 mg/5 mL
Tablet, as hydrochloride: 250 mg

halofantrine hydrochloride *see* halofantrine *on this page*

Halog® *see* halcinonide *on previous page*

Halog®**-E** *see* halcinonide *on previous page*

haloperidol (ha loe PER i dole)
Synonyms haloperidol decanoate; haloperidol lactate
Brand Names Haldol®; Haldol® Decanoate
Therapeutic Category Butyrophenone Derivative (Antipsychotic)
Use Treatment of psychoses, Tourette's disorder, and severe behavioral problems in children
Usual Dosage
Children:
<3 years: Not recommended
3-6 years: Dose and indications are not well established
Control of agitation or hyperkinesia in disturbed children: Oral: 0.01-0.03 mg/kg/day once daily
Infantile autism: Oral: Daily doses of 0.5-4 mg have been reported to be helpful in this disorder
6-12 years: Dose not well established
(Continued)

haloperidol (Continued)

I.M.: 1-3 mg/dose every 4-8 hours, up to a maximum of 0.1 mg/kg/day

Acute psychosis: Oral: Begin with 0.5-1.5 mg/day and increase gradually in increments of 0.5 mg/day, to a maintenance dose of 2-4 mg/day (0.05-0.1 mg/kg/day).

Tourette's syndrome and mental retardation with hyperkinesia: Oral: Begin with 0.5 mg/day and increase by 0.5 mg/day each day until symptoms are controlled or a maximum dose of 15 mg is reached

Children >12 years and Adults:

I.M.:

Acute psychosis: 2-5 mg/dose every 1-8 hours PRN up to a total of 10-30 mg, until control of symptoms is achieved

Mental retardation with hyperkinesia: Begin with 20 mg/day in divided doses, then increase slowly, up to a maximum of 60 mg/day; change to oral administration as soon as symptoms are controlled

Oral:

Acute psychosis: Begin with 1-15 mg/day in divided doses, then gradually increase until symptoms are controlled, up to a maximum of 100 mg/day; after control of symptoms is achieved, reduce dose to the minimal effective dose

Tourette's syndrome: Begin with 6-15 mg/day in divided doses, increase in increments of 2-10 mg/day until symptoms are controlled or adverse reactions become disabling; when symptoms are controlled, reduce to approximately 9 mg/day for maintenance

Dosage Forms

Concentrate, oral, as lactate: 2 mg/mL (5 mL, 10 mL, 15 mL, 120 mL, 240 mL)

Injection:

As decanoate: 50 mg/mL (1 mL, 5 mL); 100 mg/mL (1 mL, 5 mL)

As lactate: 5 mg/mL (1 mL, 2 mL, 2.5 mL, 10 mL)

Tablet: 0.5 mg, 1 mg, 2 mg, 5 mg, 10 mg, 20 mg

haloperidol decanoate see haloperidol on previous page

haloperidol lactate see haloperidol on previous page

haloprogin (ha loe PROE jin)

Brand Names Halotex®

Therapeutic Category Antifungal Agent

Use Topical treatment of tinea pedis, tinea cruris, tinea corporis, tinea manuum caused by Trichophyton rubrum, Trichophyton tonsurans, Trichophyton mentagrophytes, Microsporum canis, or Epidermophyton floccosum

Usual Dosage Children and Adults: Topical: Twice daily for 2-3 weeks; intertriginous areas may require up to 4 weeks of treatment

Dosage Forms

Cream: 1% (15 g, 30 g)

Solution, topical: 1% with alcohol 75% (10 mL, 30 mL)

Halotestin® see fluoxymesterone on page 230

Halotex® see haloprogin on this page

halothane (HA loe thane)

Brand Names Fluothane®

Therapeutic Category General Anesthetic

Use General induction and maintenance of anesthesia (inhalation)

Usual Dosage Maintenance concentration varies from 0.5% to 1.5%

Dosage Forms Liquid: 125 mL, 250 mL

Halotussin® [OTC] see guaifenesin on page 247

Halotussin® DAC see guaifenesin, pseudoephedrine, and codeine on page 251

Halotussin® DM [OTC] see guaifenesin and dextromethorphan on page 248

Halotussin® PE [OTC] *see* guaifenesin and pseudoephedrine *on page 250*

Haltran® [OTC] *see* ibuprofen *on page 278*

hamamelis water *see* witch hazel *on page 557*

Havrix® *see* hepatitis a vaccine *on next page*

Hayfebrol® Liquid [OTC] *see* chlorpheniramine and pseudoephedrine *on page 114*

hbig *see* hepatitis b immune globulin *on page 259*

H-BIG® *see* hepatitis b immune globulin *on page 259*

hcg *see* chorionic gonadotropin *on page 122*

hctz *see* hydrochlorothiazide *on page 264*

HD 85® *see* radiological/contrast media (ionic) *on page 457*

HD 200 Plus® *see* radiological/contrast media (ionic) *on page 457*

hdcv *see* rabies virus vaccine *on page 457*

hdrs *see* rabies virus vaccine *on page 457*

Head & Shoulders® [OTC] *see* pyrithione zinc *on page 454*

Head & Shoulders® Intensive Treatment [OTC] *see* selenium sulfide *on page 476*

Healon® *see* sodium hyaluronate *on page 485*

Healon® GV *see* sodium hyaluronate *on page 485*

Heartline® [OTC] *see* aspirin *on page 44*

Helistat® *see* microfibrillar collagen hemostat *on page 349*

Helixate® *see* antihemophilic factor (recombinant) *on page 37*

Hemabate™ *see* carboprost tromethamine *on page 92*

hemiacidrin *see* citric acid bladder mixture *on page 125*

hemin (HEE min)

Brand Names Panhematin®

Therapeutic Category Blood Modifiers

Use Treatment of recurrent attacks of acute intermittent porphyria (AIP) only after an appropriate period of alternate therapy has been tried

Usual Dosage I.V.: 1-4 mg/kg/day administered over 10-15 minutes for 3-14 days; may be repeated no earlier than every 12 hours; not to exceed 6 mg/kg in any 24-hour period

Dosage Forms Powder for injection, preservative free: 313 mg/vial [hematin 7 mg/mL] (43 mL)

Hemocyte® [OTC] *see* ferrous fumarate *on page 220*

Hemofil® M *see* antihemophilic factor (human) *on page 37*

Hemotene® *see* microfibrillar collagen hemostat *on page 349*

Hemril-HC® Uniserts® *see* hydrocortisone *on page 268*

heparin (HEP a rin)

Synonyms heparin lock flush; heparin sodium

Brand Names Hep-Lock®

Therapeutic Category Anticoagulant

Use Prophylaxis and treatment of thromboembolic disorders

Usual Dosage Note: For full-dose heparin (ie, nonlow-dose), the dose should be titrated according to PTT results. For anticoagulation, an APTT 1.5-2.5 times normal is usually desired. APTT is usually measured prior to heparin therapy, 6-8 hours after initiation of a continuous infusion (following a loading dose), and 6-8 hours after changes in the infusion rate; increase or decrease infusion by 2-4 units/kg/hour dependent on PTT. (Continued)

heparin *(Continued)*

Continuous I.V. infusion is preferred vs I.V. intermittent injections. For intermittent I.V. injections, PTT is measured 3.5-4 hours after I.V. injection.

Children:
Intermittent I.V.: Initial: 50-100 units/kg, then 50-100 units/kg every 4 hours
I.V. infusion: Initial: 50 units/kg, then 15-25 units/kg/hour; increase dose by 2-4 units/kg/hour every 6-8 hours as required

Adults:
Prophylaxis (low-dose heparin): S.C.: 5000 units every 8-12 hours
Intermittent I.V.: Initial: 10,000 units, then 50-70 units/kg (5000-10,000 units) every 4-6 hours
I.V. infusion: Initial: 75-100 units/kg, then 15 units/kg/hour with dose adjusted according to PTT results; usual range: 10-30 units/kg/hour

Dosage Forms

Heparin sodium:
Lock flush injection:
Beef lung source: 10 units/mL (1 mL, 2 mL, 2.5 mL, 3 mL, 5 mL, 10 mL, 30 mL); 100 units/mL (1 mL, 2 mL, 2.5 mL, 3 mL, 5 mL, 10 mL, 30 mL)
Porcine intestinal mucosa source: 10 units/mL (1 mL, 2 mL, 10 mL, 30 mL); 100 units/mL (1 mL, 2 mL, 10 mL, 30 mL)
Porcine intestinal mucosa source, preservative free: 10 units/mL (1 mL); 100 units/mL (1 mL)

Multiple-dose vial injection:
Beef lung source, with preservative: 1000 units/mL (5 mL, 10 mL, 30 mL); 5000 units/mL (10 mL); 10,000 units/mL (4 mL, 5 mL, 10 mL); 20,000 units/mL (2 mL, 5 mL, 10 mL); 40,000 units/mL (5 mL)
Porcine intestinal mucosa source, with preservative: 1000 units/mL (10 mL, 30 mL); 5000 units/mL (10 mL); 10,000 units/mL (4 mL); 20,000 units/mL (2 mL, 5 mL)

Single-dose vial injection:
Beef lung source: 1000 units/mL (1 mL); 5000 units/mL (1 mL); 10,000 units/mL (1 mL); 20,000 units/mL (1 mL); 40,000 units/mL (1 mL)
Porcine intestinal mucosa: 1000 units/mL (1 mL); 5000 units/mL (1 mL); 10,000 units/mL (1 mL); 20,000 units/mL (1 mL); 40,000 units/mL (1 mL)

Unit dose injection:
Porcine intestinal mucosa source, with preservative: 1000 units/dose (1 mL, 2 mL); 2500 units/dose (1 mL); 5000 units/dose (0.5 mL, 1 mL); 7500 units/dose (1 mL); 10,000 units/dose (1 mL); 15,000 units/dose (1 mL); 20,000 units/dose (1 mL)

Heparin sodium infusion, porcine intestinal mucosa source:
D_5W: 40 units/mL (500 mL); 50 units/mL (250 mL, 500 mL); 100 units/mL (100 mL, 250 mL)
NaCl 0.45%: 2 units/mL (500 mL, 1000 mL); 50 units/mL (250 mL); 100 units/mL (250 mL)
NaCl 0.9%: 2 units/mL (500 mL, 1000 mL); 5 units/mL (1000 mL); 50 units/mL (250 mL, 500 mL, 1000 mL)

Heparin calcium: Unit dose injection, porcine intestinal mucosa, preservative free: 5000 units/dose (0.2 mL); 12,500 units/dose (0.5 mL); 20,000 units/dose (0.8 mL)

heparin cofactor I *see* antithrombin III *on page 38*

heparin lock flush *see* heparin *on previous page*

heparin sodium *see* heparin *on previous page*

hepatitis a vaccine *(hep a TYE tis aye vak SEEN)*

Brand Names Havrix®

Therapeutic Category Vaccine, Inactivated Virus

Use For populations desiring protection against hepatitis A or for populations at high risk of exposure to hepatitis A virus (travelers to developing countries, household and sexual contacts of persons infected with hepatitis A), child day care employees, illicit drug users, male homosexuals, institutional workers (eg, institutions for the mentally and physically handicapped persons, prisons, etc), and healthcare workers who may be exposed to hepatitis A virus (eg, laboratory employees)

Usual Dosage I.M.:
Children: 0.5 mL (360 units) on days 1 and 30, with a booster dose 6-12 months later (completion of the first 2 doses [ie, the primary series] should be accomplished at least 2 weeks before anticipated exposure to hepatitis A)
Adults: 1 mL (1440 units), with a booster dose at 6-12 months

Dosage Forms
Injection: 360 ELISA units/0.5 mL (0.5 mL); 1440 ELISA units/mL (1 mL)
Injection, pediatric: 720 ELISA units/0.5 mL (0.5 mL)

hepatitis b immune globulin (hep a TYE tis bee i MYUN GLOB yoo lin)

Synonyms hbig
Brand Names H-BIG®; HyperHep®
Therapeutic Category Immune Globulin
Use Provide prophylactic passive immunity to hepatitis B infection to those individuals exposed. Hepatitis B immune globulin is not indicated for treatment of active hepatitis B infections and is ineffective in the treatment of chronic active hepatitis B infection.

Usual Dosage I.M.:
Newborns: Hepatitis B: 0.5 mL as soon after birth as possible (within 12 hours)
Adults: Postexposure prophylaxis: 0.06 mL/kg; usual dose: 3-5 mL; repeat at 28-30 days after exposure

Dosage Forms Injection:
H-BIG®: 4 mL, 5 mL
Hep-B-Gammagee®: 5 mL
HyperHep®: 0.5 mL, 1 mL, 5 mL

hepatitis B inactivated virus vaccine (plasma derived) *see* hepatitis b vaccine *on this page*

hepatitis B inactivated virus vaccine (recombinant DNA) *see* hepatitis b vaccine *on this page*

hepatitis b vaccine (hep a TYE tis bee vak SEEN)

Synonyms hepatitis B inactivated virus vaccine (plasma derived); hepatitis B inactivated virus vaccine (recombinant DNA)
Brand Names Engerix-B®; Recombivax HB®
Therapeutic Category Vaccine, Inactivated Virus
Use Immunization against infection caused by all known subtypes of hepatitis B virus in individuals considered at high risk of potential exposure to hepatitis B virus or HB$_s$Ag-positive materials

Usual Dosage I.M.:
Children:
≤11 years: 2.5 mcg doses
11-19 years: 5 mcg doses
Adults >20 years: 10 mcg doses

Dosage Forms Injection:
Recombinant DNA (Engerix-B®): Hepatitis B surface antigen 20 mcg/mL (1 mL)
Pediatric, recombinant DNA (Engerix-B®): Hepatitis B surface antigen 10 mcg/0.5 mL (0.5 mL)
Recombinant DNA (Recombivax HB®): Hepatitis B surface antigen 10 mcg/mL (1 mL, 3 mL)
Dialysis formulation, recombinant DNA (Recombivax HB®): Hepatitis B surface antigen 40 mcg/mL (1 mL)

Hep-Lock® *see* heparin *on page 257*

Heptalac® *see* lactulose *on page 300*
Herplex® **Ophthalmic** *see* idoxuridine *on page 279*
hes *see* hetastarch *on this page*
Hespan® *see* hetastarch *on this page*

hetastarch (HET a starch)
    Synonyms hes; hydroxyethyl starch
    Brand Names Hespan®
    Therapeutic Category Plasma Volume Expander
    Use Blood volume expander used in treatment of shock or impending shock when blood or blood products are not available; does not have oxygen-carrying capacity and is not a substitute for blood or plasma; an adjunct in leukapheresis to enhance the yield of granulocytes by centrifugal means
    Usual Dosage I.V.: Up to 1500 mL/day
    Dosage Forms Infusion, in sodium chloride 0.9%: 6% (500 mL)

Hexabrix™ *see* radiological/contrast media (ionic) *on page 457*
hexachlorocyclohexane *see* lindane *on page 309*

hexachlorophene (heks a KLOR oh feen)
    Brand Names pHisoHex®; Septisol®
    Therapeutic Category Antibacterial, Topical
    Use Surgical scrub and as a bacteriostatic skin cleanser; to control an outbreak of gram-positive staphylococcal infection when other infection control procedures have been unsuccessful
    Usual Dosage Children and Adults: Topical: Apply 5 mL cleanser and water to area to be cleansed; lather and rinse thoroughly under running water
    Dosage Forms
    Foam (Septisol®): 0.23% with alcohol 56% (180 mL, 600 mL)
    Liquid, topical (pHisoHex®): 3% (8 mL, 150 mL, 500 mL, 3840 mL)

Hexadrol® *see* dexamethasone *on page 156*
Hexadrol® **Phosphate** *see* dexamethasone *on page 156*
Hexalen® *see* altretamine *on page 20*
hexamethylenetetramine *see* methenamine *on page 336*
hexamethylmelamine *see* altretamine *on page 20*

hexylresorcinol (heks il re ZOR si nole)
    Brand Names Sucrets® Sore Throat [OTC]
    Therapeutic Category Local Anesthetic
    Use Minor antiseptic and local anesthetic for sore throat
    Usual Dosage May be used as needed, allow to dissolve slowly in mouth
    Dosage Forms Lozenge: 2.4 mg

Hibiclens® **Topical [OTC]** *see* chlorhexidine gluconate *on page 109*
Hibistat® **Topical [OTC]** *see* chlorhexidine gluconate *on page 109*
Hib polysaccharide conjugate *see* haemophilus b conjugate vaccine *on page 254*
HibTITER® *see* haemophilus b conjugate vaccine *on page 254*
Hi-Cor® **1.0** *see* hydrocortisone *on page 268*
Hi-Cor® **2.5** *see* hydrocortisone *on page 268*
Hiprex® *see* methenamine *on page 336*
Hismanal® *see* astemizole *on page 45*

Histalet Forte® Tablet *see* chlorpheniramine, pyrilamine, phenylephrine, and phenylpropanolamine *on page 118*

Histalet® Syrup [OTC] *see* chlorpheniramine and pseudoephedrine *on page 114*

Histalet® X *see* guaifenesin and pseudoephedrine *on page 250*

Histatab® Plus Tablet [OTC] *see* chlorpheniramine and phenylephrine *on page 113*

Hista-Vadrin® Tablet *see* chlorpheniramine, phenylephrine, and phenylpropanolamine *on page 116*

Histerone® Injection *see* testosterone *on page 507*

Histolyn-CYL® Injection *see* histoplasmin *on this page*

histoplasmin (his toe PLAZ min)

Synonyms histoplasmosis skin test antigen
Brand Names Histolyn-CYL® Injection
Therapeutic Category Diagnostic Agent
Use Diagnosing histoplasmosis; to assess cell-mediated immunity
Usual Dosage Adults: Intradermally: 0.1 mL of 1:100 dilution 5-10 cm apart into volar surface of forearm; induration of ≥5 mm in diameter indicates a positive reaction
Dosage Forms Injection: 1:100 (0.1 mL, 1.3 mL)

histoplasmosis skin test antigen *see* histoplasmin *on this page*

Histor-D® Syrup *see* chlorpheniramine and phenylephrine *on page 113*

Histor-D® Timecelles® *see* chlorpheniramine, phenylephrine, and methscopolamine *on page 116*

histrelin (his TREL in)

Brand Names Supprelin™ Injection
Therapeutic Category Gonadotropin Releasing Hormone Analog
Use Central idiopathic precocious puberty; also used to treat estrogen-associated gynecological disorders (ie, endometriosis, intermittent porphyria, possibly premenstrual syndrome, leiomyomata uteri [uterine fibroids])
Usual Dosage
Central idiopathic precocious puberty: S.C.: Usual dose is 10 mcg/kg/day administered as a single daily dose at the same time each day
Acute intermittent porphyria in women:
S.C.: 5 mcg/day
Intranasal: 400-800 mcg/day
Endometriosis: S.C.: 100 mcg/day
Leiomyomata uteri: S.C.: 20-50 mcg/day or 4 mcg/kg/day
Dosage Forms Injection: 7-day kits of single use: 120 mcg/0.6 mL; 300 mcg/0.6 mL; 600 mcg/0.6 mL

Hi-Vegi-Lip® *see* pancreatin *on page 394*

Hivid® *see* zalcitabine *on page 559*

HMS Liquifilm® *see* medrysone *on page 326*

HN₂ *see* mechlorethamine *on page 324*

Hold® DM [OTC] *see* dextromethorphan *on page 160*

homatropine (hoe MA troe peen)

Synonyms homatropine hydrobromide
Brand Names AK-Homatropine® Ophthalmic; Isopto® Homatropine Ophthalmic
Therapeutic Category Anticholinergic Agent
Use Producing cycloplegia and mydriasis for refraction; treatment of acute inflammatory conditions of the uveal tract
(Continued)

homatropine *(Continued)*

Usual Dosage Ophthalmic:
Children:
Mydriasis and cycloplegia for refraction: 1 drop of 2% solution immediately before the procedure; repeat at 10-minute intervals as needed
Uveitis: 1 drop of 2% solution 2-3 times/day
Adults:
Mydriasis and cycloplegia for refraction: 1-2 drops of 2% solution or 1 drop of 5% solution before the procedure; repeat at 5- to 10-minute intervals as needed
Uveitis: 1-2 drops 2-3 times/day up to every 3-4 hours as needed
Dosage Forms Solution, ophthalmic, as hydrobromide:
2% (1 mL, 5 mL); 5% (1 mL, 2 mL, 5 mL)
AK-Homatropine®: 5% (15 mL)
Isopto® Homatropine 2% (5 mL, 15 mL); 5% (5 mL, 15 mL)

homatropine and hydrocodone *see* hydrocodone and homatropine *on page 267*

homatropine hydrobromide *see* homatropine *on previous page*

horse anti-human thymocyte gamma globulin *see* lymphocyte immune globulin *on page 316*

H.P. Acthar® Gel *see* corticotropin *on page 138*

Humalog® *see* insulin preparations *on page 284*

human growth hormone (HYU man grothe HOR mone)

Synonyms somatrem; somatropin
Brand Names Genotropin® Injection; Humatrope® Injection; Norditropin® Injection; Nutropin® AQ Injection; Nutropin® Injection; Protropin® Injection; Serostim® Injection
Therapeutic Category Growth Hormone
Use Long-term treatment of growth failure from lack of adequate endogenous growth hormone secretion
Usual Dosage Children: I.M., S.C.:
Somatrem: Up to 0.1 mg (0.26 units)/kg/dose 3 times/week
Somatropin: Up to 0.06 mg (0.16 units)/kg/dose 3 times/week
Therapy should be discontinued when patient has reached satisfactory adult height, when epiphyses have fused, or when the patient ceases to respond
Dosage Forms Powder for injection (lyophilized):
Somatropin:
Genotropin®: 1.5 mg ~4 units (5 mL); 5.8 mg ~15 units (5 mL)
Humatrope®: 5 mg ~13 units (5 mL)
Norditropin®: 4 mg ~12 units; 8 mg ~24 units
Nutropin®: 5 mg ~13 units (5 mL); 10 mg ~26 units (10 mL)
Nutropin® AQ: 10 mg ~30 units (2 mL)
Serostim®: 5 mg ~13 units or 6 mg ~15.6 units
Somatrem, Protropin®: 5 mg ~13 units (10 mL)

Humate-P® *see* antihemophilic factor (human) *on page 37*

Humatin® *see* paromomycin *on page 397*

Humatrope® Injection *see* human growth hormone *on this page*

Humegon® *see* menotropins *on page 328*

Humibid® DM [OTC] *see* guaifenesin and dextromethorphan *on page 248*

Humibid® L.A. *see* guaifenesin *on page 247*

Humibid® Sprinkle *see* guaifenesin *on page 247*

HuMist® Nasal Mist [OTC] *see* sodium chloride *on page 483*

Humorsol® Ophthalmic *see* demecarium *on page 152*

Humulin® 50/50 *see* insulin preparations *on page 284*

Humulin® 70/30 *see* insulin preparations *on page 284*

Humulin® L *see* insulin preparations *on page 284*

Humulin® N *see* insulin preparations *on page 284*

Hurricaine® *see* benzocaine *on page 59*

hyaluronic acid *see* sodium hyaluronate *on page 485*

hyaluronidase (hye al yoor ON i dase)
Brand Names Wydase® Injection
Therapeutic Category Antidote
Use Increase the dispersion and absorption of other drugs; increase rate of absorption of parenteral fluids administered by hypodermoclysis; management of I.V. extravasations
Usual Dosage
Infants and Children:
Management of I.V. extravasation: Reconstitute the 150 unit vial of lyophilized powder with 1 mL normal saline; administer 0.1 mL of this solution and dilute with 0.9 mL normal saline to yield 15 units/mL; using a 25- or 26-gauge needle, five 0.2 mL injections are made subcutaneously or intradermally into the extravasation site at the leading edge, changing the needle after each injection
Hypodermoclysis: S.C.: 15 units is added to each 100 mL of I.V. fluid to be administered
Adults: Absorption and dispersion of drugs: 150 units is added to the vehicle containing the drug
Dosage Forms
Injection, stabilized solution: 150 units/mL (1 mL, 10 mL)
Powder for injection, lyophilized: 150 units, 1500 units

Hyate®:C *see* factor viii:c (porcine) *on page 215*

Hybolin™ Decanoate Injection *see* nandrolone *on page 364*

Hybolin™ Improved Injection *see* nandrolone *on page 364*

Hycamptamine *see* topotecan *on page 524*

Hycamtin® *see* topotecan *on page 524*

HycoClear Tuss® *see* hydrocodone and guaifenesin *on page 267*

Hycodan® *see* hydrocodone and homatropine *on page 267*

Hycomine® *see* hydrocodone and phenylpropanolamine *on page 267*

Hycomine® Compound *see* hydrocodone, chlorpheniramine, phenylephrine, acetaminophen, and caffeine *on page 268*

Hycomine® Pediatric *see* hydrocodone and phenylpropanolamine *on page 267*

Hycort® *see* hydrocortisone *on page 268*

Hycotuss® Expectorant Liquid *see* hydrocodone and guaifenesin *on page 267*

Hydeltrasol® Injection *see* prednisolone *on page 434*

Hydergine® *see* ergoloid mesylates *on page 198*

Hydergine® LC *see* ergoloid mesylates *on page 198*

hydralazine (hye DRAL a zeen)
Synonyms hydralazine hydrochloride
Brand Names Apresoline®
Therapeutic Category Vasodilator
Use Management of moderate to severe hypertension, congestive heart failure, hypertension secondary to pre-eclampsia/eclampsia, primary pulmonary hypertension
(Continued)

hydralazine *(Continued)*

Usual Dosage
Children:
Oral: Initial: 0.75-1 mg/kg/day in 2-4 divided doses, not to exceed 25 mg/dose; increase over 3-4 weeks to maximum of 7.5 mg/kg/day in 2-4 divided doses; maximum daily dose: 200 mg/day
I.M., I.V.: 0.1-0.5 mg/kg/dose (initial dose not to exceed 20 mg) every 4-6 hours as needed
Adults:
Oral: Initial: 10 mg 4 times/day, increase by 10-25 mg/dose every 2-5 days to maximum of 300 mg/day
I.M., I.V.:
Hypertensive initial: 10-20 mg/dose every 4-6 hours as needed, may increase to 40 mg/dose
Pre-eclampsia/eclampsia: 5 mg/dose then 5-10 mg every 20-30 minutes as needed
Dosage Forms
Injection, as hydrochloride: 20 mg/mL (1 mL)
Tablet, as hydrochloride: 10 mg, 25 mg, 50 mg, 100 mg

hydralazine and hydrochlorothiazide

(hye DRAL a zeen & hye droe klor oh THYE a zide)
Synonyms hydrochlorothiazide and hydralazine
Brand Names Apresazide®
Therapeutic Category Antihypertensive, Combination
Use Management of moderate to severe hypertension and treatment of congestive heart failure
Usual Dosage Adults: Oral: 1 capsule twice daily
Dosage Forms Capsule:
25/25: Hydralazine hydrochloride 25 mg and hydrochlorothiazide 25 mg
50/50: Hydralazine hydrochloride 50 mg and hydrochlorothiazide 50 mg
100/50: Hydralazine hydrochloride 100 mg and hydrochlorothiazide 50 mg

hydralazine hydrochloride *see* hydralazine *on previous page*

hydralazine, hydrochlorothiazide, and reserpine

(hye DRAL a zeen, hye droe klor oh THYE a zide, & re SER peen)
Brand Names Hydrap-ES®; Marpres®; Ser-Ap-Es®
Therapeutic Category Antihypertensive, Combination
Use Hypertensive disorders
Usual Dosage Adults: Oral: 1-2 tablets 3 times/day
Dosage Forms Tablet: Hydralazine 25 mg, hydrochlorothiazide 15 mg, and reserpine 0.1 mg

Hydramyn® Syrup [OTC] *see* diphenhydramine *on page 173*

Hydrap-ES® *see* hydralazine, hydrochlorothiazide, and reserpine *on this page*

hydrated chloral *see* chloral hydrate *on page 107*

Hydrate® Injection *see* dimenhydrinate *on page 171*

Hydrea® *see* hydroxyurea *on page 274*

Hydrobexan® *see* hydroxocobalamin *on page 272*

Hydrocet® *see* hydrocodone and acetaminophen *on page 266*

hydrochlorothiazide (hye droe klor oh THYE a zide)

Synonyms hctz
Brand Names Esidrix®; Ezide®; HydroDIURIL®; Hydro-Par®; Microzide®; Oretic®
Therapeutic Category Diuretic, Thiazide

Use Management of mild to moderate hypertension; treatment of edema in congestive heart failure and nephrotic syndrome

Usual Dosage Oral:

Children (daily dosages should be decreased if used with other antihypertensives):
<6 months: 2-3 mg/kg/day in 2 divided doses
>6 months: 2 mg/kg/day in 2 divided doses
Adults: 25-50 mg/day in 1-2 doses; maximum: 200 mg/day

Dosage Forms
Capsule: 12.5 mg
Solution, oral (mint flavor): 50 mg/5 mL (50 mL)
Tablet: 25 mg, 50 mg, 100 mg

hydrochlorothiazide and amiloride *see* amiloride and hydrochlorothiazide *on page 24*

hydrochlorothiazide and hydralazine *see* hydralazine and hydrochlorothiazide *on previous page*

hydrochlorothiazide and methyldopa *see* methyldopa and hydrochlorothiazide *on page 341*

hydrochlorothiazide and reserpine

(hye droe klor oh THYE a zide & re SER peen)

Synonyms reserpine and hydrochlorothiazide

Brand Names Hydropres®; Hydro-Serp®; Hydroserpine®

Therapeutic Category Antihypertensive, Combination

Use Management of mild to moderate hypertension; treatment of edema in congestive heart failure and nephrotic syndrome

Usual Dosage Adults: Oral: 1-2 tablets once or twice daily

Dosage Forms Tablet: 50: Hydrochlorothiazide 50 mg and reserpine 0.125 mg

hydrochlorothiazide and spironolactone

(hye droe klor oh THYE a zide & speer on oh LAK tone)

Synonyms spironolactone and hydrochlorothiazide

Brand Names Aldactazide®

Therapeutic Category Antihypertensive, Combination

Use Management of mild to moderate hypertension; treatment of edema in congestive heart failure and nephrotic syndrome

Usual Dosage Oral:

Children: 1.66-3.3 mg/kg/day (of spironolactone) in 2-4 divided doses
Adults: 1-8 tablets in 1-2 divided doses

Dosage Forms Tablet:
25/25: Hydrochlorothiazide 25 mg and spironolactone 25 mg
50/50: Hydrochlorothiazide 50 mg and spironolactone 50 mg

hydrochlorothiazide and triamterene

(hye droe klor oh THYE a zide & trye AM ter een)

Synonyms triamterene and hydrochlorothiazide

Brand Names Dyazide®; Maxzide®

Therapeutic Category Antihypertensive, Combination

Use Management of mild to moderate hypertension; treatment of edema in congestive heart failure and nephrotic syndrome

Usual Dosage Adults: Oral: 1-2 capsules twice daily after meals

Dosage Forms
Capsule (Dyazide®): Hydrochlorothiazide 25 mg and triamterene 37.5 mg
Tablet:
Maxzide®-25: Hydrochlorothiazide 25 mg and triamterene 37.5 mg
Maxzide®: Hydrochlorothiazide 50 mg and triamterene 75 mg

Hydrocil® [OTC] *see* psyllium *on page 451*

Hydro Cobex® *see* hydroxocobalamin *on page 272*

hydrocodone and acetaminophen
(hye droe KOE done & a seet a MIN oh fen)

Synonyms acetaminophen and hydrocodone

Brand Names Anexsia®; Anodynos-DHC®; Bancap HC®; Co-Gesic®; Dolacet®; DuoCet™; Hydrocet®; Hydrogesic®; Hy-Phen®; Lorcet®-HD; Lorcet® Plus; Lortab®; Margesic® H; Medipain 5®; Norcet®; Norco®; Stagesic®; T-Gesic®; Vicodin®; Vicodin® ES; Vicodin® HP; Zydone®

Therapeutic Category Analgesic, Narcotic

Controlled Substance C-III

Use Relief of moderate to severe pain; antitussive (hydrocodone)

Usual Dosage Doses should be titrated to appropriate analgesic effect

Adults: Oral: 1-2 tablets or capsules every 4-6 hours

Dosage Forms

Capsule:

Bancap HC®, Dolacet®, Hydrocet®, Hydrogesic®, Lorcet®-HD, Margesic® H, Medipain 5®, Norcet®, Stagesic®, T-Gesic®, Zydone®: Hydrocodone bitartrate 5 mg and acetaminophen 500 mg

Elixir (tropical fruit punch flavor) (Lortab®): Hydrocodone bitartrate 2.5 mg and acetaminophen 167 mg per 5 mL with alcohol 7% (480 mL)

Solution, oral (tropical fruit punch flavor) (Lortab®): Hydrocodone bitartrate 2.5 mg and acetaminophen 167 mg per 5 mL with alcohol 7% (480 mL)

Tablet:

Lortab® 2.5/500: Hydrocodone bitartrate 2.5 mg and acetaminophen 500 mg

Anexsia® 5/500, Anodynos-DHC®, Co-Gesic®, DuoCet™, DHC®; Hy-Phen®, Lortab®® 5/500, Vicodin®: Hydrocodone bitartrate 5 mg and acetaminophen 500 mg

Lortab® 7.5/500: Hydrocodone bitartrate 7.5 mg and acetaminophen 500 mg

Anexsia® 7.5/650, Lorcet® Plus: Hydrocodone bitartrate 7.5 mg and acetaminophen 650 mg

Vicodin® ES: Hydrocodone bitartrate 7.5 mg and acetaminophen 750 mg

Norco®: Hydrocodone bitartrate 10 mg and acetaminophen 325 mg

Lortab® 10/500: Hydrocodone bitartrate 10 mg and acetaminophen 500 mg

Lorcet® 10/650: Hydrocodone bitartrate 10 mg and acetaminophen 650 mg

Vicodin® HP: Hydrocodone bitartrate 10 mg and acetaminophen 660 mg

hydrocodone and aspirin (hye droe KOE done & AS pir in)

Brand Names Alor® 5/500; Azdone®; Damason-P®; Lortab® ASA; Panasal® 5/500

Therapeutic Category Analgesic, Narcotic

Controlled Substance C-III

Use Relief of moderate to moderately severe pain

Usual Dosage Adults: Oral: 1-2 tablets every 4-6 hours as needed for pain

Dosage Forms Tablet: Hydrocodone bitartrate 5 mg and aspirin 500 mg

hydrocodone and chlorpheniramine
(hye droe KOE done & klor fen IR a meen)

Brand Names Tussionex®

Therapeutic Category Antihistamine/Antitussive

Controlled Substance C-III

Use Symptomatic relief of cough

Usual Dosage Oral:

Children 6-12 years: 2.5 mL every 12 hours; do not exceed 5 mL/24 hours

Adults: 5 mL every 12 hours; do not exceed 10 mL/24 hours

Dosage Forms Syrup, alcohol free: Hydrocodone polistirex 10 mg and chlorpheniramine polistirex 8 mg per 5 mL (480 mL, 900 mL)

hydrocodone and guaifenesin (hye droe KOE done & gwye FEN e sin)
Synonyms guaifenesin and hydrocodone
Brand Names Codiclear® DH; HycoClear Tuss®; Hycotuss® Expectorant Liquid; Kwelcof®
Therapeutic Category Antitussive/Expectorant
Controlled Substance C-III
Use Symptomatic relief of nonproductive coughs associated with upper and lower respiratory tract congestion
Usual Dosage Oral:
Children:
<2 years: 0.3 mg/kg/day (hydrocodone) in 4 divided doses
2-12 years: 2.5 mL every 4 hours, after meals and at bedtime
>12 years: 5 mL every 4 hours, after meals and at bedtime
Adults: 5 mL every 4 hours, after meals and at bedtime, up to 30 mL/24 hours
Dosage Forms Liquid: Hydrocodone bitartrate 5 mg and guaifenesin 100 mg per 5 mL (120 mL, 480 mL)

hydrocodone and homatropine (hye droe KOE done & hoe MA troe peen)
Synonyms homatropine and hydrocodone
Brand Names Hycodan®; Hydromet®; Oncet®; Tussigon®
Therapeutic Category Antitussive
Controlled Substance C-III
Use Symptomatic relief of cough
Usual Dosage Oral (based on hydrocodone component):
Children: 0.6 mg/kg/day in 3-4 divided doses; do not administer more frequently than every 4 hours
A single dose should not exceed 10 mg in children >12 years, 5 mg in children 2-12 years, and 1.25 mg in children <2 years of age
Adults: 5-10 mg every 4-6 hours, a single dose should not exceed 15 mg; do not administer more frequently than every 4 hours
Dosage Forms
Syrup (Hycodan®, Hydromet®): Hydrocodone bitartrate 5 mg and homatropine methylbromide 1.5 mg per 5 mL (120 mL, 480 mL, 4000 mL)
Tablet (Hycodan®, Oncet®, Tussigon®): Hydrocodone bitartrate 5 mg and homatropine methylbromide 1.5 mg

hydrocodone and ibuprofen (hye droe KOE done & eye byoo PROE fen)
Brand Names Vicoprofen®
Therapeutic Category Analgesic, Narcotic
Controlled Substance C-III
Use Relief of moderate to moderately severe pain
Usual Dosage Adults: Oral: 1-2 tablets every 4-6 hours as needed for pain
Dosage Forms Tablet: Hydrocodone bitratrate 7.5 mg and ibuprofen 200 mg

hydrocodone and phenylpropanolamine
(hye droe KOE done & fen il proe pa NOLE a meen)
Synonyms phenylpropanolamine and hydrocodone
Brand Names Codamine®; Codamine® Pediatric; Hycomine®; Hycomine® Pediatric; Hydrocodone PA® Syrup
Therapeutic Category Antitussive/Decongestant
Controlled Substance C-III
Use Symptomatic relief of cough and nasal congestion
Usual Dosage Oral:
Children 6-12 years: 2.5 mL every 4 hours, up to 6 doses/24 hours
Adults: 5 mL every 4 hours, up to 6 doses/24 hours
(Continued)

hydrocodone and phenylpropanolamine *(Continued)*
Dosage Forms Syrup:
Codamine®, Hycomine®: Hydrocodone bitartrate 5 mg and phenylpropanolamine hydrochloride 25 mg per 5 mL (480 mL, 3780 mL)
Codamine® Pediatric, Hycomine® Pediatric: Hydrocodone bitartrate 2.5 mg and phenylpropanolamine hydrochloride 12.5 mg per 5 mL (480 mL, 3780 mL)

Hydrocodone and Phenyltoloxamine *see* hydrocodone and chlorpheniramine *on page 266*

hydrocodone, chlorpheniramine, phenylephrine, acetaminophen, and caffeine
(hye droe KOE done, klor fen IR a meen, fen il EF rin, a seet a MIN oh fen, & KAF een)
Brand Names Hycomine® Compound
Therapeutic Category Antitussive
Use Symptomatic relief of cough and symptoms of upper respiratory infections
Usual Dosage Adults: Oral: 1 tablet every 4 hours, up to 4 times/day
Dosage Forms Tablet: Hydrocodone bitartrate 5 mg, chlorpheniramine maleate 2 mg, phenylephrine hydrochloride 10 mg, acetaminophen 250 mg, and caffeine 30 mg

Hydrocodone PA® Syrup *see* hydrocodone and phenylpropanolamine *on previous page*

hydrocodone, phenylephrine, pyrilamine, phenindamine, chlorpheniramine, and ammonium chloride
(hye droe KOE done, fen il EF rin, peer IL a meen, fen IN da meen, klor fen IR a meen, & a MOE nee um KLOR ide)
Brand Names P-V-Tussin®
Therapeutic Category Antihistamine/Decongestant/Antitussive
Use Symptomatic relief of cough and nasal congestion
Usual Dosage Adults: Oral: 10 mL every 4-6 hours, up to 40 mL/day
Dosage Forms Syrup: Hydrocodone bitartrate 2.5 mg, phenylephrine hydrochloride 5 mg, pyrilamine maleate 6 mg, phenindamine tartrate 5 mg, chlorpheniramine maleate 2 mg, and ammonium chloride 50 mg per 5 mL with alcohol 5% (480 mL, 3780 mL)

hydrocodone, pseudoephedrine, and guaifenesin
(hye droe KOE done, soo doe e FED rin & gwye FEN e sin)
Brand Names Cophene XP®; Detussin® Expectorant; SRC® Expectorant; Tussafin® Expectorant
Therapeutic Category Antitussive/Decongestant/Expectorant
Controlled Substance C-III
Use Symptomatic relief of irritating, nonproductive cough associated with respiratory conditions such as bronchitis, bronchial asthma, tracheobronchitis, and the common cold
Usual Dosage Adults: Oral: 5 mL every 4-6 hours
Dosage Forms Liquid: Hydrocodone bitartrate 5 mg, pseudoephedrine hydrochloride 60 mg, and guaifenesin 200 mg per 5 mL with alcohol 12.5% (480 mL)

Hydrocort® *see* hydrocortisone *on this page*

hydrocortisone (hye droe KOR ti sone)
Synonyms compound f; cortisol hydrocortisone acetate; hydrocortisone buteprate; hydrocortisone butyrate; hydrocortisone cypionate; hydrocortisone sodium phosphate; hydrocortisone sodium succinate; hydrocortisone valerate
Brand Names Aeroseb-HC®; A-hydroCort®; Ala-Cort®; Ala-Scalp®; Anucort-HC® Suppository; Anuprep HC® Suppository; Anusol® HC 1 [OTC]; Anusol® HC 2.5% [OTC];

Anusol-HC® Suppository; Caldecort®; Caldecort® Anti-Itch Spray; Clocort® Maximum Strength; CortaGel® [OTC]; Cortaid® Maximum Strength [OTC]; Cortaid® with Aloe [OTC]; Cort-Dome®; Cortef®; Cortef® Feminine Itch; Cortenema®; Cortifoam®; Cortizone®-5 [OTC]; Cortizone®-10 [OTC]; Delcort®; Dermacort®; Dermarest Dricort®; DermiCort®; Dermolate® [OTC]; Dermtex® HC with Aloe; Eldecort®; Gynecort® [OTC]; Hemril-HC® Uniserts®; Hi-Cor® 1.0; Hi-Cor® 2.5; Hycort®; Hydrocort®; Hydrocortone® Acetate; Hydrocortone® Phosphate; HydroTex® [OTC]; Hytone®; LactiCare-HC®; Lanacort® [OTC]; Locoid®; Nutracort®; Orabase® HCA; Pandel®; Penecort®; Procort® [OTC]; Proctocort™; Scalpicin®; Solu-Cortef®; S-T Cort®; Synacort®; Tegrin®-HC [OTC]; Westcort®

Therapeutic Category Adrenal Corticosteroid; Corticosteroid, Topical

Use Management of adrenocortical insufficiency; relief of inflammation of corticosteroid-responsive dermatoses; adjunctive treatment of ulcerative colitis

Usual Dosage Dose should be based on severity of disease and patient response
Acute adrenal insufficiency: I.M., I.V.:
Infants and young Children: Succinate: 1-2 mg/kg/dose bolus, then 25-150 mg/day in divided doses every 6-8 hours
Older Children: Succinate: 1-2 mg/kg bolus then 150-250 mg/day in divided doses every 6-8 hours
Adults: Succinate: 100 mg I.V. bolus, then 300 mg/day in divided doses every 8 hours or as a continuous infusion for 48 hours; once patient is stable change to oral, 50 mg every 8 hours for 6 doses, then taper to 30-50 mg/day in divided doses
Chronic adrenal corticoid insufficiency: Adults: Oral: 20-30 mg/day

Anti-inflammatory or immunosuppressive:
Infants and Children:
Oral: 2.5-10 mg/kg/day **or** 75-300 mg/m^2/day every 6-8 hours
I.M., I.V.: Succinate: 1-5 mg/kg/day **or** 30-150 mg/m^2/day divided every 12-24 hours
Adolescents and Adults: Oral, I.M., I.V.: Succinate: 15-240 mg every 12 hours
Congenital adrenal hyperplasia: Oral: Initial: 30-36 mg/m^2/day with $1/3$ of dose every morning and $2/3$ every evening or $1/4$ every morning and mid-day and $1/2$ every evening; maintenance: 20-25 mg/m^2/day in divided doses
Physiologic replacement: Children:
Oral: 0.5-0.75 mg/kg/day **or** 20-25 mg/m^2/day every 8 hours
I.M.: Succinate: 0.25-0.35 mg/kg/day **or** 12-15 mg/m^2/day once daily
Shock: I.M., I.V.: Succinate:
Children: Initial: 50 mg/kg, then repeated in 4 hours and/or every 24 hours as needed
Adolescents and Adults: 500 mg to 2 g every 2-6 hours
Status asthmaticus: Children and Adults: I.V.: Succinate: 1-2 mg/kg/dose every 6 hours for 24 hours, then maintenance of 0.5-1 mg/kg every 6 hours
Rheumatic diseases:
Adults: Intralesional, intra-articular, soft tissue injection: Acetate:
Large joints: 25 mg (up to 37.5 mg)
Small joints: 10-25 mg
Tendon sheaths: 5-12.5 mg
Soft tissue infiltration: 25-50 mg (up to 75 mg)
Bursae: 25-37.5 mg
Ganglia: 12.5-25 mg
Dermatosis: Children >2 years and Adults: Topical: Apply to affected area 3-4 times/day (Buteprate: Apply once or twice daily)

Ulcerative colitis: Adults: Rectal: 10-100 mg 1-2 times/day for 2-3 weeks

Dosage Forms
Acetate:
Aerosol, rectal (Cortifoam®): 10% [90 mg/applicatorful] 20 g
Cream:
Caldecort®, Gynecort®, Cortaid® with Aloe, Cortef® Feminine Itch, Lanacort®: 0.5% (15 g, 22.5 g, 30 g)
Anusol-HC-1®, Caldecort®, Clocort® Maximum Strength, Cortaid® Maximum Strength, Dermarest Dricort®: 1% (15 g, 21 g, 30 g, 120 g)
(Continued)

hydrocortisone *(Continued)*

Ointment, topical:
 Cortaid® with Aloe, Lanacort® 5: 0.5% (15 g, 30 g)
 Gynecort® 10, Lanacort® 10: 1% (15 g, 30 g)
Injection, suspension (Hydrocortone® Acetate): 25 mg/mL (5 mL, 10 mL); 50 mg/mL (5 mL, 10 mL)
Paste (Orabase® HCA): 0.5% (5 g)
Solution, topical (Scalpicin®): 1%
Suppository, rectal (Anucort-HC®, Anuprep HC®, Anusol-HC®, Hemril-HC® Uniserts®): 25 mg
Base:
Aerosol, topical:
 Aeroseb-HC®, CaldeCORT® Anti-Itch Spray, Cortaid®: 0.5% (45 g, 58 g)
 Cortaid® Maximum Strength: 1% (45 mL)
Cream:
 Cort-Dome®, Cortizone®-5, DermiCort®, Dermolate®, Dermtex® HC with Aloe, HydroTex®: 0.5% (15 g, 30 g, 120 g, 454 g)
 Ala-Cort®, Cort-Dome®, Delcort®, Dermacort®, DermiCort®, Eldecort®, Hi-Cor® 1.0, Hycort®, Hytone®, Nutracort®, Penecort®, Synacort®: 1% (15 g, 20 g, 30 g, 60 g, 120 g, 240 g, 454 g)
 Anusol-HC-2.5%®, Eldecort®, Hi-Cor® 2.5, Hydrocort®, Hytone®, Synacort®: 2.5% (15 g, 20 g, 30 g, 60 g, 120 g, 240 g, 454 g)
 Rectal (Proctocort™): 1% (30 g)
Gel:
 CortaGel®: 0.5% (15 g, 30 g)
 CortaGel® Extra Strength: 1% (15 g, 30 g)
Lotion:
 Cetacort®, DermiCort®, HydroSKIN®, S-T Cort®: 0.5% (60 mL, 120 mL)
 Acticort 100®, Cetacort®, Cortizone-10®, Dermacort®, HydroSKIN® Maximum Strength, Hytone®, LactiCare-HC®, Nutracort®: 1% (60 mL, 120 mL)
 Ala-Scalp®: 2% (30 mL)
 Hytone®, LactiCare-HC®, Nutracort®: 2.5% (60 mL, 120 mL)
Ointment, topical:
 Cortizone®-5, HydroSKIN®: 0.5% (30 g)
 Cortizone®-10, Hycort®, HydroSKIN®, Hydro-Tex®, Hytone®, Tegrin®-HC: 1% (15 g, 20 g, 30 g, 60 g, 120 g, 240 g, 454 g)
 Hytone®: 2.5% (20 g, 30 g)
Suspension, rectal (Cortenema®): 100 mg/60 mL (7s)
Tablet:
 Cortef®: 5 mg, 10 mg, 20 mg
 Hydrocortone®: 10 mg, 20 mg
Buteprate (Pandel®): Cream: 1% (15 g, 45 g)
Butyrate (Locoid®):
 Cream: 0.1% (15 g, 45 g)
 Ointment, topical: 0.1% (15 g, 45 g)
 Solution, topical: 0.1% (20 mL, 60 mL)
Cypionate: Suspension, oral (Cortef®): 10 mg/5 mL (120 mL)
Sodium phosphate: Injection (Hydrocortone® Phosphate): 50 mg/mL (2 mL, 10 mL)
Sodium succinate: Injection (A-hydroCort®, Solu-Cortef®): 100 mg, 250 mg, 500 mg, 1000 mg
Valerate (Westcort®):
 Cream: 0.2% (15 g, 45 g, 60 g)
 Ointment, topical: 0.2% (15 g, 45 g, 60 g, 120 g)

hydrocortisone and clioquinol *see* clioquinol and hydrocortisone *on page 128*

hydrocortisone and dibucaine *see* dibucaine and hydrocortisone *on page 164*

hydrocortisone and pramoxine *see* pramoxine and hydrocortisone *on page 433*

hydrocortisone and urea *see* urea and hydrocortisone *on page 542*
hydrocortisone buteprate *see* hydrocortisone *on page 268*
hydrocortisone butyrate *see* hydrocortisone *on page 268*
hydrocortisone cypionate *see* hydrocortisone *on page 268*
hydrocortisone sodium phosphate *see* hydrocortisone *on page 268*
hydrocortisone sodium succinate *see* hydrocortisone *on page 268*
hydrocortisone valerate *see* hydrocortisone *on page 268*
Hydrocortone® Acetate *see* hydrocortisone *on page 268*
Hydrocortone® Phosphate *see* hydrocortisone *on page 268*
Hydro-Crysti-12® *see* hydroxocobalamin *on next page*
HydroDIURIL® *see* hydrochlorothiazide *on page 264*

hydroflumethiazide (hye droe floo meth EYE a zide)

Brand Names Diucardin®; Saluron®
Therapeutic Category Diuretic, Thiazide
Use Management of mild to moderate hypertension; treatment of edema in congestive heart failure and nephrotic syndrome
Usual Dosage Oral: 1 tablet 1-2 times/day
Dosage Forms Tablet: 50 mg

hydroflumethiazide and reserpine

(hye droe floo meth EYE a zide & re SER peen)
Brand Names Salutensin®
Therapeutic Category Antihypertensive, Combination
Use Management of hypertension
Usual Dosage Oral: Determined by individual titration, usually 1 tablet once or twice daily
Dosage Forms Tablet: Hydroflumethiazide 50 mg and reserpine 0.125 mg

hydrogenated ergot alkaloids *see* ergoloid mesylates *on page 198*

Hydrogesic® *see* hydrocodone and acetaminophen *on page 266*

hydromagnesium aluminate *see* magaldrate *on page 317*

Hydromet® *see* hydrocodone and homatropine *on page 267*

hydromorphone (hye droe MOR fone)

Synonyms dihydromorphinone; hydromorphone hydrochloride
Brand Names Dilaudid®; Dilaudid-5®; Dilaudid-HP®; HydroStat IR®
Therapeutic Category Analgesic, Narcotic
Controlled Substance C-II
Use Management of moderate to severe pain; antitussive at lower doses
Usual Dosage Doses should be titrated to appropriate analgesic effects; when changing routes of administration, note that oral doses are less than half as effective as parenteral doses (may be only $1/_5$ as effective)

Pain: Older Children and Adults: Oral, I.M., I.V., S.C.: 1-4 mg/dose every 4-6 hours as needed; usual adult dose: 2 mg/dose
Antitussive: Oral:
Children 6-12 years: 0.5 mg every 3-4 hours as needed
Children >12 years and Adults: 1 mg every 3-4 hours as needed
Dosage Forms
Injection, as hydrochloride:
Dilaudid®: 1 mg/mL (1 mL); 2 mg/mL (1 mL, 20 mL); 3 mg/mL (1 mL); 4 mg/mL (1 mL)
Dilaudid-HP®: 10 mg/mL (1 mL, 2 mL, 5 mL)
Liquid, as hydrochloride: 5 mg/5 mL (480 mL)
(Continued)

hydromorphone *(Continued)*

Powder for injection, as hydrochloride: (Dilaudid-HP®): 250 mg
Suppository, rectal, as hydrochloride: 3 mg (6s)
Tablet, as hydrochloride: 1 mg, 2 mg, 3 mg, 4 mg, 8 mg

hydromorphone hydrochloride *see* hydromorphone *on previous page*

Hydromox® *see* quinethazone *on page 455*

Hydro-Par® *see* hydrochlorothiazide *on page 264*

Hydrophed® *see* theophylline, ephedrine, and hydroxyzine *on page 513*

Hydropres® *see* hydrochlorothiazide and reserpine *on page 265*

hydroquinol *see* hydroquinone *on this page*

hydroquinone (HYE droe kwin one)

Synonyms hydroquinol; quinol
Brand Names Ambi® Skin Tone [OTC]; Eldopaque® [OTC]; Eldopaque Forte®; Eldoquin® [OTC]; Eldoquin® Forte®; Esoterica® Facial [OTC]; Esoterica® Regular [OTC]; Esoterica® Sensitive Skin Formula [OTC]; Esoterica® Sunscreen [OTC]; Melanex®; Porcelana® [OTC]; Porcelana® Sunscreen [OTC]; Solaquin® [OTC]; Solaquin Forte®
Therapeutic Category Topical Skin Product
Use Gradual bleaching of hyperpigmented skin conditions
Usual Dosage Topical: Apply thin layer and rub in twice daily
Dosage Forms
Cream:
Topical:
Esoterica® Sensitive Skin Formula: 1.5% (85 g)
Eldopaque®, Eldoquin®, Esoterica® Facial, Esoterica® Regular, Porcelana®: 2% (14.2 g, 28.4 g, 60 g, 85 g, 120 g)
Eldopaque Forte®, Eldoquin® Forte®, Melquin HP®: 4% (14.2 g, 28.4 g)
Topical, with sunscreen:
Esoterica® Sunscreen, Porcelana®, Solaquin®: 2% (28.4 g, 120 g)
Melpaque HP®, Nuquin HP®, Solaquin Forte®: 4% (14.2 g, 28.4 g)
Gel, topical, with sunscreen (Solaquin Forte®): 4% (14.2 g, 28.4 g)
Solution, topical (Melanex®): 3% (30 mL)

Hydro-Serp® *see* hydrochlorothiazide and reserpine *on page 265*

Hydroserpine® *see* hydrochlorothiazide and reserpine *on page 265*

HydroStat IR® *see* hydromorphone *on previous page*

HydroTex® [OTC] *see* hydrocortisone *on page 268*

hydroxocobalamin (hye droks oh koe BAL a min)

Synonyms vitamin b_{12a}
Brand Names Hydrobexan®; Hydro Cobex®; Hydro-Crysti-12®; LA-12®
Therapeutic Category Vitamin, Water Soluble
Use Pernicious anemia, vitamin B_{12} deficiency, increased B_{12} requirements due to pregnancy, thyrotoxicosis, hemorrhage, malignancy, liver or kidney disease
Usual Dosage
Children:
Congenital pernicious anemia (if evidence of neurologic involvement): I.M.: 1000 mcg/day for at least 2 weeks; maintenance: 50 mcg/month
Vitamin B_{12} deficiency: I.M., S.C.: 1-5 mg administered in single or S.C. doses of 100 mcg over 2 or more weeks
Adults:
Pernicious anemia: I.M., S.C.: 100 mcg/day for 6-7 days

Vitamin B$_{12}$ deficiency:
Oral: Usually not recommended, maximum absorbed from a single oral dose is 2-3 mcg
I.M., S.C.: 30 mcg/day for 5-10 days, followed by 100-200 mcg/month
Dosage Forms Injection: 1000 mcg/mL (10 mL, 30 mL)

hydroxyamphetamine (hye droks ee am FET a meen)
Synonyms hydroxyamphetamine hydrobromide
Brand Names Paredrine®
Therapeutic Category Adrenergic Agonist Agent
Use Produce mydriasis in diagnostic eye examination
Usual Dosage Instill 1-2 drops into conjunctival sac
Dosage Forms Solution, as hydrobromide: 1%

hydroxyamphetamine and tropicamide
(hye droks ee am FET a meen & troe PIK a mide)
Brand Names Paremyd® Ophthalmic
Therapeutic Category Adrenergic Agonist Agent
Use Mydriasis with cycloplegia
Usual Dosage Adults: Ophthalmic: Instill 1-2 drops into conjunctival sac(s)
Dosage Forms Solution, ophthalmic: Hydroxyamphetamine hydrobromide 1% and tropicamide 0.25% (5 mL, 15 mL)

hydroxyamphetamine hydrobromide *see* hydroxyamphetamine *on this page*

hydroxycarbamide *see* hydroxyurea *on next page*

hydroxychloroquine (hye droks ee KLOR oh kwin)
Synonyms hydroxychloroquine sulfate
Brand Names Plaquenil®
Therapeutic Category Aminoquinoline (Antimalarial)
Use Suppression or chemoprophylaxis of malaria caused by susceptible *P. vivax*, *P. ovale*, *P. malariae*, and some strains of *P. falciparum* (not active against pre-erythrocytic or exoerythrocytic tissue stages of *Plasmodium*); treatment of systemic lupus erythematosus (SLE) and rheumatoid arthritis
Usual Dosage Oral:
Children:
Chemoprophylaxis of malaria: 5 mg/kg (base) once weekly; should not exceed the recommended adult dose; begin 2 weeks before exposure; continue for 8 weeks after leaving endemic area
Acute attack: 10 mg/kg (base) initial dose; followed by 5 mg/kg in 6 hours on day 1; 5 mg/kg in 1 dose on day 2 and on day 3
Juvenile rheumatoid arthritis or SLE: 3-5 mg/kg/day divided 1-2 times/day to a maximum of 400 mg/day; not to exceed 7 mg/kg/day
Adults:
Chemoprophylaxis of malaria: 2 tablets weekly on same day each week; begin 2 weeks before exposure; continue for 6-8 weeks after leaving epidemic area
Acute attack: 4 tablets first dose day 1; 2 tablets in 6 hours day 1; 2 tablets in 1 dose day 2; and 2 tablets in 1 dose on day 3
Rheumatoid arthritis: 2-3 tablets/day to start with food or milk; increase dose until optimum response level is reached; usually after 4-12 weeks dose should be reduced by 1/2 and a maintenance dose of 1-2 tablets/day
Lupus erythematosus: 2 tablets every day or twice daily for several weeks depending on response; 1-2 tablets/day for prolonged maintenance therapy
Dosage Forms Tablet, as sulfate: 200 mg [base 155 mg]

hydroxychloroquine sulfate *see* hydroxychloroquine *on this page*

25-hydroxycholecalciferol *see* calcifediol *on page 80*

hydroxydaunomycin hydrochloride *see* doxorubicin *on page 183*

hydroxyethyl starch *see* hetastarch *on page 260*

hydroxyprogesterone caproate
(hye droks ee proe JES te rone KAP roe ate)
Brand Names Hylutin® Injection; Hyprogest® 250 Injection
Therapeutic Category Progestin
Use Treatment of amenorrhea, abnormal uterine bleeding, submucous fibroids, endometriosis, uterine carcinoma, and testing of estrogen production
Usual Dosage Adults: I.M.:
Amenorrhea: 375 mg; if no bleeding, begin cyclic treatment with estradiol valerate
Endometriosis: Start cyclic therapy with estradiol valerate
Uterine carcinoma: 1 g one or more times/day (1-7 g/week) for up to 12 weeks
Test for endogenous estrogen production: 250 mg anytime; bleeding 7-14 days after injection indicate positive test
Dosage Forms
Injection: 125 mg/mL (10 mL)
Hylutin®, Hyprogest®: 250 mg/mL (5 mL)

hydroxypropyl cellulose (hye droks ee PROE pil SEL yoo lose)
Brand Names Lacrisert®
Therapeutic Category Ophthalmic Agent, Miscellaneous
Use Dry eyes
Usual Dosage Ophthalmic: Adults: Apply once daily into the inferior cul-de-sac beneath the base of tarsus, not in apposition to the cornea nor beneath the eyelid at the level of the tarsal plate
Dosage Forms Insert, ophthalmic: 5 mg

hydroxypropyl methylcellulose
(hye droks ee PROE pil meth il SEL yoo lose)
Synonyms gonioscopic ophthalmic solution
Brand Names Gonak™ [OTC]; Goniosol® [OTC]
Therapeutic Category Ophthalmic Agent, Miscellaneous
Use Ophthalmic surgical aid in cataract extraction and intraocular implantation; gonioscopic examinations
Usual Dosage Introduced into anterior chamber of eye with 20-gauge or larger cannula
Dosage Forms Solution: 2.5% (15 mL)

hydroxyurea (hye droks ee yoor EE a)
Synonyms hydroxycarbamide
Brand Names Hydrea®
Therapeutic Category Antineoplastic Agent
Use Treatment of chronic myelocytic leukemia (CML), melanoma, and ovarian carcinomas; also used with radiation in treatment of tumors of the head and neck; adjunct in the management of sickle cell patients
Usual Dosage Oral (refer to individual protocols):
Children: No dosage regimens have been established. Dosages of 1500-3000 mg/m^2 as a single dose in combination with other agents every 4-6 weeks have been used in the treatment of pediatric astrocytoma, medulloblastoma and primitive neuroectodermal tumors
Adults:
Solid tumors: Intermittent therapy: 80 mg/kg as a single dose every third day; continuous therapy: 20-30 mg/kg/day administered as a single dose/day
Concomitant therapy with irradiation: 80 mg/kg as a single dose every third day starting at least 7 days before initiation of irradiation
Resistant chronic myelocytic leukemia: 20-30 mg/kg/day divided daily
Dosage Forms Capsule: 500 mg

25-hydroxyvitamin d₃ *see* calcifediol *on page 80*

hydroxyzine (hye DROKS i zeen)

Synonyms hydroxyzine hydrochloride; hydroxyzine pamoate
Brand Names Anxanil®; Atarax®; E-Vista®; Hyzine-50®; QYS®; Vistacon®; Vistaject-25®; Vistaject-50®; Vistaquel®; Vistaril®; Vistazine®
Therapeutic Category Antiemetic; Antihistamine
Use Treatment of anxiety; preoperative sedative; antipruritic; antiemetic
Usual Dosage
Children:
Oral: 2 mg/kg/day divided every 6-8 hours
I.M.: 0.5-1 mg/kg/dose every 4-6 hours as needed
Adults:
Antiemetic: I.M.: 25-100 mg/dose every 4-6 hours as needed
Anxiety: Oral: 25-100 mg 4 times/day; maximum dose: 600 mg/day
Preoperative sedation:
Oral: 50-100 mg
I.M.: 25-100 mg
Management of pruritus: Oral: 25 mg 3-4 times/day
Dosage Forms
Hydroxyzine hydrochloride:
Injection: 25 mg/mL (1 mL, 2 mL, 10 mL); 50 mg/mL (1 mL, 2 mL, 10 mL)
Syrup: 10 mg/5 mL (120 mL, 480 mL, 4000 mL)
Tablet: 10 mg, 25 mg, 50 mg, 100 mg
Hydroxyzine pamoate:
Capsule: 25 mg, 50 mg, 100 mg
Suspension, oral: 25 mg/5 mL (120 mL, 480 mL)

hydroxyzine hydrochloride *see* hydroxyzine *on this page*

hydroxyzine pamoate *see* hydroxyzine *on this page*

Hygroton® *see* chlorthalidone *on page 120*

Hylorel® *see* guanadrel *on page 253*

Hylutin® Injection *see* hydroxyprogesterone caproate *on previous page*

hyoscine *see* scopolamine *on page 475*

hyoscyamine (hye oh SYE a meen)

Synonyms hyoscyamine sulfate; *l*-hyoscyamine sulfate
Brand Names Anaspaz®; A-Spas® S/L; Cystospaz®; Cystospaz-M®; Donnamar®; ED-SPAZ®; Gastrosed™; Levbid®; Levsin®; Levsinex®; Levsin/SL®
Therapeutic Category Anticholinergic Agent
Use GI tract disorders caused by spasm, adjunctive therapy for peptic ulcers
Usual Dosage
Children:
<2 years: ¼ adult dosage
2-10 years: ½ adult dosage
Adults:
Oral, S.L.: 0.125-0.25 mg 3-4 times/day before meals or food and at bedtime; 0.375-0.75 mg (timed release) every 12 hours
I.M., I.V., S.C.: 0.25-0.5 mg every 6 hours
Dosage Forms
Capsule, as sulfate, timed release (Cystospaz-M®, Levsinex®): 0.375 mg
Elixir, as sulfate (Levsin®): 0.125 mg/5 mL with alcohol 20% (480 mL)
Injection, as sulfate (Levsin®): 0.5 mg/mL (1 mL, 10 mL)
Solution, oral (Gastrosed™, Levsin®): 0.125 mg/mL (15 mL)
Tablet, as sulfate:
Anaspaz®, Gastrosed™, Levsin®, Neoquess®: 0.125 mg
(Continued)

hyoscyamine *(Continued)*

Cystospaz®: 0.15 mg
Extended release (Levbid®): 0.375 mg

hyoscyamine, atropine, scopolamine, and phenobarbital

(hye oh SYE a meen, A troe peen, skoe POL a meen & fee noe BAR bi tal)

Brand Names Barbidonna®; Donnatal®; Hyosophen®; Malatal®; Spasmolin®

Therapeutic Category Anticholinergic Agent

Use Adjunct in treatment of peptic ulcer disease, irritable bowel, spastic colitis, spastic bladder, and renal colic

Usual Dosage Oral:

Children 2-12 years:
Kinesed® dose: $^1/_2$ to 1 tablet 3-4 times/day
Donnatal®: 0.1 mL/kg/dose every 4 hours; maximum dose: 5 mL

Adults: 0.125-0.25 mg (1-2 capsules or tablets) 3-4 times/day; or 0.375-0.75 mg (1 Donnatal® Extentab®) in sustained release form every 12 hours; or 5-10 mL elixir 3-4 times/day or every 8 hours

Dosage Forms

Capsule (Donnatal®, Spasmolin®): Hyoscyamine sulfate 0.1037 mg, atropine sulfate 0.0194 mg, scopolamine hydrobromide 0.0065 mg, and phenobarbital 16.2 mg

Elixir (Donnatal®, Hyosophen®, Spasmophen®): Hyoscyamine sulfate 0.1037 mg, atropine sulfate 0.0194 mg, scopolamine hydrobromide 0.0065 mg, and phenobarbital 16.2 mg per 5 mL (120 mL, 480 mL, 4000 mL)

Tablet:

Barbidonna®: Hyoscyamine hydrobromide 0.1286 mg, atropine sulfate 0.025 mg, scopolamine hydrobromide 0.0074 mg, and phenobarbital 16 mg

Barbidonna® No. 2: Hyoscyamine hydrobromide 0.1286 mg, atropine sulfate 0.025 mg, scopolamine hydrobromide 0.0074 mg, and phenobarbital 32 mg

Donnatal®, Hyosophen®: Hyoscyamine sulfate 0.1037 mg, atropine sulfate 0.0194 mg, scopolamine hydrobromide 0.0065 mg, and phenobarbital 16.2 mg

Long-acting (Donnatal®): Hyoscyamine sulfate 0.3111 mg, atropine sulfate 0.0582 mg, scopolamine hydrobromide 0.0195 mg, and phenobarbital 48.6 mg

Spasmophen®: Hyoscyamine sulfate 0.1037 mg, atropine sulfate 0.0194 mg, scopolamine hydrobromide 0.0065 mg, and phenobarbital 15 mg

hyoscyamine, atropine, scopolamine, kaolin, and pectin

(hye oh SYE a meen, A troe peen, skoe POL a meen, KAY oh lin & PEK tin)

Therapeutic Category Anticholinergic Agent

Use Antidiarrheal; also used in gastritis, enteritis, colitis, and acute gastrointestinal upsets, and nausea which may accompany any of these conditions

Usual Dosage Oral:

Children:
10-20 lb: 2.5 mL
20-30 lb: 5 mL
>30 lb: 5-10 mL

Adults:
Diarrhea: 30 mL at once and 15-30 mL with each loose stool
Other conditions: 15 mL every 3 hours as needed

Dosage Forms Suspension, oral: Hyoscyamine sulfate 0.1037 mg, atropine sulfate 0.0194 mg, scopolamine hydrobromide 0.0065 mg, kaolin 6 g, and pectin 142.8 mg per 30 mL

hyoscyamine, atropine, scopolamine, kaolin, pectin, and opium

(hye oh SYE a meen, A troe peen, skoe POL a meen, KAY oh lin, PEK tin, & OH pee um)

Brand Names Donnapectolin-PG®; Kapectolin PG®

Therapeutic Category Anticholinergic Agent

Controlled Substance C-V

Use Treatment of diarrhea

Usual Dosage Oral:

Children 6-12 years: Initial: 10 mL, then 5-10 mL every 3 hours thereafter

Dosage recommendations (body weight/dosage): 10 lb/2.5 mL; 20 lb/5 mL; 30 lb and over/5-10 mL. Do not administer more than 4 doses in any 24-hour period

Children >12 years and Adults: Initial: 30 mL (1 fluid oz) followed by 15 mL every 3 hours

Dosage Forms Suspension, oral: Hyoscyamine sulfate 0.1037 mg, atropine sulfate 0.0194 mg, scopolamine hydrobromide 0.0065 mg, kaolin 6 g, pectin 142.8 mg, and powdered opium 24 mg per 30 mL with alcohol 5%

hyoscyamine sulfate *see* hyoscyamine *on page 275*

Hyosophen® *see* hyoscyamine, atropine, scopolamine, and phenobarbital *on previous page*

Hypaque-Cysto® *see* radiological/contrast media (ionic) *on page 457*

Hypaque® Meglumine *see* radiological/contrast media (ionic) *on page 457*

Hypaque® Sodium *see* radiological/contrast media (ionic) *on page 457*

Hyperab® *see* rabies immune globulin (human) *on page 457*

HyperHep® *see* hepatitis b immune globulin *on page 259*

Hyperstat® I.V. *see* diazoxide *on page 163*

Hyper-Tet® *see* tetanus immune globulin (human) *on page 508*

Hy-Phen® *see* hydrocodone and acetaminophen *on page 266*

HypoTears PF Solution [OTC] *see* artificial tears *on page 42*

HypoTears Solution [OTC] *see* artificial tears *on page 42*

HypRho®-D *see* $Rh_o(D)$ immune globulin *on page 463*

HypRho®-D Mini-Dose *see* $Rh_o(D)$ immune globulin *on page 463*

Hyprogest® 250 Injection *see* hydroxyprogesterone caproate *on page 274*

Hyrexin-50® Injection *see* diphenhydramine *on page 173*

Hytakerol® *see* dihydrotachysterol *on page 169*

Hytinic® [OTC] *see* polysaccharide-iron complex *on page 424*

Hytone® *see* hydrocortisone *on page 268*

Hytrin® *see* terazosin *on page 504*

Hytuss® [OTC] *see* guaifenesin *on page 247*

Hytuss-2X® [OTC] *see* guaifenesin *on page 247*

Hyzaar® *see* losartan and hydrochlorothiazide *on page 315*

Hyzine-50® *see* hydroxyzine *on page 275*

ibenzmethyzin *see* procarbazine *on page 439*

Iberet-Folic-500® *see* ferrous sulfate, ascorbic acid, vitamin b-complex, and folic acid *on page 222*

Iberet-Folic-500® *see* vitamins, multiple (oral, adult) *on page 556*

Iberet®-Liquid [OTC] *see* ferrous sulfate, ascorbic acid, and vitamin b-complex *on page 221*

ibidomide hydrochloride *see* labetalol *on page 299*

IBU® *see* ibuprofen *on next page*

Ibuprin® [OTC] *see* ibuprofen *on next page*

ibuprofen (eye byoo PROE fen)

Synonyms *p*-isobutylhydratropic acid

Brand Names Advil® [OTC]; Bayer® Select® Pain Relief Formula [OTC]; Children's Advil® Oral Suspension [OTC]; Children's Motrin® Oral Suspension [OTC]; Dynafed® IB [OTC]; Genpril® [OTC]; Haltran® [OTC]; IBU®; Ibuprin® [OTC]; Ibuprohm® [OTC]; Junior Strength Motrin® [OTC]; Menadol® [OTC]; Midol® IB [OTC]; Motrin®; Motrin® IB [OTC]; Nuprin® [OTC]; Saleto-200® [OTC]; Saleto-400®; Saleto-600®; Saleto-800®

Therapeutic Category Analgesic, Non-narcotic; Antipyretic; Nonsteroidal Anti-Inflammatory Agent (NSAID)

Use Inflammatory diseases and rheumatoid disorders including juvenile rheumatoid arthritis (JRA); mild to moderate pain; fever; dysmenorrhea; gout

Usual Dosage Oral:

Children:

Antipyretic: 6 months to 12 years: Temperature <102.5°F (39°C): 5 mg/kg/dose; temperature >102.5°F: 10 mg/kg/dose administered every 6-8 hours; maximum daily dose: 40 mg/kg/day

Juvenile rheumatoid arthritis: 30-50 mg/kg/day in 4 divided doses; start at lower end of dosing range and titrate upward; maximum: 2.4 g/day

Analgesic: 4-10 mg/kg/dose every 6-8 hours

Adults:

Inflammatory disease: 400-800 mg/dose 3-4 times/day; maximum dose: 3.2 g/day

Pain/fever/dysmenorrhea: 200-400 mg/dose every 4-6 hours; maximum daily dose: 1.2 g

Dosage Forms

Caplet: 100 mg

Drops, oral (berry flavor): 40 mg/mL (15 mL)

Suppository, rectal: 80 mg

Suspension, oral: 100 mg/5 mL [OTC] (60 mL, 120 mL, 480 mL)

Drops: 40 mg/mL [OTC]

Tablet: 100 mg [OTC], 200 mg [OTC], 300 mg, 400 mg, 600 mg, 800 mg

Chewable: 50 mg, 100 mg

Ibuprohm® [OTC] *see* ibuprofen *on this page*

ibutilide (i BYOO ti lide)

Synonyms ibutilide fumarate

Brand Names Corvert®

Therapeutic Category Antiarrhythmic Agent, Class III

Use Acute termination of atrial fibrillation or flutter of recent onset; the effectiveness of ibutilide has not been determined in patients with arrhythmias of >90 days in duration

Usual Dosage I.V.: Initial:

<60 kg: 0.01 mg/kg over 10 minutes

≥60 kg: 1 mg over 10 minutes

If the arrhythmia does not terminate within 10 minutes after the end of the initial infusion, a second infusion of equal strength may be infused over a 10-minute period

Dosage Forms Injection, as fumarate: 0.1 mg/mL (10 mL)

ibutilide fumarate *see* ibutilide *on this page*

ICRF-187 *see* dexrazoxane *on page 158*

Idamycin® *see* idarubicin *on this page*

idarubicin (eye da ROO bi sin)

Synonyms 4-demethoxydaunorubicin; 4-dmdr; idarubicin hydrochloride

Brand Names Idamycin®

Therapeutic Category Antineoplastic Agent

Use In combination with other antineoplastic agents for treatment of acute myelogenous leukemia (AML) in adults and acute lymphocytic leukemia (ALL) in children

Usual Dosage I.V.:
Children:
Leukemia: 10-12 mg/m² once daily for 3 days and repeat every 3 weeks
Solid tumors: 5 mg/m² once daily for 3 days and repeat every 3 weeks
Adults: 12 mg/m²/day for 3 days by slow I.V. injection (10-15 minutes) in combination with Ara-C. The Ara-C may be given as 100 mg/m²/day by continuous infusion for 7 days or 25 mg/m² bolus followed by Ara-C 200 mg/m²/day for 5 days continuous infusion.
Dosage Forms Powder for injection, lyophilized, as hydrochloride: 5 mg, 10 mg

idarubicin hydrochloride *see* idarubicin *on previous page*

idoxuridine (eye doks YOOR i deen)
Synonyms idu; iudr
Brand Names Herplex® Ophthalmic
Therapeutic Category Antiviral Agent
Use Treatment of herpes simplex keratitis
Usual Dosage Adults: Ophthalmic:
Ointment: Instill 5 times/day (every 4 hours) in the conjunctival sac with last dose at bedtime; continue therapy for 5-7 days after healing appears complete
Solution: Instill 1 drop in eye(s) every hour during day and every 2 hours at night, continue until definite improvement is noted, then reduce daytime dose to 1 drop every 2 hours and every 4 hours at night; continue for 5-7 days after healing appears complete
Dosage Forms Solution, ophthalmic: 0.1% (15 mL)

idu *see* idoxuridine *on this page*

Ifex® *see* ifosfamide *on this page*

IFLrA *see* interferon alfa-2a *on page 285*

ifosfamide (eye FOSS fa mide)
Brand Names Ifex®
Therapeutic Category Antineoplastic Agent
Use In combination with other antineoplastics in treatment of lung cancer, Hodgkin's and non-Hodgkin's lymphoma, breast cancer, acute and chronic lymphocytic leukemia, ovarian cancer, testicular cancer, and sarcomas
Usual Dosage I.V. (refer to individual protocols):
Children: 1800 mg/m²/day for 3-5 days every 21-28 days or 5000 mg/m² as a single 24-hour infusion or 3 g/m²/day for 2 days
Adults: 700-2000 mg/m²/day for 5 days or 2400 mg/m²/day for 3 days every 21-28 days; 5000 mg/m² as a single dose over 24 hours
Dosage Forms Powder for injection: 1 g, 3 g

ig *see* immune globulin, intramuscular *on page 281*

igim *see* immune globulin, intramuscular *on page 281*

igiv *see* immune globulin, intravenous *on page 281*

Ilopan-Choline® Oral *see* dexpanthenol *on page 158*

Ilopan® Injection *see* dexpanthenol *on page 158*

Ilosone® Oral *see* erythromycin *on page 199*

Ilotycin® Ophthalmic *see* erythromycin, topical *on page 201*

Ilozyme® *see* pancrelipase *on page 394*

Imdur™ *see* isosorbide mononitrate *on page 292*

imidazole carboxamide *see* dacarbazine *on page 147*

imiglucerase (imi GLOO ser ase)
Brand Names Cerezyme®
Therapeutic Category Enzyme
Use Long-term enzyme replacement therapy for patients with Type 1 Gaucher's disease
Usual Dosage I.V.: 2.5 units/kg 3 times a week up to as much as 60 units/kg administered as frequently as once a week or as infrequently as every 4 weeks; 60 units/kg administered every 2 weeks is the most common dose
Dosage Forms Powder for injection, preservative free (lyophilized): 212 units [equivalent to a withdrawal dose of 200 units]

imipemide *see* imipenem and cilastatin *on this page*

imipenem and cilastatin (i mi PEN em & sye la STAT in)
Synonyms imipemide
Brand Names Primaxin®
Therapeutic Category Carbapenem (Antibiotic)
Use Treatment of documented multidrug resistant gram-negative infection due to organisms proven or suspected to be susceptible to imipenem/cilastatin; treatment of multiple organism infection in which other agents have an insufficient spectrum of activity or are contraindicated due to toxic potential; therapeutic alternative for treatment of gram negative sepsis in immunocompromised patients
Usual Dosage I.V. infusion (dosage recommendation based on imipenem component):
Children: 60-100 mg/kg/day in 4 divided doses
Adults:
Serious infection: 2-4 g/day in 3-4 divided doses
Mild to moderate infection: 1-2 g/day in 3-4 divided doses
Dosage Forms Powder for injection:
I.M.:
Imipenem 500 mg and cilastatin 500 mg
Imipenem 750 mg and cilastatin 750 mg
I.V.:
Imipenem 250 mg and cilastatin 250 mg
Imipenem 500 mg and cilastatin 500 mg

imipramine (im IP ra meen)
Synonyms imipramine hydrochloride; imipramine pamoate
Brand Names Janimine®; Tofranil®; Tofranil-PM®
Therapeutic Category Antidepressant, Tricyclic (Tertiary Amine)
Use Treatment of various forms of depression, often in conjunction with psychotherapy; enuresis in children; analgesic for certain chronic and neuropathic pain
Usual Dosage
Children: Oral (safety and efficacy of imipramine therapy for treatment of depression in children <12 years have not been established):
Enuresis: ≥6 years: Initial: 10-25 mg at bedtime, if inadequate response still seen after 1 week of therapy, increase by 25 mg/day; dose should not exceed 2.5 mg/kg/day or 50 mg at bedtime if 6-12 years of age or 75 mg at bedtime if ≥12 years of age
Adjunct in the treatment of cancer pain: Initial: 0.2-0.4 mg/kg at bedtime; dose may be increased by 50% every 2-3 days up to 1-3 mg/kg/dose at bedtime
Adolescents: Oral: Initial: 25-50 mg/day; increase gradually; maximum: 100 mg/day in single or divided doses
Adults:
Oral: Initial: 25 mg 3-4 times/day, increase dose gradually, total dose may be administered at bedtime; maximum: 300 mg/day
I.M.: Initial: Up to 100 mg/day in divided doses; change to oral as soon as possible
Dosage Forms
Capsule, as pamoate (Tofranil-PM®): 75 mg, 100 mg, 125 mg, 150 mg
Injection, as hydrochloride (Tofranil®): 12.5 mg/mL (2 mL)

Tablet, as hydrochloride (Janimine®, Tofranil®): 10 mg, 25 mg, 50 mg

imipramine hydrochloride *see* imipramine *on previous page*

imipramine pamoate *see* imipramine *on previous page*

imiquimod (i mi KWI mod)
Brand Names Aldara®
Therapeutic Category Immune Response Modifier
Use Genital and perianal warts (condyloma acuminata)
Usual Dosage Adults: Topical: Apply three times/week, prior to bedtime, leave on for 6-10 hours, remove cream by washing area with mild soap and water
Dosage Forms Cream: 5% (250 mg single dose packets)

Imitrex® *see* sumatriptan succinate *on page 500*

immune globulin, intramuscular
(i MYUN GLOB yoo lin, IN tra MUS kyoo ler)
Synonyms gamma globulin; ig; igim; immune serum globulin; isg
Therapeutic Category Immune Globulin
Use Prophylaxis against hepatitis A, measles, varicella, and possibly rubella and immunoglobulin deficiency, idiopathic thrombocytopenia purpura, Kawasaki syndrome, lymphocytic leukemia
Usual Dosage I.M.:
Hepatitis A: 0.02 mL/kg
IgG: 1.3 mL/kg then 0.66 mL/kg in 3-4 weeks
Measles: 0.25 mL/kg
Rubella: 0.55 mL/kg
Varicella: 0.6-1.2 mL/kg
Dosage Forms Injection: I.M.: 165±15 mg (of protein)/mL (2 mL, 10 mL)

immune globulin, intravenous (i MYUN GLOB yoo lin, IN tra VEE nus)
Synonyms igiv; ivig
Brand Names Gamimune® N; Gammagard®; Gammagard® S/D; Gammar-P® I.V.; Polygam®; Polygam® S/D; Sandoglobulin®; Venoglobulin®-I; Venoglobulin®-S
Therapeutic Category Immune Globulin
Use Immunodeficiency syndrome, idiopathic thrombocytopenic purpura (ITP) and B-cell chronic lymphocytic leukemia (CLL); used in conjunction with appropriate anti-infective therapy to prevent or modify acute bacterial or viral infections in patients with iatrogenically-induced or disease-associated immunodepression; autoimmune neutropenia, bone marrow transplantation patients, Kawasaki disease, Guillain-Barré syndrome, demyelinating polyneuropathies
Usual Dosage Children and Adults: I.V. infusion:
Immunodeficiency syndrome: 100-200 mg/kg/dose every month; may increase to 400 mg/kg/dose as needed
Idiopathic thrombocytopenic purpura: 400-1000 mg/kg/dose for 2-5 consecutive days; maintenance dose: 400-1000 mg/kg/dose every 3-6 weeks based on clinical response and platelet count
Kawasaki disease: 400 mg/kg/day for 4 days or 2 g/kg as a single dose
Congenital and acquired antibody deficiency syndrome: 100-400 mg/kg/dose every 3-4 weeks
Bone marrow transplant: 500 mg/kg/week
Severe systemic viral and bacterial infections: Children: 500-1000 mg/kg/week
Dosage Forms
Injection: Gamimune® N: 5% [50 mg/mL] (10 mL, 50 mL, 100 mL); 10% [100 mg/mL] (50 mL, 100 mL, 200 mL)
Powder for injection, lyophilized:
Gammagard®, Polygam®: 0.5 g, 2.5 g, 5 g, 10 g
Gammar®-P I.V.: 1 g, 2.5 g, 5 g
(Continued)

immune globulin, intravenous *(Continued)*

Polygam®: 0.5 g, 2.5 g, 5 g, 10 g
Sandoglobulin®: 1 g, 3 g, 6 g
Venoglobulin®-I: 2.5 g, 5 g
Detergent treated:
 Gammagard® S/D: 2.5 g, 5 g, 10 g
 Polygam® S/D: 2.5 g, 5 g, 10 g
 Venoglobulin®-S: 2.5 g, 5 g, 10 g

immune serum globulin *see* immune globulin, intramuscular *on previous page*

Imodium® *see* loperamide *on page 313*

Imodium® A-D [OTC] *see* loperamide *on page 313*

Imogam® *see* rabies immune globulin (human) *on page 457*

Imovax® Rabies I.D. Vaccine *see* rabies virus vaccine *on page 457*

Imovax® Rabies Vaccine *see* rabies virus vaccine *on page 457*

Imuran® *see* azathioprine *on page 50*

I-Naphline® Ophthalmic *see* naphazoline *on page 364*

Inapsine® *see* droperidol *on page 185*

indapamide (in DAP a mide)
Brand Names Lozol®
Therapeutic Category Diuretic, Miscellaneous
Use Management of mild to moderate hypertension; treatment of edema in congestive heart failure and nephrotic syndrome
Usual Dosage Adults: Oral: 2.5-5 mg/day
Dosage Forms Tablet: 1.25 mg, 2.5 mg

Inderal® *see* propranolol *on page 446*

Inderal® LA *see* propranolol *on page 446*

Inderide® *see* propranolol and hydrochlorothiazide *on page 447*

indinavir (in DIN a veer)
Brand Names Crixivan®
Therapeutic Category Antiviral Agent
Use Treatment of HIV infection, especially advanced disease; usually administered as part of a three-drug regimen (two nucleosides plus a protease inhibitor) or double therapy (one nucleoside plus a protease inhibitor)
Usual Dosage Adults: Oral: 800 mg every 8 hours
Dosage Forms Capsule: 200 mg, 400 mg

Indochron E-R® *see* indomethacin *on next page*

Indocin® *see* indomethacin *on next page*

Indocin® I.V. *see* indomethacin *on next page*

Indocin® SR *see* indomethacin *on next page*

indocyanine green (in doe SYE a neen green)
Brand Names Cardio-Green®
Therapeutic Category Diagnostic Agent
Use Determining hepatic function, cardiac output and liver blood flow and for ophthalmic angiography
Usual Dosage Dilute dose in sterile water for injection or 0.9% NaCl to final volume of 1 mL if necessary doses may be repeated periodically; total dose should not exceed 2 mg/kg

Infants: 1.25 mg
Children: 2.5 mg
Adults: 5 mg
Dosage Forms Injection: 25 mg, 50 mg

indometacin *see* indomethacin *on this page*

indomethacin (in doe METH a sin)

Synonyms indometacin; indomethacin sodium trihydrate
Brand Names Indochron E-R®; Indocin®; Indocin® I.V.; Indocin® SR
Therapeutic Category Analgesic, Non-narcotic; Nonsteroidal Anti-Inflammatory Agent (NSAID)
Use Management of inflammatory diseases and rheumatoid disorders; moderate pain; acute gouty arthritis; I.V. form used as alternative to surgery for closure of patent ductus arteriosus (PDA) in neonates
Usual Dosage
Patent ductus arteriosus: Neonates: I.V.: Initial: 0.2 mg/kg; followed with: 2 doses of 0.1 mg/kg at 12- to 24-hour intervals if age <48 hours at time of first dose; 0.2 mg/kg 2 times if 2-7 days old at time of first dose; or 0.25 mg/kg 2 times if over 7 days at time of first dose; discontinue if significant adverse effects occur. Dose should be withheld if patient has anuria or oliguria.
Analgesia:
Children: Oral: Initial: 1-2 mg/kg/day in 2-4 divided doses; maximum: 4 mg/kg/day; not to exceed 150-200 mg/day
Adults: Oral, rectal: 25-50 mg/dose 2-3 times/day; maximum dose: 200 mg/day; extended release capsule should be administered on a 1-2 times/day schedule
Dosage Forms
Capsule: 25 mg, 50 mg
Indocin®: 25 mg, 50 mg
Capsule, sustained release (Indocin® SR): 75 mg
Powder for injection, as sodium trihydrate (Indocin® I.V.): 1 mg
Suppository, rectal (Indocin®): 50 mg
Suspension, oral (Indocin®): 25 mg/5 mL (5 mL, 10 mL, 237 mL, 500 mL)

indomethacin sodium trihydrate *see* indomethacin *on this page*

INF-alpha 2 *see* interferon alfa-2b *on page 286*

Infanrix® *see* diphtheria, tetanus toxoids, and acellular pertussis vaccine *on page 175*

Infants Feverall™ [OTC] *see* acetaminophen *on page 3*

Infants' Silapap® [OTC] *see* acetaminophen *on page 3*

InFeD™ Injection *see* iron dextran complex *on page 289*

Inflamase® Forte Ophthalmic *see* prednisolone *on page 434*

Inflamase® Mild Ophthalmic *see* prednisolone *on page 434*

influenza virus vaccine (in floo EN za VYE rus vak SEEN)

Brand Names Fluogen®; Fluzone®
Therapeutic Category Vaccine, Inactivated Virus
Use Provide active immunity to influenza virus strains contained in the vaccine
Usual Dosage Annual vaccination with current vaccine; either whole- or split-virus vaccine may be used
Dosage Forms Injection:
Purified surface antigen (Flu-Imune®): 5 mL
Split-virus (Fluogen®, Fluzone®): 0.5 mL, 5 mL
Whole-virus (Fluzone®): 5 mL

Infumorph™ Injection *see* morphine sulfate *on page 356*

inh *see* isoniazid *on page 290*

Innovar® *see* droperidol and fentanyl *on page 186*

Inocor® *see* amrinone *on page 34*

insect sting kit (IN sekt sting kit)
Brand Names Ana-Kit®
Therapeutic Category Antidote
Use Anaphylaxis emergency treatment of insect bites or stings by the sensitive patient that may occur within minutes of insect sting or exposure to an allergic substance
Usual Dosage Children and Adults:
Epinephrine:
<2 years: 0.05-0.1 mL
2-6 years: 0.15 mL
6-12 years: 0.2 mL
>12 years : 0.3 mL
Chlorpheniramine:
<6 years: 1 tablet
6-12 years: 2 tablets
>12 years: 4 tablets
Dosage Forms Kit: Epinephrine hydrochloride 1:1000 (1 mL syringe), chlorpheniramine maleate chewable tablet 2 mg (4), sterile alcohol pads (2), tourniquet

Insta-Char® **[OTC]** *see* charcoal *on page 105*

Insta-Glucose® **[OTC]** *see* glucose, instant *on page 242*

insulin preparations (IN su lin prep a RAY shuns)
Brand Names Humalog®; Humulin® 50/50; Humulin® 70/30; Humulin® L; Humulin® N; Lente® Iletin® I; Lente® Iletin® II; Lente® Insulin; Lente® L; Novolin® 70/30; Novolin® L; Novolin® N; Novolin® R; NPH Iletin® I; NPH-N; Pork NPH Iletin® II; Pork Regular Iletin® II; Regular (Concentrated) Iletin® II U-500; Regular Iletin® I; Regular Insulin; Regular Purified Pork Insulin; Velosulin® Human
Therapeutic Category Antidiabetic Agent, Parenteral
Use Treatment of insulin-dependent diabetes mellitus, also noninsulin-dependent diabetes mellitus unresponsive to treatment with diet and/or oral hypoglycemics; to assure proper utilization of glucose and reduce glucosuria in nondiabetic patients receiving parenteral nutrition whose glucosuria cannot be adequately controlled with infusion rate adjustments or those who require assistance in achieving optimal caloric intakes
Usual Dosage Dose requires continuous medical supervision; only regular insulin may be administered I.V. The daily dose should be divided up depending upon the product used and the patient's response, eg, regular insulin every 4-6 hours; NPH insulin every 8-12 hours.

Children and Adults: S.C.: 0.5-1 unit/kg/day
Adolescents (during growth spurt) S.C.: 0.8-1.2 units/kg/day

Diabetic ketoacidosis: Children: I.V. loading dose: 0.1 unit/kg, then maintenance continuous infusion: 0.1 unit/kg/hour (range: 0.05-0.2 units/kg/hour depending upon the rate of decrease of serum glucose - too rapid decrease of serum glucose may lead to cerebral edema)
Optimum rate of decrease (serum glucose): 80-100 mg/dL/hour

Note: Newly diagnosed patients with JODM presenting in DKA and patients with blood sugars <800 mg/dL may be relatively "sensitive" to insulin and should receive loading and initial maintenance doses approximately 1/2 of those indicated above.

Note: The term "purified" refers to insulin preparations containing no more than 10 ppm proinsulin (purified and human insulins are less immunogenic)

Dosage Forms All insulins are 100 units/mL (10 mL) except where indicated:

RAPID ACTING:

Insulin lispro rDNA origin: Humalog® [*Lilly*] (1.5 mL, 10 mL)

Insulin Injection (Regular Insulin)

Beef and pork: Regular Iletin® I [*Lilly*]

Human:

rDNA: Humulin® R [*Lilly*], Novolin® R [*Novo Nordisk*]

Semisynthetic: Velosulin® Human [*Novo Nordisk*]

Pork: Regular Insulin [*Novo Nordisk*]

Purified pork:

Pork Regular Iletin® II [*Lilly*], Regular Purified Pork Insulin [*Novo Nordisk*]

Regular (Concentrated) Iletin® II U-500 (*Lilly*): 500 units/mL

INTERMEDIATE-ACTING:

Insulin Zinc Suspension (Lente)

Beef and pork: Lente® Iletin® I [*Lilly*]

Human, rDNA: Humulin® L [*Lilly*], Novolin® L [*Novo Nordisk*]

Purified pork: Lente® Iletin® II [*Lilly*], Lente® L [*Novo Nordisk*]

Isophane Insulin Suspension (NPH)

Beef and pork: NPH Iletin® I [*Lilly*]

Human, rDNA: Humulin® N [*Lilly*], Novolin® N [*Novo Nordisk*]

Purified pork: Pork NPH Iletin® II [*Lilly*], NPH-N [*Novo Nordisk*]

LONG-ACTING:

Insulin zinc suspension, extended (Ultralente®)

Human, rDNA: Humulin® U [Lilly]

COMBINATIONS:

Isophane Insulin Suspension and Insulin Injection

Isophane insulin suspension (50%) and insulin injection (50%) human (rDNA): Humulin® 50/50 [*Lilly*]

Isophane insulin suspension (70%) and insulin injection (30%) human (rDNA): Humulin® 70/30 [*Lilly*], Novolin® 70/30 [*Novo Nordisk*]

Intal® Inhalation Capsule *see* cromolyn sodium *on page 141*

Intal® Nebulizer Solution *see* cromolyn sodium *on page 141*

Intal® Oral Inhaler *see* cromolyn sodium *on page 141*

α-2-interferon *see* interferon alfa-2b *on next page*

interferon alfa-2a (in ter FEER on AL fa too aye)

Synonyms IFLrA; rIFN-A

Brand Names Roferon-A®

Therapeutic Category Biological Response Modulator

Use Hairy cell leukemia, AIDS-related Kaposi's sarcoma in patients >18 years of age, multiple unlabeled uses

Usual Dosage

Children: S.C.: Pulmonary hemangiomatosis: 1-3 million units/m²/day once daily

Adults >18 years:

Hairy cell leukemia: I.M., S.C.: Induction dose is 3 million units/day for 16-24 weeks; maintenance: 3 million units 3 times/week

AIDS-related Kaposi's sarcoma: I.M., S.C.: Induction dose is 36 million units for 10-12 weeks; maintenance: 36 million units 3 times/week (may begin with dose escalation from 3-9-18 million units each day over 3 consecutive days followed by 36 million units daily for the remainder of the 10-12 weeks of induction)

Dosage Forms

Injection: 3 million units/mL (1 mL); 6 million units/mL (3 mL); 9 million units/mL (0.9 mL, 3 mL); 36 million units/mL (1 mL)

Powder for injection: 6 million units/mL when reconstituted

interferon alfa-2b (in ter FEER on AL fa too bee)
Synonyms INF-alpha 2; α-2-interferon; rLFN-α2
Brand Names Intron® A
Therapeutic Category Biological Response Modulator
Use Induce hairy cell leukemia remission; treatment of AIDS-related Kaposi's sarcoma; condylomata acuminata; chronic hepatitis C
Usual Dosage Adults (refer to individual protocols):
Hairy cell leukemia: I.M., S.C.: 2 million units/m^2 3 times/week
AIDS-related Kaposi's sarcoma: I.M., S.C.: 30 million units/m^2 3 times/week or 50 million units/m^2 I.V. 5 days/week every other week
Condylomata acuminata: Intralesionally: 1 million units/lesion 3 times/week for 3 weeks; not to exceed 5 million units per treatment (maximum: 5 lesions at one time)
Chronic hepatitis C: I.M., S.C.: 3 million units 3 times/week for approximately a 6-month course
Dosage Forms
Injection, albumin free: 3 million units (0.5 mL); 5 million units (0.5 mL); 10 million units (1 mL); 25 million units
Powder for injection, lyophilized: 18 million units, 50 million units

interferon alfa-n3 (in ter FEER on AL fa en three)
Brand Names Alferon® N
Therapeutic Category Biological Response Modulator
Use Intralesional treatment of refractory or recurring genital or venereal warts; useful in patients who do not respond or are not candidates for usual treatments; indications and dosage regimens are specific for a particular brand of interferon
Usual Dosage Adults: Inject 250,000 units (0.05 mL) in each wart twice weekly for a maximum of 8 weeks; therapy should not be repeated for at least 3 months after the initial 8-week course of therapy
Dosage Forms Injection: 5 million units (1 mL)

interferon beta-1a (in ter FEER on BAY ta won aye)
Brand Names Avonex®
Therapeutic Category Biological Response Modulator
Use Treatment of relapsing forms of multiple sclerosis (MS); to slow the accumulation of physical disability and decrease the frequency of clinical exacerbations
Usual Dosage Adults >18 years: I.M.: 30 mcg once weekly
Dosage Forms Powder for injection, lyophilized: 33 mcg [6.6 million units]

interferon beta-1b (in ter FEER on BAY ta won bee)
Synonyms rlfn-b
Brand Names Betaseron®
Therapeutic Category Biological Response Modulator
Use Reduce the frequency of clinical exacerbations in ambulatory patients with relapsing-remitting multiple sclerosis
Usual Dosage Adults: S.C.: 0.25 mg every other day
Dosage Forms Powder for injection, lyophilized: 0.3 mg [9.6 million units]

interferon gamma-1b (in ter FEER on GAM ah won bee)
Brand Names Actimmune®
Therapeutic Category Biological Response Modulator
Use Reduce the frequency and severity of serious infections associated with chronic granulomatous disease
Usual Dosage Adults: S.C. (dosing is based on body surface (m^2)):
≤0.5: 1.5 mcg/kg/dose
>0.5: 50 mcg/m^2 (1.5 million units/m^2) 3 times/week
Dosage Forms Injection: 100 mcg [3 million units]

interleukin-2 *see* aldesleukin *on page 15*

Intralipid® *see* fat emulsion *on page 216*

Intron® **A** *see* interferon alfa-2b *on previous page*

Intropin® **Injection** *see* dopamine *on page 181*

Inversine® *see* mecamylamine *on page 324*

Invirase® *see* saquinavir *on page 474*

Iobid DM® *see* guaifenesin and dextromethorphan *on page 248*

Iodex® **[OTC]** *see* povidone-iodine *on page 431*

Iodex-p® **[OTC]** *see* povidone-iodine *on page 431*

iodine (EYE oh dyne)
Therapeutic Category Topical Skin Product
Use Topically as an antiseptic in the management of minor, superficial skin wounds and has been used to disinfect the skin preoperatively
Usual Dosage Topical: Apply as necessary to affected areas of skin
Dosage Forms
Solution: 2%
Tincture: 2%

iodochlorhydroxyquin *see* clioquinol *on page 128*

iodochlorhydroxyquin and hydrocortisone *see* clioquinol and hydrocortisone *on page 128*

Iodopen® *see* trace metals *on page 525*

iodoquinol (eye oh doe KWIN ole)
Synonyms diiodohydroxyquin
Brand Names Yodoxin®
Therapeutic Category Amebicide
Use Treatment of acute and chronic intestinal amebiasis due to *Entamoeba histolytica*; asymptomatic cyst passers; *Blastocystis hominis* infections; iodoquinol alone is ineffective for amebic hepatitis or hepatic abscess
Usual Dosage Oral:
Children: 30-40 mg/kg/day in 3 divided doses for 20 days; not to exceed 1.95 g/day
Adults: 650 mg 3 times/day after meals for 20 days; not to exceed 2 g/day
Dosage Forms
Powder: 25 g
Tablet: 210 mg, 650 mg

iodoquinol and hydrocortisone
(eye oh doe KWIN ole & hye droe KOR ti sone)
Brand Names Vytone® Topical
Therapeutic Category Antifungal/Corticosteroid
Use Treatment of eczema; infectious dermatitis; chronic eczematoid otitis externa; mycotic dermatoses
Usual Dosage Topical: Apply 3-4 times/day
Dosage Forms Cream: Iodoquinol 1% and hydrocortisone 1% (30 g)

Iofed® *see* brompheniramine and pseudoephedrine *on page 74*

Iofed® **PD** *see* brompheniramine and pseudoephedrine *on page 74*

Iopidine® *see* apraclonidine *on page 39*

I-Paracaine® *see* proparacaine *on page 444*

ipecac syrup (IP e kak SIR up)
Therapeutic Category Antidote
Use Treatment of acute oral drug overdosage and certain poisonings
Usual Dosage Oral:
Children:
6-12 months: 5-10 mL followed by 10-20 mL/kg of water; repeat dose one time if vomiting does not occur within 20 minutes
1-12 years: 15 mL followed by 10-20 mL/kg of water; repeat dose one time if vomiting does not occur within 20 minutes
Adults: 30 mL followed by 200-300 mL of water; repeat dose one time if vomiting does not occur within 20 minutes
Dosage Forms Syrup: 70 mg/mL (15 mL, 30 mL, 473 mL, 4000 mL)

I-Pentolate® see cyclopentolate on page 143

I-Phrine® **Ophthalmic Solution** see phenylephrine on page 411

IPOL™ see poliovirus vaccine, inactivated on page 422

ipratropium (i pra TROE pee um)
Synonyms ipratropium bromide
Brand Names Atrovent®
Therapeutic Category Anticholinergic Agent
Use Bronchodilator used in bronchospasm associated with asthma, COPD, bronchitis, and emphysema; nasal spray used for symptomatic relief of rhinorrhea
Usual Dosage Children >12 years and Adults: 2 inhalations 4 times/day up to 12 inhalations/24 hours
Dosage Forms Solution, as bromide:
Inhalation: 18 mcg/actuation (14 g)
Nasal spray: 0.03% (30 mL)
Nebulizing: 0.02% (2.5 mL)

ipratropium and albuterol (i pra TROE pee um & al BYOO ter ole)
Brand Names Combivent®
Therapeutic Category Bronchodilator
Use Treatment of chronic obstructive pulmonary disease (COPD) in those patients that are currently on a regular bronchodilator who continue to have bronchospasms and require a second bronchodilator
Usual Dosage Adults: 2 inhalations 4 times/day, maximum of 12 inhalations/24 hours
Dosage Forms Aerosol: Ipratropium bromide 21 mcg and albuterol sulfate 120 mcg per actuation [200 doses] (14.7 g)

ipratropium bromide see ipratropium on this page

iproveratril hydrochloride see verapamil on page 548

ipv see poliovirus vaccine, inactivated on page 422

Ircon® **[OTC]** see ferrous fumarate on page 220

irinotecan (eye rye no TEE kan)
Brand Names Camptosar®
Therapeutic Category Antineoplastic Agent
Use Treatment of patients with metastatic carcinoma of the colon or rectum whose disease has progressed following 5-FU based therapy
Usual Dosage Adults: I.V.: The recommended starting dose is 125 mg/m^2 (I.V. infusion over 90 minutes) once a week for 4 weeks, followed by a 2-week rest period; additional 6-week cycles of treatment may be repeated indefinitely in patients who remain stable or do not develop intolerable toxicities
Dosage Forms Injection: 20 mg/mL (5 mL)

iron dextran complex (EYE ern DEKS tran KOM pleks)
Brand Names Dexferrum® Injection; InFeD™ Injection
Therapeutic Category Electrolyte Supplement
Use Treatment of microcytic, hypochromic anemia resulting from iron deficiency when oral iron administration is infeasible or ineffective
Usual Dosage I.M., I.V.:
A 0.5 mL test dose (0.25 mL in infants) should be administered prior to starting iron dextran therapy

Total replacement dosage of iron dextran (mL) = 0.0476 x weight (kg) x $(Hb_n - Hb_o)$ + 1 mL/per 5 kg body weight (up to maximum of 14 mL)
Hb_n = desired hemoglobin (g/dL)
Hb_o = measured hemoglobin (g/dL)

Maximum daily dose:
Infants <5 kg: 25 mg iron
Children:
5-10 kg: 50 mg iron
10-50 kg: 100 mg iron
Adults >50 kg: 100 mg iron
Dosage Forms Injection: 50 mg/mL (2 mL, 10 mL)

isd *see* isosorbide dinitrate *on page 292*

isdn *see* isosorbide dinitrate *on page 292*

isg *see* immune globulin, intramuscular *on page 281*

Ismelin® *see* guanethidine *on page 253*

ismn *see* isosorbide mononitrate *on page 292*

ISMO™ *see* isosorbide mononitrate *on page 292*

Ismotic® *see* isosorbide *on page 291*

isoamyl nitrite *see* amyl nitrite *on page 34*

isobamate *see* carisoprodol *on page 93*

Isobamate *see* carisoprodol, aspirin, and codeine *on page 93*

Isocaine® **HCl** *see* mepivacaine *on page 329*

Isocal® **[OTC]** *see* enteral nutritional products *on page 194*

Isoclor® **Expectorant** *see* guaifenesin, pseudoephedrine, and codeine *on page 251*

Isocom® *see* acetaminophen, isometheptene, and dichloralphenazone *on page 6*

isoetharine (eye soe ETH a reen)
Synonyms isoetharine hydrochloride; isoetharine mesylate
Brand Names Arm-a-Med® Isoetharine; Beta-2®; Bronkometer®; Bronkosol®; Dey-Lute® Isoetharine
Therapeutic Category Adrenergic Agonist Agent
Use Bronchodilator used in asthma and for the reversible bronchospasm occurring with bronchitis and emphysema
Usual Dosage Treatments are usually not repeated more often than every 4 hours, except in severe cases, and may be repeated up to 5 times/day if necessary
Nebulizer: Children: 0.1-0.2 mg/kg/dose every 2-6 hours as needed; adult: 0.5 mL diluted in 2-3 mL normal saline or 4 inhalations of undiluted 1% solution
Dosage Forms
Aerosol, oral, as mesylate: 340 mcg/metered spray
Solution, inhalation, as hydrochloride: 0.062% (4 mL); 0.08% (3.5 mL); 0.1% (2.5 mL, 5 mL); 0.125% (4 mL); 0.167% (3 mL); 0.17% (3 mL); 0.2% (2.5 mL); 0.25% (2 mL, 3.5 mL); 0.5% (0.5 mL); 1% (0.5 mL, 0.25 mL, 10 mL, 14 mL, 30 mL)

isoetharine hydrochloride *see* isoetharine *on previous page*

isoetharine mesylate *see* isoetharine *on previous page*

isoflurane (eye soe FLURE ane)

Brand Names Forane®
Therapeutic Category General Anesthetic
Use General induction and maintenance of anesthesia (inhalation)
Usual Dosage 1.5% to 3%
Dosage Forms Solution: 100 mL, 125 mL, 250 mL

isoflurophate (eye soe FLURE oh fate)

Synonyms dfp; diisopropyl fluorophosphate; dyflos; fluostigmin
Brand Names Floropryl® Ophthalmic
Therapeutic Category Cholinergic Agent
Use Treat primary open-angle glaucoma and conditions that obstruct aqueous outflow and to treat accommodative convergent strabismus
Usual Dosage Adults: Ophthalmic:
Glaucoma: Instill 1/4" strip in eye every 8-72 hours
Strabismus: Instill 1/4" strip to each eye every night for 2 weeks then reduce to 1/4" every other night to once weekly for 2 months
Dosage Forms Ointment, ophthalmic: 0.025% in polyethylene mineral oil gel (3.5 g)

Isollyl® Improved *see* butalbital compound and aspirin *on page 78*

isoniazid (eye soe NYE a zid)

Synonyms inh; isonicotinic acid hydrazide
Brand Names Laniazid® Oral; Nydrazid® Injection
Therapeutic Category Antitubercular Agent
Use Treatment of susceptible mycobacterial infection due to *M. tuberculosis* and prophylactically to those individuals exposed to tuberculosis
Usual Dosage Oral, I.M.:
Children: 10-20 mg/kg/day in 1-2 divided doses (maximum: 300 mg total dose)
Prophylaxis: 10 mg/kg/day administered daily (up to 300 mg total dose) for 12 months
Adults: 5 mg/kg/day administered daily (usual dose: 300 mg)
Disseminated disease: 10 mg/kg/day in 1-2 divided doses
Treatment should be continued for 9 months with rifampin or for 6 months with rifampin and pyrazinamide
Prophylaxis: 300 mg/day administered daily for 12 months

American Thoracic Society and CDC currently recommend twice weekly therapy as part of a short-course regimen which follows 1-2 months of daily treatment for uncomplicated pulmonary tuberculosis in compliant patients
Children: 20-40 mg/kg/dose (up to 900 mg) twice weekly
Adults: 15 mg/kg/dose (up to 900 mg) twice weekly
Dosage Forms
Injection: 100 mg/mL (10 mL)
Syrup (orange flavor): 50 mg/5 mL (473 mL)
Tablet: 50 mg, 100 mg, 300 mg

isonicotinic acid hydrazide *see* isoniazid *on this page*

isonipecaine hydrochloride *see* meperidine *on page 328*

Isopap® *see* acetaminophen, isometheptene, and dichloralphenazone *on page 6*

isoprenaline hydrochloride *see* isoproterenol *on next page*

isoproterenol (eye soe proe TER e nole)

Synonyms isoprenaline hydrochloride

Brand Names Arm-a-Med® Isoproterenol; Dey-Dose® Isoproterenol; Isuprel®; Medihaler-Iso®

Therapeutic Category Adrenergic Agonist Agent

Use Asthma or COPD (reversible airway obstruction); ventricular arrhythmias due to A-V nodal block; hemodynamically compromised bradyarrhythmias or atropine-resistant bradyarrhythmias, temporary use in third degree A-V block until pacemaker insertion; low cardiac output or vasoconstrictive shock states

Usual Dosage

Children:

Bronchodilation: Inhalation 1-2 metered doses up to 5 times/day

Nebulization: 0.01 mL/kg; minimum dose: 0.1 mL; maximum dose: 0.5 mL diluted in 2-3 mL normal saline

I.V. infusion: 0.05-2 mcg/kg/minute; rate (mL/hour) = dose (mcg/kg/minute) x weight (kg) x 60 minutes/hour divided by concentration (mcg/mL)

Adults:

Bronchodilation: 1-2 inhalations 4-6 times/day

A-V nodal block: I.V. infusion: 2-20 mcg/minute

Dosage Forms

Inhalation:

Aerosol: 0.2% (1:500) (15 mL, 22.5 mL); 0.25% (1:400) (15 mL)

Solution for nebulization: 0.031% (4 mL); 0.062% (4 mL); 0.25% (0.5 mL, 30 mL); 0.5% (0.5 mL, 10 mL, 60 mL); 1% (10 mL)

Injection: 0.2 mg/mL (1:5000) (1 mL, 5 mL, 10 mL)

Tablet, sublingual: 10 mg, 15 mg

isoproterenol and phenylephrine (eye soe proe TER e nole & fen il EF rin)

Brand Names Duo-Medihaler® Aerosol

Therapeutic Category Adrenergic Agonist Agent

Use Treatment of bronchospasm associated with acute and chronic bronchial asthma, bronchitis, pulmonary emphysema, and bronchiectasis

Usual Dosage Daily maintenance: 1-2 inhalations 4-6 times/day, no more than 2 inhalations at any one time or more than 6 in any 1 hour within 24 hours

Dosage Forms Aerosol: Each actuation releases isoproterenol hydrochloride 0.16 mg and phenylephrine bitartrate 0.24 mg (15 mL, 22.5 mL)

Isoptin® *see* verapamil *on page 548*

Isoptin® SR *see* verapamil *on page 548*

Isopto® Atropine *see* atropine *on page 47*

Isopto® Carbachol Ophthalmic *see* carbachol *on page 89*

Isopto® Carpine Ophthalmic *see* pilocarpine *on page 417*

Isopto® Cetamide® Ophthalmic *see* sulfacetamide sodium *on page 496*

Isopto® Cetapred® Ophthalmic *see* sulfacetamide sodium and prednisolone *on page 497*

Isopto® Homatropine Ophthalmic *see* homatropine *on page 261*

Isopto® Hyoscine Ophthalmic *see* scopolamine *on page 475*

Isopto® Plain Solution [OTC] *see* artificial tears *on page 42*

Isopto® Tears Solution [OTC] *see* artificial tears *on page 42*

Isordil® *see* isosorbide dinitrate *on next page*

isosorbide (eye soe SOR bide)

Brand Names Ismotic®

Therapeutic Category Diuretic, Osmotic

(Continued)

isosorbide *(Continued)*

Use Short-term emergency treatment of acute angle-closure glaucoma
Usual Dosage Adults: Oral: Initial: 1.5 g/kg; usual range: 1-3 g/kg 2-4 times/day
Dosage Forms Solution: 45% [450 mg/mL] (220 mL)

isosorbide dinitrate (eye soe SOR bide dye NYE trate)

Synonyms isd; isdn
Brand Names Dilatrate®-SR; Isordil®; Sorbitrate®
Therapeutic Category Vasodilator
Use Prevention and treatment of angina pectoris; for congestive heart failure; to relieve pain, dysphagia, and spasm in esophageal spasm with GE reflux
Usual Dosage Adults:
Oral: 5-30 mg 4 times/day or 40 mg every 6-12 hours in sustained-released dosage form
Chewable: 5-10 mg every 2-3 hours
Sublingual: 2.5-10 mg every 4-6 hours
Dosage Forms
Capsule, sustained release: 40 mg
Tablet:
Chewable: 5 mg, 10 mg
Oral: 5 mg, 10 mg, 20 mg, 30 mg
Sublingual: 2.5 mg, 5 mg, 10 mg
Sustained release: 40 mg

isosorbide mononitrate (eye soe SOR bide mon oh NYE trate)

Synonyms ismn
Brand Names Imdur™; ISMO™; Monoket®
Therapeutic Category Vasodilator
Use Long-acting metabolite of the vasodilator isosorbide dinitrate used for the prophylactic treatment of angina pectoris
Usual Dosage Adults: Oral:
Regular tablet: 20 mg twice daily separated by 7 hours
Extended-release tablet: 30 mg ($1/2$ of 60 mg tablet) or 60 mg (administered as a single tablet) once daily; after several days the dosage may be increased to 120 mg (administered as two 60 mg tablets) once daily; the daily dose should be administered in the morning upon arising
Dosage Forms
Tablet (Ismo™, Monoket®): 10 mg, 20 mg
Tablet, extended release (Imdur™): 30 mg, 60 mg, 120 mg

isotretinoin (eye soe TRET i noyn)

Synonyms 13-*cis*-retinoic acid
Brand Names Accutane®
Therapeutic Category Retinoic Acid Derivative
Use Treatment of severe recalcitrant cystic and/or conglobate acne unresponsive to conventional therapy

Investigational use: Treatment of children with metastatic neuroblastoma or leukemia that does not respond to conventional therapy
Usual Dosage Oral:
Children: Maintenance therapy for neuroblastoma: 100-250 mg/m^2/day in 2 divided doses has been used investigationally
Children and Adults: 0.5-2 mg/kg/day in 2 divided doses for 15-20 weeks
Dosage Forms Capsule: 10 mg, 20 mg, 40 mg

Isovue® *see* radiological/contrast media (non-ionic) *on page 459*

isoxsuprine (eye SOKS syoo preen)
Synonyms isoxsuprine hydrochloride
Brand Names Vasodilan®
Therapeutic Category Vasodilator
Use Treatment of peripheral vascular diseases, such as arteriosclerosis obliterans and Raynaud's disease
Usual Dosage Adults: Oral: 10-20 mg 3-4 times/day
Dosage Forms Tablet, as hydrochloride: 10 mg, 20 mg

isoxsuprine hydrochloride *see* isoxsuprine *on this page*

isradipine (iz RA di peen)
Brand Names DynaCirc®
Therapeutic Category Calcium Channel Blocker
Use Management of hypertension, alone or concurrently with thiazide-type diuretics
Usual Dosage Adults: Oral: Initial: 2.5 mg twice daily, if satisfactory response does not occur after 2-4 weeks the dose may be adjusted in increments of 5 mg/day at 2- to 4-week intervals up to a maximum of 20 mg/day
Dosage Forms Capsule: 2.5 mg, 5 mg

Isuprel® *see* isoproterenol *on page 291*
Itch-X® **[OTC]** *see* pramoxine *on page 432*

itraconazole (i tra KOE na zole)
Brand Names Sporanox®
Therapeutic Category Antifungal Agent
Use Treatment of systemic fungal infections in immunocompromised and nonimmunocompromised patients including the treatment of susceptible blastomycosis, histoplasmosis, and aspergillosis in patients who do not respond to or cannot tolerate amphotericin B; it also has activity against *Cryptococcus*, *Coccidioides*, and sporotrichosis species; has also been used for prophylaxis against aspergillosis infection
Usual Dosage Adults: Oral: 200 mg once daily, if no obvious improvement or there is evidence of progressive fungal disease, increase the dose in 100 mg increments to a maximum of 400 mg/day; doses >200 mg/day are administered in 2 divided doses
Life-threatening: Loading dose: 200 mg administered 3 times/day (600 mg/day) should be administered for the first 3 days
Dosage Forms
Capsule: 100 mg
Solution, oral: 100 mg/10 mL (150 mL)

I-Tropine® *see* atropine *on page 47*
iudr *see* idoxuridine *on page 279*

ivermectin (eye ver MEK tin)
Brand Names Stromectol®
Therapeutic Category Antibiotic, Miscellaneous
Use Treatment of the following infections: Strongylodiasis of the intestinal tract due the nematode parasite *Strongyloides stercoralis*. Onchocerciasis due to the nematode parasite *Onchocerca volvulus*. Note: Ivermectin is ineffective against adult *Onchocerca volvulus* parasites because they reside in subcutaneous nodules which are infrequently palpable. Surgical excision of these nodules may be considered in the management of patients with onchocerciasis.
Usual Dosage Oral:
Children >5 years of age and older: 150 mcg/kg as a single dose once every 12 months
Adults: 150 mcg/kg as a single dose; may be repeated every 6-12 **months**
Dosage Forms Tablet: 6 mg

ivig *see* immune globulin, intravenous *on page 281*

IvyBlock® *see* bentoquatam *on page 58*

Janimine® *see* imipramine *on page 280*

Japanese encephalitis virus vaccine, inactivated
(jap a NEESE en sef a LYE tis VYE rus vak SEEN, in ak ti VAY ted)
Brand Names JE-VAX®
Therapeutic Category Vaccine, Inactivated Virus
Use Active immunization against Japanese encephalitis for persons spending a month or longer in endemic areas, especially if travel will include rural areas
Usual Dosage S.C. (administered on days 0, 7, and 30):
Children 1-3 years: 3 doses of 0.5 mL; booster doses of 0.5 mL may administer 2 years after primary immunization series
Children >3 years and Adults: 3 doses of 1 mL; booster doses of 1 mL may be administered 2 years after primary immunization series
Dosage Forms Powder for injection, lyophilized: 1 mL, 10 mL

Jenamicin® Injection *see* gentamicin *on page 240*

Jenest-28™ *see* ethinyl estradiol and norethindrone *on page 209*

JE-VAX® *see* Japanese encephalitis virus vaccine, inactivated *on this page*

Junior Strength Motrin® [OTC] *see* ibuprofen *on page 278*

Junior Strength Panadol® [OTC] *see* acetaminophen *on page 3*

Just Tears® Solution [OTC] *see* artificial tears *on page 42*

K+ 10® *see* potassium chloride *on page 427*

Kabikinase® *see* streptokinase *on page 492*

Kadian® Capsule *see* morphine sulfate *on page 356*

Kalcinate® *see* calcium gluconate *on page 84*

kanamycin (kan a MYE sin)
Synonyms kanamycin sulfate
Brand Names Kantrex®
Therapeutic Category Aminoglycoside (Antibiotic)
Use
Oral: Preoperative bowel preparation in the prophylaxis of infections and adjunctive treatment of hepatic coma (oral kanamycin is not indicated in the treatment of systemic infections)
Parenteral: Initial therapy of severe infections where the strain is thought to be susceptible in patients allergic to other antibiotics, or in mixed staphylococcal or gram-negative infections
Usual Dosage
Children: Infections: I.M., I.V.: 15 mg/kg/day in divided doses every 8-12 hours
Adults:
Infections: I.M., I.V.: 15 mg/kg/day in divided doses every 8-12 hours
Preoperative intestinal antisepsis: Oral: 1 g every 4-6 hours for 36-72 hours
Dosage Forms
Capsule, as sulfate: 500 mg
Injection, as sulfate:
Pediatric: 75 mg (2 mL)
Adults: 500 mg (2 mL); 1 g (3 mL)

kanamycin sulfate *see* kanamycin *on this page*

Kantrex® *see* kanamycin *on this page*

Kaochlor® *see* potassium chloride *on page 427*

Kaochlor-Eff® *see* potassium bicarbonate, potassium chloride, and potassium citrate *on page 427*

Kaochlor® **SF** *see* potassium chloride *on page 427*

Kaodene® **[OTC]** *see* kaolin and pectin *on this page*

kaolin and pectin (KAY oh lin & PEK tin)

Synonyms pectin and kaolin
Brand Names Kaodene® [OTC]; Kao-Spen® [OTC]; Kapectolin® [OTC]
Therapeutic Category Antidiarrheal
Use Treatment of uncomplicated diarrhea
Usual Dosage Oral:
  Children:
    <6 years: Do not use
    6-12 years: 30-60 mL after each loose stool
  Adults: 60-120 mL after each loose stool
Dosage Forms Suspension, oral: Kaolin 975 mg and pectin 22 mg per 5 mL

kaolin and pectin with opium (KAY oh lin & PEK tin with OH pee um)

Brand Names Parepectolin®
Therapeutic Category Antidiarrheal
Controlled Substance C-V
Use Symptomatic relief of diarrhea
Usual Dosage Oral:
  Children:
    3-6 years: 7.5 mL with each loose bowel movement, not to exceed 30 mL in 12 hours
    6-12 years: 5-10 mL with each loose bowel movement, not to exceed 40 mL in 12 hours
    Children >12 years and Adults: 15-30 mL with each loose bowel movement, not to exceed 120 mL in 12 hours
Dosage Forms Suspension, oral: Kaolin 5.5 g, pectin 162 mg, and opium 15 mg per 30 mL [3.7 mL paregoric] (240 mL)

Kaon® *see* potassium gluconate *on page 429*

Kaon-Cl® *see* potassium chloride *on page 427*

Kaon-Cl-10® *see* potassium chloride *on page 427*

Kaopectate® **Advanced Formula [OTC]** *see* attapulgite *on page 48*

Kaopectate® **II [OTC]** *see* loperamide *on page 313*

Kaopectate® **Maximum Strength Caplets** *see* attapulgite *on page 48*

Kao-Spen® **[OTC]** *see* kaolin and pectin *on this page*

Kapectolin® **[OTC]** *see* kaolin and pectin *on this page*

Kapectolin PG® *see* hyoscyamine, atropine, scopolamine, kaolin, pectin, and opium *on page 276*

Karidium® *see* fluoride *on page 228*

Karigel® *see* fluoride *on page 228*

Karigel®**-N** *see* fluoride *on page 228*

Kasof® **[OTC]** *see* docusate *on page 179*

Kay Ciel® *see* potassium chloride *on page 427*

Kayexalate® *see* sodium polystyrene sulfonate *on page 488*

K+ Care® *see* potassium chloride *on page 427*

K+ Care® **Effervescent** *see* potassium bicarbonate *on page 426*

KCl *see* potassium chloride *on page 427*

K-Dur® 10 *see* potassium chloride *on page 427*

K-Dur® 20 *see* potassium chloride *on page 427*

Keflex® *see* cephalexin *on page 103*

Keftab® *see* cephalexin *on page 103*

Kefurox® Injection *see* cefuroxime *on page 101*

Kefzol® *see* cefazolin *on page 96*

K-Electrolyte® Effervescent *see* potassium bicarbonate *on page 426*

Kemadrin® *see* procyclidine *on page 440*

Kenacort® *see* triamcinolone *on page 528*

Kenaject-40® *see* triamcinolone *on page 528*

Kenalog® *see* triamcinolone *on page 528*

Kenalog-10® *see* triamcinolone *on page 528*

Kenalog-40® *see* triamcinolone *on page 528*

Kenalog® H *see* triamcinolone *on page 528*

Kenalog® in Orabase® *see* triamcinolone *on page 528*

Kenonel® *see* triamcinolone *on page 528*

Keralyt® Gel *see* salicylic acid and propylene glycol *on page 472*

Kerlone® Oral *see* betaxolol *on page 66*

Kestrone® *see* estrone *on page 205*

Ketalar® Injection *see* ketamine *on this page*

ketamine (KEET a meen)
Synonyms ketamine hydrochloride
Brand Names Ketalar® Injection
Therapeutic Category General Anesthetic
Controlled Substance C-III
Use Anesthesia, short surgical procedures, dressing changes
Usual Dosage
  Children:
  I.M.: 3-7 mg/kg
  I.V.: Range: 0.5-2 mg/kg, use smaller doses (0.5-1 mg/kg) for sedation for minor procedures; usual induction dosage: 1-2 mg/kg
  Adults:
  I.M.: 3-8 mg/kg
  I.V.: Range: 1-4.5 mg/kg; usual induction dosage: 1-2 mg/kg
  Children and Adults: Maintenance: Supplemental doses of $1/3$ to $1/2$ of initial dose
Dosage Forms Injection, as hydrochloride: 10 mg/mL (20 mL, 25 mL, 50 mL); 50 mg/mL (10 mL); 100 mg/mL (5 mL)

ketamine hydrochloride *see* ketamine *on this page*

ketoconazole (kee toe KOE na zole)
Brand Names Nizoral®
Therapeutic Category Antifungal Agent
Use Treatment of susceptible fungal infections, including candidiasis, oral thrush, blastomycosis, histoplasmosis, coccidioidomycosis, paracoccidioidomycosis, chronic mucocutaneous candidiasis, as well as certain recalcitrant cutaneous dermatophytoses; used topically for treatment of tinea corporis, tinea cruris, tinea versicolor, and cutaneous candidiasis; shampoo is used for dandruff
Usual Dosage
  Children: Oral: 5-10 mg/kg/day divided every 12-24 hours until lesions clear

Adults:
Oral: 200-400 mg/day as a single daily dose
Topical: Rub gently into the affected area once daily to twice daily for two weeks
Dosage Forms
Cream: 2% (15 g, 30 g, 60 g)
Shampoo: 2% (120 mL)
Tablet: 200 mg

ketoprofen (kee toe PROE fen)

Brand Names Actron® [OTC]; Orudis®; Orudis® KT [OTC]; Oruvail®
Therapeutic Category Analgesic, Non-narcotic; Nonsteroidal Anti-Inflammatory Agent (NSAID)
Use Acute or long-term treatment of rheumatoid arthritis and osteoarthritis; primary dysmenorrhea; mild to moderate pain
Usual Dosage Oral:
Children 3 months to 14 years: Fever: 0.5-1 mg/kg
Children >12 years and Adults:
Rheumatoid arthritis or osteoarthritis: 50-75 mg 3-4 times/day up to a maximum of 300 mg/day
Mild to moderate pain: 25-50 mg every 6-8 hours up to a maximum of 300 mg/day
Dosage Forms
Capsule: 25 mg, 50 mg, 75 mg
Orudis®: 25 mg, 50 mg, 75 mg
Actron®, Orudis® KT [OTC]: 12.5 mg
Capsule, extended release (Oruvail®): 100 mg, 200 mg

ketorolac tromethamine (KEE toe role ak troe METH a meen)

Brand Names Acular® Ophthalmic; Toradol® Injection; Toradol® Oral
Therapeutic Category Analgesic, Non-narcotic; Nonsteroidal Anti-Inflammatory Agent (NSAID)
Use
Oral, I.M., I.V.,: Short-term (≤5 days) management of moderate to severe pain, including postoperative pain, visceral pain associated with cancer, pain associated with trauma, acute renal colic
Ophthalmic: Ocular itch associated with seasonal allergic conjunctivitis
Usual Dosage Adults (pain relief usually begins within 10 minutes with parenteral forms):
Oral: 10 mg every 4-6 hours as needed for a maximum of 40 mg/day; on day of transition from I.M. to oral: maximum oral dose: 40 mg (or 120 mg combined oral and I.M.); maximum 5 days administration
I.M.: Initial: 30-60 mg, then 15-30 mg every 6 hours as needed for up to 5 days maximum; maximum dose in the first 24 hours: 150 mg with 120 mg/24 hours for up to 5 days total
I.V.: Initial: 30 mg, then 15-30 mg every 6 hours as needed for up to 5 days **maximum**; maximum daily dose: 120 mg for up to 5 days total
Ophthalmic: Instill 1 drop in eye(s) 4 times/day
Dosage Forms
Injection: 15 mg/mL (1 mL); 30 mg/mL (1 mL, 2 mL)
Solution, ophthalmic: 0.5% (5 mL)
Tablet: 10 mg

Key-Pred® Injection see prednisolone on page 434

Key-Pred-SP® Injection see prednisolone on page 434

K-G® see potassium gluconate on page 429

K-Gen® Effervescent see potassium bicarbonate on page 426

KI see potassium iodide on page 430

K-Ide® *see* potassium bicarbonate and potassium citrate, effervescent *on page 427*

Kinevac® *see* sincalide *on page 480*

Klaron® **Lotion** *see* sulfacetamide sodium *on page 496*

K-Lease® *see* potassium chloride *on page 427*

Klerist-D® **Tablet [OTC]** *see* chlorpheniramine and pseudoephedrine *on page 114*

Klonopin™ *see* clonazepam *on page 130*

K-Lor™ *see* potassium chloride *on page 427*

Klor-Con® *see* potassium chloride *on page 427*

Klor-Con® **8** *see* potassium chloride *on page 427*

Klor-Con® **10** *see* potassium chloride *on page 427*

Klor-Con/25® *see* potassium chloride *on page 427*

Klor-con®**/EF** *see* potassium bicarbonate and potassium citrate, effervescent *on page 427*

Klorvess® *see* potassium chloride *on page 427*

Klorvess® **Effervescent** *see* potassium bicarbonate and potassium chloride, effervescent *on page 426*

Klotrix® *see* potassium chloride *on page 427*

K-Lyte® *see* potassium bicarbonate and potassium citrate, effervescent *on page 427*

K/Lyte/CL® *see* potassium bicarbonate and potassium chloride, effervescent *on page 426*

K-Lyte®**/Cl** *see* potassium chloride *on page 427*

K-Lyte® **Effervescent** *see* potassium bicarbonate *on page 426*

K-Norm® *see* potassium chloride *on page 427*

Koāte®**-HP** *see* antihemophilic factor (human) *on page 37*

Koāte®**-HS** *see* antihemophilic factor (human) *on page 37*

Kogenate® *see* antihemophilic factor (recombinant) *on page 37*

Kolephrin® **GG/DM [OTC]** *see* guaifenesin and dextromethorphan *on page 248*

Kolyum® *see* potassium chloride and potassium gluconate *on page 428*

Konakion® **Injection** *see* phytonadione *on page 416*

Kondon's Nasal® **[OTC]** *see* ephedrine *on page 194*

Konsyl® **[OTC]** *see* psyllium *on page 451*

Konsyl-D® **[OTC]** *see* psyllium *on page 451*

Konȳne® **80** *see* factor ix complex (human) *on page 215*

Koromex® **[OTC]** *see* nonoxynol 9 *on page 377*

K-Phos® **Neutral** *see* potassium phosphate and sodium phosphate *on page 431*

K-Phos® **Original** *see* potassium acid phosphate *on page 426*

K-Tab® *see* potassium chloride *on page 427*

Ku-Zyme® **HP** *see* pancrelipase *on page 394*

K-Vescent® *see* potassium bicarbonate and potassium citrate, effervescent *on page 427*

Kwelcof® *see* hydrocodone and guaifenesin *on page 267*

Kytril™ **Injection** *see* granisetron *on page 246*

L-**3-hydroxytyrosine** *see* levodopa *on page 305*

LA-12® *see* hydroxocobalamin *on page 272*

labetalol (la BET a lole)
Synonyms ibidomide hydrochloride; labetalol hydrochloride
Brand Names Normodyne®; Trandate®
Therapeutic Category Alpha-/Beta- Adrenergic Blocker
Use Treatment of mild to severe hypertension; I.V. for hypertensive emergencies
Usual Dosage
Children: Limited information regarding labetalol use in pediatric patients is currently available in literature. Some centers recommend initial oral doses of 4 mg/kg/day in 2 divided doses. Reported oral doses have started at 3 mg/kg/day and 20 mg/kg/day and have increased up to 40 mg/kg/day.

I.V., intermittent bolus doses of 0.3-1 mg/kg/dose have been reported

For treatment of pediatric hypertensive emergencies, initial continuous infusions of 0.4-1 mg/kg/hour with a maximum of 3 mg/kg/hour have been used.

Due to limited documentation of its use, labetalol should be initiated cautiously in pediatric patients with careful dosage adjustment and blood pressure monitoring
Adults:
Oral: Initial: 100 mg twice daily, may increase as needed every 2-3 days by 100 mg until desired response is obtained; usual dose: 200-400 mg twice daily; not to exceed 2.4 g/day
I.V.: 20 mg or 1-2 mg/kg whichever is lower, IVP over 2 minutes, may administer 40-80 mg at 10-minute intervals, up to 300 mg total dose
I.V. infusion: Initial: 2 mg/minute; titrate to response
Dosage Forms
Injection, as hydrochloride: 5 mg/mL (20 mL, 40 mL, 60 mL)
Tablet, as hydrochloride: 100 mg, 200 mg, 300 mg

labetalol hydrochloride *see labetalol on this page*
Lac-Hydrin® *see lactic acid with ammonium hydroxide on next page*
Lacril® Ophthalmic Solution [OTC] *see artificial tears on page 42*
Lacrisert® *see hydroxypropyl cellulose on page 274*
LactAid® [OTC] *see lactase on this page*

lactase (LAK tase)
Brand Names Dairy Ease® [OTC]; LactAid® [OTC]; Lactrase® [OTC]
Therapeutic Category Nutritional Supplement
Use Help digest lactose in milk for patients with lactose intolerance
Usual Dosage Oral:
Capsule: 1-2 capsules administered with milk or meal; pretreat milk with 1-2 capsules per quart of milk
Liquid: 5-15 drops per quart of milk
Tablet: 1-3 tablets with meals
Dosage Forms
Caplet: 3000 FCC lactase units
Capsule: 250 mg
Liquid: 1250 neutral lactase units/5 drops
Tablet, chewable: 3300 FCC lactase units

lactic acid and salicylic acid *see salicylic acid and lactic acid on page 472*

lactic acid and sodium-PCA (LAK tik AS id & SOW dee um-pee see aye)
Synonyms sodium-pca and lactic acid
Brand Names LactiCare® [OTC]
Therapeutic Category Topical Skin Product
Use Lubricate and moisturize the skin counteracting dryness and itching
Usual Dosage Topical: Apply as needed
(Continued)

lactic acid and sodium-PCA *(Continued)*

Dosage Forms Lotion, topical: Lactic acid 5% and sodium-PCA 2.5% (240 mL)

lactic acid with ammonium hydroxide
(LAK tik AS id with a MOE nee um hye DROKS ide)
Synonyms ammonium lactate
Brand Names Lac-Hydrin®
Therapeutic Category Topical Skin Product
Use Treatment of moderate to severe xerosis and ichthyosis vulgaris
Usual Dosage Topical: Shake well; apply to affected areas, use twice daily, rub in well
Dosage Forms Lotion: Lactic acid 12% with ammonium hydroxide (150 mL)

LactiCare® [OTC] *see* lactic acid and sodium-PCA *on previous page*

LactiCare-HC® *see* hydrocortisone *on page 268*

Lactinex® [OTC] *see* Lactobacillus acidophilus *and* Lactobacillus bulgaricus *on this page*

Lactobacillus acidophilus **and** *Lactobacillus bulgaricus*
(lak toe ba SIL us as i DOF fil us & lak toe ba SIL us bul GAR i cus)
Brand Names Bacid® [OTC]; Lactinex® [OTC]; More-Dophilus® [OTC]
Therapeutic Category Gastrointestinal Agent, Miscellaneous
Use Uncomplicated diarrhea particularly that caused by antibiotic therapy; re-establish normal physiologic and bacterial flora of the intestinal tract
Usual Dosage Children and Adults: Oral:
Capsule: 2 capsules 2-4 times/day
Granules: 1 packet added to or administered with cereal, food, milk, fruit juice, or water, 3-4 times/day
Tablet, chewable: 4 tablets 3-4 times/day; may follow each dose with a small amount of milk, fruit juice, or water
Recontamination protocol for BMT unit: 1 packet 3 times/day for 6 doses for those patients who refuse yogurt.
Dosage Forms
Capsule: 50s, 100s
Granules: 1 g/packet (12 packets/box)
Powder: 12 oz
Tablet, chewable: 50s

lactoflavin *see* riboflavin *on page 465*

Lactrase® [OTC] *see* lactase *on previous page*

lactulose (LAK tyoo lose)
Brand Names Cephulac®; Cholac®; Chronulac®; Constilac®; Constulose®; Duphalac®; Enulose®; Evalose®; Heptalac®; Lactulose PSE®
Therapeutic Category Ammonium Detoxicant; Laxative
Use Adjunct in the prevention and treatment of portal-systemic encephalopathy (PSE); treatment of chronic constipation
Usual Dosage Oral:
Infants: 2.5-10 mL/day divided 3-4 times/day
Children: 40-90 mL/day divided 3-4 times/day
Adults:
Acute episodes of portal systemic encephalopathy: 30-45 mL at 1- to 2-hour intervals until laxative effect observed
Chronic therapy: 30-45 mL/dose 3-4 times/day; titrate dose to produce 2-3 soft stools per day
Rectal: 300 mL diluted with 700 mL of water or normal saline, and administered via a rectal balloon catheter and retained for 30-60 minutes; may administer every 4-6 hours

Dosage Forms Syrup: 10 g/15 mL (15 mL, 30 mL, 237 mL, 473 mL, 946 mL, 1890 mL)

Lactulose PSE® *see* lactulose *on previous page*

ladakamycin *see* azacitidine *on page 49*

Lamictal® *see* lamotrigine *on this page*

Lamisil® **Cream** *see* terbinafine, topical *on page 505*

Lamisil® **Oral** *see* terbinafine, oral *on page 504*

lamivudine (la MI vyoo deen)
Synonyms 3TC
Brand Names Epivir®
Therapeutic Category Antiviral Agent
Use In combination with zidovudine for treatment of HIV infection when therapy is warranted based on clinical and/or immunological evidence of disease progression
Usual Dosage Adults: Oral: 150 mg twice daily
Dosage Forms
Solution, oral: 10 mg/mL (240 mL)
Tablet: 150 mg

lamotrigine (la MOE tri jeen)
Synonyms ltg
Brand Names Lamictal®
Therapeutic Category Anticonvulsant
Use Adjunctive treatment of partial seizures, with or without secondary generalized seizures; investigations for absence, generalized tonic-clonic, atypical absence, myoclonic seizures, and Lennox-Gastaut syndrome are in progress
Usual Dosage Oral:
Initial dose: 50-100 mg/day then titrate to daily maintenance dose of 100-400 mg/day in 1-2 divided daily doses
With concomitant valproic acid therapy: Start initial dose at 25 mg/day then titrate to maintenance dose of 50-200 mg/day in 1-2 divided daily doses
Dosage Forms Tablet: 25 mg, 100 mg, 150 mg, 200 mg

Lamprene® *see* clofazimine *on page 129*

Lanacane® **[OTC]** *see* benzocaine *on page 59*

Lanacort® **[OTC]** *see* hydrocortisone *on page 268*

Lanaphilic® **Topical [OTC]** *see* urea *on page 542*

Laniazid® **Oral** *see* isoniazid *on page 290*

lanolin, cetyl alcohol, glycerin, and petrolatum
(LAN oh lin, SEE til AL koe hol, GLIS er in, & pe troe LAY tum)
Brand Names Lubriderm® [OTC]
Therapeutic Category Topical Skin Product
Use Treatment of dry skin
Usual Dosage Topical: Apply to skin as necessary
Dosage Forms Lotion: 480 mL

Lanophyllin® *see* theophylline *on page 511*

Lanorinal® *see* butalbital compound and aspirin *on page 78*

Lanoxicaps® *see* digoxin *on page 168*

Lanoxin® *see* digoxin *on page 168*

lansoprazole (lan SOE pra zole)
Brand Names Prevacid®
Therapeutic Category Gastric Acid Secretion Inhibitor
Use Short-term treatment (up to 4 weeks) for healing and symptom relief of active duodenal ulcers (should not be used for maintenance therapy of duodenal ulcers); up to 8 weeks of treatment for all grades of erosive esophagitis (8 additional weeks can be given for incompletely healed esophageal erosions or for recurrence); and long-term treatment of pathological hypersecretory conditions, including Zollinger-Ellison syndrome
Usual Dosage Oral:
Duodenal or gastric ulcer: 30 mg once daily for 4-8 weeks
Erosive esophagitis: 30 mg once daily for 4-8 weeks
Hypersecretory conditions: 30-180 mg once daily, titrated to reduce acid secretion to <10 mEq/hour (5 mEq/hour in patients with prior gastric surgery)
Dosage Forms Capsule, delayed release: 15 mg, 30 mg

Largon® Injection see propiomazine on page 444

Lariam® see mefloquine on page 326

Larodopa® see levodopa on page 305

Lasix® see furosemide on page 236

Lassar's zinc paste see zinc oxide on page 561

latanoprost (la TAN oh prost)
Brand Names Xalatan®
Therapeutic Category Prostaglandin
Use Prostaglandin analog to reduce intraocular pressure that occurs in patients with glaucoma who cannot tolerate or have not responded to any other available treatments
Usual Dosage Ophthalmic:
Children: Not recommended
Adults: 1 drop in affected eye(s) once daily in the evening
Dosage Forms Solution, ophthalmic: 0.005% (2.5 mL)

***Latrodectus mactans* antivenin** see antivenin (*Latrodectus mactans*) on page 39

Lavacol® [OTC] see alcohol, ethyl on page 14

l-bunolol hydrochloride see levobunolol on page 304

l-carnitine see levocarnitine on page 304

lcd see coal tar on page 132

lcr see vincristine on page 550

l-deprenyl see selegiline on page 476

l-dopa see levodopa on page 305

Lederplex® [OTC] see vitamin b complex on page 553

Lente® Iletin® I see insulin preparations on page 284

Lente® Iletin® II see insulin preparations on page 284

Lente® Insulin see insulin preparations on page 284

Lente® L see insulin preparations on page 284

Lescol® see fluvastatin on page 233

leucovorin (loo koe VOR in)
Synonyms calcium leucovorin; citrovorum factor; folinic acid; 5-formyl tetrahydrofolate; leucovorin calcium
Brand Names Wellcovorin®

Therapeutic Category Folic Acid Derivative
Use Antidote for folic acid antagonists; treatment of folate deficient megaloblastic anemias of infancy, sprue, pregnancy; nutritional deficiency when oral folate therapy is not possible
Usual Dosage Children and Adults:
Adjunctive therapy with antimicrobial agents (pyrimethamine): Oral: 2-15 mg/day for 3 days or until blood counts are normal or 5 mg every 3 days; doses of 6 mg/day are needed for patients with platelet counts <100,000/mm^3
Folate deficient megaloblastic anemia: I.M.: 1 mg/day
Megaloblastic anemia secondary to congenital deficiency of dihydrofolate reductase: I.M.: 3-6 mg/day
Rescue dose: I.V.: 10 mg/m^2 to start, then 10 mg/m^2 every 6 hours orally for 72 hours; if serum creatinine 24 hours after methotrexate is elevated 50% or more **or** the serum MTX concentration is >5 x 10^{-6}M, increase dose to 100 mg/m^2/dose every 3 hours until serum methotrexate level is less than 1 x 10^{-8}M
Dosage Forms
Injection, as calcium: 3 mg/mL (1 mL)
Powder:
For injection, as calcium: 25 mg, 50 mg, 100 mg, 350 mg
For oral solution, as calcium: 1 mg/mL (60 mL)
Tablet, as calcium: 5 mg, 10 mg, 15 mg, 25 mg

leucovorin calcium *see* leucovorin *on previous page*

Leukeran® *see* chlorambucil *on page 107*

Leukine™ *see* sargramostim *on page 474*

leuprolide acetate (loo PROE lide AS e tate)

Synonyms leuprorelin acetate
Brand Names Lupron®; Lupron Depot®; Lupron Depot-3® Month; Lupron Depot-4® Month; Lupron Depot-Ped™
Therapeutic Category Antineoplastic Agent; Luteinizing Hormone-Releasing Hormone Analog
Use Treatment of precocious puberty; palliative treatment of advanced prostate carcinoma
Usual Dosage
Children: S.C.: Precocious puberty: 20-45 mcg/kg/day
Adults:
Advanced prostatic carcinoma:
S.C.: 1 mg/day **or**
I.M. (suspension): 7.5 mg/dose administered monthly
Endometriosis: ≥18 years: I.M.: 3.75 mg/month for 6 months
Dosage Forms
Injection: 5 mg/mL (2.8 mL)
Powder for injection (depot):
Depot®: 3.75 mg, 7.5 mg
Depot-3® Month: 11.25 mg, 22.5 mg
Depot-4® Month: 30 mg
Depot-Ped™: 7.5 mg, 11.25 mg, 15 mg

leuprorelin acetate *see* leuprolide acetate *on this page*

leurocristine *see* vincristine *on page 550*

Leustatin™ *see* cladribine *on page 125*

levamisole (lee VAM i sole)

Synonyms levamisole hydrochloride
Brand Names Ergamisol®
Therapeutic Category Immune Modulator
(Continued)

levamisole *(Continued)*

Use Adjuvant treatment with fluorouracil in Dukes stage C colon cancer

Usual Dosage Oral: Initial: 50 mg every 8 hours for 3 days, then 50 mg every 8 hours for 3 days every 2 weeks (fluorouracil is always administered concomitantly)

Dosage Forms Tablet, as base: 50 mg

levamisole hydrochloride *see* levamisole *on previous page*

Levaquin® *see* levofloxacin *on next page*

levarterenol bitartrate *see* norepinephrine *on page 378*

Levatol® *see* penbutolol *on page 399*

Levbid® *see* hyoscyamine *on page 275*

Levlen® *see* ethinyl estradiol and levonorgestrel *on page 208*

levobunolol (lee voe BYOO noe lole)

Synonyms *l*-bunolol hydrochloride; levobunolol hydrochloride

Brand Names AKBeta®; Betagan® Liquifilm®

Therapeutic Category Beta-Adrenergic Blocker

Use To lower intraocular pressure in chronic open-angle glaucoma or ocular hypertension

Usual Dosage Adults: Ophthalmic: 1-2 drops of 0.5% solution in eye(s) once daily or 1-2 drops of 0.25% solution twice daily

Dosage Forms Solution, ophthalmic, as hydrochloride: 0.25% (5 mL, 10 mL, 15 mL); 0.5% (2 mL, 5 mL, 10 mL, 15 mL)

levobunolol hydrochloride *see* levobunolol *on this page*

levocabastine (LEE voe kab as teen)

Synonyms levocabastine hydrochloride

Brand Names Livostin®

Therapeutic Category Antihistamine

Use Temporary relief of the signs and symptoms of seasonal allergic conjunctivitis

Usual Dosage Adults: Ophthalmic: Instill 1 drop in affected eye 4 times/day for up to 2 weeks

Dosage Forms Suspension, ophthalmic, as hydrochloride: 0.05% (2.5 mL, 5 mL, 10 mL)

levocabastine hydrochloride *see* levocabastine *on this page*

levocarnitine (lee voe KAR ni teen)

Synonyms l-carnitine

Brand Names Carnitor® Injection; Carnitor® Oral; VitaCarn® Oral

Therapeutic Category Dietary Supplement

Use Treatment of primary or secondary carnitine deficiency

Usual Dosage Oral:

Children: 50-100 mg/kg/day divided 2-3 times/day, maximum: 3 g/day; dosage must be individualized based upon patient response; higher dosages have been used

Adults: 1-3 g/day for 50 kg subject; start at 1 g/day, increase slowly assessing tolerance and response

Dosage Forms

Capsule: 250 mg

Injection: 1 g/5 mL (5 mL)

Liquid (cherry flavor): 100 mg/mL (10 mL)

Tablet: 330 mg

levodopa (lee voe DOE pa)

Synonyms L-3-hydroxytyrosine; l-dopa

Brand Names Dopar®; Larodopa®

Therapeutic Category Diagnostic Agent; Dopaminergic Agent (Antiparkinson's)

Use Diagnostic agent for growth hormone deficiency

Usual Dosage Children: Oral (administered as a single dose to evaluate growth hormone deficiency): 0.5 g/m²

or

<30 lbs: 125 mg
30-70 lbs: 250 mg
>70 lbs: 500 mg

Dosage Forms

Capsule: 100 mg, 250 mg, 500 mg
Tablet: 100 mg, 250 mg, 500 mg

levodopa and carbidopa (lee voe DOE pa & kar bi DOE pa)

Synonyms carbidopa and levodopa

Brand Names Sinemet®

Therapeutic Category Anti-Parkinson's Agent; Dopaminergic Agent (Antiparkinson's)

Use Treatment of Parkinsonian syndrome

Usual Dosage Adults: Oral (carbidopa/levodopa): 75/300 to 150/1500 mg/day in 3-4 divided doses; can increase up to 200/2000 mg/day

Dosage Forms Tablet:

10/100: Carbidopa 10 mg and levodopa 100 mg
25/100: Carbidopa 25 mg and levodopa 100 mg
25/250: Carbidopa 25 mg and levodopa 250 mg
Sustained release: Carbidopa 25 mg and levodopa 100 mg; carbidopa 50 mg and levodopa 200 mg

Levo-Dromoran® *see* levorphanol *on next page*

levofloxacin (lee voe FLOKS a sin)

Brand Names Levaquin®

Therapeutic Category Quinolone

Use Treatment of bacterial respiratory tract infections

Usual Dosage Adults: Oral, I.V.: 500 mg every 24 hours for at least 7 days (dose and duration varies with indication); at least 2 hours before or 2 hours after antacids containing magnesium or aluminum

Dosage Forms

Infusion, in D₅W: 5 mg/mL (50 mL, 100 mL)
Injection: 25 mg/mL (20 mL)
Tablet: 250 mg, 500 mg

levomepromazine *see* methotrimeprazine *on page 338*

levomethadyl acetate hydrochloride

(lee voe METH a dil AS e tate hye droe KLOR ide)

Brand Names ORLAAM®

Therapeutic Category Analgesic, Narcotic

Controlled Substance C-II

Use Management of opiate dependence

Usual Dosage Adults: Oral: 20-40 mg 3 times/week; range: 10 mg to as high as 140 mg 3 times/week

Dosage Forms Solution, oral: 10 mg/mL (474 mL)

levonorgestrel (LEE voe nor jes trel)
Brand Names Norplant® Implant
Therapeutic Category Contraceptive, Implant; Contraceptive, Progestin Only
Use Prevention of pregnancy
Usual Dosage Each Norplant® silastic capsule releases 80 mcg of drug/day for 6-18 months, following which a rate of release of 25-30 mcg/day is maintained for ≤5 years
Dosage Forms Capsule, subdermal implantation: 36 mg (6s)

levonorgestrel and ethinyl estradiol *see* ethinyl estradiol and levonorgestrel *on page 208*

Levophed® Injection *see* norepinephrine *on page 378*

Levoprome® *see* methotrimeprazine *on page 338*

Levora® *see* ethinyl estradiol and levonorgestrel *on page 208*

levorphanol (lee VOR fa nole)
Synonyms levorphanol tartrate; levorphan tartrate
Brand Names Levo-Dromoran®
Therapeutic Category Analgesic, Narcotic
Controlled Substance C-II
Use Relief of moderate to severe pain; also used parenterally for preoperative sedation and an adjunct to nitrous oxide/oxygen anesthesia
Usual Dosage Adults: Oral, S.C.: 2 mg, up to 3 mg if necessary
Dosage Forms
Injection, as tartrate: 2 mg/mL (1 mL, 10 mL)
Tablet, as tartrate: 2 mg

levorphanol tartrate *see* levorphanol *on this page*

levorphan tartrate *see* levorphanol *on this page*

Levo-T™ *see* levothyroxine *on this page*

Levothroid® *see* levothyroxine *on this page*

levothyroxine (lee voe thye ROKS een)
Synonyms levothyroxine sodium; *L*-thyroxine sodium; t_4 thyroxine sodium
Brand Names Eltroxin®; Levo-T™; Levothroid®; Levoxyl™; Synthroid®
Therapeutic Category Thyroid Product
Use Replacement or supplemental therapy in hypothyroidism; management of nontoxic goiter, chronic lymphocytic thyroiditis, as an adjunct to thyrotoxicosis
Usual Dosage
Children:
Oral:
0-6 months: 8-10 mcg/kg/day
6-12 months: 6-8 mcg/kg/day
1-5 years: 5-6 mcg/kg/day
6-12 years: 4-5 mcg/kg/day
>12 years: 2-3 mcg/kg/day
I.M., I.V.: 75% of the oral dose
Adults:
Oral: 12.5-50 mcg/day to start, then increase by 25-50 mcg/day at intervals of 2-4 weeks; average adult dose: 100-200 mcg/day
I.M., I.V.: 50% of the oral dose

Myxedema coma or stupor: I.V.: 200-500 mcg one time, then 100-300 mcg the next day if necessary
Dosage Forms
Powder for injection, as sodium, lyophilized: 200 mcg/vial (6 mL, 10 mL); 500 mcg/vial (6 mL, 10 mL)

Tablet, as sodium: 25 mcg, 50 mcg, 75 mcg, 88 mcg, 100 mcg, 112 mcg, 125 mcg, 150 mcg, 175 mcg, 200 mcg, 300 mcg

levothyroxine sodium *see* levothyroxine *on previous page*

Levoxyl™ *see* levothyroxine *on previous page*

Levsin® *see* hyoscyamine *on page 275*

Levsinex® *see* hyoscyamine *on page 275*

Levsin/SL® *see* hyoscyamine *on page 275*

levulose, dextrose and phosphoric acid *see* phosphorated carbohydrate solution *on page 415*

Lexxel® *see* enalapril and felodipine *on page 193*

LH-RH *see* gonadorelin *on page 245*

l-hyoscyamine sulfate *see* hyoscyamine *on page 275*

Librax® *see* clidinium and chlordiazepoxide *on page 127*

Libritabs® *see* chlordiazepoxide *on page 109*

Librium® *see* chlordiazepoxide *on page 109*

Lice-Enz® Shampoo [OTC] *see* pyrethrins *on page 452*

Lida-Mantle HC® Topical *see* lidocaine and hydrocortisone *on next page*

Lidex® *see* fluocinonide *on page 227*

Lidex-E® *see* fluocinonide *on page 227*

lidocaine (LYE doe kane)

Synonyms lidocaine hydrochloride; lignocaine hydrochloride

Brand Names Anestacon®; Dermaflex® Gel; Dilocaine®; Dr Scholl's® Cracked Heel Relief Cream [OTC]; Duo-Trach®; LidoPen® Auto-Injector; Nervocaine®; Octocaine®; Solarcaine® Aloe Extra Burn Relief [OTC]; Xylocaine®; Zilactin-L® [OTC]

Therapeutic Category Analgesic, Topical; Antiarrhythmic Agent, Class I-B; Local Anesthetic

Use Drug of choice for ventricular ectopy, ventricular tachycardia (VT), ventricular fibrillation (VF); for pulseless VT or VF preferably administer **after** defibrillation and epinephrine; control of premature ventricular contractions, wide-complex PSVT; local anesthetic

Usual Dosage

Topical: Apply to affected area as needed; maximum: 3 mg/kg/dose; do not repeat within 2 hours

Injectable local anesthetic: Varies with procedure, degree of anesthesia needed, vascularity of tissue, duration of anesthesia required, and physical condition of patient; maximum: 4.5 mg/kg/dose; do not repeat within 2 hours

Children: Endotracheal, I.O., I.V.: Loading dose: 1 mg/kg; may repeat in 10-15 minutes to a maximum total dose of 5 mg/kg; after loading dose, start I.V. continuous infusion 20-50 mcg/kg/minute. Use 20 mcg/kg/minute in patients with shock, hepatic disease, mild congestive heart failure (CHF); moderate to severe CHF may require 1/2 loading dose and lower infusion rates to avoid toxicity. Endotracheal doses should be diluted to 1-2 mL with normal saline prior to endotracheal administration and may need 2-3 times the I.V. dose.

Adults: Antiarrhythmic:

Endotracheal: Total dose: 5 mg/kg; follow with 0.5 mg/kg in 10 minutes if effective

I.M.: 300 mg may be repeated in 1-1½ hours

I.V.: Loading dose: 1 mg/kg/dose, then 50-100 mg bolus over 2-3 minutes; may repeat in 5-10 minutes up to 200-300 mg in a 1-hour period; continuous infusion of 20-50 mcg/kg/minute or 1-4 mg/minute; decrease the dose in patients with CHF, shock, or hepatic disease

Dosage Forms

Cream, as hydrochloride: 2% (56 g)

(Continued)

lidocaine *(Continued)*

Injection, as hydrochloride: 0.5% [5 mg/mL] (50 mL); 1% [10 mg/mL] (2 mL, 5 mL, 10 mL, 20 mL, 30 mL, 50 mL); 1.5% [15 mg/mL] (20 mL); 2% [20 mg/mL] (2 mL, 5 mL, 10 mL, 20 mL, 30 mL, 50 mL); 4% [40 mg/mL] (5 mL); 10% [100 mg/mL] (10 mL); 20% [200 mg/mL] (10 mL, 20 mL)

Injection, as hydrochloride:

I.M. use: 10% [100 mg/mL] (3 mL, 5 mL)

Direct I.V.: 1% [10 mg/mL] (5 mL, 10 mL); 20 mg/mL (5 mL)

I.V. admixture, preservative free: 4% [40 mg/mL] (25 mL, 30 mL); 10% [100 mg/mL] (10 mL); 20% [200 mg/mL] (5 mL, 10 mL)

I.V. infusion, in D_5W: 0.2% [2 mg/mL] (500 mL); 0.4% [4 mg/mL] (250 mL, 500 mL, 1000 mL); 0.8% [8 mg/mL] (250 mL, 500 mL)

Gel, as hydrochloride, topical: 2% (30 mL); 2.5% (15 mL)

Liquid, as hydrochloride:

Topical: 2.5% (7.5 mL)

Viscous: 2% (20 mL, 100 mL)

Ointment, as hydrochloride, topical: 2.5% [OTC]; 5% (35 g)

Solution, as hydrochloride, topical: 2% (15 mL, 240 mL); 4% (50 mL)

lidocaine and epinephrine (LYE doe kane & ep i NEF rin)

Brand Names Octocaine® Injection; Xylocaine® With Epinephrine

Therapeutic Category Local Anesthetic

Use Local infiltration anesthesia

Usual Dosage Children (dosage varies with the anesthetic procedure): Use lidocaine concentrations of 0.5% or 1% (or even more dilute) to decrease possibility of toxicity; lidocaine dose should not exceed 4.5 mg/kg/dose; do not repeat within 2 hours

Dosage Forms Injection with epinephrine:

1:200,000: Lidocaine hydrochloride 0.5% [5 mg/mL] (50 mL); 1% [10 mg/mL] (30 mL); 1.5% [15 mg/mL] (5 mL, 10 mL, 30 mL); 2% [20 mg/mL] (20 mL)

1:100,000: Lidocaine hydrochloride 1% [10 mg/mL] (20 mL, 50 mL); 2% [20 mg/mL] (1.8 mL, 20 mL, 50 mL)

1:50,000: Lidocaine hydrochloride 2% [20 mg/mL] (1.8 mL)

lidocaine and hydrocortisone (LYE doe kane & hye droe KOR ti sone)

Brand Names Lida-Mantle HC® Topical

Therapeutic Category Anesthetic/Corticosteroid

Use Topical anti-inflammatory and anesthetic for skin disorders

Usual Dosage Topical: Apply 2-4 times/day

Dosage Forms Cream: Lidocaine 3% and hydrocortisone 0.5% (15 g, 30 g)

lidocaine and prilocaine (LYE doe kane & PRIL oh kane)

Brand Names EMLA®

Therapeutic Category Analgesic, Topical

Use Topical anesthetic for use on normal intact skin to provide local analgesia for minor procedures such as I.V. cannulation or venipuncture; has also been used for painful procedures such as lumbar puncture and skin graft harvesting

Usual Dosage Children and Adults: Topical: Apply a thick layer of cream to intact skin and cover with an occlusive dressing; for minor procedures, apply 2.5 g/site for at least 60 minutes; for painful procedures, apply 2 g/10 cm^2 of skin and leave on for at least 2 hours

Dosage Forms Cream: Lidocaine 2.5% and prilocaine 2.5% [2 Tegaderm® dressings] (5 g, 30 g)

lidocaine hydrochloride *see* lidocaine *on previous page*

LidoPen® Auto-Injector *see* lidocaine *on previous page*

lignocaine hydrochloride *see* lidocaine *on previous page*

Limbitrol® DS 10-25 *see* amitriptyline and chlordiazepoxide *on page 27*

Lincocin® Injection *see* lincomycin *on this page*

Lincocin® Oral *see* lincomycin *on this page*

lincomycin (lin koe MYE sin)

Synonyms lincomycin hydrochloride

Brand Names Lincocin® Injection; Lincocin® Oral; Lincorex® Injection

Therapeutic Category Macrolide (Antibiotic)

Use Treatment of susceptible bacterial infections, mainly those caused by streptococci and staphylococci

Usual Dosage

Children >1 month:
Oral: 30-60 mg/kg/day in 3-4 divided doses
I.M.: 10 mg/kg every 12-24 hours
I.V.: 10-20 mg/kg/day in divided doses 2-3 times/day

Adults:
Oral: 500 mg every 6-8 hours
I.M.: 600 mg every 12-24 hours
I.V.: 600-1 g every 8-12 hours up to 8 g/day

Dosage Forms

Capsule, as hydrochloride: 250 mg, 500 mg
Injection, as hydrochloride: 300 mg/mL (2 mL, 10 mL)

lincomycin hydrochloride *see* lincomycin *on this page*

Lincorex® Injection *see* lincomycin *on this page*

lindane (LIN dane)

Synonyms benzene hexachloride; gamma benzene hexachloride; hexachlorocyclo-hexane

Brand Names G-well®; Scabene®

Therapeutic Category Scabicides/Pediculicides

Use Treatment of scabies (*Sarcoptes scabiei*), *Pediculus capitis* (head lice), and *Pediculus pubis* (crab lice)

Usual Dosage Children and Adults: Topical:

Scabies: Apply a thin layer of lotion and massage it on skin from the neck to the toes. For adults, bathe and remove the drug after 8-12 hours; for children, wash off 6 hours after application.

Pediculosis: 15-30 mL of shampoo is applied and lathered for 4-5 minutes; rinse hair thoroughly and comb with a fine tooth comb to remove nits; repeat treatment in 7 days if lice or nits are still present

Dosage Forms

Cream: 1% (60 g, 454 g)
Lotion: 1% (60 mL, 473 mL, 4000 mL)
Shampoo: 1% (60 mL, 473 mL, 4000 mL)

Lioresal® *see* baclofen *on page 54*

liothyronine (lye oh THYE roe neen)

Synonyms liothyronine sodium; sodium *l*-triiodothyronine; t_3 thyronine sodium

Brand Names Cytomel® Oral; Triostat™ Injection

Therapeutic Category Thyroid Product

Use Replacement or supplemental therapy in hypothyroidism, management of nontoxic goiter, chronic lymphocytic thyroiditis, as an adjunct in thyrotoxicosis and as a diagnostic aid; levothyroxine is recommended for chronic therapy; (if rapid correction of thyroid is needed, T_3 is preferred, but use cautiously and with lower recommended doses)

(Continued)

liothyronine *(Continued)*

Usual Dosage

Mild hypothyroidism: 25 mcg/day; daily dosage may then be increased by 12.5 or 25 mcg/day every 1 or 2 weeks; maintenance: 25-75 mcg/day

Myxedema: 5mcg/day; may be increased by 5-10 mcg/day every 1-2 weeks; when 25 mcg is reached, dosage may often be increased by 12.5 or 25 mcg every 1 or 2 weeks; maintenance: 50-100 mcg/day

Cretinism: 5 mcg/day with a 5 mcg increment every 3-4 days until the desired response is achieved

Simple (nontoxic) goiter: 5 mcg/day; may be increased every week or two by 5 or 10 mcg; when 25 mcg/day is reached, dosage may be increased every week or two by 12.5 or 25 mcg; maintenance: 75 mcg/day

T_3 suppression test: I^{131} thyroid uptake is in the borderline-high range, administer 75-100 mcg/day for 7 days then repeat I^{131} thyroid uptake test

Children and Elderly: Start therapy with 5 mcg/day; increase only by 5 mcg increments at the recommended intervals

Dosage Forms

Injection, as sodium: 10 mcg/mL (1 mL)

Tablet, as sodium: 5 mcg, 25 mcg, 50 mcg

liothyronine sodium *see* liothyronine *on previous page*

liotrix *(LYE oh triks)*

Synonyms t_3/t_4 liotrix

Brand Names Thyrolar®

Therapeutic Category Thyroid Product

Use Replacement or supplemental therapy in hypothyroidism

Usual Dosage Congenital hypothyroidism: Oral:

Children (dose/day):

0-6 months: 8-10 mcg/kg

6-12 months: 6-8 mcg/kg

1-5 years: 5-6 mcg/kg

6-12 years: 4-5 mcg/kg

>12 years: 2-3 mcg/kg

Adults: 30 mg/day, increasing by 15 mg/day at 2- to 3-week intervals to a maximum of 180 mg/day

Dosage Forms Tablet: 30 mg, 60 mg, 120 mg, 180 mg [thyroid equivalent]

lipancreatin *see* pancrelipase *on page 394*

lipase, protease, and amylase *see* pancrelipase *on page 394*

Lipidil® *see* fenofibrate *on page 218*

Lipitor® *see* atorvastatin *on page 46*

Liposyn® *see* fat emulsion *on page 216*

Lipovite® [OTC] *see* vitamin b complex *on page 553*

Liquibid® *see* guaifenesin *on page 247*

Liqui-Char® [OTC] *see* charcoal *on page 105*

liquid antidote *see* charcoal *on page 105*

Liquid Barosperse® *see* radiological/contrast media (ionic) *on page 457*

Liquid Pred® *see* prednisone *on page 436*

Liqui-E® *see* tocophersolan *on page 522*

Liquifilm® Forte Solution [OTC] *see* artificial tears *on page 42*

Liquifilm® Tears Solution [OTC] *see* artificial tears *on page 42*

Liquipake® *see* radiological/contrast media (ionic) *on page 457*

Liquiprin® **[OTC]** *see* acetaminophen *on page 3*

lisinopril (lyse IN oh pril)
Brand Names Prinivil®; Zestril®
Therapeutic Category Angiotensin-Converting Enzyme (ACE) Inhibitors
Use Treatment of hypertension, either alone or in combination with other antihypertensive agents
Usual Dosage Adults: Oral: 10-40 mg/day in a single dose
Dosage Forms Tablet: 2.5 mg, 5 mg, 10 mg, 20 mg, 40 mg

lisinopril and hydrochlorothiazide
(lyse IN oh pril & hye droe klor oh THYE a zide)
Brand Names Prinzide®; Zestoretic®
Therapeutic Category Antihypertensive, Combination
Use Treatment of hypertension
Usual Dosage Adults: Oral: Dosage is individualized; see each component for appropriate dosing suggestions
Dosage Forms Tablet:
Lisinopril 10 mg and hydrochlorothiazide 12.5 mg
[12.5]-Lisinopril 20 mg and hydrochlorothiazide 12.5 mg
[25]-lisinopril 20 mg and hydrochlorothiazide 25 mg

Listermint® **with Fluoride [OTC]** *see* fluoride *on page 228*

Lithane® *see* lithium *on this page*

lithium (LITH ee um)
Synonyms lithium carbonate; lithium citrate
Brand Names Eskalith®; Lithane®; Lithobid®; Lithonate®; Lithotabs®
Therapeutic Category Antimanic Agent
Use Management of acute manic episodes, bipolar disorders, and depression
Usual Dosage Oral: Monitor serum concentrations and clinical response (efficacy and toxicity) to determine proper dose

Children: 15-60 mg/kg/day in 3-4 divided doses; dose not to exceed usual adult dosage
Adults: 300 mg 3-4 times/day; usual maximum maintenance dose: 2.4 g/day
Dosage Forms
Capsule, as carbonate: 150 mg, 300 mg, 600 mg
Syrup, as citrate: 300 mg/5 mL (5 mL, 10 mL, 480 mL)
Tablet, as carbonate: 300 mg
Controlled release, as carbonate: 450 mg
Slow release, as carbonate: 300 mg

lithium carbonate *see* lithium *on this page*

lithium citrate *see* lithium *on this page*

Lithobid® *see* lithium *on this page*

Lithonate® *see* lithium *on this page*

Lithostat® *see* acetohydroxamic acid *on page 8*

Lithotabs® *see* lithium *on this page*

Livostin® *see* levocabastine *on page 304*

LKV-Drops® **[OTC]** *see* vitamin, multiple (pediatric) *on page 554*

l-lysine (el LYE seen)
Synonyms l-lysine hydrochloride
Brand Names Enisyl® [OTC]; Lycolan® Elixir [OTC]
Therapeutic Category Dietary Supplement
(Continued)

l-lysine *(Continued)*
Use Improves utilization of vegetable proteins
Usual Dosage Adults: Oral: 334-1500 mg/day
Dosage Forms
Capsule, as hydrochloride: 500 mg
Elixir, as hydrochloride: 100 mg/15 mL with glycine 1800 mg/15 mL and alcohol 12%
Tablet, as hydrochloride: 312 mg, 334 mg, 500 mg, 1000 mg

l-lysine hydrochloride *see* l-lysine *on previous page*

8-L-lysine vasopressin *see* lypressin *on page 317*

LMD® *see* dextran *on page 159*

Locoid® *see* hydrocortisone *on page 268*

Lodine® *see* etodolac *on page 212*

Lodine® **XL** *see* etodolac *on page 212*

Lodosyn® *see* carbidopa *on page 90*

Iodoxamide tromethamine (loe DOKS a mide troe METH a meen)
Brand Names Alomide® Ophthalmic
Therapeutic Category Mast Cell Stabilizer
Use Symptomatic treatment of vernal keratoconjunctivitis, vernal conjunctivitis, and vernal keratitis
Usual Dosage Children >2 years and Adults: Ophthalmic: Instill 1-2 drops in eye(s) 4 times/day for up to 3 months
Dosage Forms Solution, ophthalmic: 0.1% (10 mL)

Loestrin® *see* ethinyl estradiol and norethindrone *on page 209*

Logen® *see* diphenoxylate and atropine *on page 174*

Lomanate® *see* diphenoxylate and atropine *on page 174*

lomefloxacin (loe me FLOKS a sin)
Synonyms lomefloxacin hydrochloride
Brand Names Maxaquin®
Therapeutic Category Quinolone
Use Quinolone antibiotic for skin and skin structure, lower respiratory and urinary tract infections, and sexually transmitted diseases
Usual Dosage Adults: Oral: 400 mg once daily for 10-14 days
Dosage Forms Tablet, as hydrochloride: 400 mg

lomefloxacin hydrochloride *see* lomefloxacin *on this page*

Lomotil® *see* diphenoxylate and atropine *on page 174*

lomustine (loe MUS teen)
Synonyms ccnu
Brand Names CeeNU®
Therapeutic Category Antineoplastic Agent
Use Treatment of brain tumors, Hodgkin's and non-Hodgkin's lymphomas, melanoma, renal carcinoma, lung cancer, colon cancer
Usual Dosage Refer to individual protocol. Oral:
Children: 75-150 mg/m^2 as a single dose every 6 weeks. Subsequent doses are readjusted after initial treatment according to platelet and leukocyte counts
Adults: 100-130 mg/m^2 as a single dose every 6 weeks; readjust after initial treatment according to platelet and leukocyte counts
Dosage Forms
Capsule: 10 mg, 40 mg, 100 mg

Dose Pack: 10 mg (2s); 100 mg (2s); 40 mg (2s)

Loniten® *see* minoxidil *on page 352*
Lonox® *see* diphenoxylate and atropine *on page 174*
Lo/Ovral® *see* ethinyl estradiol and norgestrel *on page 210*

loperamide (loe PER a mide)
Synonyms loperamide hydrochloride
Brand Names Diar-aid® [OTC]; Imodium®; Imodium® A-D [OTC]; Kaopectate® II [OTC]; Pepto® Diarrhea Control [OTC]
Therapeutic Category Antidiarrheal
Use Treatment of acute diarrhea and chronic diarrhea associated with inflammatory bowel disease; chronic functional diarrhea (idiopathic), chronic diarrhea caused by bowel resection or organic lesions; to decrease the volume of ileostomy discharge
Usual Dosage Oral:
Children:
Acute diarrhea: 0.4-0.8 mg/kg/day divided every 6-12 hours, maximum: 2 mg/dose
Chronic diarrhea: 0.08-0.24 mg/kg/day divided 2-3 times/day, maximum: 2 mg/dose
Adults: 4 mg (2 capsules) initially, followed by 2 mg after each loose stool, up to 16 mg/day (8 capsules)
Dosage Forms
Caplet, as hydrochloride: 2 mg
Capsule, as hydrochloride: 2 mg
Liquid, oral, as hydrochloride: 1 mg/5 mL (60 mL, 90 mL, 120 mL)
Tablet, as hydrochloride: 2 mg

loperamide hydrochloride *see* loperamide *on this page*
Lopid® *see* gemfibrozil *on page 239*
lopremone *see* protirelin *on page 448*
Lopressor® *see* metoprolol *on page 346*
Loprox® *see* ciclopirox *on page 122*
Lorabid™ *see* loracarbef *on this page*

loracarbef (lor a KAR bef)
Brand Names Lorabid™
Therapeutic Category Antibiotic, Carbacephem
Use Treatment of mild to moderate community-acquired infections of the respiratory tract, skin and skin structure, and urinary tract that are caused by susceptible *S. pneumoniae*, *H. influenzae*, *B. catarrhalis*, *S. aureus*, and *E. coli*
Usual Dosage Oral:
Acute otitis media: Children: 15 mg/kg twice a day for 10 days
Urinary tract infections: Women: 200 mg once a day for 7 days
Dosage Forms
Capsule: 200 mg, 400 mg
Suspension, oral: 100 mg/5 mL (50 mL, 100 mL); 200 mg/5 mL (50 mL, 100 mL)

loratadine (lor AT a deen)
Brand Names Claritin®
Therapeutic Category Antihistamine
Use Perennial and seasonal allergic rhinitis and other allergic symptoms including urticaria
Usual Dosage Adults: Oral: 10 mg/day on an empty stomach
Dosage Forms
Syrup: 1 mg/mL (480 mL)
Tablet: 10 mg
Rapid-disintegrating tablets: 10 mg (RediTabs®)

loratadine and pseudoephedrine (lor AT a deen & soo doe e FED rin)
Brand Names Claritin-D®; Claritin-D® 24-Hour
Therapeutic Category Antihistamine/Decongestant Combination
Use Temporary relief of symptoms of seasonal and perennial allergic rhinitis, and vaso-motor rhinitis, including nasal obstruction
Usual Dosage Adults: Oral: 1 tablet every 12 hours
Dosage Forms
Tablet: Loratadine 5 mg and pseudoephedrine sulfate 120 mg
Tablet, extended release: Loratadine 10 mg and pseudoephedrine sulfate 240 mg

lorazepam (lor A ze pam)
Brand Names Ativan®
Therapeutic Category Benzodiazepine
Controlled Substance C-IV
Use Management of anxiety; status epilepticus; preoperative sedation and amnesia
Usual Dosage
Anxiety and sedation:
Infants and Children: Oral, I.V.: Usual: 0.05 mg/kg/dose (range: 0.02-0.09 mg/kg) every 4-8 hours
Adults: Oral: 1-10 mg/day in 2-3 divided doses; usual dose: 2-6 mg/day in divided doses
Insomnia: Adults: Oral: 2-4 mg at bedtime

Preoperative: Adults:
I.M.: 0.05 mg/kg administered 2 hours before surgery; maximum: 4 mg/dose
I.V.: 0.044 mg/kg 15-20 minutes before surgery; usual maximum: 2 mg/dose
Operative amnesia: Adults: I.V.: up to 0.05 mg/kg; maximum: 4 mg/dose
Status epilepticus: I.V.:
Infants and Children: 0.1 mg/kg slow I.V. over 2-5 minutes, do not exceed 4 mg/single dose; may repeat second dose of 0.05 mg/kg slow I.V. in 10-15 minutes if needed
Adolescents: 0.07 mg/kg slow I.V. over 2-5 minutes; maximum: 4 mg/dose; may repeat in 10-15 minutes
Adults: 4 mg/dose administered slowly over 2-5 minutes; may repeat in 10-15 minutes; usual maximum dose: 8 mg
Dosage Forms
Injection: 2 mg/mL (1 mL, 10 mL); 4 mg/mL (1 mL, 10 mL)
Solution, oral concentrated, alcohol and dye free: 2 mg/mL (30 mL)
Tablet: 0.5 mg, 1 mg, 2 mg

Lorcet®-HD see hydrocodone and acetaminophen on page 266

Lorcet® Plus see hydrocodone and acetaminophen on page 266

Loroxide® [OTC] see benzoyl peroxide on page 61

Lortab® see hydrocodone and acetaminophen on page 266

Lortab® ASA see hydrocodone and aspirin on page 266

losartan (loe SAR tan)
Synonyms DuP 753; losartan potassium; MK594
Brand Names Cozaar®
Therapeutic Category Angiotensin II Antagonists
Use Treatment of hypertension alone or in combination with other antihypertensives; in considering the use of monotherapy with Cozaar®, it should be noted that in controlled trials Cozaar® had an effect on blood pressure that was notably less in black patients than in nonblacks, a finding similar to the small effect of ACE inhibitors in blacks
Usual Dosage Adults: Oral: Initial: 50 mg once daily, with 25 mg used in patients with possible depletion of intravascular volume (eg, patients treated with diuretics) and patients with a history of hepatic impairment; can be administered once or twice daily with total daily doses ranging from 25-100 mg; if the antihypertensive effect measured

at trough using once daily dosing is inadequate, a twice daily regimen at the same total daily dose or an increase in dose may give a more satisfactory response; if blood pressure is not controlled by Cozaar® alone, a low dose of a diuretic may be added; hydrochlorothiazide has been shown to have an additive effect

Dosage Forms Tablet, film coated, as potassium: 25 mg, 50 mg

losartan and hydrochlorothiazide
(loe SAR tan & hye droe klor oh THYE a zide)
Brand Names Hyzaar®
Therapeutic Category Antihypertensive, Combination
Use Treatment of hypertension
Usual Dosage Adults: Oral: 1 tablet daily
Dosage Forms Tablet: Losartan potassium 50 mg and hydrochlorothiazide 12.5 mg

losartan potassium *see* losartan *on previous page*

Losec® *see* omeprazole *on page 383*

Lotensin® *see* benazepril *on page 58*

Lotensin HCT® *see* benazepril and hydrochlorothiazide *on page 58*

Lotrel™ *see* amlodipine and benazepril *on page 28*

Lotrimin® *see* clotrimazole *on page 131*

Lotrimin® AF Cream [OTC] *see* clotrimazole *on page 131*

Lotrimin® AF Lotion [OTC] *see* clotrimazole *on page 131*

Lotrimin® AF Powder [OTC] *see* miconazole *on page 348*

Lotrimin® AF Solution [OTC] *see* clotrimazole *on page 131*

Lotrimin® AF Spray Liquid [OTC] *see* miconazole *on page 348*

Lotrimin® AF Spray Powder [OTC] *see* miconazole *on page 348*

Lotrisone® *see* betamethasone and clotrimazole *on page 65*

lovastatin (LOE va sta tin)
Synonyms mevinolin; monacolin k
Brand Names Mevacor®
Therapeutic Category HMG-CoA Reductase Inhibitor
Use Adjunct to dietary therapy to decrease elevated serum total and LDL cholesterol concentrations in primary hypercholesterolemia
Usual Dosage Adults: Oral: Initial: 20 mg with evening meal, then adjust at 4-week intervals; maximum dose: 80 mg/day
Dosage Forms Tablet: 10 mg, 20 mg, 40 mg

Lovenox® Injection *see* enoxaparin *on page 194*

loxapine (LOKS a peen)
Synonyms loxapine hydrochloride; loxapine succinate; oxilapine succinate
Brand Names Loxitane®
Therapeutic Category Antipsychotic Agent, Dibenzoxazepine
Use Management of psychotic disorders
Usual Dosage Adults:
Oral: 10 mg twice daily, increase dose until psychotic symptoms are controlled; usual dose range: 60-100 mg/day in divided doses 2-4 times/day; dosages >250 mg/day are not recommended
I.M.: 12.5-50 mg every 4-6 hours or longer as needed and change to oral therapy as soon as possible
Dosage Forms
Capsule, as succinate: 5 mg, 10 mg, 25 mg, 50 mg
Concentrate, oral, as hydrochloride: 25 mg/mL (120 mL dropper bottle)
(Continued)

loxapine (Continued)

Injection, as hydrochloride: 50 mg/mL (1 mL)

loxapine hydrochloride see loxapine on previous page

loxapine succinate see loxapine on previous page

Loxitane® see loxapine on previous page

Lozol® see indapamide on page 282

l-pam see melphalan on page 327

LRH see gonadorelin on page 245

l-sarcolysin see melphalan on page 327

ltg see lamotrigine on page 301

L-thyroxine sodium see levothyroxine on page 306

Lubriderm® [OTC] see lanolin, cetyl alcohol, glycerin, and petrolatum on page 301

LubriTears® Solution [OTC] see artificial tears on page 42

Ludiomil® see maprotiline on page 321

Lufyllin® see dyphylline on page 188

Lugol's solution see potassium iodide on page 430

Luminal® see phenobarbital on page 409

Lupron® see leuprolide acetate on page 303

Lupron Depot® see leuprolide acetate on page 303

Lupron Depot-3® Month see leuprolide acetate on page 303

Lupron Depot-4® Month see leuprolide acetate on page 303

Lupron Depot-Ped™ see leuprolide acetate on page 303

Luride® see fluoride on page 228

Luride® Lozi-Tab® see fluoride on page 228

Luride®-SF Lozi-Tab® see fluoride on page 228

luteinizing hormone releasing hormone see gonadorelin on page 245

Lutrepulse® see gonadorelin on page 245

Luvox® see fluvoxamine on page 233

LY170053 see olanzapine on page 382

Lycolan® Elixir [OTC] see l-lysine on page 311

Lymphazurin® see radiological/contrast media (ionic) on page 457

lymphocyte immune globulin (LIM foe site i MYUN GLOB yoo lin)

Synonyms antithymocyte globulin (equine); atg; horse anti-human thymocyte gamma globulin

Brand Names Atgam®

Therapeutic Category Immunosuppressant Agent

Use Prevention and treatment of acute allograft rejection; treatment of moderate to severe aplastic anemia in patients not considered suitable candidates for bone marrow transplantation; prevention of graft-vs-host disease following bone marrow transplantation

Usual Dosage An intradermal skin test is recommended prior to administration of the initial dose of ATG. Use 0.1 mL of a 1:1000 dilution of ATG in normal saline

Aplastic anemia protocol: I.V.: 10-20 mg/kg/day for 8-14 days, then administer every other day for 7 more doses

Rejection prevention: Children and Adults: I.V.: 15 mg/kg/day for 14 days, then administer every other day for 7 more doses; initial dose should be administered within 24 hours before or after transplantation

Rejection treatment: Children and Adults: I.V. 10-15 mg/kg/day for 14 days, then administer every other day for 7 more doses

Dosage Forms Injection: 50 mg/mL (5 mL)

Lyphocin® *see* vancomycin *on page 545*

lypressin (lye PRES in)
Synonyms 8-*L*-lysine vasopressin
Brand Names Diapid® Nasal Spray
Therapeutic Category Antidiuretic Hormone Analog
Use Control or prevent signs and complications of neurogenic diabetes insipidus
Usual Dosage Children and Adults: Nasal: 1-2 sprays into one or both nostrils 4 times/day; approximately 2 USP posterior pituitary pressor units per spray
Dosage Forms Spray: 0.185 mg/mL (equivalent to 50 USP posterior pituitary units/mL) (8 mL)

Lysodren® *see* mitotane *on page 353*

Maalox® **[OTC]** *see* aluminum hydroxide and magnesium hydroxide *on page 21*

Maalox Anti-Gas® **[OTC]** *see* simethicone *on page 480*

Maalox® **Plus [OTC]** *see* aluminum hydroxide, magnesium hydroxide, and simethicone *on page 22*

Maalox® **Therapeutic Concentrate [OTC]** *see* aluminum hydroxide and magnesium hydroxide *on page 21*

Macrobid® *see* nitrofurantoin *on page 375*

Macrodantin® *see* nitrofurantoin *on page 375*

Macrodex® *see* dextran *on page 159*

mafenide (MA fe nide)
Synonyms mafenide acetate
Brand Names Sulfamylon® Topical
Therapeutic Category Antibacterial, Topical
Use Adjunct in the treatment of second and third degree burns to prevent septicemia caused by susceptible organisms such as *Pseudomonas aeruginosa*
Usual Dosage Children and Adults: Topical: Apply once or twice daily with a sterile gloved hand; apply to a thickness of approximately 16 mm; the burned area should be covered with cream at all times
Dosage Forms Cream, topical, as acetate: 85 mg/g (56.7 g, 113.4 g, 411 g)

mafenide acetate *see* mafenide *on this page*

magaldrate (MAG al drate)
Synonyms hydromagnesium aluminate
Brand Names Riopan® [OTC]
Therapeutic Category Antacid
Use Symptomatic relief of hyperacidity associated with peptic ulcer, gastritis, peptic esophagitis and hiatal hernia
Usual Dosage Adults: Oral: 540-1080 mg between meals and at bedtime
Dosage Forms Suspension, oral: 540 mg/5 mL (360 mL)

magaldrate and simethicone (MAG al drate & sye METH i kone)
Synonyms simethicone and magaldrate
Brand Names Riopan Plus® [OTC]
(Continued)

magaldrate and simethicone (Continued)

Therapeutic Category Antacid; Antiflatulent

Use Relief of hyperacidity associated with peptic ulcer, gastritis, peptic esophagitis and hiatal hernia which are accompanied by symptoms of gas

Usual Dosage Adults: Oral: 5-10 mL between meals and at bedtime

Dosage Forms Suspension, oral: Magaldrate 480 mg and simethicone 20 mg per 5 mL (360 mL)

Magalox Plus® [OTC] *see* aluminum hydroxide, magnesium hydroxide, and simethicone *on page 22*

Magan® *see* magnesium salicylate *on next page*

Magnacal® [OTC] *see* enteral nutritional products *on page 194*

magnesia magma *see* magnesium hydroxide *on next page*

magnesium chloride (mag NEE zhum KLOR ide)

Brand Names Slow-Mag® [OTC]

Therapeutic Category Electrolyte Supplement

Use Correct or prevent hypomagnesemia

Usual Dosage I.V. in TPN:

Children: 2-10 mEq/day; the usual recommended pediatric maintenance intake of magnesium ranges from 0.2-0.6 mEq/kg/day. The dose of magnesium may also be based on the caloric intake; on that basis, 3-10 mEq/day of magnesium are needed; maximum maintenance dose: 8-16 mEq/day

Adults: 8-24 mEq/day

Dosage Forms

Injection: 200 mg/mL [1.97 mEq/mL] (30 mL, 50 mL)

Tablet: Elemental magnesium 64 mg

magnesium citrate (mag NEE zhum SIT rate)

Synonyms citrate of magnesia

Brand Names Evac-Q-Mag® [OTC]

Therapeutic Category Laxative

Use Evacuation of bowel prior to certain surgical and diagnostic procedures

Usual Dosage Cathartic: Oral:

Children:

<6 years: 2-4 mL/kg administered as a single daily dose or in divided doses

6-12 years: $1/3$ to $1/2$ bottle

Children ≥12 years and Adults: $1/2$ to 1 full bottle

Dosage Forms Solution, oral: 300 mL

magnesium gluconate (mag NEE zhum GLOO koe nate)

Brand Names Magonate® [OTC]

Therapeutic Category Electrolyte Supplement

Use Dietary supplement for treatment of magnesium deficiencies

Usual Dosage The recommended dietary allowance (RDA) of magnesium is 4.5 mg/kg which is a total daily allowance of 350-400 mg for adult men and 280-300 mg for adult women. During pregnancy the RDA is 300 mg and during lactation the RDA is 355 mg. Average daily intakes of dietary magnesium have declined in recent years due to processing of food. The latest estimate of the average American dietary intake was 349 mg/day.

Dietary supplement: Oral:

Children: 3-6 mg/kg/day in divided doses 3-4 times/day; maximum: 400 mg/day

Adults: 27-54 mg 2-3 times/day or 100 mg 4 times/day

Dosage Forms Tablet: 500 mg [elemental magnesium 27 mg]

magnesium hydroxide (mag NEE zhum hye DROKS ide)

Synonyms magnesia magma; milk of magnesia; mom
Brand Names Phillips'® Milk of Magnesia [OTC]
Therapeutic Category Antacid; Electrolyte Supplement; Laxative
Use Short-term treatment of occasional constipation and symptoms of hyperacidity
Usual Dosage Oral:
Laxative:
<2 years: 0.5 mL/kg/dose
2-5 years: 5-15 mL/day or in divided doses
6-12 years: 15-30 mL/day or in divided doses
≥12 years: 30-60 mL/day or in divided doses
Antacid:
Children: 2.5-5 mL as needed
Adults: 5-15 mL as needed
Dosage Forms
Liquid: 390 mg/5 mL (10 mL, 15 mL, 20 mL, 30 mL, 100 mL, 120 mL, 180 mL, 360 mL, 720 mL)
Liquid, concentrate: 10 mL equivalent to 30 mL milk of magnesia USP
Suspension, oral: 2.5 g/30 mL (10 mL, 15 mL, 30 mL)
Tablet: 300 mg, 600 mg

magnesium hydroxide and aluminum hydroxide *see* aluminum hydroxide and magnesium hydroxide *on page 21*

magnesium hydroxide and mineral oil emulsion

(mag NEE zhum hye DROKS ide & MIN er al oyl e MUL shun)
Synonyms mom/mineral oil emulsion
Brand Names Haley's M-O® [OTC]
Therapeutic Category Laxative
Use Short-term treatment of occasional constipation
Usual Dosage Adults: Oral: 5-45 mL at bedtime
Dosage Forms Suspension, oral: Equivalent to magnesium hydroxide 24 mL/mineral oil emulsion 6 mL (30 mL unit dose)

magnesium oxide (mag NEE zhum OKS ide)

Brand Names Maox®
Therapeutic Category Antacid; Electrolyte Supplement; Laxative
Use Treatment of magnesium deficiencies, short-term treatment of occasional constipation, and symptoms of hyperacidity
Usual Dosage Oral:
Antacid: 250 mg to 1.5 g with water or milk 4 times/day after meals and at bedtime
Laxative: 2-4 g at bedtime with full glass of water
Dosage Forms
Capsule: 140 mg
Tablet: 400 mg, 425 mg

magnesium salicylate (mag NEE zhum sa LIS i late)

Brand Names Doan's®, Original [OTC]; Extra Strength Doan's® [OTC]; Magan®; Mobidin®
Therapeutic Category Nonsteroidal Anti-Inflammatory Agent (NSAID)
Use Mild to moderate pain, fever, various inflammatory conditions
Usual Dosage Adults: Oral: 650 mg 4 times/day or 1090 mg 3 times/day; may increase to 3.6-4.8 mg/day in 3-4 divided doses
Dosage Forms
Caplet:
Doan's®, Original: 325 mg
Extra Strength Doan's®: 500 mg
(Continued)

magnesium salicylate *(Continued)*
Tablet:
Magan®: 545 mg
Mobidin®: 600 mg

magnesium sulfate (mag NEE zhum SUL fate)
Synonyms epsom salts
Therapeutic Category Anticonvulsant; Electrolyte Supplement; Laxative
Use Treatment and prevention of hypomagnesemia; hypertension; encephalopathy and seizures associated with acute nephritis in children; also used as a cathartic
Usual Dosage Dose represented as $MgSO_4$ unless stated otherwise
Hypomagnesemia:
Children:
I.M., I.V.: 25-50 mg/kg/dose (0.2-0.4 mEq/kg/dose) every 4-6 hours for 3-4 doses, maximum single dose: 2000 mg (16 mEq), may repeat if hypomagnesemia persists (higher dosage up to 100 mg/kg/dose $MgSO_4$ I.V. has been used)
Oral: 100-200 mg/kg/dose 4 times/day
Maintenance: I.V.: 30-60 mg/kg/day (0.25-0.5 mEq/kg/day)
Adults: I.M., I.V.: 1 g every 6 hours for 4 doses or 250 mg/kg over a 4-hour period; for severe hypomagnesemia: 8-12 g $MgSO_4$/day in divided doses has been used; Oral: 3 g every 6 hours for 4 doses as needed
Management of seizures and hypertension: Children: I.M., I.V.: 20-100 mg/kg/dose every 4-6 hours as needed; in severe cases doses as high as 200 mg/kg/dose have been used

Cathartic: Oral:
Children: 0.25 g/kg/dose
Adults: 10-30 g
Dosage Forms
Granules: ~40 mEq magnesium/5 g (240 g)
Injection: 100 mg/mL (20 mL); 125 mg/mL (8 mL); 250 mg/mL (150 mL); 500 mg/mL (2 mL, 5 mL, 10 mL, 30 mL, 50 mL)
Solution, oral: 50% [500 mg/mL] (30 mL)

Magnevist® *see* radiological/contrast media (ionic) *on page 457*

Magonate® [OTC] *see* magnesium gluconate *on page 318*

Malatal® *see* hyoscyamine, atropine, scopolamine, and phenobarbital *on page 276*

malathion (mal a THYE on)
Brand Names Ovide™ Topical
Therapeutic Category Scabicides/Pediculicides
Use Treatment of head lice and their ova
Usual Dosage Topical: Sprinkle Ovide™ lotion on dry hair and rub gently until the scalp is thoroughly moistened; pay special attention to the back of the head and neck. Allow to dry naturally, use no heat and leave uncovered. After 8-12 hours, the hair should be washed with a nonmedicated shampoo; rinse and use a fine-toothed comb to remove dead lice and eggs. If required, repeat with second application in 7-9 days. Further treatment is generally not necessary. Other family members should be evaluated to determine if infested and if so, receive treatment.
Dosage Forms Lotion: 0.5% (59 mL)

Mallamint® [OTC] *see* calcium carbonate *on page 82*

Mallazine® Eye Drops [OTC] *see* tetrahydrozoline *on page 510*

Mallisol® [OTC] *see* povidone-iodine *on page 431*

malt soup extract (malt soop EKS trakt)
Brand Names Maltsupex® [OTC]
Therapeutic Category Laxative
Use Short-term treatment of constipation
Usual Dosage Oral:
Infants >1 month:
Breast fed: 1-2 teaspoonfuls in 2-4 oz of water or fruit juice 1-2 times/day
Bottle fed: $\frac{1}{2}$ to 2 tablespoonfuls/day in formula for 3-4 days, then 1-2 teaspoonfuls/day
Children 2-11 years: 1-2 tablespoonfuls 1-2 times/day
Adults ≥12 years: 2 tablespoonfuls twice daily for 3-4 days, then 1-2 tablespoonfuls every evening
Dosage Forms
Liquid: Nondiastatic barley malt extract 16 g/15 mL
Powder: Nondiastatic barley malt extract 16 g/heaping tablespoonful
Tablet: Nondiastatic barley malt extract 750 mg

Maltsupex® [OTC] *see* malt soup extract *on this page*

Mandol® *see* cefamandole *on page 96*

mandrake *see* podophyllum resin *on page 422*

manganese injection *see* trace metals *on page 525*

mannitol (MAN i tole)
Synonyms *d*-mannitol
Brand Names Osmitrol® Injection; Resectisol® Irrigation Solution
Therapeutic Category Diuretic, Osmotic
Use Reduction of increased intracranial pressure (ICP) associated with cerebral edema; promotion of diuresis in the prevention and/or treatment of oliguria or anuria due to acute renal failure; reduction of increased intraocular pressure; promotion of urinary excretion of toxic substances
Usual Dosage
Children:
Test dose (to assess adequate renal function): 200 mg/kg over 3-5 minutes to produce a urine flow of at least 1 mL/kg/hour for 1-3 hours
Initial: 0.5-1 g/kg
Maintenance: 0.25-0.5 g/kg/hour administered every 4-6 hours
Adults:
Test dose: 12.5 g (200 mg/kg) over 3-5 minutes to produce a urine flow of at least 30-50 mL of urine per hour over the next 2-3 hours
Initial: 0.5-1 g/kg
Maintenance: 0.25-0.5 g/kg every 4-6 hours
Dosage Forms
Injection: 5% [50 mg/mL] (1000 mL); 10% [100 mg/mL] (500 mL, 1000 mL); 15% [150 mg/mL] (150 mL, 500 mL); 20% [200 mg/mL] (150 mL, 250 mL, 500 mL); 25% [250 mg/mL] (50 mL)
Solution, urogenital: 0.54% [5.4 mg/mL] (2000 mL)

Mantoux *see* tuberculin tests *on page 539*

Maolate® *see* chlorphenesin *on page 112*

Maox® *see* magnesium oxide *on page 319*

Mapap® [OTC] *see* acetaminophen *on page 3*

maprotiline (ma PROE ti leen)
Synonyms maprotiline hydrochloride
Brand Names Ludiomil®
Therapeutic Category Antidepressant, Tetracyclic
Use Treatment of depression and anxiety associated with depression
(Continued)

maprotiline *(Continued)*

Usual Dosage Oral:
Children 6-14 years: 10 mg/day, increase to a maximum daily dose of 75 mg
Adults: 75 mg/day to start, increase by 25 mg every 2 weeks up to 150-225 mg/day; administered in 3 divided doses or in a single daily dose
Dosage Forms Tablet, as hydrochloride: 25 mg, 50 mg, 75 mg

maprotiline hydrochloride *see* maprotiline *on previous page*

Maranox® [OTC] *see* acetaminophen *on page 3*

Marax® *see* theophylline, ephedrine, and hydroxyzine *on page 513*

Marcaine® *see* bupivacaine *on page 76*

Marcillin® *see* ampicillin *on page 33*

Marezine® [OTC] *see* cyclizine *on page 143*

Marezine® *see* meclizine *on page 324*

Margesic® H *see* hydrocodone and acetaminophen *on page 266*

Marinol® *see* dronabinol *on page 185*

Marpres® *see* hydralazine, hydrochlorothiazide, and reserpine *on page 264*

Marthritic® *see* salsalate *on page 473*

masoprocol *(ma SOE pro kole)*

Brand Names Actinex® Topical
Therapeutic Category Topical Skin Product
Use Treatment of actinic keratosis
Usual Dosage Adults: Topical: Wash and dry area; gently massage into affected area every morning and evening for 28 days
Dosage Forms Cream: 10% (30 g)

Massé® Breast Cream [OTC] *see* glycerin, lanolin, and peanut oil *on page 243*

Massengill® Medicated Douche w/Cepticin [OTC] *see* povidone-iodine *on page 431*

Matulane® *see* procarbazine *on page 439*

Mavik® *see* trandolapril *on page 526*

Maxair™ Inhalation Aerosol *see* pirbuterol *on page 420*

Maxaquin® *see* lomefloxacin *on page 312*

Maxidex® *see* dexamethasone *on page 156*

Maxiflor® *see* diflorasone *on page 167*

Maximum Strength Anbesol® [OTC] *see* benzocaine *on page 59*

Maximum Strength Desenex® Antifungal Cream [OTC] *see* miconazole *on page 348*

Maximum Strength Dex-A-Diet® [OTC] *see* phenylpropanolamine *on page 413*

Maximum Strength Dexatrim® [OTC] *see* phenylpropanolamine *on page 413*

Maximum Strength Nytol® [OTC] *see* diphenhydramine *on page 173*

Maximum Strength Orajel® [OTC] *see* benzocaine *on page 59*

Maxipime® *see* cefepime *on page 97*

Maxitrol® *see* neomycin, polymyxin b, and dexamethasone *on page 369*

Maxivate® *see* betamethasone *on page 64*

Maxolon® *see* metoclopramide *on page 344*

Maxzide® *see* hydrochlorothiazide and triamterene *on page 265*

may apple *see* podophyllum resin *on page 422*

Mazanor® *see* mazindol *on this page*

mazindol (MAY zin dole)
Brand Names Mazanor®; Sanorex®
Therapeutic Category Anorexiant
Controlled Substance C-IV
Use Short-term adjunct in exogenous obesity
Usual Dosage Adults: Oral: Initial: 1 mg once daily and adjust to patient response; usual dose is 1 mg 3 times daily, 1 hour before meals, or 2 mg once daily, 1 hour before lunch; administer with meals to avoid GI discomfort
Dosage Forms Tablet:
Mazanor®: 1 mg
Sanorex®: 1 mg, 2 mg

mch *see* microfibrillar collagen hemostat *on page 349*

m-cresyl acetate (em-KREE sil AS e tate)
Brand Names Cresylate®
Therapeutic Category Otic Agent, Anti-infective
Use Provides an acid medium; for external otitis infections caused by susceptible bacteria or fungus
Usual Dosage Otic: Instill 2-4 drops as required
Dosage Forms Solution: 25% with isopropanol 25%, chlorobutanol 1%, benzyl alcohol 1%, and castor oil 5% in propylene glycol (15 mL dropper bottle)

MCT Oil® **[OTC]** *see* medium chain triglycerides *on page 325*

MD-Gastroview® *see* radiological/contrast media (ionic) *on page 457*

measles and rubella vaccines, combined
(MEE zels & roo BEL a vak SEENS, kom BINED)
Synonyms rubella and measles vaccines, combined
Brand Names M-R-VAX® II
Therapeutic Category Vaccine, Live Virus
Use Simultaneous immunization against measles and rubella
Usual Dosage S.C.: Inject into outer aspect of upper arm
Dosage Forms Injection: 1000 $TCID_{50}$ each of live attenuated measles virus vaccine and live rubella virus vaccine

measles, mumps and rubella vaccines, combined
(MEE zels, mumpz & roo BEL a vak SEENS, kom BINED)
Synonyms mmr
Brand Names M-M-R® II
Therapeutic Category Vaccine, Live Virus
Use Measles, mumps, and rubella prophylaxis
Usual Dosage S.C.: Inject in outer aspect of the upper arm to children ≥15 months of age; each dose contains 1000 $TCID_{50}$ (tissue culture infectious doses) of live attenuated measle virus vaccine, 5000 $TCID_{50}$ of live mumps virus vaccine and 1000 $TCID_{50}$ of live rubella virus vaccine
Dosage Forms Injection: 1000 $TCID_{50}$ each of measles virus vaccine and rubella virus vaccine, 5000 $TCID_{50}$ mumps virus vaccine

measles virus vaccine, live (MEE zels VYE rus vak SEEN, live)
Synonyms more attenuated enders strain; rubeola vaccine
Brand Names Attenuvax®
Therapeutic Category Vaccine, Live Virus
Use Immunization against measles (rubeola) in persons ≥15 months of age
(Continued)

measles virus vaccine, live *(Continued)*

Usual Dosage Children >15 months and Adults: S.C.: 0.5 mL in outer aspect of the upper arm

Dosage Forms Injection: 1000 $TCID_{50}$ per dose

Mebaral® *see* mephobarbital *on page 329*

mebendazole (me BEN da zole)

Brand Names Vermox®

Therapeutic Category Anthelmintic

Use Treatment of enterobiasis (pinworm infection), trichuriasis (whipworm infections), ascariasis (roundworm infection), and hookworm infections caused by *Necator americanus* or *Ancylostoma duodenale*; drug of choice in the treatment of capillariasis

Usual Dosage Children and Adults: Oral:

Pinworms: Single chewable tablet; may need to repeat after 2 weeks

Whipworms, roundworms, hookworms: 1 tablet twice daily, morning and evening on 3 consecutive days; if patient is not cured within 3-4 weeks, a second course of treatment may be administered

Dosage Forms Tablet, chewable: 100 mg

mecamylamine (mek a MIL a meen)

Synonyms mecamylamine hydrochloride

Brand Names Inversine®

Therapeutic Category Ganglionic Blocking Agent

Use Treatment of moderately severe to severe hypertension and in uncomplicated malignant hypertension

Usual Dosage Adults: Oral: 2.5 mg twice daily after meals for 2 days; increased by increments of 2.5 mg at intervals of ≥2 days until desired blood pressure response is achieved

Dosage Forms Tablet, as hydrochloride: 2.5 mg

mecamylamine hydrochloride *see* mecamylamine *on this page*

mechlorethamine (me klor ETH a meen)

Synonyms HN_2; mechlorethamine hydrochloride; mustine; nitrogen mustard

Brand Names Mustargen® Hydrochloride

Therapeutic Category Antineoplastic Agent

Use Combination therapy of Hodgkin's disease, brain tumors, non-Hodgkin's lymphoma, and malignant lymphomas; palliative treatment of bronchogenic, breast, and ovarian carcinoma; sclerosing agent in intracavitary therapy of pleural, pericardial, and other malignant effusions

Usual Dosage Refer to individual protocols

Children: MOPP: I.V.: 6 mg/m^2 on days 1 and 8 of a 28-day cycle

Adults:

I.V.: 0.4 mg/kg or 12-16 mg/m^2 for one dose or divided into 0.1 mg/kg/day for 4 days

Intracavitary: 10-20 mg or 0.2-0.4 mg/kg

Dosage Forms Powder for injection, as hydrochloride: 10 mg

mechlorethamine hydrochloride *see* mechlorethamine *on this page*

Meclan® **Topical** *see* meclocycline *on next page*

meclizine (MEK li zeen)

Synonyms meclizine hydrochloride; meclozine hydrochloride

Brand Names Antivert®; Antrizine®; Bonine® [OTC]; Dizmiss® [OTC]; Dramamine® II [OTC]; Marezine®; Meni-D®; Ru-Vert-M®; Vergon® [OTC]

Therapeutic Category Antihistamine

Use Prevention and treatment of motion sickness; management of vertigo

Usual Dosage Children >12 years and Adults: Oral:
Motion sickness: 25-50 mg 1 hour before travel, repeat dose every 24 hours if needed
Vertigo: 25-100 mg/day in divided doses
Dosage Forms
Capsule, as hydrochloride: 15 mg, 25 mg, 30 mg
Tablet, as hydrochloride: 12.5 mg, 25 mg, 50 mg
Chewable: 25 mg
Film coated: 25 mg

meclizine hydrochloride *see* meclizine *on previous page*

meclocycline (me kloe SYE kleen)
Synonyms meclocycline sulfosalicylate
Brand Names Meclan® Topical
Therapeutic Category Antibiotic, Topical
Use Topical treatment of inflammatory acne vulgaris
Usual Dosage Topical: Apply to affected areas twice daily
Dosage Forms Cream, topical, as sulfosalicylate: 1% (20 g, 45 g)

meclocycline sulfosalicylate *see* meclocycline *on this page*

meclofenamate (me kloe fen AM ate)
Synonyms meclofenamate sodium
Therapeutic Category Analgesic, Non-narcotic; Nonsteroidal Anti-Inflammatory Agent (NSAID)
Use Treatment of inflammatory disorders
Usual Dosage Adults: Oral: 200-300 mg 3-4 times/day
Dosage Forms Capsule, as sodium: 50 mg, 100 mg

meclofenamate sodium *see* meclofenamate *on this page*

meclozine hydrochloride *see* meclizine *on previous page*

medicinal carbon *see* charcoal *on page 105*

Medigesic® *see* butalbital compound and acetaminophen *on page 78*

Medihaler-Iso® *see* isoproterenol *on page 291*

Medipain 5® *see* hydrocodone and acetaminophen *on page 266*

Mediplast® Plaster [OTC] *see* salicylic acid *on page 472*

Medi-Quick® Topical Ointment [OTC] *see* bacitracin, neomycin, and polymyxin b *on page 53*

Medi-Tuss® [OTC] *see* guaifenesin *on page 247*

medium chain triglycerides (mee DEE um chane trye GLIS er ides)
Synonyms triglycerides, medium chain
Brand Names MCT Oil® [OTC]
Therapeutic Category Nutritional Supplement
Use Dietary supplement for those who cannot digest long chain fats; malabsorption associated with disorders such as pancreatic insufficiency, bile salt deficiency, and bacterial overgrowth of the small bowel; induce ketosis as a prevention for seizures (akinetic, clonic, and petit mal)
Usual Dosage Oral: 15 mL 3-4 times/day
Dosage Forms Oil: 14 g/15 mL (960 mL)

Medralone® Injection *see* methylprednisolone *on page 343*

Medrol® Oral *see* methylprednisolone *on page 343*

medroxyprogesterone acetate (me DROKS ee proe JES te rone AS e tate)
Synonyms acetoxymethylprogesterone; methylacetoxyprogesterone
Brand Names Amen® Oral; Curretab® Oral; Cycrin® Oral; Depo-Provera® Injection; Provera® Oral
Therapeutic Category Contraceptive, Progestin Only; Progestin
Use Secondary amenorrhea or abnormal uterine bleeding due to hormonal imbalance
Usual Dosage
　Adolescents and Adults: Oral:
　　Amenorrhea: 5-10 mg/day for 5-10 days or 2.5 mg/day
　　Abnormal uterine bleeding: 5-10 mg for 5-10 days starting on day 16 or 21 of cycle
　　Accompanying cyclic estrogen therapy, postmenopausal: 2.5-10 mg the last 10-13 days of estrogen dosing each month
　Adults:
　　Contraception: Deep I.M.: 150 mg every 3 months or 450 mg every 6 months
　　Endometrial or renal carcinoma: I.M.: 400-1000 mg/week
Dosage Forms
　Injection, suspension: 100 mg/mL (5 mL); 150 mg/mL (1 mL); 400 mg/mL (1 mL, 2.5 mL, 10 mL)
　Tablet: 2.5 mg, 5 mg, 10 mg

medrysone (ME dri sone)
Brand Names HMS Liquifilm®
Therapeutic Category Adrenal Corticosteroid
Use Treatment of allergic conjunctivitis, vernal conjunctivitis, episcleritis, ophthalmic epinephrine sensitivity reaction
Usual Dosage Children and Adults: Ophthalmic: 1 drop in conjunctival sac 2-4 times/day up to every 4 hours; may use every 1-2 hours during first 1-2 days
Dosage Forms Solution, ophthalmic: 1% (5 mL, 10 mL)

mefenamic acid (me fe NAM ik AS id)
Brand Names Ponstel®
Therapeutic Category Analgesic, Non-narcotic; Nonsteroidal Anti-Inflammatory Agent (NSAID)
Use Short-term relief of mild to moderate pain including primary dysmenorrhea
Usual Dosage Children >14 years and Adults: Oral: 500 mg to start then 250 mg every 4 hours as needed; maximum therapy: 1 week
Dosage Forms Capsule: 250 mg

mefloquine (ME floe kwin)
Synonyms mefloquine hydrochloride
Brand Names Lariam®
Therapeutic Category Antimalarial Agent
Use Treatment of acute malarial infections and prevention of malaria
Usual Dosage Adults: Oral:
　Mild to moderate malaria infection: 5 tablets (1250 mg) as a single dose with at least 8 oz of water
　Malaria prophylaxis: 1 tablet (250 mg) weekly starting 1 week before travel, continuing weekly during travel and for 4 weeks after leaving endemic area
Dosage Forms Tablet, as hydrochloride: 250 mg

mefloquine hydrochloride *see* mefloquine *on this page*

Mefoxin® *see* cefoxitin *on page 99*

Mega B® [OTC] *see* vitamin b complex *on page 553*

Mega-B® [OTC] *see* vitamins, multiple (oral, adult) *on page 556*

Megace® *see* megestrol acetate *on next page*

Megaton™ **[OTC]** *see* vitamin b complex *on page 553*

megestrol acetate (me JES trole AS e tate)

Brand Names Megace®

Therapeutic Category Antineoplastic Agent; Progestin

Use Palliative treatment of breast and endometrial carcinomas, appetite stimulation and promotion of weight gain in cachexia

Usual Dosage Adults: Oral:
Breast carcinoma: 40 mg 4 times/day
Endometrial: 40-320 mg/day in divided doses

Dosage Forms
Suspension, oral: 40 mg/mL with alcohol 0.06% (240 mL)
Tablet: 20 mg, 40 mg

Melanex® *see* hydroquinone *on page 272*

Mellaril® *see* thioridazine *on page 516*

Mellaril-S® *see* thioridazine *on page 516*

melphalan (MEL fa lan)

Synonyms l-pam; l-sarcolysin; phenylalanine mustard

Brand Names Alkeran®

Therapeutic Category Antineoplastic Agent

Use Palliative treatment of multiple myeloma and nonresectable epithelial ovarian carcinoma; neuroblastoma, rhabdomyosarcoma, breast cancer, sarcoma; I.V. formulation: Use in patients in whom oral therapy is not appropriate

Usual Dosage Refer to individual protocols
Children: I.V. (investigational, distributed under the auspices of the NCI for authorized studies):
Pediatric rhabdomyosarcoma: 10-35 mg/m^2 bolus every 21-28 days
Chemoradiotherapy supported by marrow infusions for neuroblastoma: 70-140 mg/m^2 on day 7 and 6 before BMT
Adults: Oral:
Multiple myeloma: 6 mg/day or 10 mg/day for 7-10 days, or 0.15 mg/kg/day for 7 days
Ovarian carcinoma: 0.2 mg/kg/day for 5 days, repeat in 4-5 weeks

Dosage Forms
Powder for injection: 50 mg
Tablet: 2 mg

Menadol® **[OTC]** *see* ibuprofen *on page 278*

Menest® *see* estrogens, esterified *on page 205*

Meni-D® *see* meclizine *on page 324*

meningococcal polysaccharide vaccine, groups A, C, Y and W-135

(me NIN joe kok al pol i SAK a ride vak SEEN groops aye, see, why & dubl yoo won thur tee fyve)

Brand Names Menomune®-A/C/Y/W-135

Therapeutic Category Vaccine, Live Bacteria

Use Immunization against infection caused by *Neisseria meningitidis* groups A,C,Y, and W-135 in persons ≥2 years

Usual Dosage S.C.: 0.5 mL; do not inject intradermally or I.V.

Dosage Forms Injection: 10 dose, 50 dose

Menomune®**-A/C/Y/W-135** *see* meningococcal polysaccharide vaccine, groups A, C, Y and W-135 *on this page*

menotropins (men oh TROE pins)

Brand Names Humegon®; Pergonal®; Repronex®

Therapeutic Category Gonadotropin

Use Sequentially with hCG to induce ovulation and pregnancy in the infertile woman with functional anovulation; used with hCG in men to stimulate spermatogenesis in those with primary hypogonadotropic hypogonadism

Usual Dosage I.M.:

Male: Following pretreatment with hCG, 1 ampul 3 times/week and hCG 2000 units twice weekly until sperm is detected in the ejaculate (4-6 months) then may be increased to 2 ampuls of menotropins 3 times/week

Female: 1 ampul/day (75 units of FSH and LH) for 9-12 days followed by 10,000 units hCG 1 day after the last dose; repeated at least twice at same level before increasing dosage to 2 ampuls

Dosage Forms Injection: Follicle stimulating hormone activity 75 units and luteinizing hormone activity 75 units per 2 mL ampul; follicle stimulating hormone activity 150 units and luteinizing hormone activity 150 units per 2 mL ampul

Mentax® *see* butenafine *on page 79*

mepenzolate (me PEN zoe late)

Synonyms mepenzolate bromide

Brand Names Cantil®

Therapeutic Category Anticholinergic Agent

Use Management of peptic ulcer disease; inhibit salivation and excessive secretions in respiratory tract preoperatively

Usual Dosage Adults: Oral: 25-50 mg 4 times/day with meal and at bedtime

Dosage Forms Tablet, as bromide: 25 mg

mepenzolate bromide *see* mepenzolate *on this page*

Mepergan® *see* meperidine and promethazine *on this page*

meperidine (me PER i deen)

Synonyms isonipecaine hydrochloride; meperidine hydrochloride; pethidine hydrochloride

Brand Names Demerol®

Therapeutic Category Analgesic, Narcotic

Controlled Substance C-II

Use Management of moderate to severe pain; adjunct to anesthesia and preoperative sedation

Usual Dosage Doses should be titrated to appropriate analgesic effect; when changing route of administration, note that oral doses are about half as effective as parenteral dose

Oral, I.M., I.V., S.C.:

Children: 1-1.5 mg/kg/dose every 3-4 hours as needed; 1-2 mg/kg as a single dose preoperative medication may be used; maximum 100 mg/dose

Adults: 50-150 mg/dose every 3-4 hours as needed

Dosage Forms

Injection, as hydrochloride:

Multiple-dose vials: 50 mg/mL (30 mL); 100 mg/mL (20 mL)

Single-dose: 10 mg/mL (5 mL, 10 mL, 30 mL); 25 mg/dose (0.5 mL, 1 mL); 50 mg/dose (1 mL); 75 mg/dose (1 mL, 1.5 mL); 100 mg/dose (1 mL)

Syrup, as hydrochloride: 50 mg/5 mL (500 mL)

Tablet, as hydrochloride: 50 mg, 100 mg

meperidine and promethazine (me PER i deen & proe METH a zeen)

Brand Names Mepergan®

Therapeutic Category Analgesic, Narcotic

Use Management of moderate to severe pain
Usual Dosage Adults:
Oral: 1 capsule every 4-6 hours
I.M.: 1-2 mL every 3-4 hours
Dosage Forms
Capsule: Meperidine hydrochloride 50 mg and promethazine hydrochloride 25 mg
Injection: Meperidine hydrochloride 25 mg and promethazine hydrochloride 25 per mL (2 mL, 10 mL)

meperidine hydrochloride *see* meperidine *on previous page*

mephentermine (me FEN ter meen)
Synonyms mephentermine sulfate
Brand Names Wyamine® Sulfate Injection
Therapeutic Category Adrenergic Agonist Agent
Use Treatment of hypotension secondary to ganglionic blockade or spinal anesthesia; may be used as an emergency measure to maintain blood pressure until whole blood replacement becomes available
Usual Dosage
Hypotension: I.M., I.V.:
Children: 0.4 mg/kg
Adults: 0.5 mg/kg
Hypotensive emergency: I.V. infusion: 20-60 mg
Dosage Forms Injection, as sulfate: 15 mg/mL (2 mL, 10 mL); 30 mg/mL (10 mL)

mephentermine sulfate *see* mephentermine *on this page*

mephenytoin (me FEN i toyn)
Synonyms methoin; methylphenylethylhydantoin; phenantoin
Brand Names Mesantoin®
Therapeutic Category Anticonvulsant
Use Treatment of tonic-clonic and partial seizures in patients who are uncontrolled with less toxic anticonvulsants
Usual Dosage Oral:
Children: 3-15 mg/kg/day in 3 divided doses; usual maintenance dose: 100-400 mg/day in 3 divided doses
Adults: Initial dose: 50-100 mg/day administered daily; increase by 50-100 mg at weekly intervals; usual maintenance dose: 200-600 mg/day in 3 divided doses; maximum: 800 mg/day
Dosage Forms Tablet: 100 mg

mephobarbital (me foe BAR bi tal)
Synonyms methylphenobarbital
Brand Names Mebaral®
Therapeutic Category Barbiturate
Controlled Substance C-IV
Use Treatment of generalized tonic-clonic and simple partial seizures
Usual Dosage Epilepsy: Oral:
Children: 4-10 mg/kg/day in 2-4 divided doses
Adults: 200-600 mg/day in 2-4 divided doses
Dosage Forms Tablet: 32 mg, 50 mg, 100 mg

Mephyton® Oral *see* phytonadione *on page 416*

mepivacaine (me PIV a kane)
Synonyms mepivacaine hydrochloride
Brand Names Carbocaine®; Isocaine® HCl; Polocaine®
Therapeutic Category Local Anesthetic
(Continued)

mepivacaine *(Continued)*
Use Local anesthesia by nerve block; infiltration in dental procedures
Usual Dosage
Injectable local anesthetic: Varies with procedure, degree of anesthesia needed, vascularity of tissue, duration of anesthesia required, and physical condition of patient
Topical: Apply to affected area as needed
Dosage Forms Injection, as hydrochloride: 1% [10 mg/mL] (30 mL, 50 mL); 1.5% [15 mg/mL] (30 mL); 2% [20 mg/mL] (20 mL, 50 mL); 3% [30 mg/mL] (1.8 mL)

mepivacaine hydrochloride *see mepivacaine on previous page*

meprobamate (me proe BA mate)
Brand Names Equanil®; Miltown®; Neuramate®
Therapeutic Category Antianxiety Agent, Miscellaneous
Controlled Substance C-IV
Use Management of anxiety disorders
Usual Dosage Oral:
Children 6-12 years: 100-200 mg 2-3 times/day
Sustained release: 200 mg twice daily
Adults: 400 mg 3-4 times/day, up to 2400 mg/day
Sustained release: 400-800 mg twice daily
Dosage Forms
Capsule, sustained release: 200 mg, 400 mg
Tablet: 200 mg, 400 mg, 600 mg

meprobamate and aspirin *see aspirin and meprobamate on page 45*

Mepron™ *see atovaquone on page 46*

merbromin (mer BROE min)
Brand Names Mercurochrome®
Therapeutic Category Topical Skin Product
Use Topical antiseptic
Usual Dosage Topical: Apply freely, until injury has healed
Dosage Forms Solution, topical: 2%

mercaptopurine (mer kap toe PYOOR een)
Synonyms 6-mercaptopurine; 6-mp
Brand Names Purinethol®
Therapeutic Category Antineoplastic Agent
Use Treatment of acute leukemias (ALL, CML)
Usual Dosage Oral (refer to individual protocols):
Induction: 2.5 mg/kg/day for several weeks or more; if, after 4 weeks there is no improvement and no myelosuppression, increase dosage up to 5 mg/kg/day
Maintenance: 1.5-2.5 mg/kg/day
Dosage Forms Tablet: 50 mg

6-mercaptopurine *see mercaptopurine on this page*

mercapturic acid *see acetylcysteine on page 8*

mercuric oxide (mer KYOOR ik OKS ide)
Synonyms yellow mercuric oxide
Therapeutic Category Antibiotic, Ophthalmic
Use Treatment of irritation and minor infections of the eyelids
Usual Dosage Ophthalmic: Apply small amount to inner surface of lower eyelid once or twice daily
Dosage Forms Ointment, ophthalmic: 1%, 2% [OTC]

Mercurochrome® *see* merbromin *on previous page*

meropenem (mer oh PEN em)
Brand Names Merrem® I.V.
Therapeutic Category Carbapenem (Antibiotic)
Use Meropenem is indicated as single agent therapy for the treatment of intra-abdominal infections including complicated appendicitis and peritonitis in adults and bacterial meningitis in pediatric patients >3 months of age caused by *S. pneumoniae, H. influenzae,* and *N. meningitidis* (penicillin-resistant pneumococci have not been studied in clinical trials); it is better tolerated than imipenem and highly effective against a broad range of bacteria
Usual Dosage
Children:
Intra-abdominal infections: 20 mg/kg every 8 hours (maximum dose: 1 g every 8 hours)
Meningitis: 40 mg/kg every 8 hours (maximum dose: 2 g every 8 hours)
Adults: 1 g every 8 hours
Dosage Forms
Infusion: 500 mg (100 mL); 1 g (100 mL)
ADD-vantage®: 500 mg (15 mL); 1 g (15 mL)
Injection: 25 mg/mL (20 mL); 33.3 mg/mL (30 mL)

Merrem® **I.V.** *see* meropenem *on this page*
Mersol® **[OTC]** *see* thimerosal *on page 515*
Merthiolate® **[OTC]** *see* thimerosal *on page 515*
Meruvax® **II** *see* rubella virus vaccine, live *on page 471*

mesalamine (me SAL a meen)
Synonyms 5-aminosalicylic acid; 5-asa; fisalamine; mesalazine
Brand Names Asacol® Oral; Pentasa® Oral; Rowasa® Rectal
Therapeutic Category 5-Aminosalicylic Acid Derivative
Use Treatment of ulcerative colitis, proctosigmoiditis, and proctitis
Usual Dosage Adults (usual course of therapy is 3-6 weeks): Oral: 800 mg 3 times/day
Retention enema: 60 mL (4 g) at bedtime, retained over night, approximately 8 hours
Rectal suppository: Insert 1 suppository in rectum twice daily
Dosage Forms
Capsule, controlled release (Pentasa®): 250 mg
Suppository, rectal (Rowasa®): 500 mg
Suspension, rectal (Rowasa®): 4 g/60 mL (7s)
Tablet, enteric coated (Asacol®): 400 mg

mesalazine *see* mesalamine *on this page*
Mesantoin® *see* mephenytoin *on page 329*

mesna (MES na)
Synonyms sodium 2-mercaptoethane sulfonate
Brand Names Mesnex™
Therapeutic Category Antidote
Use Detoxifying agent used as a protectant against hemorrhagic cystitis induced by ifosfamide and cyclophosphamide
Usual Dosage Children and Adults (refer to individual protocols):
Ifosfamide: I.V.: 20% W/W of ifosfamide dose at time of administration and 4 and 8 hours after each dose of ifosfamide
Cyclophosphamide: I.V.: 20% W/W of cyclophosphamide dose prior to administration and 3, 6, 9, 12 hours after cyclophosphamide dose (total daily dose: 120% to 180% of cyclophosphamide dose)
Oral dose: 40% W/W of the antineoplastic agent dose in 3 doses at 4-hour intervals
(Continued)

mesna *(Continued)*
Dosage Forms Injection: 100 mg/mL (2 mL, 4 mL, 10 mL)

Mesnex™ *see mesna on previous page*

mesoridazine (mez oh RID a zeen)
Synonyms mesoridazine besylate
Brand Names Serentil®
Therapeutic Category Phenothiazine Derivative
Use Symptomatic management of psychotic disorders, including schizophrenia, behavioral problems, alcoholism as well as reducing anxiety and tension occurring in neurosis
Usual Dosage Initial: 25 mg for most patients; may repeat dose in 30-60 minutes, if necessary; the usual optimum dosage range is 25-200 mg/day. Concentrate may be diluted just prior to administration with distilled water, acidified tap water, orange or grape juice; do not prepare and store bulk dilutions.
Dosage Forms
Injection, as besylate: 25 mg/mL (1 mL)
Liquid, oral, as besylate: 25 mg/mL (118 mL)
Tablet, as besylate: 10 mg, 25 mg, 50 mg, 100 mg

mesoridazine besylate *see mesoridazine on this page*
Mestinon® Injection *see pyridostigmine on page 452*
Mestinon® Oral *see pyridostigmine on page 452*

mestranol and norethindrone (MES tra nole & nor eth IN drone)
Synonyms norethindrone and mestranol
Brand Names Genora® 1/50; Nelova® 1/50M; Norethin 1/50M; Norinyl® 1+50; Ortho-Novum® 1/50
Therapeutic Category Contraceptive, Oral
Use Prevention of pregnancy; treatment of hypermenorrhea, endometriosis, female hypogonadism
Usual Dosage Contraception: Oral: 1 tablet daily, beginning on day 5 of menstrual cycle (first day of menstrual flow is day 1). With 20-tablet and 21-tablet packages, new dosing cycle begins 7 days after last tablet taken; with 28-tablet packages, dosage is 1 tablet daily without interruption; extra tablets are placebos or contain iron. If next menstrual period does not begin on schedule, rule out pregnancy before starting new dosing cycle; if menstrual period begins, start new dosing cycle 7 days after last tablet was taken. If all doses have been taken on schedule and 1 menstrual period is missed, continue dosing cycle; if 2 consecutive menstrual periods are missed, pregnancy test is required before new dosing cycle is started.
Dosage Forms Tablet: Mestranol 0.05 mg and norethindrone 1 mg (21s and 28s)

metacortandralone prednisolone acetate *see prednisolone on page 434*
Metahydrin® *see trichlormethiazide on page 530*
Metamucil® [OTC] *see psyllium on page 451*
Metamucil® Instant Mix [OTC] *see psyllium on page 451*
Metaprel® *see metaproterenol on this page*

metaproterenol (met a proe TER e nol)
Synonyms metaproterenol sulfate; orciprenaline sulfate
Brand Names Alupent®; Arm-a-Med® Metaproterenol; Dey-Dose® Metaproterenol; Metaprel®; Prometa®
Therapeutic Category Adrenergic Agonist Agent
Use Bronchodilator in reversible airway obstruction due to asthma or COPD

Usual Dosage
Oral:
Children:
<2 years: 0.4 mg/kg/dose administered 3-4 times/day; in infants, the dose can be administered every 8-12 hours
2-6 years: 1-2.6 mg/kg/day divided every 6-8 hours
6-9 years: 10 mg/dose administered 3-4 times/day
Children >9 years and Adults: 20 mg/dose administered 3-4 times/day
Inhalation: Children >12 years and Adults: 2-3 inhalations every 3-4 hours, up to 12 inhalations in 24 hours
Nebulizer:
Infants: 6 mg/dose administered over 5 minutes
Children <12 years: 0.01-0.02 mL/kg of 5% solution; diluted in 2-3 mL normal saline every 4-6 hours (may be administered more frequently according to need), maximum dose: 15 mg/dose every 4-6 hours
Adolescents and Adults: 5-20 breaths of full strength 5% metaproterenol or 0.2-0.3 mL of 5% metaproterenol in 2.5-3 mL normal saline nebulized every 4-6 hours (can be administered more frequently according to need)

Dosage Forms
Aerosol, oral, as sulfate: 0.65 mg/dose (5 mL, 10 mL)
Solution for inhalation, as sulfate, preservative free: 0.4% [4 mg/mL] (2.5 mL); 0.6% [6 mg/mL] (2.5 mL); 5% [50 mg/mL] (10 mL, 30 mL)
Syrup, as sulfate: 10 mg/5 mL (480 mL)
Tablet, as sulfate: 10 mg, 20 mg

metaproterenol sulfate *see* metaproterenol *on previous page*

metaraminol (met a RAM i nole)
Synonyms metaraminol bitartrate
Brand Names Aramine®
Therapeutic Category Adrenergic Agonist Agent
Use Acute hypotensive crisis in the treatment of shock
Usual Dosage Adults:
Prevention of hypotension: I.M., S.C.: 2-10 mg
Adjunctive treatment of hypotension: I.V.: 15-100 mg in 250-500 mL NS or 5% dextrose in water
Severe shock: I.V.: 0.5-5 mg direct I.V. injection then use I.M. dose
Dosage Forms Injection, as bitartrate: 10 mg/mL (10 mL)

metaraminol bitartrate *see* metaraminol *on this page*

Metasep® [OTC] *see* parachlorometaxylenol *on page 396*

Metastron® Injection *see* strontium-89 *on page 493*

metaxalone (me TAKS a lone)
Brand Names Skelaxin®
Therapeutic Category Skeletal Muscle Relaxant
Use Relief of discomfort associated with acute, painful musculoskeletal conditions
Usual Dosage Children >12 years and Adults: Oral: 800 mg 3-4 times/day
Dosage Forms Tablet: 400 mg

metformin (met FOR min)
Synonyms metformin hydrochloride
Brand Names Glucophage®
Therapeutic Category Antidiabetic Agent (Oral)
Use Management of noninsulin-dependent diabetes mellitus (type II) as monotherapy when hyperglycemia cannot be managed on diet alone. May be used concomitantly with
(Continued)

metformin *(Continued)*

a sulfonylurea when diet and metformin or sulfonylurea alone do not result in adequate glycemic control.

Usual Dosage Oral (allow 1-2 weeks between dose titrations):

Adults:

500 mg tablets: Initial: 500 mg twice daily (administered with the morning and evening meals). Dosage increases should be made in increments of one tablet every week, administered in divided doses, up to a maximum of 2,500 mg/day. Doses of up to 2000 mg/day may be administered twice daily. If a dose of 2,500 mg/day is required, it may be better tolerated 3 times/day (with meals).

850 mg tablets: Initial: 850 mg once daily (administered with the morning meal). Dosage increases should be made in increments of one tablet every OTHER week, administered in divided doses, up to a maximum of 2550 mg/day. The usual maintenance dose is 850 mg twice daily (with the morning and evening meals). Some patients may be administered 850 mg 3 times/day (with meals).

Elderly patients: The initial and maintenance dosing should be conservative, due to the potential for decreased renal function. Generally, elderly patients should not be titrated to the maximum dose of metformin.

Transfer from other antidiabetic agents: No transition period is generally necessary except when transferring from chlorpropamide. When transferring from chlorpropamide, care should be exercised during the first 2 weeks because of the prolonged retention of chlorpropamide in the body, leading to overlapping drug effects and possible hypoglycemia.

Concomitant metformin and oral sulfonylurea therapy: If patients have not responded to 4 weeks of the maximum dose of metformin monotherapy, consideration to a gradually addition of an oral sulfonylurea while continuing metformin at the maximum dose, even if prior primary or secondary failure to a sulfonylurea has occurred.

Dosage Forms Tablet, as hydrochloride: 500 mg, 850 mg

metformin hydrochloride *see* metformin *on previous page*

methacholine (meth a KOLE leen)

Synonyms methacholine chloride

Brand Names Provocholine®

Therapeutic Category Diagnostic Agent

Use Diagnosis of bronchial airway hyperactivity in subjects who do not have clinically apparent asthma

Usual Dosage The following is a suggested schedule for administration of methacholine challenge. Calculate cumulative units by multiplying number of breaths by concentration given. Total cumulative units is the sum of cumulative units for each concentration given.

Vial	Serial Concentration (mg/mL)	No. of Breaths	Cumulative Units per Concentration	Total Cumulative Units
E	0.025	5	0.125	0.125
D	0.25	5	1.25	1.375
C	2.5	5	12.5	13.88
B	10	5	50	63.88
A	25	5	125	188.88

Dosage Forms Powder for reconstitution, inhalation, as chloride: 100 mg/5 mL

methacholine chloride *see* methacholine *on this page*

methadone (METH a done)
Synonyms methadone hydrochloride
Brand Names Dolophine®
Therapeutic Category Analgesic, Narcotic
Controlled Substance C-II
Use Management of severe pain, used in narcotic detoxification maintenance programs and for the treatment of iatrogenic narcotic dependency
Usual Dosage Doses should be titrated to appropriate effects:
Children: Analgesia:
Oral, I.M., S.C.: 0.7 mg/kg/24 hours divided every 4-6 hours as needed or 0.1-0.2 mg/kg every 4-12 hours as needed; maximum: 10 mg/dose
I.V.: 0.1 mg/kg every 4 hours initially for 2-3 doses, then every 6-12 hours as needed; maximum: 10 mg/dose
Adults:
Analgesia: Oral, I.M., S.C.: 2.5-10 mg every 3-8 hours as needed, up to 5-20 mg every 6-8 hours
Detoxification: Oral: 15-40 mg/day
Maintenance of opiate dependence: Oral: 20-120 mg/day
Dosage Forms
Injection, as hydrochloride: 10 mg/mL (1 mL, 10 mL, 20 mL)
Solution, as hydrochloride:
Oral: 5 mg/5 mL (5 mL, 500 mL); 10 mg/5 mL (500 mL)
Oral, concentrate: 10 mg/mL (30 mL)
Tablet, as hydrochloride: 5 mg, 10 mg
Tablet, dispersible, as hydrochloride: 40 mg

methadone hydrochloride *see* methadone *on this page*

methaminodiazepoxide hydrochloride *see* chlordiazepoxide *on page 109*

methamphetamine (meth am FET a meen)
Synonyms desoxyephedrine hydrochloride; methamphetamine hydrochloride
Brand Names Desoxyn®
Therapeutic Category Amphetamine
Controlled Substance C-II
Use Narcolepsy; exogenous obesity; abnormal behavioral syndrome in children (minimal brain dysfunction)
Usual Dosage Oral:
Attention deficit disorder: Children >6 years: 2.5-5 mg 1-2 times/day, may increase by 5 mg increments weekly until optimum response is achieved, usually 20-25 mg/day
Exogenous obesity: Children >12 years and Adults: 5 mg, 30 minutes before each meal, 10-15 mg in morning; treatment duration should not exceed a few weeks
Dosage Forms Tablet:
As hydrochloride: 5 mg
Extended release, as hydrochloride (Gradumet®): 5 mg, 10 mg, 15 mg

methamphetamine hydrochloride *see* methamphetamine *on this page*

methantheline (meth AN tha leen)
Synonyms methantheline bromide; methanthelinium bromide
Brand Names Banthine®
Therapeutic Category Anticholinergic Agent
Use Adjunctive treatment of peptic ulcer, irritable bowel syndrome, pancreatitis, ureteral and urinary bladder spasm; to reduce duodenal motility during diagnostic radiologic procedures and treatment of an uninhibited neurogenic bladder
Usual Dosage Oral:
Children:
<1 year: 12.5-25 mg 4 times/day
(Continued)

methantheline *(Continued)*
>1 year: 12.5-50 mg 4 times/day
Adults: 50-100 mg every 6 hours
Dosage Forms Tablet, as bromide: 50 mg

methantheline bromide *see* methantheline *on previous page*
methanthelinium bromide *see* methantheline *on previous page*

methazolamide (meth a ZOE la mide)
Brand Names GlaucTabs®; Neptazane®
Therapeutic Category Carbonic Anhydrase Inhibitor
Use Adjunctive treatment of open-angle or secondary glaucoma; short-term therapy of narrow-angle glaucoma when delay of surgery is desired
Usual Dosage Adults: Oral: 50-100 mg 2-3 times/day
Dosage Forms Tablet: 25 mg, 50 mg

methenamine (meth EN a meen)
Synonyms hexamethylenetetramine; methenamine hippurate; methenamine mandelate
Brand Names Hiprex®; Urex®
Therapeutic Category Antibiotic, Miscellaneous
Use Prophylaxis or suppression of recurrent urinary tract infections
Usual Dosage Oral:
Children:
Hippurate: 6-12 years: 25-50 mg/kg/day divided every 12 hours
Mandelate: 50-75 mg/kg/day divided every 6 hours
Adults:
Hippurate: 1 g twice daily
Mandelate: 1 g 4 times/day after meals and at bedtime
Dosage Forms Tablet:
As hippurate (Hiprex®, Urex®): 1 g (Hiprex® contains tartrazine dye)
As mandelate, enteric coated: 250 mg, 500 mg, 1 g

methenamine hippurate *see* methenamine *on this page*
methenamine mandelate *see* methenamine *on this page*
Methergine® *see* methylergonovine *on page 342*

methicillin (meth i SIL in)
Synonyms dimethoxyphenyl penicillin sodium; methicillin sodium; sodium methicillin
Brand Names Staphcillin®
Therapeutic Category Penicillin
Use Treatment of susceptible bacterial infections such as osteomyelitis, septicemia, endocarditis, and CNS infections due to penicillinase-producing strains of *Staphylococcus*
Usual Dosage I.M., I.V.:
Children: 150-200 mg/kg/day divided every 6 hours; 200-400 mg/kg/day divided every 4-6 hours has been used for treatment of severe infections; maximum dose: 12 g/day
Adults: 4-12 g/day in divided doses every 4-6 hours
Dosage Forms Powder for injection, as sodium: 1 g, 4 g, 6 g, 10 g

methicillin sodium *see* methicillin *on this page*

methimazole (meth IM a zole)
Synonyms thiamazole
Brand Names Tapazole®
Therapeutic Category Antithyroid Agent

Use Palliative treatment of hyperthyroidism, to return the hyperthyroid patient to a normal metabolic state prior to thyroidectomy, and to control thyrotoxic crisis that may accompany thyroidectomy

Usual Dosage Oral:
Children: Initial: 0.4 mg/kg/day in 3 divided doses; maintenance: 0.2 mg/kg/day in 3 divided doses
Adults: Initial: 10 mg every 8 hours; maintenance dose ranges from 5-30 mg/day

Dosage Forms Tablet: 5 mg, 10 mg

methionine (me THYE oh neen)

Brand Names Pedameth®

Therapeutic Category Dietary Supplement

Use Treatment of diaper rash and control of odor, dermatitis and ulceration caused by ammoniacal urine

Usual Dosage Oral:
Children: Control of diaper rash: 75 mg in formula or other liquid 3-4 times/day for 3-5 days
Adults:
Control of odor in incontinent adults: 200-400 mg 3-4 times/day
Dietary supplement: 500 mg/day

Dosage Forms
Capsule: 200 mg, 300 mg, 500 mg
Liquid: 75 mg/5 mL (473 mL)
Tablet: 500 mg

methocarbamol (meth oh KAR ba mole)

Brand Names Robaxin®

Therapeutic Category Skeletal Muscle Relaxant

Use Treatment of muscle spasm associated with acute painful musculoskeletal conditions; supportive therapy in tetanus

Usual Dosage
Children: Recommended **only** for use in tetanus I.V.: 15 mg/kg/dose or 500 mg/m^2/dose, may repeat every 6 hours if needed; maximum dose: 1.8 g/m^2/day for 3 days only
Adults: Muscle spasm:
Oral: 1.5 g 4 times/day for 2-3 days, then decrease to 4-4.5 g/day in 3-6 divided doses
I.M., I.V.: 1 g every 8 hours if oral not possible

Dosage Forms
Injection: 100 mg/mL in polyethylene glycol 50% (10 mL)
Tablet: 500 mg, 750 mg

methocarbamol and aspirin (meth oh KAR ba mole & AS pir in)

Brand Names Robaxisal®

Therapeutic Category Skeletal Muscle Relaxant

Use Adjunct to rest, physical therapy, and other measures for the relief of discomfort associated with acute, painful musculoskeletal disorders

Usual Dosage Children >12 years and Adults: Oral: 2 tablets 4 times/day

Dosage Forms Tablet: Methocarbamol 400 mg and aspirin 325 mg

methohexital (meth oh HEKS i tal)

Synonyms methohexital sodium

Brand Names Brevital® Sodium

Therapeutic Category Barbiturate

Controlled Substance C-IV

Use Induction and maintenance of general anesthesia for short procedures

Usual Dosage Doses must be titrated to effect
(Continued)

methohexital *(Continued)*

Children:
I.M.: Preop: 5-10 mg/kg/dose
I.V.: Induction: 1-2 mg/kg/dose
Rectal: Preop/induction: 20-35 mg/kg/dose; usual: 25 mg/kg/dose; administer as 10% aqueous solution
Adults: I.V.: Induction: 50-120 mg to start; 20-40 mg every 4-7 minutes
Dosage Forms Injection, as sodium: 500 mg, 2.5 g, 5 g

methohexital sodium *see* methohexital *on previous page*

methoin *see* mephenytoin *on page 329*

methotrexate *(meth oh TREKS ate)*

Synonyms amethopterin; methotrexate sodium; MTX
Brand Names Folex® PFS; Rheumatrex®
Therapeutic Category Antineoplastic Agent
Use Treatment of trophoblastic neoplasms, leukemias, osteosarcoma, non-Hodgkin's lymphoma; psoriasis, rheumatoid arthritis
Usual Dosage Refer to individual protocols
Children:
High-dose MTX for acute lymphocytic leukemia: I.V.: Loading dose of 200 mg/m^2 and a 24-hour infusion of 1200 mg/m^2/day
Induction of remission in acute lymphoblastic leukemias: Oral, I.M., I.V.: 3.3 mg/m^2/day for 4-6 weeks
Leukemia: Remission maintenance: Oral, I.M.: 20-30 mg/m^2 2 times/week
Juvenile rheumatoid arthritis: Oral: 5-15 mg/m^2/week as a single dose or as 3 divided doses administered 12 hours apart
Osteosarcoma:
I.T.: 10-15 mg/m^2 (maximum dose: 15 mg) by protocol
I.V.: <12 years: 12 g/m^2 (12-18 g); >12 years: 8 g/m^2 (maximum dose: 18 g)
Non-Hodgkin's lymphoma: I.V.: 200-300 mg/m^2
Adults:
Trophoblastic neoplasms: Oral, I.M.: 15-30 mg/day for 5 days, repeat in 7 days for 3-5 courses
Rheumatoid arthritis: Oral: 7.5 mg once weekly or 2.5 mg every 12 hours for 3 doses/week; not to exceed 20 mg/week
Dosage Forms
Injection, as sodium: 2.5 mg/mL (2 mL); 25 mg/mL (2 mL, 4 mL, 8 mL, 10 mL)
Preservative free: 25 mg (2 mL, 4 mL, 8 mL, 10 mL)
Powder, for injection: 20 mg, 25 mg, 50 mg, 100 mg, 250 mg, 1 g
Tablet, as sodium: 2.5 mg
Dose pack: 2.5 mg (4 cards with 2, 3, 4, 5, or 6 tablets each)

methotrexate sodium *see* methotrexate *on this page*

methotrimeprazine *(meth oh trye MEP ra zeen)*

Synonyms levomepromazine; methotrimeprazine hydrochloride
Brand Names Levoprome®
Therapeutic Category Analgesic, Non-narcotic
Use Relief of moderate to severe pain in nonambulatory patients; for analgesia and sedation when respiratory depression is to be avoided, as in obstetrics; preanesthetic for producing sedation, somnolence and relief of apprehension and anxiety
Usual Dosage Adults: I.M.:
Sedation analgesia: 10-20 mg every 4-6 hours as needed
Preoperative medication: 2-20 mg, 45 minutes to 3 hours before surgery
Postoperative analgesia: 2.5-7.5 mg every 4-6 hours is suggested as necessary since residual effects of anesthetic may be present

Pre- and postoperative hypotension: I.M.: 5-10 mg
Dosage Forms Injection, as hydrochloride: 20 mg/mL (10 mL)

methotrimeprazine hydrochloride *see* methotrimeprazine *on previous page*

methoxamine (meth OKS a meen)
Synonyms methoxamine hydrochloride
Brand Names Vasoxyl®
Therapeutic Category Adrenergic Agonist Agent
Use Treatment of hypotension occurring during general anesthesia; to terminate episodes of supraventricular tachycardia; treatment of shock
Usual Dosage Adults:
Emergencies: I.V.: 3-5 mg
Supraventricular tachycardia: I.V.: 10 mg
During spinal anesthesia: I.M.: 10-20 mg
Dosage Forms Injection, as hydrochloride: 20 mg/mL (1 mL)

methoxamine hydrochloride *see* methoxamine *on this page*

methoxsalen (meth OKS a len)
Synonyms methoxypsoralen; 8-mop
Brand Names 8-MOP®; Oxsoralen®; Oxsoralen-Ultra®
Therapeutic Category Psoralen
Use Symptomatic control of severe, recalcitrant, disabling psoriasis in conjunction with long wave ultraviolet radiation; induce repigmentation in vitiligo topical repigmenting agent in conjunction with controlled doses of ultraviolet A (UVA) or sunlight
Usual Dosage
Psoriasis: Adults: Oral: 10-70 mg 1½-2 hours before exposure to ultraviolet light, 2-3 times at least 48 hours apart; dosage is based upon patient's body weight and skin type
Vitiligo: Children >12 years and Adults:
Oral: 20 mg 2-4 hours before exposure to UVA light or sunlight
Topical: Apply lotion 1-2 hours before exposure to UVA light, no more than once weekly
Dosage Forms
Capsule: 10 mg
Lotion: 1% (30 mL)

methoxycinnamate and oxybenzone
(meth OKS ee SIN a mate & oks i BEN zone)
Synonyms sunscreen (paba-free)
Brand Names PreSun® 29 [OTC]; Ti-Screen® [OTC]
Therapeutic Category Sunscreen
Use Reduce the chance of premature aging of the skin and skin cancer from overexposure to the sun
Usual Dosage Topical: Adults: Apply liberally to all exposed areas at least 30 minutes prior to sun exposure
Dosage Forms Lotion:
SPF 15: 120 mL
SPF 29: 120 mL

methoxyflurane (meth oks ee FLOO rane)
Brand Names Penthrane®
Therapeutic Category General Anesthetic
Use Adjunct to provide anesthesia procedures <4 hours in duration
Usual Dosage 0.3% to 0.8% for analgesia and anesthesia, with 0.1% to 2% for maintenance when used with nitrous oxide
(Continued)

339

methoxyflurane *(Continued)*
Dosage Forms Liquid: 15 mL, 125 mL

methoxypsoralen *see methoxsalen on previous page*

methscopolamine (meth skoe POL a meen)
Synonyms methscopolamine bromide
Brand Names Pamine®
Therapeutic Category Anticholinergic Agent
Use Adjunctive therapy in the treatment of peptic ulcer
Usual Dosage Oral: 2.5 mg 30 minutes before meals or food and 2.5-5 mg at bedtime
Dosage Forms Tablet, as bromide: 2.5 mg

methscopolamine bromide *see methscopolamine on this page*

methsuximide (meth SUKS i mide)
Brand Names Celontin®
Therapeutic Category Anticonvulsant
Use Control of absence (petit mal) seizures; useful adjunct in refractory, partial complex (psychomotor) seizures
Usual Dosage Oral:
Children: Initial: 10-15 mg/kg/day in 3-4 divided doses; increase weekly up to maximum of 30 mg/kg/day
Adults: 300 mg/day for the first week; may increase by 300 mg/day at weekly intervals up to 1.2 g in 2-4 divided doses/day
Dosage Forms Capsule: 150 mg, 300 mg

methyclothiazide (meth i kloe THYR a zide)
Brand Names Aquatensen®; Enduron®
Therapeutic Category Diuretic, Thiazide
Use Management of mild to moderate hypertension; treatment of edema in congestive heart failure and nephrotic syndrome
Usual Dosage Adults: Oral:
Edema: 2.5-10 mg/day
Hypertension: 2.5-5 mg/day
Dosage Forms Tablet: 2.5 mg, 5 mg

methyclothiazide and deserpidine
(meth i kloe THYE a zide & de SER pi deen)
Brand Names Enduronyl®; Enduronyl® Forte
Therapeutic Category Antihypertensive, Combination
Use Management of mild to moderately severe hypertension
Usual Dosage Oral: Individualized, normally 1-4 tablets/day
Dosage Forms Tablet: Methyclothiazide 5 mg and deserpidine 0.25 mg; methyclothiazide 5 mg and deserpidine 0.5 mg

methyclothiazide and pargyline (meth i kloe THYE a zide & PAR gi leen)
Synonyms pargyline and methyclothiazide
Brand Names Eutron®
Therapeutic Category Antihypertensive, Combination
Use Management of hypertension
Usual Dosage Oral: Individualized, normally 1-4 tablets/day
Dosage Forms Tablet: Methyclothiazide 5 mg and pargyline hydrochloride 25 mg

methylacetoxyprogesterone *see medroxyprogesterone acetate on page 326*

methylbenzethonium chloride (meth il ben ze THOE nee um KLOR ide)
Brand Names Diaparene® [OTC]; Puri-Clens™ [OTC]; Sween Cream® [OTC]
Therapeutic Category Topical Skin Product
Use Treatment of diaper rash and ammonia dermatitis
Usual Dosage Topical: Apply to area as needed
Dosage Forms
Cream: 0.1% (30 g, 60 g, 120 g)
Ointment, topical: 0.1% (30 g, 60 g, 120 g)
Powder: 0.055% (120 g, 270 g, 420 g)

methylcellulose (meth il SEL yoo lose)
Brand Names Citrucel® [OTC]
Therapeutic Category Laxative
Use Adjunct in treatment of constipation
Usual Dosage Oral:
Children: 5-10 mL 1-2 times/day
Adults: 5-20 mL 3 times/day
Dosage Forms Powder: 105 mg/g

methyldopa (meth il DOE pa)
Synonyms methyldopate hydrochloride
Brand Names Aldomet®
Therapeutic Category Alpha-Adrenergic Blocking Agent
Use Management of moderate to severe hypertension
Usual Dosage
Children:
Oral: Initial: 10 mg/kg/day in 2-4 divided doses; increase every 2 days as needed to maximum dose of 65 mg/kg/day; do not exceed 3 g/day
I.V.: 5-10 mg/kg/dose every 6-8 hours
Adults:
Oral: Initial: 250 mg 2-3 times/day; increase every 2 days as needed; usual dose 1-1.5 g/day in 2-4 divided doses; maximum dose: 3 g/day
I.V.: 250-1000 mg every 6-8 hours
Dosage Forms
Injection, as methyldopate hydrochloride: 50 mg/mL (5 mL, 10 mL)
Suspension, oral: 250 mg/5 mL (5 mL, 473 mL)
Tablet: 125 mg, 250 mg, 500 mg

methyldopa and chlorothiazide *see* chlorothiazide and methyldopa *on* *page 111*

methyldopa and hydrochlorothiazide
(meth il DOE pa & hye droe klor oh THYE a zide)
Synonyms hydrochlorothiazide and methyldopa
Brand Names Aldoril®
Therapeutic Category Antihypertensive, Combination
Use Management of moderate to severe hypertension
Usual Dosage Oral: 1 tablet 2-3 times/day for first 48 hours, then decrease or increase at intervals of not less than 2 days until an adequate response is achieved
Dosage Forms Tablet:
15: Methyldopa 250 mg and hydrochlorothiazide 15 mg
25: Methyldopa 250 mg and hydrochlorothiazide 25 mg
D50: Methyldopa 500 mg and hydrochlorothiazide 50 mg

methyldopate hydrochloride *see* methyldopa *on this page*

methylene blue (METH i leen bloo)
Brand Names Urolene Blue®
Therapeutic Category Antidote
Use Antidote for cyanide poisoning and drug-induced methemoglobinemia, indicator dye, bacteriostatic genitourinary antiseptic
Usual Dosage
Children:
NADH-methemoglobin reductase deficiency: Oral: 1.5-5 mg/kg/day (maximum: 300 mg/day) administered with 5-8 mg/kg/day of ascorbic acid
Methemoglobinemia: I.V.: 1-2 mg/kg over several minutes
Adults:
Genitourinary antiseptic: Oral: 55-130 mg 3 times/day (maximum: 390 mg/day)
Methemoglobinemia: I.V.: 1-2 mg/kg over several minutes; may be repeated in 1 hour if necessary
Dosage Forms
Injection: 10 mg/mL (1 mL, 10 mL)
Tablet: 65 mg

methylergometrine maleate *see* methylergonovine *on this page*

methylergonovine (meth il er goe NOE veen)
Synonyms methylergometrine maleate; methylergonovine maleate
Brand Names Methergine®
Therapeutic Category Ergot Alkaloid
Use Prevention and treatment of postpartum and postabortion hemorrhage caused by uterine atony or subinvolution
Usual Dosage Adults:
Oral: 0.2-0.4 mg every 6-12 hours for 2-7 days
I.M., I.V.: 0.2 mg every 2-4 hours for 5 doses then change to oral dosage
Dosage Forms
Injection, as maleate: 0.2 mg/mL (1 mL)
Tablet, as maleate: 0.2 mg

methylergonovine maleate *see* methylergonovine *on this page*

methylmorphine *see* codeine *on page 134*

methylphenidate (meth il FEN i date)
Synonyms methylphenidate hydrochloride
Brand Names Ritalin®; Ritalin-SR®
Therapeutic Category Central Nervous System Stimulant, Nonamphetamine
Controlled Substance C-II
Use Attention deficit disorder with hyperactivity (ADDH); narcolepsy
Usual Dosage Oral:
Children ≥6 years: Attention deficit disorder: Initial: 0.3 mg/kg/dose or 2.5-5 mg/dose administered before breakfast and lunch; increase by 0.1 mg/kg/dose or by 5-10 mg/day at weekly intervals; usual dose: 0.5-1 mg/kg/day; maximum dose: 2 mg/kg/day or 60 mg/day
Adults: Narcolepsy: 10 mg 2-3 times/day, up to 60 mg/day
Dosage Forms
Tablet, as hydrochloride: 5 mg, 10 mg, 20 mg
Sustained release: 20 mg

methylphenidate hydrochloride *see* methylphenidate *on this page*

methylphenobarbital *see* mephobarbital *on page 329*

methylphenylethylhydantoin *see* mephenytoin *on page 329*

methylphenyl isoxazolyl penicillin *see* oxacillin *on page 387*

methylphytyl napthoquinone *see* phytonadione *on page 416*

methylprednisolone (meth il pred NIS oh lone)

Synonyms 6-α-methylprednisolone; methylprednisolone acetate; methylprednisolone sodium succinate

Brand Names Adlone® Injection; A-methaPred® Injection; depMedalone® Injection; Depoject® Injection; Depo-Medrol® Injection; Depopred® Injection; D-Med® Injection; Duralone® Injection; Medralone® Injection; Medrol® Oral; M-Prednisol® Injection; Solu-Medrol® Injection

Therapeutic Category Adrenal Corticosteroid

Use Anti-inflammatory or immunosuppressant agent in the treatment of a variety of diseases including those of hematologic, allergic, inflammatory, neoplastic, and autoimmune origin

Usual Dosage Methylprednisolone sodium succinate is highly soluble and has a rapid effect by I.M. and I.V. routes. Methylprednisolone acetate has a low solubility and has a sustained I.M. effect.

Children:
Anti-inflammatory or immunosuppressive: Oral, I.M., I.V. (sodium succinate): 0.16-0.8 mg/kg/day or 5-25 mg/m²/day in divided doses every 6-12 hours
Status asthmaticus: I.V. (sodium succinate): Loading dose: 2 mg/kg/dose, then 0.5-1 mg/kg/dose every 6 hours for up to 5 days
Lupus nephritis: I.V. (sodium succinate): 30 mg/kg every other day for 6 doses
Adults:
Anti-inflammatory or immunosuppressive: Oral: 4-48 mg/day to start, followed by gradual reduction in dosage to the lowest possible level consistent with maintaining an adequate clinical response
I.M. (sodium succinate): 10-80 mg/day once daily
I.M. (acetate): 40-120 mg every 1-2 weeks
I.V. (sodium succinate): 10-40 mg over a period of several minutes and repeated I.V. or I.M. at intervals depending on clinical response; when high dosages are needed, administer 30 mg/kg over a period of 10-20 minutes and may be repeated every 4-6 hours for 48 hours
Status asthmaticus: I.V. (sodium succinate): Loading dose: 2 mg/kg/dose, then 0.5-1 mg/kg/dose every hours for up to 5 days
Lupus nephritis:
I.V. (sodium succinate): 1 g/day for 3 days
Intra-articular (acetate):
Large joints: 20-80 mg
Small joints: 4-10 mg
Intralesional (acetate): 20-60 mg

Dosage Forms
Injection:
As acetate: 20 mg/mL (5 mL, 10 mL); 40 mg/mL (1 mL, 5 mL, 10 mL); 80 mg/mL (1 mL, 5 mL)
As sodium succinate: 40 mg (1 mL, 3 mL); 125 mg (2 mL, 5 mL); 500 mg (1 mL, 4 mL, 8 mL, 20 mL); 1000 mg (1 mL, 8 mL, 50 mL); 2000 mg (30.6 mL)
Tablet: 2 mg, 4 mg, 8 mg, 16 mg, 24 mg, 32 mg
Dose pack: 4 mg (21s)

6-α-methylprednisolone *see* methylprednisolone *on this page*

methylprednisolone acetate *see* methylprednisolone *on this page*

methylprednisolone sodium succinate *see* methylprednisolone *on this page*

methyltestosterone (meth il tes TOS te rone)

Brand Names Android®; Oreton® Methyl; Testred®; Virilon®

Therapeutic Category Androgen

(Continued)

methyltestosterone *(Continued)*

Use
Male: Hypogonadism; delayed puberty; impotence and climacteric symptoms
Female: Palliative treatment of metastatic breast cancer; postpartum breast pain and/or engorgement

Usual Dosage Adults:
Male:
Oral: 10-40 mg/day
Buccal: 5-20 mg/day
Female:
Breast pain/engorgement:
Oral: 80 mg/day for 3-5 days
Buccal: 40 mg/day for 3-5 days
Breast cancer:
Oral: 200 mg/day
Buccal: 100 mg/day

Dosage Forms
Capsule: 10 mg
Tablet: 10 mg, 25 mg
Buccal: 5 mg, 10 mg

methysergide (meth i SER jide)

Synonyms methysergide maleate
Brand Names Sansert®
Therapeutic Category Ergot Alkaloid
Use Prophylaxis of vascular headache
Usual Dosage Oral: 4-8 mg/day with meals; if no improvement is noted after 3 weeks, drug is unlikely to be beneficial; must not be administered continuously for longer than 6 months, and a drug-free interval of 3-4 weeks must follow each 6-month course; dosage should be tapered over the 2- to 3-week period before drug discontinuation to avoid rebound headaches
Dosage Forms Tablet, as maleate: 2 mg

methysergide maleate *see methysergide on this page*

Meticorten® *see prednisone on page 436*

Metimyd® **Ophthalmic** *see sulfacetamide sodium and prednisolone on page 497*

metipranolol (met i PRAN oh lol)

Synonyms metipranolol hydrochloride
Brand Names OptiPranolol® Ophthalmic
Therapeutic Category Beta-Adrenergic Blocker
Use Agent for lowering intraocular pressure
Usual Dosage Adults: Ophthalmic: 1 drop in the affected eye(s) twice daily
Dosage Forms Solution, ophthalmic, as hydrochloride: 0.3% (5 mL, 10 mL)

metipranolol hydrochloride *see metipranolol on this page*

metoclopramide (met oh kloe PRA mide)

Brand Names Clopra®; Maxolon®; Octamide® PFS; Reglan®
Therapeutic Category Gastrointestinal Agent, Prokinetic
Use Gastroesophageal reflux; prevention of nausea associated with chemotherapy; facilitates intubation of the small intestine and symptomatic treatment of diabetic gastric stasis

Usual Dosage

Children:

Gastroesophageal reflux: Oral: 0.1 mg/kg/dose up to 4 times/day; efficacy of continuing metoclopramide beyond 12 weeks in reflux has not been determined; total daily dose should not exceed 0.5 mg/kg/day

Gastrointestinal hypomotility: Oral, I.M., I.V.: 0.1 mg/kg/dose up to 4 times/day, not to exceed 0.5 mg/kg/day

Antiemetic: I.V.: 1-2 mg/kg 30 minutes before chemotherapy and every 2-4 hours

Facilitate intubation: I.V.: <6 years: 0.1 mg/kg; 6-14 years: 2.5-5 mg

Adults:

Stasis/reflux: Oral: 10-15 mg/dose up to 4 times/day 30 minutes before meals or food and at bedtime; efficacy of continuing metoclopramide beyond 12 weeks in reflux has not been determined

Gastrointestinal hypomotility: Oral, I.M., I.V.: 10 mg 30 minutes before each meal and at bedtime

Antiemetic: I.V.: 1-2 mg/kg 30 minutes before chemotherapy and every 2-4 hours

Facilitate intubation: I.V.: 10 mg

Dosage Forms

Injection: 5 mg/mL (2 mL, 10 mL, 30 mL, 50 mL, 100 mL)

Solution, oral, concentrated: 10 mg/mL (10 mL, 30 mL)

Syrup, sugar free: 5 mg/5 mL (10 mL, 480 mL)

Tablet: 5 mg, 10 mg

metocurine iodide (met oh KYOOR een EYE oh dide)

Synonyms dimethyl tubocurarine iodide

Brand Names Metubine® Iodide

Therapeutic Category Skeletal Muscle Relaxant

Use Adjunct to anesthesia to induce skeletal muscle relaxation

Usual Dosage

Children:

Chronic respiratory paralysis in neonates: Start 0.25-0.5 mg/kg/dose (repeat once if paralysis is not achieved in 3 minutes); maintenance: repeat previous dose as soon as movement is observed. The dose should be titrated to achieve a dosage interval of 3-4 hours, then plateau at 10-20 mg/kg/24 hours

Neuromuscular blockade for surgery: Initial: 0.2-0.4 mg/kg/dose; maintenance: 0.1-0.25 mg/kg/dose every 25-90 minutes

Adults:

Surgery: 0.2-0.4 mg/kg (initial); supplement dose: 0.5-1 mg; use of anesthetics that potentiate effect of neuromuscular blocking drug requires less metocurine

Electric shock therapy: 1.75-5.5 mg

Dosage Forms Injection: 2 mg/mL (20 mL)

metolazone (me TOLE a zone)

Brand Names Mykrox®; Zaroxolyn®

Therapeutic Category Diuretic, Miscellaneous

Use Management of mild to moderate hypertension; treatment of edema in congestive heart failure, nephrotic syndrome, and impaired renal function

Usual Dosage Oral:

Children: 0.2-0.4 mg/kg/day divided every 12-24 hours

Adults:

Edema: 5-20 mg/dose every 24 hours

Hypertension: 2.5-5 mg/dose every 24 hours

Dosage Forms Tablet:

Zaroxolyn® (slow acting): 2.5 mg, 5 mg, 10 mg

Mykrox® (rapidly acting): 0.5 mg

Metopirone® *see* metyrapone *on page 347*

metoprolol (me toe PROE lole)
Synonyms metoprolol tartrate
Brand Names Lopressor®; Toprol XL®
Therapeutic Category Beta-Adrenergic Blocker
Use Treatment of hypertension and angina pectoris; prevention of myocardial infarction; selective inhibitor of beta$_1$-adrenergic receptors
Usual Dosage Safety and efficacy in children have not been established.
Children: Oral: 1-5 mg/kg/24 hours divided twice daily; allow 3 days between dose adjustments
Adults:
Oral: 100-450 mg/day in 2-3 divided doses, begin with 50 mg twice daily and increase doses at weekly intervals to desired effect
I.V.: 5 mg every 2 minutes for 3 doses in early treatment of myocardial infarction; thereafter administer 50 mg orally every 6 hours 15 minutes after last I.V. dose and continue for 48 hours; then administer a maintenance dose of 100 mg twice daily
Dosage Forms
Injection, as tartrate: 1 mg/mL (5 mL)
Tablet, as tartrate: 50 mg, 100 mg
Sustained release: 50 mg, 100 mg, 200 mg

metoprolol tartrate see metoprolol on this page

Metrodin® Injection see urofollitropin on page 543

MetroGel® Topical see metronidazole on this page

MetroGel®-Vaginal see metronidazole on this page

Metro I.V.® Injection see metronidazole on this page

metronidazole (me troe NI da zole)
Synonyms metronidazole hydrochloride
Brand Names Flagyl®; MetroGel® Topical; MetroGel®-Vaginal; Metro I.V.® Injection; Protostat® Oral
Therapeutic Category Amebicide; Antibiotic, Topical; Antibiotic, Miscellaneous; Antiprotozoal
Use Treatment of susceptible anaerobic bacterial and protozoal infections in the following conditions: amebiasis (liver abscess, dysentery), giardiasis, symptomatic and asymptomatic trichomoniasis; skin and skin structure infections, CNS infections, intra-abdominal infections, and systemic anaerobic bacterial infections; topically for the treatment of acne rosacea; treatment of antibiotic-associated pseudomembranous colitis (AAPC) caused by *C. difficile*; bacterial vaginosis
Usual Dosage
Infants and Children:
Amebiasis: Oral: 35-50 mg/kg/day in divided doses every 8 hours
Other parasitic infections: Oral: 15-30 mg/kg/day in divided doses every 8 hours
Anaerobic infections: Oral, I.V.: 30 mg/kg/day in divided doses every 6 hours
Clostridium difficile (antibiotic-associated colitis): Oral: 20 mg/kg/day divided every 6 hours
Maximum dose: 2 g/day
Adults:
Amebiasis: Oral: 500-750 mg every 8 hours
Other parasitic infections: Oral: 250 mg every 8 hours or 2 g as a single dose
Anaerobic infections: Oral, I.V.: 30 mg/kg/day in divided doses every 6 hours; not to exceed 4 g/day
AAPC: Oral: 250-500 mg 3-4 times/day for 10-14 days
Topical: Apply a thin film twice daily to affected areas
Vaginal: One applicatorful in vagina each morning and evening, as needed
Dosage Forms
Capsule: 375 mg

Gel:
Topical: 0.75% [7.5 mg/mL] (30 g)
Vaginal: 0.75% (5 g applicator delivering 37.5 mg in 70 g tube)
Injection, ready-to-use: 5 mg/mL (100 mL)
Powder for injection, as hydrochloride: 500 mg
Tablet: 250 mg, 500 mg

metronidazole hydrochloride *see* metronidazole *on previous page*

Metubine® Iodide *see* metocurine iodide *on page 345*

metyrapone (me TEER a pone)

Synonyms metyrapone tartrate
Brand Names Metopirone®
Therapeutic Category Diagnostic Agent
Use Diagnostic test for hypothalamic-pituitary ACTH function
Usual Dosage Oral:
Children: 15 mg/kg every 4 hours for 6 doses; minimum dose: 250 mg
Adults: 750 mg every 4 hours for 6 doses
Dosage Forms Capsule, as tartrate: 250 mg

metyrapone tartrate *see* metyrapone *on this page*

metyrosine (me TYE roe seen)

Synonyms AMPT; OGMT
Brand Names Demser®
Therapeutic Category Tyrosine Hydroxylase Inhibitor
Use Short-term management of pheochromocytoma before surgery, long-term management when surgery is contraindicated or when malignant
Usual Dosage Children >12 years and Adults: Oral: Initial: 250 mg 4 times/day, increased by 250-500 mg/day up to 4 g/day; maintenance: 2-3 g/day in 4 divided doses; for preoperative preparation, administer optimum effective dosage for 5-7 days
Dosage Forms Capsule: 250 mg

Mevacor® *see* lovastatin *on page 315*

mevinolin *see* lovastatin *on page 315*

mexiletine (MEKS i le teen)

Brand Names Mexitil®
Therapeutic Category Antiarrhythmic Agent, Class I-B
Use Management of serious ventricular arrhythmias; suppression of PVCs
Unlabeled use: Diabetic neuropathy
Usual Dosage Oral:
Children: Range: 1.4-5 mg/kg/dose (mean: 3.3 mg/kg/dose) administered every 8 hours; start with lower initial dose and increase according to effects and serum concentrations
Adults: Initial: 200 mg every 8 hours (may load with 400 mg if necessary); adjust dose every 2-3 days; usual dose: 200-300 mg every 8 hours; maximum dose: 1.2 g/day (some patients respond to every 12-hour dosing)
Dosage Forms Capsule: 150 mg, 200 mg, 250 mg

Mexitil® *see* mexiletine *on this page*

Mezlin® *see* mezlocillin *on this page*

mezlocillin (mez loe SIL in)

Synonyms mezlocillin sodium
Brand Names Mezlin®
Therapeutic Category Penicillin
(Continued)

mezlocillin *(Continued)*

Use Treatment of infections caused by susceptible gram-negative aerobic bacilli (*Klebsiella, Proteus, Escherichia coli, Enterobacter, Pseudomonas aeruginosa, Serratia*) involving the skin and skin structure, bone and joint, respiratory tract, urinary tract, gastrointestinal tract, as well as septicemia

Usual Dosage I.M., I.V.:

Children: 200-300 mg/kg/day divided every 4-6 hours; maximum: 24 g/day

Adults:

Uncomplicated urinary tract infection: 1.5-2 g every 6 hours

Serious infections: 3-4 g every 4-6 hours

Dosage Forms Powder for injection, as sodium: 1 g, 2 g, 3 g, 4 g, 20 g

mezlocillin sodium *see* mezlocillin *on previous page*

Miacalcin® Injection *see* calcitonin *on page 81*

Miacalcin® Nasal Spray *see* calcitonin *on page 81*

mibefradil *(mi be FRA dil)*

Synonyms mibefradil dihydrochloride; mibefradilum

Brand Names Posicor®

Therapeutic Category Vasodilator

Use Treatment of hypertension, alone or in combination with other antihypertensive agents; chronic stable angina pectoris, alone or in combination with other antianginal drugs

Usual Dosage Oral: 50-100 mg/day; larger dose is, on average, more effective; doses >100 mg offer little or no additional benefit and induce a great rate of adverse reactions; can be taken with or without food

Hypertension: 50 mg once daily; titrate to 100 mg once daily based on blood pressure response; full effect of given dose level is generally seen after 1-2 weeks

Chronic stable angina pectoris: 50 mg once daily

Dosage Forms Tablet, as dihydrochloride: 50 mg, 100 mg

mibefradil dihydrochloride *see* mibefradil *on this page*

mibefradilum *see* mibefradil *on this page*

Micanol® Cream *see* anthralin *on page 36*

Micatin® Topical [OTC] *see* miconazole *on this page*

miconazole *(mi KON a zole)*

Synonyms miconazole nitrate

Brand Names Absorbine® Antifungal Foot Powder [OTC]; Breezee® Mist Antifungal [OTC]; Femizol-M® [OTC]; Fungoid® Creme; Fungoid® Tincture; Lotrimin® AF Powder [OTC]; Lotrimin® AF Spray Liquid [OTC]; Lotrimin® AF Spray Powder [OTC]; Maximum Strength Desenex® Antifungal Cream [OTC]; Micatin® Topical [OTC]; Monistat-Derm™ Topical; Monistat i.v.™ Injection; Monistat™ Vaginal; Ony-Clear® Spray; Prescription Strength Desenex® [OTC]; Zeasorb-AF® Powder [OTC]

Therapeutic Category Antifungal Agent

Use

I.V.: Treatment of severe systemic fungal infections and fungal meningitis due to susceptible *Cryptococcus* neoformans, *Candida albicans*, *Candida tropicalis*, *Candida parapsilosis*, *Coccidioides immitis*, and *Histoplasma capsulatum* that are refractory to standard treatment

Topical: Treatment of vulvovaginal candidiasis; topical treatment of superficial fungal infections

Usual Dosage

Children:

I.V.: 20-40 mg/kg/day divided every 8 hours

Topical: Apply twice daily for 2-4 weeks

Vaginal: Insert contents of one applicator of vaginal cream or 100 mg suppository at bedtime for 7 days, or 200 mg suppository at bedtime for 3 days
Adults:
I.T.: 20 mg every 3-7 days
I.V.: Candidiasis: 600-1800 mg/day divided every 8 hours
Topical: Apply twice daily for 2-4 weeks
Vaginal: Insert contents of one applicator of vaginal cream or 100 mg suppository at bedtime for 7 days, or 200 mg suppository at bedtime for 3 days
Coccidioidomycosis: 1800-3600 mg/day divided every 8 hours
Cryptococcosis: 1200-2400 mg/day divided every 8 hours
Paracoccidioidomycosis: 200-1200 mg/day divided every 8 hours
Dosage Forms
Cream:
Topical, as nitrate: 2% (15 g, 30 g, 56.7 g, 85 g)
Vaginal, as nitrate: 2% (45 g is equivalent to 7 doses)
Injection: 1% [10 mg/mL] (20 mL)
Lotion, as nitrate: 2% (30 mL, 60 mL)
Powder, topical: 2% (45 g, 90 g, 113 g)
Spray, topical: 2% (105 mL)
Suppository, vaginal, as nitrate: 100 mg (7s); 200 mg (3s)
Tincture: 2% with alcohol (7.39 mL, 29.57 mL)

miconazole nitrate *see* miconazole *on previous page*

MICRhoGAM™ *see* Rh₀(D) immune globulin *on page 463*

microfibrillar collagen hemostat
(mye kro Fl bri lar KOL la jen HEE moe stat)
Synonyms mch
Brand Names Avitene®; Helistat®; Hemotene®
Therapeutic Category Hemostatic Agent
Use Adjunct to hemostasis when control of bleeding by ligature is ineffective or impractical
Usual Dosage Apply dry directly to source of bleeding
Dosage Forms
Fibrous: 1 g, 5 g
Nonwoven web: 70 mm x 70 mm x 1 mm; 70 mm x 35 mm x 1 mm
Sponge: 1" x 2" (10s); 3" x 4" (10s); 9" x 10" (5s)

Micro-K® 10 *see* potassium chloride *on page 427*

Micro-K Extencaps® *see* potassium chloride *on page 427*

Micro-K® LS *see* potassium chloride *on page 427*

Microlipid™ [OTC] *see* enteral nutritional products *on page 194*

Micronase® *see* glyburide *on page 243*

Micronor® *see* norethindrone *on page 378*

Microzide® *see* hydrochlorothiazide *on page 264*

Midamor® *see* amiloride *on page 24*

midazolam (MID aye zoe lam)
Synonyms midazolam hydrochloride
Brand Names Versed®
Therapeutic Category Benzodiazepine
Controlled Substance C-IV
Use Preoperative sedation; conscious sedation prior to diagnostic or radiographic procedures
Usual Dosage The dose of midazolam needs to be individualized based on the patient's age, underlying diseases, and concurrent medications. Personnel and equipment
(Continued)

midazolam *(Continued)*

needed for standard respiratory resuscitation should be immediately available during midazolam administration.

Children:
Preoperative sedation:
I.M.: 0.07-0.08 mg/kg 30-60 minutes presurgery
I.V.: 0.035 mg/kg/dose, repeat over several minutes as required to achieve the desired sedative effect up to a total dose of 0.1-0.2 mg/kg
Conscious sedation during mechanical ventilation: I.V.: Loading dose: 0.05-0.2 mg/kg then follow with initial continuous infusion: 1-2 mcg/kg/minute; titrate to the desired effect; usual range: 0.4-6 mcg/kg/minute
Conscious sedation for procedures:
Oral, Intranasal: 0.2-0.4 mg/kg (maximum: 15 mg) 30-45 minutes before the procedure
I.V.: 0.05 mg/kg 3 minutes before procedure
Adolescents >12 years: I.V.: 0.5 mg every 3-4 minutes until effect achieved
Adults:
Preoperative sedation: I.M.: 0.07-0.08 mg/kg 30-60 minutes presurgery; usual dose: 5 mg
Conscious sedation: I.V.: Initial: 0.5-2 mg slow I.V. over at least 2 minutes; slowly titrate to effect by repeating doses every 2-3 minutes if needed; usual total dose: 2.5-5 mg; use decreased doses in elderly patients
Adults, healthy <60 years: Some patients respond to doses as low as 1 mg; no more than 2.5 mg should be administered over a period of 2 minutes. Additional doses of midazolam may be administered after a 2-minute waiting period and evaluation of sedation after each dose increment. A total dose >5 mg is generally not needed. If narcotics or other CNS depressants are administered concomitantly, the midazolam dose should be reduced by 30%.
Dosage Forms Injection, as hydrochloride: 1 mg/mL (2 mL, 5 mL, 10 mL); 5 mg/mL (1 mL, 2 mL, 5 mL, 10 mL)

midazolam hydrochloride *see* midazolam *on previous page*

Midchlor® *see* acetaminophen, isometheptene, and dichloralphenazone *on page 6*

midodrine (MI doe dreen)

Synonyms midodrine hydrochloride
Brand Names ProAmatine™
Therapeutic Category Alpha-Adrenergic Agonist
Use Treatment of symptomatic orthostatic hypotension in patients whose lives are considerably impaired despite standard clinical care.
Usual Dosage Adults: Oral: 10 mg 3 times/day (every 3-4 hours); dosing should take place during daytime hours, when the patient needs to be upright, pursuing activities of daily living; a suggested dosing schedule is as follows:
Dose 1: Shortly before or upon rising in the morning
Dose 2: At midday
Dose 3: In the late afternoon (not later the 6 PM)
Dosage Forms Tablet, as hydrochloride: 2.5 mg, 5 mg

midodrine hydrochloride *see* midodrine *on this page*

Midol® IB [OTC] *see* ibuprofen *on page 278*

Midol® PM [OTC] *see* acetaminophen and diphenhydramine *on page 4*

Midrin® *see* acetaminophen, isometheptene, and dichloralphenazone *on page 6*

miglitol
Brand Names Glyset®
Therapeutic Category Antidiabetic Agent (Oral)
Use As an adjunct to diet to lower blood glucose in patients with noninsulin-dependent diabetes mellitus (NIDDM)
Usual Dosage Oral: Adults: 25 mg three times/day with the first bite of food at each meal; the dose may be increased to 50 mg three times/day after 4-8 weeks; maximum recommended dose is 100 mg three times/day
Dosage Forms Tablet: 25 mg, 50 mg, 100 mg

Migratine® *see* acetaminophen, isometheptene, and dichloralphenazone *on page 6*

mih *see* procarbazine *on page 439*

Miles Nervine® Caplets [OTC] *see* diphenhydramine *on page 173*

milk of magnesia *see* magnesium hydroxide *on page 319*

Milontin® *see* phensuximide *on page 411*

Milophene® *see* clomiphene *on page 129*

milrinone (MIL ri none)
Synonyms milrinone lactate
Brand Names Primacor®
Therapeutic Category Cardiovascular Agent, Other
Use Short-term I.V. therapy of congestive heart failure
Usual Dosage Adults: I.V.: Loading dose: 50 mcg/kg administered over 10 minutes, then 0.375-0.75 mcg/kg/min as a continuous infusion for a total daily dose of 0.59-1.13 mg/kg
Dosage Forms Injection, as lactate: 1 mg/mL (5 mL, 10 mL, 20 mL)

milrinone lactate *see* milrinone *on this page*

Miltown® *see* meprobamate *on page 330*

Minidyne® [OTC] *see* povidone-iodine *on page 431*

Mini-Gamulin® Rh *see* Rh$_o$(D) immune globulin *on page 463*

Minipress® *see* prazosin *on page 433*

Minitran™ Patch *see* nitroglycerin *on page 376*

Minizide® *see* prazosin and polythiazide *on page 434*

Minocin® IV Injection *see* minocycline *on this page*

Minocin® Oral *see* minocycline *on this page*

minocycline (mi noe SYE kleen)
Synonyms minocycline hydrochloride
Brand Names Dynacin® Oral; Minocin® IV Injection; Minocin® Oral; Vectrin®
Therapeutic Category Tetracycline Derivative
Use Treatment of susceptible bacterial infections of both gram-negative and gram-positive organisms; acne
Usual Dosage
Children 8-12 years: 4 mg/kg stat, then 4 mg/kg/day (maximum: 200 mg/day) in divided doses every 12 hours
Adults:
Infection: Oral, I.V.: 200 mg stat, 100 mg every 12 hours
Acne: Oral: 50 mg 1-3 times/day
Dosage Forms
Capsule:
As hydrochloride: 50 mg, 100 mg
As hydrochloride (Dynacin®): 50 mg, 100 mg
(Continued)

minocycline *(Continued)*

Pellet-filled, as hydrochloride (Minocin®): 50 mg, 100 mg
Injection, as hydrochloride (Minocin® IV): 100 mg
Suspension, oral, as hydrochloride (Minocin®)50 mg/5 mL (60 mL)

minocycline hydrochloride *see* minocycline *on previous page*

minoxidil (mi NOKS i dil)

Brand Names Loniten®; Rogaine® for Men [OTC]; Rogaine® for Women [OTC]
Therapeutic Category Topical Skin Product; Vasodilator
Use Management of severe hypertension; topically for management of alopecia or male
pattern alopecia
Usual Dosage
Children <12 years: Hypertension: Oral: Initial: 0.1-0.2 mg/kg once daily; maximum: 5
mg/day; increase gradually every 3 days; usual dosage: 0.25-1 mg/kg/day in 1-2
divided doses; maximum: 50 mg/day
Adults:
Hypertension: Oral: Initial: 5 mg once daily, increase gradually every 3 days; usual
dose: 10-40 mg/day in 1-2 divided doses; maximum: 100 mg/day
Alopecia: Topical: Apply twice daily
Dosage Forms
Solution, topical: 2% = 20 mg/metered dose (60 mL)
Tablet: 2.5 mg, 10 mg

Mintezol® *see* thiabendazole *on page 514*

Minute-Gel® *see* fluoride *on page 228*

Miochol-E® *see* acetylcholine *on page 8*

Miostat® Intraocular *see* carbachol *on page 89*

Mirapex® *see* pramipexole *on page 432*

mirtazapine (mir TAZ a peen)

Brand Names Remeron®
Therapeutic Category Antidepressant, Selective Serotonin Reuptake Inhibitor
Use Treatment of depression, works through noradrenergic and serotonergic pharmaco-
logic action
Usual Dosage Adults: Oral: Initial: 15 mg/day, then 15-45 mg/day
Dosage Forms Tablet: 15 mg, 30 mg

misoprostol (mye soe PROST ole)

Brand Names Cytotec®
Therapeutic Category Prostaglandin
Use Prevention of NSAID-induced gastric ulcers
Usual Dosage Oral: 200 mcg 4 times/day with food
Dosage Forms Tablet: 100 mcg, 200 mcg

Mithracin® *see* plicamycin *on page 421*

mithramycin *see* plicamycin *on page 421*

mitomycin (mye toe MYE sin)

Synonyms mitomycin-c; mtc
Brand Names Mutamycin®
Therapeutic Category Antineoplastic Agent
Use Therapy of disseminated adenocarcinoma of stomach, colon, or pancreas in combi-
nation with other approved chemotherapeutic agents; bladder cancer, breast cancer

Usual Dosage Children and Adults (refer to individual protocols): I.V.: 10-20 mg/m^2/dose every 6-8 weeks, or 2 mg/m^2/day for 5 days, stop for 2 days then repeat; subsequent doses should be adjusted to platelet and leukocyte response.

Dosage Forms Powder for injection: 5 mg, 20 mg, 40 mg

mitomycin-c *see* mitomycin *on previous page*

mitotane (MYE toe tane)
Synonyms o,p'-ddd
Brand Names Lysodren®
Therapeutic Category Antineoplastic Agent
Use Treatment of inoperable adrenal cortical carcinoma
Usual Dosage Adults: Oral: 8-10 g/day in 3-4 divided doses; dose is changed based on side effects with aim of administering as high a dose as tolerated
Dosage Forms Tablet: 500 mg

mitoxantrone (mye toe ZAN trone)
Synonyms dhad; mitoxantrone hydrochloride
Brand Names Novantrone®
Therapeutic Category Antineoplastic Agent
Use FDA approved for remission-induction therapy of acute nonlymphocytic leukemia (ANLL); mitoxantrone is also active against other various leukemias, lymphoma, and breast cancer, and moderately active against pediatric sarcoma
Usual Dosage I.V. (refer to individual protocols):
Leukemias:
  Children ≤2 years: 0.4 mg/kg/day once daily for 3-5 days
  Children >2 years and Adults: 8-12 mg/m^2/day once daily for 5 days or 12 mg/m^2/day once daily for 3 days
Solid tumors:
  Children: 18-20 mg/m^2 every 3-4 weeks
  Adults: 12-14 mg/m^2 every 3-4 weeks
Dosage Forms Injection, as base: 2 mg/mL (10 mL, 12.5 mL, 15 mL)

mitoxantrone hydrochloride *see* mitoxantrone *on this page*

Mitran® Oral *see* chlordiazepoxide *on page 109*

Mitrolan® Chewable Tablet [OTC] *see* calcium polycarbophil *on page 86*

Mivacron® *see* mivacurium *on this page*

mivacurium (mye va KYOO ree um)
Synonyms mivacurium chloride
Brand Names Mivacron®
Therapeutic Category Skeletal Muscle Relaxant
Use Short-acting nondepolarizing neuromuscular blocking agent; an adjunct to general anesthesia; facilitates endotracheal intubation; provides skeletal muscle relaxation during surgery or mechanical ventilation
Usual Dosage I.V.:
Children 2-12 years: 0.2 mg/kg over 5-15 seconds; continuous infusion: 14 mcg/kg
Adults: Initial: 0.15 mg/kg administered over 5-15 seconds
Dosage Forms
Infusion, as chloride, in D$_5$W: 0.5 mg/mL (50 mL)
Injection, as chloride: 2 mg/mL (5 mL, 10 mL)

mivacurium chloride *see* mivacurium *on this page*

MK594 *see* losartan *on page 314*

mmr *see* measles, mumps and rubella vaccines, combined *on page 323*

M-M-R® II *see* measles, mumps and rubella vaccines, combined *on page 323*

Moban® see molindone on this page

Mobidin® see magnesium salicylate on page 319

Moctanin® see monoctanoin on next page

Modane® Bulk [OTC] see psyllium on page 451

Modane® Plus [OTC] see docusate and phenolphthalein on page 180

Modane® Soft [OTC] see docusate on page 179

Modicon™ see ethinyl estradiol and norethindrone on page 209

modified Dakin's solution see sodium hypochlorite solution on page 485

Moducal® [OTC] see glucose polymers on page 242

Moduretic® see amiloride and hydrochlorothiazide on page 24

moexipril (mo EKS i pril)
Synonyms moexipril hydrochloride
Brand Names Univasc®
Therapeutic Category Angiotensin-Converting Enzyme (ACE) Inhibitors
Use Treatment of hypertension, alone or in combination with thiazide diuretics
Usual Dosage Oral:
Patients not receiving diuretics: Initial: 7.5 mg 1 hour prior to meals once daily; if antihypertensive effect diminishes toward end of dosing interval, increase or divide dose; maintenance dose of 7.5-30 mg/day in 1 or 2 divided doses
Patients receiving diuretics: Discontinue diuretic 2-3 days before starting moexipril to avoid symptomatic hypotension; if blood pressure is not controlled, resume diuretic therapy; if diuretic cannot be held, initiate moexipril at 3.75 mg/day
Dosage Forms Tablet, as hydrochloride: 7.5 mg, 15 mg

moexipril and hydrochlorothiazide
(mo EKS i pril & hye droe klor oh THYE a zide)
Brand Names Uniretic®
Therapeutic Category Angiotensin-Converting Enzyme (ACE) Inhibitors; Diuretic, Thiazide
Use Treatment of hypertension
Dosage Forms Tablet: Moexipril hydrochloride 7.5 mg and hydrochlorothiazide 12.5 mg; moexipril hydrochloride 15 mg and hydrochlorothiazide 25 mg

moexipril hydrochloride see moexipril on this page

Moi-Stir® Solution [OTC] see saliva substitute on page 473

Moi-Stir® Swabsticks [OTC] see saliva substitute on page 473

Moisture® Ophthalmic Drops [OTC] see artificial tears on page 42

molindone (moe LIN done)
Synonyms molindone hydrochloride
Brand Names Moban®
Therapeutic Category Antipsychotic Agent, Dihydoindoline
Use Management of psychotic disorder
Usual Dosage Oral: 50-75 mg/day; up to 225 mg/day
Dosage Forms
Concentrate, oral, as hydrochloride: 20 mg/mL (120 mL)
Tablet, as hydrochloride: 5 mg, 10 mg, 25 mg, 50 mg, 100 mg

molindone hydrochloride see molindone on this page

Mol-Iron® [OTC] see ferrous sulfate on page 221

Mollifene® Ear Wax Removing Formula [OTC] see carbamide peroxide on page 90

molybdenum injection *see* trace metals *on page 525*

Molypen® *see* trace metals *on page 525*

mom *see* magnesium hydroxide *on page 319*

mometasone furoate (moe MET a sone FYOOR oh ate)
Brand Names Elocon® Topical
Therapeutic Category Corticosteroid, Topical
Use Relief of inflammatory and pruritic manifestations of corticosteroid-responsive dermatoses
Usual Dosage Topical: Apply to area once daily, do not use occlusive dressings
Dosage Forms
  Cream: 0.1% (15 g, 45 g)
  Lotion: 0.1% (30 mL, 60 mL)
  Ointment, topical: 0.1% (15 g, 45 g)

mom/mineral oil emulsion *see* magnesium hydroxide and mineral oil emulsion *on page 319*

monacolin k *see* lovastatin *on page 315*

Monafed® *see* guaifenesin *on page 247*

Monafed® **DM** *see* guaifenesin and dextromethorphan *on page 248*

Monilia **skin test** *see* Candida albicans (*Monilia*) *on page 87*

Monistat-Derm™ **Topical** *see* miconazole *on page 348*

Monistat i.v.™ **Injection** *see* miconazole *on page 348*

Monistat™ **Vaginal** *see* miconazole *on page 348*

monobenzone (mon oh BEN zone)
Brand Names Benoquin®
Therapeutic Category Topical Skin Product
Use Final depigmentation in extensive vitiligo
Usual Dosage Adults: Topical: Apply 2-3 times/day
Dosage Forms Cream: 20% (35.4 g)

Monocid® *see* cefonicid *on page 98*

Monoclate-P® *see* antihemophilic factor (human) *on page 37*

monoclonal antibody *see* muromonab-CD3 *on page 359*

monoctanoin (mon OK ta noyn)
Synonyms monooctanoin
Brand Names Moctanin®
Therapeutic Category Gallstone Dissolution Agent
Use Solubilize cholesterol gallstones that are retained in the biliary tract after cholecystectomy
Usual Dosage Administer via T-tube into common bile duct at rate of 3-5 mL/hour at pressure of 10 mL water for 7-21 days
Dosage Forms Solution: 120 mL

Monodox® **Oral** *see* doxycycline *on page 184*

Mono-Gesic® *see* salsalate *on page 473*

Monoket® *see* isosorbide mononitrate *on page 292*

Mononine® *see* factor ix complex (human) *on page 215*

monooctanoin *see* monoctanoin *on this page*

Monopril® *see* fosinopril *on page 234*

Monurol™ *see* fosfomycin *on page 234*

8-mop *see* methoxsalen *on page 339*

8-MOP® *see* methoxsalen *on page 339*

more attenuated enders strain *see* measles virus vaccine, live *on page 323*

More-Dophilus® **[OTC]** *see Lactobacillus acidophilus* and *Lactobacillus bulgaricus on page 300*

moricizine (mor I siz een)
Synonyms moricizine hydrochloride
Brand Names Ethmozine®
Therapeutic Category Antiarrhythmic Agent, Class I
Use Treatment of ventricular tachycardia and life-threatening ventricular arrhythmias; a Class I antiarrhythmic agent
Usual Dosage Adults: Oral: 200-300 mg every 8 hours, adjust dosage at 150 mg/day at 3-day intervals
Dosage Forms Tablet, as hydrochloride: 200 mg, 250 mg, 300 mg

moricizine hydrochloride *see* moricizine *on this page*

morphine sulfate (MOR feen SUL fate)
Synonyms ms
Brand Names Astramorph™ PF Injection; Duramorph® Injection; Infumorph™ Injection; Kadian® Capsule; MS Contin® Oral; MSIR® Oral; MS/L®; MS/S®; OMS® Oral; Oramorph SR™ Oral; RMS® Rectal; Roxanol™ Oral; Roxanol Rescudose®; Roxanol SR™ Oral
Therapeutic Category Analgesic, Narcotic
Controlled Substance C-II
Use Relief of moderate to severe acute and chronic pain; pain of myocardial infarction; relieves dyspnea of acute left ventricular failure and pulmonary edema; preanesthetic medication
Usual Dosage Doses should be titrated to appropriate effect; when changing routes of administration in chronically treated patients, please note that oral doses are approximately $1/6$ as effective as parenteral dose

Infants and Children:
Oral: Tablet and solution (prompt release): 0.2-0.5 mg/kg/dose every 4-6 hours as needed; tablet (controlled release): 0.3-0.6 mg/kg/dose every 12 hours
I.M., I.V., S.C.: 0.1-0.2 mg/kg/dose every 2-4 hours as needed; usual maximum: 15 mg/dose; may initiate at 0.05 mg/kg/dose
I.V., S.C. continuous infusion: Sickle cell or cancer pain: 0.025-2 mg/kg/hour; postoperative pain: 0.01-0.04 mg/kg/hour
Sedation/analgesia for procedures: I.V.: 0.05-0.1 mg/kg 5 minutes before the procedure
Adolescents >12 years: Sedation/analgesia for procedures: I.V.: 3-4 mg and repeat in 5 minutes if necessary
Adults:
Oral: Prompt release: 10-30 mg every 4 hours as needed; controlled release: 15-30 mg every 8-12 hours
I.M., I.V., S.C.: 2.5-20 mg/dose every 2-6 hours as needed; usual: 10 mg/dose every 4 hours as needed
I.V., S.C. continuous infusion: 0.8-10 mg/hour; may increase depending on pain relief/adverse effects; usual range up to 80 mg/hour
Epidural: Initial: 5 mg in lumbar region; if inadequate pain relief within 1 hour, administer 1-2 mg, maximum dose: 10 mg/24 hours
Intrathecal ($1/10$ of epidural dose): 0.2-1 mg/dose; repeat doses **not** recommended
Dosage Forms
Capsule (MSIR®): 15 mg, 30 mg
Capsule, sustained release (Kadian®): 20 mg, 50 mg, 100 mg
Injection: 0.5 mg/mL (10 mL); 1 mg/mL (10 mL, 30 mL, 60 mL); 2 mg/mL (1 mL, 2 mL, 60 mL); 3 mg/mL (50 mL); 4 mg/mL (1 mL, 2 mL); 5 mg/mL (1 mL, 30 mL); 8 mg/mL (1

mL, 2 mL); 10 mg/mL (1 mL, 2 mL, 10 mL); 15 mg/mL (1 mL, 2 mL, 20 mL); 25 mg/mL (4 mL, 10 mL, 20 mL, 40 mL); 50 mg/mL (10 mL, 20 mL, 40 mL)
Injection:
  Preservative free (Astramorph™ PF, Duramorph®): 0.5 mg/mL (2 mL, 10 mL); 1 mg/mL (2 mL, 10 mL); 10 mg/mL (20 mL); 25 mg/mL (20 mL)
  I.V. via PCA pump: 1 mg/mL (10 mL, 30 mL, 60 mL); 5 mg/mL (30 mL)
  I.V. infusion preparation: 25 mg/mL (4 mL, 10 mL, 20 mL)
Solution, oral: 10 mg/5 mL (5 mL, 10 mL, 100 mL, 120 mL, 500 mL); 20 mg/5 mL (5 mL, 100 mL, 120 mL, 500 mL)
  MSIR®: 10 mg/5 mL (5 mL, 120 mL, 500 mL); 20 mg/5 mL (5 mL 120 mL, 500 mL); 20 mg/mL (30 mL, 120 mL)
  MS/L®: 100 mg/5 mL (120 mL) 20 mg/5 mL
  OMS®: 20 mg/mL (30 mL, 120 mL)
  Roxanol™: 10 mg/2.5 mL (2.5 mL); 20 mg/mL (1 mL, 1.5 mL, 30 mL, 120 mL, 240 mL)
Suppository, rectal: 5 mg, 10 mg, 20 mg, 30 mg
  MS/S®, RMS®, Roxanol™: 5 mg, 10 mg, 20 mg, 30 mg
Tablet: 15 mg, 30 mg
  MSIR®: 15 mg, 30 mg
Controlled release:
  MS Contin®: 15 mg, 30 mg, 60 mg, 100 mg, 200 mg
  Roxanol™ SR: 30 mg
Soluble: 10 mg, 15 mg, 30 mg
Sustained release (Oramorph SR™): 30 mg, 60 mg, 100 mg

morrhuate sodium (MOR yoo ate SOW dee um)
Brand Names Scleromate™
Therapeutic Category Sclerosing Agent
Use Treatment of small, uncomplicated varicose veins of the lower extremities
Usual Dosage I.V.:
  Children 1-18 years: Esophageal hemorrhage: 2, 3, or 4 mL of 5% solution repeated every 3-4 days until bleeding is controlled, then every 6 weeks until varices obliterated
  Adults: 50-250 mg, repeated at 5- to 7-day intervals (50-100 mg for small veins, 150-250 mg for large veins)
Dosage Forms Injection: 50 mg/mL (5 mL)

Mosco® Liquid [OTC] see salicylic acid on page 472

Motofen® see difenoxin and atropine on page 167

Motrin® see ibuprofen on page 278

Motrin® IB [OTC] see ibuprofen on page 278

Motrin® IB Sinus [OTC] see pseudoephedrine and ibuprofen on page 450

Mouthkote® Solution [OTC] see saliva substitute on page 473

6-mp see mercaptopurine on page 330

M-Prednisol® Injection see methylprednisolone on page 343

M-R-VAX® II see measles and rubella vaccines, combined on page 323

ms see morphine sulfate on previous page

MS Contin® Oral see morphine sulfate on previous page

MSIR® Oral see morphine sulfate on previous page

MS/L® see morphine sulfate on previous page

MS/S® see morphine sulfate on previous page

msta see mumps skin test antigen on next page

mtc see mitomycin on page 352

M.T.E.-4® see trace metals on page 525

M.T.E.-5® see trace metals on page 525

M.T.E.-6® *see* trace metals *on page 525*

MTX *see* methotrexate *on page 338*

Muco-Fen-DM® *see* guaifenesin and dextromethorphan *on page 248*

Muco-Fen-LA® *see* guaifenesin *on page 247*

Mucomyst® *see* acetylcysteine *on page 8*

Mucoplex® [OTC] *see* vitamin b complex *on page 553*

Mucosil™ *see* acetylcysteine *on page 8*

MulTE-PAK-4® *see* trace metals *on page 525*

MulTE-PAK-5® *see* trace metals *on page 525*

multiple sulfonamides *see* sulfadiazine, sulfamethazine, and sulfamerazine *on page 498*

Multitest CMI® *see* skin test antigens, multiple *on page 481*

multivitamins/fluoride *see* vitamin, multiple (pediatric) *on page 554*

Multi Vit® Drops [OTC] *see* vitamin, multiple (pediatric) *on page 554*

mumps skin test antigen (mumpz skin test AN ti jen)
Synonyms msta
Therapeutic Category Diagnostic Agent
Use Assess the status of cell-mediated immunity
Usual Dosage Children and Adults: 0.1 mL intradermally into flexor surface of the forearm; examine reaction site in 24-48 hours; a positive reaction is ≥1.5 mm diameter induration
Dosage Forms Injection: 1 mL (10 tests)

Mumpsvax® *see* mumps virus vaccine, live, attenuated *on this page*

mumps virus vaccine, live, attenuated
(mumpz VYE rus vak SEEN, live, a ten YOO ate ed)
Brand Names Mumpsvax®
Therapeutic Category Vaccine, Live Virus
Use Immunization against mumps in children ≥12 months and adults
Usual Dosage S.C.: 1 vial (5000 units) in outer aspect of the upper arm
Dosage Forms Injection: Single dose

mupirocin (myoo PEER oh sin)
Synonyms mupirocin calcium; pseudomonic acid a
Brand Names Bactroban®; Bactroban® Nasal
Therapeutic Category Antibiotic, Topical
Use Topical treatment of impetigo caused by *Staphylococcus aureus* and *Streptococcus pyogenes*; also effective for the topical treatment of folliculitis, furunculosis, minor wounds, burns, and ulcers caused by susceptible organisms; used as a prophylactic agent applied to intravenous catheter exit sites; used for eradication of *S. aureus* from nasal and perineal carriage sites
Usual Dosage
Children and Adults: Topical: Apply small amount to affected area 2-5 times/day for 5-14 days
Children ≥12 years and Adults: Intranasal: ~1/2 of a single use tube (0.5 g) to each nostril twice daily for 5 days
Dosage Forms
Ointment, as calcium:
Intranasal: 2% (1 g single use tube)
Topical: 2% (15 g)

mupirocin calcium *see* mupirocin *on this page*

Murine® Ear Drops [OTC] *see* carbamide peroxide *on page 90*

Murine® Plus Ophthalmic [OTC] *see* tetrahydrozoline *on page 510*

Murine® Solution [OTC] *see* artificial tears *on page 42*

Muro 128® Ophthalmic [OTC] *see* sodium chloride *on page 483*

Murocel® Ophthalmic Solution [OTC] *see* artificial tears *on page 42*

Murocoll-2® Ophthalmic *see* phenylephrine and scopolamine *on page 412*

muromonab-CD3 (myoo roe MOE nab see dee three)
Synonyms monoclonal antibody; okt3
Brand Names Orthoclone® OKT3
Therapeutic Category Immunosuppressant Agent
Use Treatment of acute allograft rejection in renal transplant patients; effective in reversing acute hepatic, cardiac, and bone marrow transplant rejection episodes resistant to conventional treatment
Usual Dosage I.V. (refer to individual protocols):
Children <30 kg: 2.5 mg/day once daily for 10-14 days
Adults: 5 mg/day once daily for 10-14 days
Children and Adults: Methylprednisolone sodium succinate 1 mg/kg I.V. administered prior to first muromonab-CD3 administration and I.V. hydrocortisone sodium succinate 50-100 mg administered 30 minutes after administration are strongly recommended to decrease the incidence of reactions to the first dose; patient temperature should not exceed 37.8°C (100°F) at time of administration
Dosage Forms Injection: 5 mg/5 mL

Muroptic-5® [OTC] *see* sodium chloride *on page 483*

Muse® Pellet *see* alprostadil *on page 18*

Mustargen® Hydrochloride *see* mechlorethamine *on page 324*

mustine *see* mechlorethamine *on page 324*

Mutamycin® *see* mitomycin *on page 352*

M.V.C.® 9 + 3 *see* vitamin, multiple (injectable) *on page 554*

M.V.I.®-12 *see* vitamin, multiple (injectable) *on page 554*

M.V.I.® Concentrate *see* vitamin, multiple (injectable) *on page 554*

M.V.I.® Pediatric *see* vitamin, multiple (injectable) *on page 554*

Myambutol® *see* ethambutol *on page 206*

Mycelex® *see* clotrimazole *on page 131*

Mycelex®-7 *see* clotrimazole *on page 131*

Mycelex®-G *see* clotrimazole *on page 131*

Mycifradin® Sulfate Oral *see* neomycin *on page 367*

Mycifradin® Sulfate Topical *see* neomycin *on page 367*

Mycinettes® [OTC] *see* benzocaine *on page 59*

Mycitracin® Topical [OTC] *see* bacitracin, neomycin, and polymyxin b *on page 53*

Mycobutin® *see* rifabutin *on page 465*

Mycogen II Topical *see* nystatin and triamcinolone *on page 381*

Mycolog®-II Topical *see* nystatin and triamcinolone *on page 381*

Myconel® Topical *see* nystatin and triamcinolone *on page 381*

mycophenolate (mye koe FEN oh late)
Synonyms mycophenolate mofetil
Brand Names CellCept®
(Continued)

mycophenolate *(Continued)*

Therapeutic Category Immunosuppressant Agent

Use Immunosuppressant used with corticosteroids and cyclosporine to prevent organ rejection in patients receiving allogenic renal transplants

Usual Dosage Adults: Oral: 1 g twice daily (2 g daily dose), administered within 72 hours of transplantation, when administered in combination with corticosteroids and cyclosporine

Dosage Forms Capsule, as mofetil: 250 mg, 500 mg

mycophenolate mofetil *see* mycophenolate *on previous page*

Mycostatin® *see* nystatin *on page 381*

Myco-Triacet® II *see* nystatin and triamcinolone *on page 381*

Mydfrin® Ophthalmic Solution *see* phenylephrine *on page 411*

Mydriacyl® *see* tropicamide *on page 538*

Mykrox® *see* metolazone *on page 345*

Mylanta® [OTC] *see* aluminum hydroxide, magnesium hydroxide, and simethicone *on page 22*

Mylanta Gas® [OTC] *see* simethicone *on page 480*

Mylanta® Gelcaps® *see* calcium carbonate and magnesium carbonate *on page 83*

Mylanta®-II [OTC] *see* aluminum hydroxide, magnesium hydroxide, and simethicone *on page 22*

Myleran® *see* busulfan *on page 77*

Mylicon® [OTC] *see* simethicone *on page 480*

Mylosar® *see* azacitidine *on page 49*

Myminic® Expectorant [OTC] *see* guaifenesin and phenylpropanolamine *on page 249*

Myoflex® [OTC] *see* triethanolamine salicylate *on page 532*

Myotonachol™ *see* bethanechol *on page 66*

Myphetane DC® *see* brompheniramine, phenylpropanolamine, and codeine *on page 74*

Mysoline® *see* primidone *on page 437*

Mytelase® Caplets® *see* ambenonium *on page 23*

Mytrex® F Topical *see* nystatin and triamcinolone *on page 381*

Mytussin® [OTC] *see* guaifenesin *on page 247*

Mytussin® AC *see* guaifenesin and codeine *on page 247*

Mytussin® DAC *see* guaifenesin, pseudoephedrine, and codeine *on page 251*

Mytussin® DM [OTC] *see* guaifenesin and dextromethorphan *on page 248*

nabumetone *(na BYOO me tone)*

Brand Names Relafen®

Therapeutic Category Analgesic, Non-narcotic; Nonsteroidal Anti-Inflammatory Agent (NSAID)

Use Management of osteoarthritis and rheumatoid arthritis

Usual Dosage Adults: Oral: 1000 mg/day; an additional 500-1000 mg may be needed in some patients to obtain more symptomatic relief; may be administered once or twice daily

Dosage Forms Tablet: 500 mg, 750 mg

NAC *see* acetylcysteine *on page 8*

N-acetylcysteine *see* acetylcysteine *on page 8*

N-acetyl-L-cysteine *see* acetylcysteine *on page 8*
n-acetyl-p-aminophenol *see* acetaminophen *on page 3*
NaCl *see* sodium chloride *on page 483*

nadolol (nay DOE lole)
Brand Names Corgard®
Therapeutic Category Beta-Adrenergic Blocker
Use Treatment of hypertension and angina pectoris; prevention of myocardial infarction; prophylaxis of migraine headaches
Usual Dosage Adults: Oral: Initial: 40 mg once daily; increase gradually; usual dosage: 40-80 mg/day; may need up to 240-320 mg/day; doses as high as 640 mg/day have been used
Dosage Forms Tablet: 20 mg, 40 mg, 80 mg, 120 mg, 160 mg

nafarelin (NAF a re lin)
Synonyms nafarelin acetate
Brand Names Synarel®
Therapeutic Category Hormone, Posterior Pituitary
Use Treatment of endometriosis, including pain and reduction of lesions; treatment of central precocious puberty (gonadotropin-dependent precocious puberty) in children of both sexes
Usual Dosage Adults: 1 spray in 1 nostril each morning and evening for 6 months
Dosage Forms Solution, nasal, as acetate: 2 mg/mL (10 mL)

nafarelin acetate *see* nafarelin *on this page*
Nafazair® Ophthalmic *see* naphazoline *on page 364*
Nafcil™ Injection *see* nafcillin *on this page*

nafcillin (naf SIL in)
Synonyms ethoxynaphthamido penicillin sodium; nafcillin sodium
Brand Names Nafcil™ Injection; Nallpen® Injection; Unipen® Injection; Unipen® Oral
Therapeutic Category Penicillin
Use Treatment of bacterial infections such as osteomyelitis, septicemia, endocarditis, and CNS infections due to susceptible penicillinase-producing strains of *Staphylococcus*
Usual Dosage
Children: I.M., I.V.:
Mild to moderate infections: 50-100 mg/kg/day in divided doses every 6 hours
Severe infections: 100-200 mg/kg/day in divided doses every 4-6 hours
Maximum dose: 12 g/day
Oral: 50-100 mg/kg/day divided every 6 hours
Adults:
Oral: 250-500 mg every 4-6 hours, up to 1 g every 4-6 hours for more severe infections
I.M.: 500 mg every 4-6 hours
I.V.: 500-2000 mg every 4-6 hours
Dosage Forms
Capsule, as sodium: 250 mg
Powder for injection, as sodium: 500 mg, 1 g, 2 g, 4 g, 10 g
Solution, as sodium: 250 mg/5 mL (100 mL)
Tablet, as sodium: 500 mg

nafcillin sodium *see* nafcillin *on this page*

naftifine (NAF ti feen)
Synonyms naftifine hydrochloride
Brand Names Naftin®
(Continued)

naftifine *(Continued)*

Therapeutic Category Antifungal Agent
Use Topical treatment of tinea cruris and tinea corporis
Usual Dosage Adults: Topical: Apply twice daily
Dosage Forms
Cream, as hydrochloride: 1% (15 g, 30 g, 60 g)
Gel, topical, as hydrochloride: 1% (20 g, 40 g, 60 g)

naftifine hydrochloride *see* naftifine *on previous page*

Naftin® *see* naftifine *on previous page*

NaHCO₃ *see* sodium bicarbonate *on page 483*

nalbuphine (NAL byoo feen)

Synonyms nalbuphine hydrochloride
Brand Names Nubain®
Therapeutic Category Analgesic, Narcotic
Use Relief of moderate to severe pain
Usual Dosage I.M., I.V., S.C.: 10 mg/70 kg every 3-6 hours
Dosage Forms Injection, as hydrochloride: 10 mg/mL (1 mL, 10 mL); 20 mg/mL (1 mL, 10 mL)

nalbuphine hydrochloride *see* nalbuphine *on this page*

Naldecon® *see* chlorpheniramine, phenyltoloxamine, phenylpropanolamine, and phenylephrine *on page 117*

Naldecon® **DX Adult Liquid [OTC]** *see* guaifenesin, phenylpropanolamine, and dextromethorphan *on page 251*

Naldecon-EX® **Children's Syrup [OTC]** *see* guaifenesin and phenylpropanolamine *on page 249*

Naldecon® **Senior DX [OTC]** *see* guaifenesin and dextromethorphan *on page 248*

Naldecon® **Senior EX [OTC]** *see* guaifenesin *on page 247*

Naldelate® *see* chlorpheniramine, phenyltoloxamine, phenylpropanolamine, and phenylephrine *on page 117*

Nalfon® *see* fenoprofen *on page 218*

Nalgest® *see* chlorpheniramine, phenyltoloxamine, phenylpropanolamine, and phenylephrine *on page 117*

nalidixic acid (nal i DIKS ik AS id)

Synonyms nalidixinic acid
Brand Names NegGram®
Therapeutic Category Quinolone
Use Lower urinary tract infections due to susceptible gram-negative organisms including *E. coli*, *Enterobacter*, *Klebsiella*, and *Proteus* (inactive against *Pseudomonas*)
Usual Dosage Oral:
Children: 55 mg/kg/day divided every 6 hours; suppressive therapy is 33 mg/kg/day divided every 6 hours
Adults: 1 g 4 times/day for 2 weeks; then suppressive therapy of 500 mg 4 times/day
Dosage Forms
Suspension, oral (raspberry flavor): 250 mg/5 mL (473 mL)
Tablet: 250 mg, 500 mg, 1 g

nalidixinic acid *see* nalidixic acid *on this page*

Nallpen® **Injection** *see* nafcillin *on previous page*

***n*-allylnoroxymorphone hydrochloride** *see* naloxone *on next page*

nalmefene (NAL me feen)

Synonyms nalmefene hydrochloride
Brand Names Revex®
Therapeutic Category Antidote
Use Complete or partial of opioid drug effects; management of known or suspected opioid overdose
Usual Dosage Titrate to reverse the undesired effects of opioids; once adequate reversal has been established, additional administration is not required and may actually be harmful due to unwanted reversal of analgesia or precipitated withdrawal; the recommended initial dose for nonopioid dependent patient is 0.5 mg/70 kg, a second dose of 1 mg/70 kg 2-5 minutes later may be administered, after a total dose of 1.5 mg/70 kg has been administered with no clinical response, additional nalmefene is not likely to have an effect
Dosage Forms Injection, as hydrochloride: 100 mcg/mL [blue label] (1 mL); 1000 mcg/mL [green label] (2 mL)

nalmefene hydrochloride see nalmefene on this page

naloxone (nal OKS one)

Synonyms n-allylnoroxymorphone hydrochloride; naloxone hydrochloride
Brand Names Narcan® Injection
Therapeutic Category Antidote
Use Reverses CNS and respiratory depression in suspected narcotic overdose; neonatal opiate depression; coma of unknown etiology

Investigational use: Shock, phencyclidine, and alcohol ingestion
Usual Dosage I.M., I.V. (preferred), intratracheal, S.C. (administer undiluted injection):
Infants and Children:
Postanesthesia narcotic reversal: 0.01 mg/kg; may repeat every 2-3 minutes as needed based on response
Opiate intoxication:
Birth (including premature infants) to 5 years or <20 kg: 0.1 mg/kg; repeat every 2-3 minutes if needed; may need to repeat doses every 20-60 minutes
>5 years or ≥20 kg: 2 mg/dose; if no response, repeat every 2-3 minutes; may need to repeat doses every 20-60 minutes
Children and Adults: Continuous infusion: I.V.: If continuous infusion is required, calculate dosage/hour based on effective intermittent dose used and duration of adequate response seen, titrate dose
Adults: 0.4-2 mg every 2-3 minutes as needed; may need to repeat doses every 20-60 minutes; if no response is observed for a total of 10 mg, re-evaluate patient for possibility of a drug or disease process unresponsive to naloxone. **Note:** Use 0.1-0.2 mg increments in patients who are opioid dependent and in postoperative patients to avoid large cardiovascular changes
Dosage Forms
Injection, as hydrochloride: 0.4 mg/mL (1 mL, 2 mL, 10 mL); 1 mg/mL (2 mL, 10 mL)
Injection, neonatal, as hydrochloride: 0.02 mg/mL (2 mL)

naloxone hydrochloride see naloxone on this page

Nalspan® see chlorpheniramine, phenyltoloxamine, phenylpropanolamine, and phenylephrine on page 117

naltrexone (nal TREKS one)

Synonyms naltrexone hydrochloride
Brand Names ReVia®
Therapeutic Category Antidote
Use Adjunct to the maintenance of an opioid-free state in detoxified individual
Usual Dosage Do not administer until patient is opioid-free for 7-10 days as required by urine analysis
(Continued)

naltrexone *(Continued)*

Adults: Oral: 25 mg; if no withdrawal signs within 1 hour administer another 25 mg; maintenance regimen is flexible, variable and individualized (50 mg/day to 100-150 mg 3 times/week)

Dosage Forms Tablet, as hydrochloride: 50 mg

naltrexone hydrochloride *see* naltrexone *on previous page*

nandrolone (NAN droe lone)

Synonyms nandrolone decanoate; nandrolone phenpropionate

Brand Names Anabolin® Injection; Androlone®-D Injection; Androlone® Injection; Deca-Durabolin® Injection; Hybolin™ Decanoate Injection; Hybolin™ Improved Injection; Neo-Durabolic Injection

Therapeutic Category Androgen

Controlled Substance C-III

Use Control of metastatic breast cancer; management of anemia of renal insufficiency

Usual Dosage

Children 2-13 years: 25-50 mg every 3-4 weeks

Adults:

Male: 100-200 mg/week

Female: 50-100 mg/week

Dosage Forms Injection:

As phenpropionate, in oil: 25 mg/mL (5 mL); 50 mg/mL (2 mL)

As decanoate, in oil: 50 mg/mL (1 mL, 2 mL); 100 mg/mL (1 mL, 2 mL); 200 mg/mL (1 mL)

Repository, as decanoate: 50 mg/mL (2 mL); 100 mg/mL (2 mL); 200 mg/mL (2 mL)

nandrolone decanoate *see* nandrolone *on this page*

nandrolone phenpropionate *see* nandrolone *on this page*

naphazoline (naf AZ oh leen)

Synonyms naphazoline hydrochloride

Brand Names AK-Con® Ophthalmic; Albalon® Liquifilm® Ophthalmic; Allerest® Eye Drops [OTC]; Clear Eyes® [OTC]; Comfort® Ophthalmic [OTC]; Degest® 2 Ophthalmic [OTC]; Estivin® II Ophthalmic [OTC]; I-Naphline® Ophthalmic; Nafazair® Ophthalmic; Naphcon Forte® Ophthalmic; Naphcon® Ophthalmic [OTC]; Opcon® Ophthalmic; Privine® Nasal [OTC]; VasoClear® Ophthalmic [OTC]; Vasocon Regular® Ophthalmic

Therapeutic Category Adrenergic Agonist Agent

Use Topical ocular vasoconstrictor (to soothe, refresh, moisturize, and relieve redness due to minor eye irritation); temporarily relieves nasal congestion associated with rhinitis, sinusitis, hay fever, or the common cold

Usual Dosage

Nasal:

Children:

<6 years: Not recommended (especially infants) due to CNS depression

6-12 years: 1 spray of 0.05% into each nostril, repeat in 3 hours if necessary

Children >12 years and Adults: 0.05%, instill 2 drops or sprays every 3-6 hours if needed; therapy should not exceed 3-5 days or more frequently than every 3 hours

Ophthalmic:

Children <6 years: Not recommended for use due to CNS depression (especially in infants)

Children >6 years and Adults: Instill 1-2 drops into conjunctival sac of affected eye(s) every 3-4 hours; therapy generally should not exceed 3-4 days

Dosage Forms Solution, as hydrochloride:

Nasal:

Drops: 0.05% (20 mL)

Spray: 0.05% (15 mL)

Ophthalmic: 0.012% (7.5 mL, 30 mL); 0.02% (15 mL); 0.03% (15 mL); 0.1% (15 mL)

naphazoline and antazoline (naf AZ oh leen & an TAZ oh leen)
Brand Names Albalon-A® Ophthalmic; Antazoline-V® Ophthalmic; Vasocon-A® [OTC] Ophthalmic
Therapeutic Category Antihistamine/Decongestant Combination
Use Topical ocular congestion, irritation, and itching
Usual Dosage Ophthalmic: 1-2 drops every 3-4 hours
Dosage Forms Solution: Naphazoline hydrochloride 0.05% and antazoline phosphate 0.5% (15 mL)

naphazoline and pheniramine (naf AZ oh leen & fen NIR a meen)
Synonyms pheniramine and naphazoline
Brand Names Naphcon-A® Ophthalmic [OTC]
Therapeutic Category Antihistamine/Decongestant Combination
Use Topical ocular vasoconstrictor
Usual Dosage Ophthalmic: 1-2 drops every 3-4 hours
Dosage Forms Solution, ophthalmic: Naphazoline hydrochloride 0.025% and pheniramine 0.3% (15 mL)

naphazoline hydrochloride *see* naphazoline *on previous page*

Naphcon-A® Ophthalmic [OTC] *see* naphazoline and pheniramine *on this page*

Naphcon Forte® Ophthalmic *see* naphazoline *on previous page*

Naphcon® Ophthalmic [OTC] *see* naphazoline *on previous page*

Naprelan® *see* naproxen *on this page*

Naprosyn® *see* naproxen *on this page*

naproxen (na PROKS en)
Synonyms naproxen sodium
Brand Names Aleve® [OTC]; Anaprox®; Naprelan®; Naprosyn®
Therapeutic Category Analgesic, Non-narcotic; Antipyretic; Nonsteroidal Anti-Inflammatory Agent (NSAID)
Use Management of inflammatory disease and rheumatoid disorders (including juvenile rheumatoid arthritis); acute gout; mild to moderate pain; dysmenorrhea; fever
Usual Dosage Oral (as naproxen):
Children >2 years:
  Antipyretic or analgesic: 5-7 mg/kg/dose every 8-12 hours
  Juvenile rheumatoid arthritis: 10 mg/kg/day, up to a maximum of 1000 mg/day divided twice daily
Adults:
  Rheumatoid arthritis, osteoarthritis, and ankylosing spondylitis: 500-1000 mg/day in 2 divided doses
  Mild to moderate pain or dysmenorrhea: Initial: 500 mg, then 250 mg every 6-8 hours; maximum: 1250 mg/day
Dosage Forms
Suspension, oral: 125 mg/5 mL (15 mL, 30 mL, 480 mL)
Tablet, as sodium: 220 mg (200 mg base)
Anaprox®: 220 mg (200 mg base); 275 mg (250 mg base); 550 mg (500 mg base)
Tablet:
Aleve®: 200 mg
Naprosyn®: 250 mg, 375 mg, 500 mg
Tablet, controlled release (Naprelan®): 375 mg, 500 mg

naproxen sodium *see* naproxen *on this page*

Naqua® *see* trichlormethiazide *on page 530*

Narcan® Injection *see* naloxone *on page 363*

Nardil® *see* phenelzine *on page 408*

Naropin™ *see* ropivacaine *on page 470*

Nasabid™ *see* guaifenesin and pseudoephedrine *on page 250*

Nasacort® *see* triamcinolone *on page 528*

Nasacort® AQ *see* triamcinolone *on page 528*

Nasahist B® *see* brompheniramine *on page 73*

NāSal™ [OTC] *see* sodium chloride *on page 483*

Nasalcrom® Nasal Solution [OTC] *see* cromolyn sodium *on page 141*

Nasalide® Nasal Aerosol *see* flunisolide *on page 226*

Nasal Moist® [OTC] *see* sodium chloride *on page 483*

Nasarel® Nasal Spray *see* flunisolide *on page 226*

Natabec® [OTC] *see* vitamin, multiple (prenatal) *on page 554*

Natabec® FA [OTC] *see* vitamin, multiple (prenatal) *on page 554*

Natabec® Rx *see* vitamin, multiple (prenatal) *on page 554*

Natacyn® *see* natamycin *on this page*

Natalins® [OTC] *see* vitamin, multiple (prenatal) *on page 554*

Natalins® Rx *see* vitamin, multiple (prenatal) *on page 554*

natamycin (na ta MYE sin)
Synonyms pimaricin
Brand Names Natacyn®
Therapeutic Category Antifungal Agent
Use Treatment of blepharitis, conjunctivitis, and keratitis caused by susceptible fungi (*Aspergillus*, *Candida*), *Cephalosporium*, *Curvularia*, *Fusarium*, *Penicillium*, *Microsporum*, *Epidermophyton*, *Blastomyces dermatitidis*, *Coccidioides immitis*, *Cryptococcus neoformans*, *Histoplasma capsulatum*, *Sporothrix schenckii*, *Trichomonas vaginalis*
Usual Dosage Adults: Ophthalmic: 1 drop in conjunctival sac every 1-2 hours, after 3-4 days dose may be reduced to one drop 6-8 times/day; usual course of therapy: 2-3 weeks
Dosage Forms Suspension, ophthalmic: 5% (15 mL)

natural lung surfactant *see* beractant *on page 63*

Nature's Tears® Solution [OTC] *see* artificial tears *on page 42*

Naturetin® *see* bendroflumethiazide *on page 58*

Naus-A-Way® [OTC] *see* phosphorated carbohydrate solution *on page 415*

Nausetrol® [OTC] *see* phosphorated carbohydrate solution *on page 415*

Navane® *see* thiothixene *on page 517*

Navelbine® *see* vinorelbine *on page 551*

ND-Stat® *see* brompheniramine *on page 73*

Nebcin® Injection *see* tobramycin *on page 521*

NebuPent™ Inhalation *see* pentamidine *on page 403*

nedocromil sodium (ne doe KROE mil SOW dee um)
Brand Names Tilade® Inhalation Aerosol
Therapeutic Category Mast Cell Stabilizer
Use Maintenance therapy in patients with mild to moderate bronchial asthma
Usual Dosage Adults: Inhalation: 2 inhalations 4 times/day
Dosage Forms Aerosol: 1.75 mg/activation (16.2 g)

N.E.E.® **1/35** *see* ethinyl estradiol and norethindrone *on page 209*

nefazodone (nef AY zoe done)
Synonyms nefazodone hydrochloride
Brand Names Serzone®
Therapeutic Category Antidepressant, Miscellaneous
Use Treatment of depression
Usual Dosage Adults: Oral: Initial: 200 mg/day administered in two divided doses with a range of 300-600 mg/day in two divided doses thereafter
Dosage Forms Tablet, as hydrochloride: 50 mg, 100 mg, 150 mg, 200 mg, 250 mg

nefazodone hydrochloride *see* nefazodone *on this page*

NegGram® *see* nalidixic acid *on page 362*

nelfinavir (nel FIN a veer)
Brand Names Viracept®
Therapeutic Category Antiviral Agent
Use As monotherapy or preferably in combination with nucleoside analogs in the treatment of HIV infection, in adults and children, when antiretroviral therapy is warranted
Usual Dosage Oral:
Children 2-13 years: 20-30 mg/kg 3 times/day with a meal or light snack; if tablets are unable to be taken, use oral powder in small amount of water, milk, formula, or dietary supplements; do not use acidic food/juice or store for >6 hours
Adults: 750 mg 3 times/day with meals
Dosage Forms
Powder, oral: 50 mg/g (contains 11.2 mg phenylalanine)
Tablet: 250 mg

Nelova™ **0.5/35E** *see* ethinyl estradiol and norethindrone *on page 209*

Nelova® **1/50M** *see* mestranol and norethindrone *on page 332*

Nelova™ **10/11** *see* ethinyl estradiol and norethindrone *on page 209*

Nembutal® *see* pentobarbital *on page 404*

Neo-Calglucon® **[OTC]** *see* calcium glubionate *on page 84*

Neo-Cortef® *see* neomycin and hydrocortisone *on next page*

NeoDecadron® **Ophthalmic** *see* neomycin and dexamethasone *on next page*

NeoDecadron® **Topical** *see* neomycin and dexamethasone *on next page*

Neo-Dexameth® **Ophthalmic** *see* neomycin and dexamethasone *on next page*

Neo-Durabolic Injection *see* nandrolone *on page 364*

Neo-fradin® **Oral** *see* neomycin *on this page*

Neoloid® **[OTC]** *see* castor oil *on page 95*

Neomixin® **Topical [OTC]** *see* bacitracin, neomycin, and polymyxin b *on page 53*

neomycin (nee oh MYE sin)
Synonyms neomycin sulfate
Brand Names Mycifradin® Sulfate Oral; Mycifradin® Sulfate Topical; Neo-fradin® Oral; Neo-Tabs® Oral
Therapeutic Category Aminoglycoside (Antibiotic); Antibiotic, Topical
Use Administered orally to prepare GI tract for surgery; treat minor skin infections; treat diarrhea caused by *E. coli*; adjunct in the treatment of hepatic encephalopathy
(Continued)

neomycin *(Continued)*

Usual Dosage
Children: Oral:

Preoperative intestinal antisepsis: 90 mg/kg/day divided every 4 hours for 2 days; or 25 mg/kg at 1 PM, 2 PM, and 11 PM on the day preceding surgery as an adjunct to mechanical cleansing of the intestine and in combination with erythromycin base

Hepatic coma: 50-100 mg/kg/day in divided doses every 6-8 hours or 2.5-7 g/m^2/day divided every 4-6 hours for 5-6 days not to exceed 12 g/day

Children and Adults: Topical: Apply ointment 1-4 times/day; topical solutions containing 0.1% to 1% neomycin have been used for irrigation

Adults: Oral:

Preoperative intestinal antisepsis: 1 g each hour for 4 doses then 1 g every 4 hours for 5 doses; or 1 g at 1 PM, 2 PM, and 11 PM on day preceding surgery as an adjunct to mechanical cleansing of the bowel and oral erythromycin; or 6 g/day divided every 4 hours for 2-3 days

Hepatic coma: 500-2000 mg every 6-8 hours or 4-12 g/day divided every 4-6 hours for 5-6 days

Chronic hepatic insufficiency: Oral: 4 g/day for an indefinite period

Dosage Forms
Cream, as sulfate: 0.5% (15 g)

Injection, as sulfate: 500 mg

Ointment, topical, as sulfate: 0.5% (15 g, 30 g, 120 g)

Solution, oral, as sulfate: 125 mg/5 mL (480 mL)

Tablet, as sulfate: 500 mg [base 300 mg]

neomycin and dexamethasone (nee oh MYE sin & deks a METH a sone)

Synonyms dexamethasone and neomycin

Brand Names AK-Neo-Dex® Ophthalmic; NeoDecadron® Ophthalmic; NeoDecadron® Topical; Neo-Dexameth® Ophthalmic

Therapeutic Category Antibiotic/Corticosteroid, Ophthalmic; Antibiotic/Corticosteroid, Topical

Use Treatment of steroid responsive inflammatory conditions of the palpebral and bulbar conjunctiva, lid, cornea, and anterior segment of the globe

Usual Dosage

Ophthalmic: Instill 1-2 drops in eye(s) every 3-4 hours

Topical: Apply thin coat 3-4 times/day until favorable response is observed, then reduce dose to one application/day

Dosage Forms

Cream: Neomycin sulfate 0.5% [5 mg/g] and dexamethasone 0.1% [1 mg/g] (15 g, 30 g)

Ointment, ophthalmic: Neomycin sulfate 0.35% [3.5 mg/g] and dexamethasone 0.05% [0.5 mg/g] (3.5 g)

Solution, ophthalmic: Neomycin sulfate 0.35% [3.5 mg/mL] and dexamethasone 0.1% [1 mg/mL] (5 mL)

neomycin and hydrocortisone (nee oh MYE sin & hye droe KOR ti sone)

Brand Names Neo-Cortef®

Therapeutic Category Antibiotic/Corticosteroid, Ophthalmic; Antibiotic/Corticosteroid, Topical

Use Treatment of susceptible topical bacterial infections with associated inflammation

Usual Dosage Topical: Apply to area in a thin film 2-4 times/day

Dosage Forms

Cream: Neomycin sulfate 0.5% and hydrocortisone 1% (20 g)

Solution, ophthalmic: Neomycin sulfate 0.5% and hydrocortisone 0.5% (5 mL)

neomycin and polymyxin b (nee oh MYE sin & pol i MIKS in bee)

Synonyms polymyxin b and neomycin

Brand Names Neosporin® Cream [OTC]; Neosporin® G.U. Irrigant

Therapeutic Category Antibiotic, Topical; Genitourinary Irrigant

Use Short-term use as a continuous irrigant or rinse in the urinary bladder to prevent bacteriuria and gram-negative rod septicemia associated with the use of indwelling catheters; to help prevent infection in minor cuts, scrapes, and burns

Usual Dosage Children and Adults:

Topical: Apply cream 2-4 times/day

Bladder irrigation: Continuous irrigant or rinse in the urinary bladder for up to 10 days where 1 mL is added to 1 L of normal saline with administration rate adjusted to patient's urine output; usually no more than 1 L of irrigant is used per day

Dosage Forms

Cream: Neomycin sulfate 3.5 mg and polymyxin B sulfate 10,000 units per g (0.94 g, 15 g)

Solution, irrigant: Neomycin sulfate 40 mg and polymyxin B sulfate 200,000 units per mL (1 mL, 20 mL)

neomycin, polymyxin b, and dexamethasone

(nee oh MYE sin, pol i MIKS in bee, & deks a METH a sone)

Brand Names AK-Trol®; Dexacidin®; Dexasporin®; Maxitrol®

Therapeutic Category Antibiotic/Corticosteroid, Ophthalmic

Use Steroid-responsive inflammatory ocular conditions in which a corticosteroid is indicated and where bacterial infection or a risk of bacterial infection exists

Usual Dosage Children and Adults: Ophthalmic:

Ointment: Place a small amount ($\sim \frac{1}{2}$") in the affected eye 3-4 times/day or apply at bedtime as an adjunct with drops

Solution: Instill 1-2 drops into affected eye(s) every 4-6 hours; in severe disease, drops may be used hourly and tapered to discontinuation

Dosage Forms

Ointment, ophthalmic: Neomycin sulfate 3.5 mg, polymyxin B sulfate 10,000 units, and dexamethasone 0.1% per g (3.5 g)

Suspension, ophthalmic: Neomycin sulfate 3.5 mg, polymyxin B sulfate 10,000 units, and dexamethasone 0.1% per mL (5 mL)

neomycin, polymyxin b, and gramicidin

(nee oh MYE sin, pol i MIKS in bee, & gram i SYE din)

Brand Names AK-Spore® Ophthalmic Solution; Neosporin® Ophthalmic Solution

Therapeutic Category Antibiotic, Ophthalmic

Use Treatment of superficial ocular infection, infection prophylaxis in minor skin abrasions

Usual Dosage Ophthalmic: Drops: 1-2 drops 4-6 times/day or more frequently as required for severe infections

Dosage Forms Solution, ophthalmic: Neomycin sulfate 1.75 mg, polymyxin B sulfate 10,000 units, and gramicidin 0.025 mg per mL (2 mL, 10 mL)

neomycin, polymyxin b, and hydrocortisone

(nee oh MYE sin, pol i MIKS in bee, & hye droe KOR ti sone)

Brand Names AK-Spore H.C.® Ophthalmic Suspension; AK-Spore H.C.® Otic; Antibi-Otic® Otic; Cortatrigen® Otic; Cortisporin® Ophthalmic Suspension; Cortisporin® Otic; Cortisporin® Topical Cream; Octicair® Otic; Otic-Care® Otic; Otocort® Otic; Otosporin® Otic; Pediotic® Otic; UAD Otic®

Therapeutic Category Antibiotic/Corticosteroid, Ophthalmic; Antibiotic/Corticosteroid, Otic; Antibiotic/Corticosteroid, Topical

Use Steroid-responsive inflammatory condition for which a corticosteroid is indicated and where bacterial infection or a risk of bacterial infection exists

Usual Dosage Duration of use should be limited to 10 days unless otherwise directed by the physician

Ophthalmic: Adults and Children:

Ointment: Apply to the affected eye every 3-4 hours

(Continued)

neomycin, polymyxin b, and hydrocortisone *(Continued)*

Suspension: 1 drop every 3-4 hours
Otic: Solution/suspension:
Children: 3 drops into affected ear 3-4 times/day
Adults: 4 drops into affected ear 3-4 times/day
Dosage Forms
Cream, topical: Neomycin sulfate 5 mg, polymyxin B sulfate 10,000 units, and hydrocortisone 10 mg per mL (7.5 g)
Solution, otic: Neomycin sulfate 5 mg, polymyxin B sulfate 10,000 units, and hydrocortisone 10 mg per mL (10 mL)
Suspension:
Ophthalmic: Neomycin sulfate 5 mg, polymyxin B sulfate 10,000 units, and hydrocortisone 10 mg per mL (7.5 mL)
Otic: Neomycin sulfate 5 mg, polymyxin B sulfate 10,000 units, and hydrocortisone 10 mg per mL (10 mL)

neomycin, polymyxin b, and prednisolone

(nee oh MYE sin, pol i MIKS in bee, & pred NIS oh lone)
Brand Names Poly-Pred® Ophthalmic Suspension
Therapeutic Category Antibiotic/Corticosteroid, Ophthalmic
Use Steroid-responsive inflammatory ocular condition in which bacterial infection or a risk of bacterial ocular infection exists
Usual Dosage Children and Adults: Ophthalmic: Instill 1-2 drops every 3-4 hours; acute infections may require every 30-minute instillation initially with frequency of administration reduced as the infection is brought under control. To treat the lids: Instill 1-2 drops every 3-4 hours, close the eye and rub the excess on the lids and lid margins.
Dosage Forms Suspension, ophthalmic: Neomycin sulfate 0.35%, polymyxin B sulfate 10,000 units, and prednisolone acetate 0.5% per mL (5 mL, 10 mL)

neomycin sulfate *see* neomycin *on page 367*

neonatal trace metals *see* trace metals *on page 525*

Neopap® [OTC] *see* acetaminophen *on page 3*

Neoral® Oral *see* cyclosporine *on page 145*

Neosar® Injection *see* cyclophosphamide *on page 144*

Neosporin® Cream [OTC] *see* neomycin and polymyxin b *on page 368*

Neosporin® G.U. Irrigant *see* neomycin and polymyxin b *on page 368*

Neosporin® Ophthalmic Ointment *see* bacitracin, neomycin, and polymyxin b *on page 53*

Neosporin® Ophthalmic Solution *see* neomycin, polymyxin b, and gramicidin *on previous page*

Neosporin® Topical Ointment [OTC] *see* bacitracin, neomycin, and polymyxin b *on page 53*

neostigmine (nee oh STIG meen)

Synonyms neostigmine bromide; neostigmine methylsulfate
Brand Names Prostigmin®
Therapeutic Category Cholinergic Agent
Use Treatment of myasthenia gravis; prevention and treatment of postoperative bladder distention and urinary retention; reversal of the effects of nondepolarizing neuromuscular blocking agents after surgery
Usual Dosage
Myasthenia gravis: Diagnosis: I.M.:
Children: 0.04 mg/kg as a single dose
Adults: 0.02 mg/kg as a single dose

Myasthenia gravis: Treatment:
Children:
Oral: 2 mg/kg/day divided every 3-4 hours
I.M., I.V., S.C.: 0.01-0.04 mg/kg every 2-4 hours
Adults:
Oral: 15 mg/dose every 3-4 hours
I.M., I.V., S.C.: 0.5-2.5 mg every 1-3 hours
Reversal of nondepolarizing neuromuscular blockade after surgery in conjunction with atropine or glycopyrrolate: I.V.:
Infants: 0.025-0.1 mg/kg/dose
Children: 0.025-0.08 mg/kg/dose
Adults: 0.5-2.5 mg; total dose not to exceed 5 mg
Bladder atony: Adults: I.M., S.C.:
Prevention: 0.25 mg every 4-6 hours for 2-3 days
Treatment: 0.5-1 mg every 3 hours for 5 doses after bladder has emptied
Dosage Forms
Injection, as methylsulfate: 0.25 mg/mL (1 mL); 0.5 mg/mL (1 mL, 10 mL); 1 mg/mL (10 mL)
Tablet, as bromide: 15 mg

neostigmine bromide *see* neostigmine *on previous page*

neostigmine methylsulfate *see* neostigmine *on previous page*

Neo-Synephrine® 12 Hour Nasal Solution [OTC] *see* oxymetazoline *on page 390*

Neo-Synephrine® Nasal Solution [OTC] *see* phenylephrine *on page 411*

Neo-Synephrine® Ophthalmic Solution *see* phenylephrine *on page 411*

Neo-Tabs® Oral *see* neomycin *on page 367*

Neotrace-4® *see* trace metals *on page 525*

Neotricin HC® Ophthalmic Ointment *see* bacitracin, neomycin, polymyxin b, and hydrocortisone *on page 53*

NeoVadrin® [OTC] *see* vitamin, multiple (prenatal) *on page 554*

NeoVadrin® B Complex [OTC] *see* vitamin b complex *on page 553*

Nephro-Calci® [OTC] *see* calcium carbonate *on page 82*

Nephrocaps® *see* vitamin b complex with vitamin c and folic acid *on page 553*

Nephro-Fer™ [OTC] *see* ferrous fumarate *on page 220*

Nephrox Suspension [OTC] *see* aluminum hydroxide *on page 21*

Neptazane® *see* methazolamide *on page 336*

Nervocaine® *see* lidocaine *on page 307*

Nesacaine® *see* chloroprocaine *on page 110*

Nesacaine®-MPF *see* chloroprocaine *on page 110*

Nestrex® *see* pyridoxine *on page 453*

1-*n*-ethyl sisomicin *see* netilmicin *on this page*

netilmicin (ne til MYE sin)

Synonyms 1-*n*-ethyl sisomicin; netilmicin sulfate
Brand Names Netromycin® Injection
Therapeutic Category Aminoglycoside (Antibiotic)
Use Short-term treatment of serious or life-threatening infections including septicemia, peritonitis, intra-abdominal abscess, lower respiratory tract infections, urinary tract infections, skin, bone and joint infections caused by sensitive *Pseudomonas aeruginosa, Escherichia coli, Proteus, Klebsiella, Serratia, Enterobacter, Citrobacter,* and *Staphylococcus*
(Continued)

netilmicin (Continued)

Usual Dosage I.M., I.V.:
Children 6 weeks to 12 years: 1-2.5 mg/kg/dose every 8 hours
Children >12 years and Adults: 1.5-2 mg/kg/dose every 8-12 hours
Dosage Forms
Injection, as sulfate: 100 mg/mL (1.5 mL)
Neonatal: 10 mg/mL (2 mL)
Pediatric: 25 mg/mL (2 mL)

netilmicin sulfate see netilmicin on previous page

Netromycin® Injection see netilmicin on previous page

Neupogen® see filgrastim on page 223

Neuramate® see meprobamate on page 330

Neurontin® see gabapentin on page 236

Neut® Injection see sodium bicarbonate on page 483

Neutra-Phos® see potassium phosphate and sodium phosphate on page 431

Neutra-Phos®-K see potassium phosphate on page 430

Neutrexin™ Injection see trimetrexate glucuronate on page 535

Neutrogena® Acne Mask [OTC] see benzoyl peroxide on page 61

Neutrogena® T/Derm see coal tar on page 132

nevirapine (ne VYE ra peen)

Brand Names Viramune®
Therapeutic Category Antiviral Agent
Use In combination therapy with nucleoside antiretroviral agents in HIV-1 infected adults previously treated for whom current therapy is deemed inadequate
Usual Dosage Adults: Oral: 200 mg once daily for 2 weeks followed by 200 mg twice daily
Dosage Forms Tablet: 200 mg

New Decongestant® see chlorpheniramine, phenyltoloxamine, phenylpropanolamine, and phenylephrine on page 117

N.G.T.® Topical see nystatin and triamcinolone on page 381

niacin (NYE a sin)

Synonyms nicotinic acid; vitamin b_3
Brand Names Niaspan®; Nicobid® [OTC]; Nicolar® [OTC]; Nicotinex [OTC]; Slo-Niacin® [OTC]
Therapeutic Category Vitamin, Water Soluble
Use Adjunctive treatment of hyperlipidemias; peripheral vascular disease and circulatory disorders; treatment of pellagra; dietary supplement
Usual Dosage
Children: Pellagra: Oral, I.M., I.V.: 50-100 mg/dose 3 times/day
Oral: Recommended daily allowances:
0-1 year: 6-8 mg/day
2-6 years: 9-11 mg/day
7-10 years: 16 mg/day
>10 years: 15-18 mg/day
Adults: Oral:
Hyperlipidemia: 1.5-6 g/day in 3 divided doses with or after meals
Pellagra: 50 mg 3-10 times/day, maximum: 500 mg/day
Niacin deficiency: 10-20 mg/day, maximum: 100 mg/day
Dosage Forms
Capsule, timed release: 125 mg, 250 mg, 300 mg, 400 mg, 500 mg

Elixir: 50 mg/5 mL (473 mL, 4000 mL)
Injection: 100 mg/mL (30 mL)
Tablet: 25 mg, 50 mg, 100 mg, 250 mg, 500 mg
  Extended release: 500 mg, 750 mg, 1000 mg
  Timed release: 150 mg, 250 mg, 500 mg, 750 mg

niacinamide (nye a SIN a mide)
Synonyms nicotinamide
Therapeutic Category Vitamin, Water Soluble
Use Prophylaxis and treatment of pellagra
Usual Dosage Oral:
  Children: Pellagra: 100-300 mg/day
  Adults: 50 mg 3-10 times/day
  Pellagra: 300-500 mg/day
  Hyperlipidemias: 1-2 g 3 times/day
Dosage Forms Tablet: 50 mg, 100 mg, 125 mg, 250 mg, 500 mg

Niaspan® *see niacin* *on previous page*

nicardipine (nye KAR de peen)
Synonyms nicardipine hydrochloride
Brand Names Cardene®; Cardene® SR
Therapeutic Category Calcium Channel Blocker
Use Chronic stable angina; management of essential hypertension
Usual Dosage Adults:
  Oral: 40 mg 3 times/day (allow 3 days between dose increases)
  Oral, sustained release: Initial: 30 mg twice daily, titrate up to 60 mg twice daily
  I.V.: (Dilute to 0.1 mg/mL) Initial: 5 mg/hour increased by 2.5 mg/hour every 15 minutes
  to a maximum of 15 mg/hour
  Oral to I.V. dose:
    20 mg every 8 hours = I.V. 0.5 mg/hour
    30 mg every 8 hours = I.V. 1.2 mg/hour
    40 mg every 8 hours = I.V. 2.2 mg/hour
Dosage Forms
  Capsule, as hydrochloride: 20 mg, 30 mg
  Sustained release: 30 mg, 45 mg, 60 mg
  Injection, as hydrochloride: 2.5 mg/mL (10 mL)

nicardipine hydrochloride *see nicardipine* *on this page*

N'ice® **Vitamin C Drops [OTC]** *see ascorbic acid* *on page 42*

Nicobid® **[OTC]** *see niacin* *on previous page*

Nicoderm® **Patch** *see nicotine* *on this page*

Nicolar® **[OTC]** *see niacin* *on previous page*

Nicorette® **DS Gum** *see nicotine* *on this page*

Nicorette® **Gum** *see nicotine* *on this page*

nicotinamide *see niacinamide* *on this page*

nicotine (nik oh TEEN)
Brand Names Habitrol™ Patch; Nicoderm® Patch; Nicorette® DS Gum; Nicorette® Gum;
  Nicotrol® NS Nasal Spray; Nicotrol® Patch [OTC]; ProStep® Patch
Therapeutic Category Smoking Deterrent
Use Treatment aid to giving up smoking while participating in a behavioral modification
  program, under medical supervision
Usual Dosage
  Gum: Chew 1 piece of gum when urge to smoke, up to 30 pieces/day; most patients
  require 10-12 pieces of gum/day
  (Continued)

nicotine *(Continued)*

Transdermal patches: Apply new patch every 24 hours to nonhairy, clean, dry skin on the upper body or upper outer arm; each patch should be applied to a different site; start with the 21 mg/day or 22 mg/day patch, except those patients with stable coronary artery disease should start with 14 mg/day; most patients the dosage can be reduced after 6-8 weeks; progressively lower doses are used every 2 weeks, with complete nicotine elimination achieved after 10 weeks

Dosage Forms

Patch, transdermal:
Habitrol™: 21 mg/day; 14 mg/day; 7 mg/day (30 systems/box)
Nicoderm®: 21 mg/day; 14 mg/day; 7 mg/day (14 systems/box)
Nicotrol® [OTC]: 15 mg/day (gradually released over 16 hours)
ProStep®: 22 mg/day; 11 mg/day (7 systems/box)
Pieces, chewing gum, as polacrilex: 2 mg/square [OTC] (96 pieces/box); 4 mg/square (96 pieces/box)
Spray, nasal: 0.5 mg/actuation [10 mg/mL-200 actuations] (10 mL)

Nicotinex [OTC] *see* niacin *on page 372*

nicotinic acid *see* niacin *on page 372*

Nicotrol® NS Nasal Spray *see* nicotine *on previous page*

Nicotrol® Patch [OTC] *see* nicotine *on previous page*

nifedipine (nye FED i peen)

Brand Names Adalat®; Adalat® CC; Procardia®; Procardia XL®
Therapeutic Category Calcium Channel Blocker
Use Angina, hypertrophic cardiomyopathy, hypertension
Usual Dosage
Children: Oral, S.L.:
Hypertensive emergencies: 0.25-0.5 mg/kg/dose
Hypertrophic cardiomyopathy: 0.6-0.9 mg/kg/24 hours in 3-4 divided doses
Adults: Initial: 10 mg 3 times/day as capsules or 30-60 mg once daily as sustained release tablet; maintenance: 10-30 mg 3-4 times/day (capsules); maximum: 180 mg/24 hours (capsules) or 120 mg/day (sustained release)
Dosage Forms
Capsule, liquid-filled (Adalat®, Procardia®): 10 mg, 20 mg
Tablet:
Extended release (Adalat® CC): 30 mg, 60 mg, 90 mg
Sustained release (Procardia XL®): 30 mg, 60 mg, 90 mg

Niferex® [OTC] *see* polysaccharide-iron complex *on page 424*

Niferex®-PN *see* vitamin, multiple (prenatal) *on page 554*

Nilandron™ *see* nilutamide *on this page*

Nilstat® *see* nystatin *on page 381*

nilutamide (ni LU ta mide)

Brand Names Nilandron™
Therapeutic Category Antineoplastic Agent
Use With orchiectomy (surgical castration) for the treatment of metastatic prostate cancer
Usual Dosage Adults: Oral: 300 mg (6-50 mg tablets) once daily for 30 days, then 150 mg (3-50 mg tablets) once daily; starting on the same day or day after surgical castration
Dosage Forms Tablet: 50 mg

Nimbex® *see* cisatracurium *on page 124*

nimodipine (nye MOE di peen)
Brand Names Nimotop®
Therapeutic Category Calcium Channel Blocker
Use Improvement of neurological deficits due to spasm following subarachnoid hemorrhage from ruptured congenital intracranial aneurysms who are in good neurological condition postictus
Usual Dosage Adults: Oral: 60 mg every 4 hours for 21 days, start therapy within 96 hours after subarachnoid hemorrhage
Dosage Forms Capsule, liquid-filled: 30 mg

Nimotop® *see* nimodipine *on this page*
Nipent™ *see* pentostatin *on page 405*

nisoldipine (NYE sole di peen)
Brand Names Sular™
Therapeutic Category Calcium Channel Blocker
Use Management of hypertension, may be used alone or in combination with other antihypertensive agents
Usual Dosage Adults: Oral: Initial: 20 mg once daily, then increase by 10 mg per week (or longer intervals) to attain adequate control of blood pressure; doses >60 mg once daily are not recommended
Dosage Forms Tablet, extended release: 10 mg, 20 mg, 30 mg, 40 mg

Nitrek® Patch *see* nitroglycerin *on next page*
Nitro-Bid® I.V. Injection *see* nitroglycerin *on next page*
Nitro-Bid® Ointment *see* nitroglycerin *on next page*
Nitrodisc® Patch *see* nitroglycerin *on next page*
Nitro-Dur® Patch *see* nitroglycerin *on next page*
nitrofural *see* nitrofurazone *on this page*

nitrofurantoin (nye troe fyoor AN toyn)
Brand Names Furadantin®; Macrobid®; Macrodantin®
Therapeutic Category Antibiotic, Miscellaneous
Use Prevention and treatment of urinary tract infections caused by susceptible gram-negative and some gram-positive organisms including *E. coli*, *Klebsiella*, *Enterobacter*, *Enterococa*, and *S. aureus*; *Pseudomonas*, *Serratia*, and most species of *Proteus* are generally resistant to nitrofurantoin
Usual Dosage Oral:
Children >1 month: 5-7 mg/kg/day divided every 6 hours; maximum: 400 mg/day
Chronic therapy: 1-2 mg/kg/day in divided doses every 12-24 hours; maximum dose: 400 mg/day
Adults: 50-100 mg/dose every 6 hours (not to exceed 400 mg/24 hours)
Prophylaxis: 50-100 mg/dose at bedtime
Dosage Forms
Capsule: 50 mg, 100 mg
Macrocrystal: 25 mg, 50 mg, 100 mg
Macrocrystal/monohydrate: 100 mg
Suspension, oral: 25 mg/5 mL (470 mL)

nitrofurazone (nye troe FYOOR a zone)
Synonyms nitrofural
Brand Names Furacin® Topical
Therapeutic Category Antibacterial, Topical
Use Antibacterial agent used in second and third degree burns and skin grafting
(Continued)

nitrofurazone *(Continued)*

Usual Dosage Children and Adults: Topical: Apply once daily or every few days to lesion or place on gauze

Dosage Forms
Cream: 0.2% (4 g, 28 g)
Ointment, soluble dressing: 0.2% (28 g, 56 g, 454 g, 480 g)
Solution, topical: 0.2% (480 mL, 3780 mL)

Nitrogard® Buccal *see* nitroglycerin *on this page*

nitrogen mustard *see* mechlorethamine *on page 324*

nitroglycerin (nye troe GLI ser in)

Synonyms glyceryl trinitrate; nitroglycerol; ntg

Brand Names Deponit® Patch; Minitran™ Patch; Nitrek® Patch; Nitro-Bid® I.V. Injection; Nitro-Bid® Ointment; Nitrodisc® Patch; Nitro-Dur® Patch; Nitrogard® Buccal; Nitroglyn® Oral; Nitrolingual® Translingual Spray; Nitrol® Ointment; Nitrong® Oral Tablet; Nitrostat® Sublingual; Transdermal-NTG® Patch; Transderm-Nitro® Patch; Tridil® Injection

Therapeutic Category Vasodilator

Use Angina pectoris; I.V. for congestive heart failure (especially when associated with acute myocardial infarction); pulmonary hypertension; hypertensive emergencies occurring perioperatively (especially during cardiovascular surgery)

Usual Dosage Note: Hemodynamic and antianginal tolerance often develops within 24-48 hours of continuous nitrate administration

Children: Pulmonary hypertension: Continuous infusion: Start 0.25-0.5 mcg/kg/minute and titrate by 1 mcg/kg/minute at 20- to 60-minute intervals to desired effect; usual dose: 1-3 mcg/kg/minute; maximum: 5 mcg/kg/minute

Adults:
Oral: 2.5-9 mg 2-4 times/day (up to 26 mg 4 times/day)
I.V.: 5 mcg/minute, increase by 5 mcg/minute every 3-5 minutes to 20 mcg/minute; if no response at 20 mcg/minute increase by 10 mcg/minute every 3-5 minutes, up to 200 mcg/minute
Sublingual: 0.2-0.6 mg every 5 minutes for maximum of 3 doses in 15 minutes; may also use prophylactically 5-10 minutes prior to activities which may provoke an attack
Ointment: 1" to 2" every 8 hours up to 4" to 5" every 4 hours
Patch, transdermal: 0.2-0.4 mg/hour initially and titrate to doses of 0.4-0.8 mg/hour; tolerance is minimized by using a patch on period of 12-14 hours and patch off period of 10-12 hours
Translingual: 1-2 sprays into mouth under tongue every 3-5 minutes for maximum of 3 doses in 15 minutes, may also be used 5-10 minutes prior to activities which may provoke an attack prophylactically
Buccal: Initial: 1 mg every 3-5 hours while awake (3 times/day); titrate dosage upward if angina occurs with tablet in place

May need to use nitrate-free interval (10-12 hours/day) to avoid tolerance development; tolerance may possibly be reversed with acetylcysteine; gradually decrease dose in patients receiving NTG for prolonged period to avoid withdrawal reaction

Dosage Forms
Capsule, sustained release: 2.5 mg, 6.5 mg, 9 mg
Injection: 0.5 mg/mL (10 mL); 0.8 mg/mL (10 mL); 5 mg/mL (1 mL, 5 mL, 10 mL, 20 mL); 10 mg/mL (5 mL, 10 mL)
Ointment, topical (Nitrol®): 2% [20 mg/g] (30 g, 60 g)
Patch, transdermal, topical: Systems designed to deliver 2.5, 5, 7.5, 10, or 15 mg NTG over 24 hours
Spray, translingual: 0.4 mg/metered spray (13.8 g)
Tablet:
Buccal, controlled release: 1 mg, 2 mg, 3 mg
Sublingual (Nitrostat®): 0.3 mg, 0.4 mg, 0.6 mg
Sustained release: 2.6 mg, 6.5 mg, 9 mg

nitroglycerol *see* nitroglycerin *on previous page*

Nitroglyn® Oral *see* nitroglycerin *on previous page*

Nitrolingual® Translingual Spray *see* nitroglycerin *on previous page*

Nitrol® Ointment *see* nitroglycerin *on previous page*

Nitrong® Oral Tablet *see* nitroglycerin *on previous page*

Nitropress® *see* nitroprusside *on this page*

nitroprusside (nye troe PRUS ide)

Synonyms nitroprusside sodium; sodium nitroferricyanide; sodium nitroprusside
Brand Names Nitropress®
Therapeutic Category Vasodilator
Use Management of hypertensive crises; congestive heart failure; used for controlled hypotension during anesthesia
Usual Dosage I.V.:
  Children: Continuous infusion:
    Initial: 1 mcg/kg/minute by continuous I.V. infusion; increase in increments of 1 mcg/kg/minute at intervals of 20-60 minutes; titrating to the desired response
    Usual dose: 3 mcg/kg/minute; rarely need >4 mcg/kg/minute
    Maximum: 10 mcg/kg/minute. Dilute 15 mg x weight (kg) to 250 mL D_5W, then dose in mcg/kg/minute = infusion rate in mL/hour
  Adults: Begin at 5 mcg/kg/minute; increase in increments of 5 mcg/kg/minute (up to 20 mcg/kg/minute), then in increments of 10-20 mcg/kg/minute; titrating to the desired hemodynamic effect or the appearance of headache or nausea. When >500 mcg/kg is administered by prolonged infusion of faster than 2 mcg/kg/minute, cyanide is generated faster than an unaided patient can handle.
Dosage Forms Injection, as sodium: 10 mg/mL (5 mL); 25 mg/mL (2 mL)

nitroprusside sodium *see* nitroprusside *on this page*

Nitrostat® Sublingual *see* nitroglycerin *on previous page*

Nix™ Creme Rinse *see* permethrin *on page 406*

nizatidine (ni ZA ti deen)

Brand Names Axid®; Axid® AR [OTC]
Therapeutic Category Histamine H_2 Antagonist
Use Treatment and maintenance of duodenal ulcer; treatment of gastroesophageal reflux disease (GERD)
Usual Dosage Adults: Active duodenal ulcer: Oral:
  Treatment: 300 mg at bedtime or 150 mg twice daily
  Maintenance: 150 mg/day
Dosage Forms
  Capsule: 150 mg, 300 mg
  Tablet: 75 mg

Nizoral® *see* ketoconazole *on page 296*

n-methylhydrazine *see* procarbazine *on page 439*

Nolahist® [OTC] *see* phenindamine *on page 409*

Nolamine® *see* chlorpheniramine, phenindamine, and phenylpropanolamine *on page 115*

Nolex® LA *see* guaifenesin and phenylpropanolamine *on page 249*

Nolvadex® *see* tamoxifen *on page 502*

nonoxynol 9 (non OKS i nole nine)

Brand Names Because® [OTC]; Delfen® [OTC]; Emko® [OTC]; Encare® [OTC]; Gynol II® [OTC]; Koromex® [OTC]; Ramses® [OTC]; Semicid® [OTC]; Shur-Seal® [OTC] (Continued)

nonoxynol 9 *(Continued)*
Therapeutic Category Spermicide
Use Spermatocide in contraception
Usual Dosage Insert into vagina at least 15 minutes before intercourse
Dosage Forms Vaginal:
Cream: 2% (103.5 g)
Foam: 12.5% (60 g)
Jelly: 2% (81 g, 126 g)

No Pain-HP® [OTC] *see* capsaicin *on page 87*

noradrenaline acid tartrate *see* norepinephrine *on this page*

Norcet® *see* hydrocodone and acetaminophen *on page 266*

Norco® *see* hydrocodone and acetaminophen *on page 266*

Norcuron® *see* vecuronium *on page 547*

nordeoxyguanosine *see* ganciclovir *on page 237*

Nordette® *see* ethinyl estradiol and levonorgestrel *on page 208*

Norditropin® Injection *see* human growth hormone *on page 262*

norepinephrine (nor ep i NEF rin)
Synonyms levarterenol bitartrate; noradrenaline acid tartrate; norepinephrine bitartrate
Brand Names Levophed® Injection
Therapeutic Category Adrenergic Agonist Agent
Use Treatment of shock which persists after adequate fluid volume replacement; severe hypotension; cardiogenic shock
Usual Dosage Note: Dose stated in terms of norepinephrine base. I.V.:
Children: Initial: 0.05-0.1 mcg/kg/minute, titrate to desired effect; rate (mL/hour) = dose (mcg/kg/minute) x weight (kg) x 60 minutes/hour divided by concentration (mcg/mL)
Adults: 8-12 mcg/minute as an infusion; initiate at 4 mcg/minute and titrate to desired response
Dosage Forms Injection, as bitartrate: 1 mg/mL (4 mL)

norepinephrine bitartrate *see* norepinephrine *on this page*

Norethin™ 1/35E *see* ethinyl estradiol and norethindrone *on page 209*

Norethin 1/50M *see* mestranol and norethindrone *on page 332*

norethindrone (nor eth IN drone)
Synonyms norethisterone
Brand Names Aygestin®; Micronor®; NOR-Q.D.®
Therapeutic Category Contraceptive, Progestin Only; Progestin
Use Treatment of amenorrhea; abnormal uterine bleeding; endometriosis
Usual Dosage Adolescents and Adults: Oral:
Amenorrhea and abnormal uterine bleeding: 2.5-10 mg on days 5-25 of menstrual cycle
Endometriosis: 5 mg/day for 14 days; increase at increments of 2.5 mg/day every 2 weeks up to 15 mg/day
Dosage Forms
Tablet: 0.35 mg, 5 mg
As acetate: 5 mg

norethindrone acetate and ethinyl estradiol *see* ethinyl estradiol and norethindrone *on page 209*

norethindrone and mestranol *see* mestranol and norethindrone *on page 332*

norethisterone *see* norethindrone *on this page*

Norflex™ *see* orphenadrine *on page 385*

norfloxacin (nor FLOKS a sin)
Brand Names Chibroxin™ Ophthalmic; Noroxin® Oral
Therapeutic Category Quinolone
Use Complicated and uncomplicated urinary tract infections caused by susceptible gram-negative and gram-positive bacteria
Usual Dosage
Children >1 year and Adults: Ophthalmic: Instill 1-2 drops in affected eye(s) 4 times/day for up to 7 days
Adults: Oral: 400 mg twice daily for 7-21 days depending on infection
Dosage Forms
Solution, ophthalmic: 0.3% [3 mg/mL] (5 mL)
Tablet: 400 mg

Norgesic™ *see* orphenadrine, aspirin and caffeine *on page 386*

Norgesic™ Forte *see* orphenadrine, aspirin and caffeine *on page 386*

norgestimate and ethinyl estradiol *see* ethinyl estradiol and norgestimate *on page 210*

norgestrel (nor JES trel)
Brand Names Ovrette®
Therapeutic Category Contraceptive, Progestin Only
Use Prevention of pregnancy; treatment of hypermenorrhea, endometriosis, female hypogonadism
Usual Dosage Oral: Administer daily, starting the first day of menstruation, administer one tablet at the same time each day, every day of the year. If one dose is missed, administer as soon as remembered, then next tablet at regular time; if two doses are missed, administer one tablet and discard the other, then administer daily at usual time; if three doses are missed, use an additional form of birth control until menses or pregnancy is ruled out
Dosage Forms Tablet: 0.075 mg

norgestrel and ethinyl estradiol *see* ethinyl estradiol and norgestrel *on page 210*

Norinyl® 1+35 *see* ethinyl estradiol and norethindrone *on page 209*

Norinyl® 1+50 *see* mestranol and norethindrone *on page 332*

normal saline *see* sodium chloride *on page 483*

Normiflo® *see* ardeparin *on page 41*

Normodyne® *see* labetalol *on page 299*

Noroxin® Oral *see* norfloxacin *on this page*

Norpace® *see* disopyramide *on page 177*

Norplant® Implant *see* levonorgestrel *on page 306*

Norpramin® *see* desipramine *on page 154*

NOR-Q.D.® *see* norethindrone *on previous page*

North American coral snake antivenin *see* antivenin (*Micrurus fulvius*) *on page 39*

North and South American antisnake-bite serum *see* antivenin (*Crotalidae*) polyvalent *on page 38*

nortriptyline (nor TRIP ti leen)
Synonyms nortriptyline hydrochloride
Brand Names Aventyl® Hydrochloride; Pamelor®
Therapeutic Category Antidepressant, Tricyclic (Secondary Amine)
Use Treatment of various forms of depression, often in conjunction with psychotherapy; nocturnal enuresis
(Continued)

nortriptyline *(Continued)*

Usual Dosage Oral:
Adults: 25 mg 3-4 times/day up to 150 mg/day
Adolescents and Elderly: 30-50 mg/day in divided doses
Dosage Forms
Capsule, as hydrochloride: 10 mg, 25 mg, 50 mg, 75 mg
Solution, as hydrochloride: 10 mg/5 mL (473 mL)

nortriptyline hydrochloride *see* nortriptyline *on previous page*

Norvasc® *see* amlodipine *on page 28*

Norvir® *see* ritonavir *on page 468*

Norzine® *see* thiethylperazine *on page 515*

Nōstrilla® [OTC] *see* oxymetazoline *on page 390*

Nostril® Nasal Solution [OTC] *see* phenylephrine *on page 411*

Novacet® Topical *see* sulfur and sulfacetamide sodium *on page 500*

Novantrone® *see* mitoxantrone *on page 353*

Novocain® Injection *see* procaine *on page 438*

Novolin® 70/30 *see* insulin preparations *on page 284*

Novolin® L *see* insulin preparations *on page 284*

Novolin® N *see* insulin preparations *on page 284*

Novolin® R *see* insulin preparations *on page 284*

NP-27® [OTC] *see* tolnaftate *on page 523*

NPH Iletin® I *see* insulin preparations *on page 284*

NPH-N *see* insulin preparations *on page 284*

NSC-106977 *see* erwinia asparaginase *on page 199*

ntg *see* nitroglycerin *on page 376*

NTZ® Long Acting Nasal Solution [OTC] *see* oxymetazoline *on page 390*

Nubain® *see* nalbuphine *on page 362*

Nucofed® *see* guaifenesin, pseudoephedrine, and codeine *on page 251*

Nucofed® Pediatric Expectorant *see* guaifenesin, pseudoephedrine, and codeine *on page 251*

Nucotuss® *see* guaifenesin, pseudoephedrine, and codeine *on page 251*

Nu-Iron® [OTC] *see* polysaccharide-iron complex *on page 424*

Nullo® [OTC] *see* chlorophyll *on page 110*

NuLytely® *see* polyethylene glycol-electrolyte solution *on page 423*

Numorphan® *see* oxymorphone *on page 391*

Numzitdent® [OTC] *see* benzocaine *on page 59*

Numzit Teething® [OTC] *see* benzocaine *on page 59*

Nupercainal® [OTC] *see* dibucaine *on page 163*

Nuprin® [OTC] *see* ibuprofen *on page 278*

Nuromax® Injection *see* doxacurium *on page 182*

Nu-Tears® II Solution [OTC] *see* artificial tears *on page 42*

Nu-Tears® Solution [OTC] *see* artificial tears *on page 42*

Nutracort® *see* hydrocortisone *on page 268*

Nutraplus® Topical [OTC] *see* urea *on page 542*

Nutrilipid® *see* fat emulsion *on page 216*

Nutropin® **AQ Injection** *see* human growth hormone *on page 262*
Nutropin® **Injection** *see* human growth hormone *on page 262*
Nydrazid® **Injection** *see* isoniazid *on page 290*

nystatin (nye STAT in)
Brand Names Mycostatin®; Nilstat®; Nystex®
Therapeutic Category Antifungal Agent
Use Treatment of susceptible cutaneous, mucocutaneous, oral cavity and vaginal fungal infections normally caused by the *Candida* species
Usual Dosage
Oral candidiasis:
Infants: 200,000 units 4 times/day or 100,000 units to each side of mouth 4 times/day
Children and Adults: 400,000-600,000 units 4 times/day; troche: 200,000-400,000 units 4-5 times/day
Cutaneous candidal infections: Children and Adults: Topical: Apply 3-4 times/day
Intestinal infections: Adults: Oral: 500,000-1,000,000 units every 8 hours
Vaginal infections: Adults: Vaginal tablets: Insert 1-2 tablets/day at bedtime for 2 weeks
Dosage Forms
Cream: 100,000 units/g (15 g, 30 g)
Ointment, topical: 100,000 units/g (15 g, 30 g)
Powder:
For preparation of oral suspension: 50 million units, 1 billion units, 2 billion units, 5 billion units
Topical: 100,000 units/g (15 g)
Suspension, oral: 100,000 units/mL (5 mL, 60 mL, 480 mL)
Tablet:
Oral: 500,000 units
Vaginal: 100,000 units (15 and 30/box with applicator)
Troche: 200,000 units

nystatin and triamcinolone (nye STAT in & trye am SIN oh lone)
Synonyms triamcinolone and nystatin
Brand Names Mycogen II Topical; Mycolog®-II Topical; Myconel® Topical; Myco-Triacet® II; Mytrex® F Topical; N.G.T.® Topical; Tri-Statin® II Topical
Therapeutic Category Antifungal/Corticosteroid
Use Treatment of cutaneous candidiasis
Usual Dosage Topical: Apply twice daily
Dosage Forms
Cream: Nystatin 100,000 units and triamcinolone acetonide 0.1% (15 g, 30 g, 45 g, 60 g, 240 g)
Ointment, topical: Nystatin 100,000 units and triamcinolone acetonide 0.1% (15 g, 30 g, 60 g, 120 g)

Nystex® *see* nystatin *on this page*
Nytol® **Oral [OTC]** *see* diphenhydramine *on page 173*
Occlusal-HP Liquid *see* salicylic acid *on page 472*
Ocean Nasal Mist [OTC] *see* sodium chloride *on page 483*
OCL® *see* polyethylene glycol-electrolyte solution *on page 423*
Octamide® **PFS** *see* metoclopramide *on page 344*
Octicair® **Otic** *see* neomycin, polymyxin b, and hydrocortisone *on page 369*
Octocaine® *see* lidocaine *on page 307*
Octocaine® **Injection** *see* lidocaine and epinephrine *on page 308*

octreotide acetate (ok TREE oh tide AS e tate)
Brand Names Sandostatin®
Therapeutic Category Somatostatin Analog
Use Control of symptoms in patients with metastatic carcinoid, vasoactive intestinal peptide-secreting tumors (VIPomas), and secretory diarrhea
Usual Dosage Adults: S.C.: Initial: 50 mcg 1-2 times/day and titrate dose based on patient tolerance and response

Carcinoid: 100-600 mcg/day in 2-4 divided doses
VIPomas: 200-300 mcg/day in 2-4 divided doses
Diarrhea: Initial: I.V.: 50-100 mcg every 8 hours; increase by 100 mcg/dose at 48-hour intervals; maximum dose: 500 mcg every 8 hours

Dosage Forms Injection: 0.05 mg/mL (1 mL); 0.1 mg/mL (1 mL); 0.2 mg/mL (5 mL); 0.5 mg/mL (1 mL); 1 mg/mL (5 mL)

OcuClear® Ophthalmic [OTC] see oxymetazoline on page 390

OcuCoat® Ophthalmic Solution [OTC] see artificial tears on page 42

OcuCoat® PF Ophthalmic Solution [OTC] see artificial tears on page 42

Ocufen® Ophthalmic see flurbiprofen on page 231

Ocuflox™ Ophthalmic see ofloxacin on this page

Ocupress® Ophthalmic see carteolol on page 94

Ocusert Pilo-20® Ophthalmic see pilocarpine on page 417

Ocusert Pilo-40® Ophthalmic see pilocarpine on page 417

Ocusulf-10® Ophthalmic see sulfacetamide sodium on page 496

Ocutricin® Topical Ointment see bacitracin, neomycin, and polymyxin b on page 53

Off-Ezy® Wart Remover [OTC] see salicylic acid on page 472

ofloxacin (oh FLOKS a sin)
Brand Names Floxin®; Ocuflox™ Ophthalmic
Therapeutic Category Quinolone
Use Quinolone antibiotic for skin and skin structure, lower respiratory and urinary tract infections and sexually transmitted diseases; pelvic inflammatory disease (PID)
Usual Dosage Adults:
Oral, I.V.: 200-400 mg every 12 hours for 7-10 days for most infections or for 6 weeks for prostatitis
Ophthalmic: Instill 1-2 drops in affected eye(s) every 2-4 hours for the first 2 days, then use 4 times/day for an additional 5 days
Dosage Forms
Injection: 200 mg (50 mL); 400 mg (10 mL, 20 mL, 100 mL)
Solution, ophthalmic: 0.3% (5 mL)
Tablet: 200 mg, 300 mg, 400 mg

Ogen® Oral see estropipate on page 206

Ogen® Vaginal see estropipate on page 206

OGMT see metyrosine on page 347

okt3 see muromonab-CD3 on page 359

olanzapine (oh LAN za peen)
Synonyms LY170053
Brand Names Zyprexa®
Therapeutic Category Antipsychotic Agent
Use Treatment of schizophrenia

Usual Dosage Adults: Oral: Usual starting dose: 10 mg/day, up to a maximum of 20 mg/day

Dosage Forms Tablet: 5 mg, 7.5 mg, 10 mg

old tuberculin *see* tuberculin tests *on page 539*

oleovitamin a *see* vitamin a *on page 552*

oleum ricini *see* castor oil *on page 95*

olopatadine (oh LOP ah tah deen)
Brand Names Patanol®
Therapeutic Category Antihistamine
Use Allergic conjunctivitis
Usual Dosage Adults: Ophthalmic: 1 drop in affected eye(s) every 6-8 hours (twice daily)
Dosage Forms Solution, ophthalmic: 0.1% (5 mL)

olsalazine (ole SAL a zeen)
Synonyms olsalazine sodium
Brand Names Dipentum®
Therapeutic Category 5-Aminosalicylic Acid Derivative
Use Maintenance of remission of ulcerative colitis in patients intolerant to sulfasalazine
Usual Dosage Adults: Oral: 1 g daily in 2 divided doses
Dosage Forms Capsule, as sodium: 250 mg

olsalazine sodium *see* olsalazine *on this page*

omeprazole (oh ME pray zol)
Brand Names Prilosec™
Therapeutic Category Gastric Acid Secretion Inhibitor
Use Short-term (4-8 weeks) treatment of erosive esophagitis (grade 2 or above), diagnosed by endoscopy; maintain healing of erosive esophagitis; short-term treatment of symptomatic gastroesophageal reflux disease (GERD) poorly responsive to customary medical treatment; short-term treatment of active duodenal ulcer; long-term treatment of pathological hypersecretory conditions
Usual Dosage Adults: Oral:
Duodenal ulcer: 20 mg/day for 4-8 weeks
GERD or erosive esophagitis: 20 mg/day for 4-8 weeks
Maintenance of healing erosive esophagitis: 20 mg/day
Pathological hypersecretory conditions: 60 mg once daily initially; doses up to 120 mg 3 times/day have been administered; administer daily doses >80 mg in divided doses; patients with Zollinger-Ellison syndrome have been treated continuously for over 5 years
Dosage Forms Capsule, delayed release: 10 mg, 20 mg

OmniHIB® *see haemophilus* b conjugate vaccine *on page 254*

Omnipaque® *see* radiological/contrast media (non-ionic) *on page 459*

Omnipen® *see* ampicillin *on page 33*

Omnipen®-N *see* ampicillin *on page 33*

OMS® Oral *see* morphine sulfate *on page 356*

Oncaspar® *see* pegaspargase *on page 398*

Oncet® *see* hydrocodone and homatropine *on page 267*

Oncovin® Injection *see* vincristine *on page 550*

ondansetron (on DAN se tron)
Synonyms ondansetron hydrochloride
Brand Names Zofran®
(Continued)

ondansetron *(Continued)*

Therapeutic Category Selective 5-HT$_3$ Receptor Antagonist

Use Prevention of nausea and vomiting associated with initial and repeat courses of emetogenic cancer chemotherapy and prevention of postoperative nausea and vomiting

Usual Dosage I.V. (the I.V. product has been used orally successfully. Dosage should be calculated based on weight):

Children >3 years and Adults: 0.15 mg/kg/dose infused 30 minutes before the start of emetogenic chemotherapy, with subsequent doses administered 4 and 8 hours after the first dose; decreased effectiveness has been reported when administered for prolonged therapy (eg, more than 3 doses)

Adults:
>80 kg: 12 mg IVPB
45-80 kg: 8 mg IVPB
<45 kg: 0.15 mg/kg/dose IVPB

Dosage Forms
Injection, as hydrochloride: 2 mg/mL (20 mL); 32 mg (single-dose vials)
Tablet, as hydrochloride: 4 mg, 8 mg

ondansetron hydrochloride *see* ondansetron *on previous page*

Ony-Clear® Nail *see* triacetin *on page 528*

Ony-Clear® Spray *see* miconazole *on page 348*

op-cck *see* sincalide *on page 480*

Opcon® Ophthalmic *see* naphazoline *on page 364*

o,p′-ddd *see* mitotane *on page 353*

Operand® [OTC] *see* povidone-iodine *on page 431*

Ophthalgan® Ophthalmic *see* glycerin *on page 243*

Ophthetic® *see* proparacaine *on page 444*

opium alkaloids (OH pee um AL ka loyds)

Brand Names Pantopon®
Therapeutic Category Analgesic, Narcotic
Controlled Substance C-II
Use For relief of severe pain
Usual Dosage Adults: I.M., S.C.: 5-20 mg every 4-5 hours
Dosage Forms Injection: 20 mg/mL (1 mL)

opium and belladonna *see* belladonna and opium *on page 57*

opium tincture (OH pee um TING chur)

Synonyms deodorized opium tincture; dto
Therapeutic Category Analgesic, Narcotic
Controlled Substance C-II
Use Treatment of diarrhea or relief of pain; **a 25-fold dilution with water** (final concentration 0.4 mg/mL morphine) can be used to treat neonatal abstinence syndrome (opiate withdrawal)
Usual Dosage Oral:
Children:
Diarrhea: 0.005-0.01 mL/kg/dose every 3-4 hours
Analgesia: 0.01-0.02 mL/kg/dose every 3-4 hours
Adults: 0.6 mL 4 times/day
Dosage Forms Liquid: 10% [0.6 mL equivalent to morphine 6 mg] with alcohol 19%

Opticyl® *see* tropicamide *on page 538*

Optigene® Ophthalmic [OTC] *see* tetrahydrozoline *on page 510*

Optimine® *see* azatadine *on page 49*
Optimoist® **Solution [OTC]** *see* saliva substitute *on page 473*
OptiPranolol® **Ophthalmic** *see* metipranolol *on page 344*
Optiray® *see* radiological/contrast media (non-ionic) *on page 459*
opv *see* poliovirus vaccine, live, trivalent, oral *on page 423*
Orabase®**-B [OTC]** *see* benzocaine *on page 59*
Orabase® **HCA** *see* hydrocortisone *on page 268*
Orabase®**-O [OTC]** *see* benzocaine *on page 59*
Orabase® **Plain [OTC]** *see* gelatin, pectin, and methylcellulose *on page 238*
Orabase® **With Benzocaine [OTC]** *see* benzocaine, gelatin, pectin, and sodium carboxymethylcellulose *on page 61*
Oragrafin® **Calcium** *see* radiological/contrast media (ionic) *on page 457*
Oragrafin® **Sodium** *see* radiological/contrast media (ionic) *on page 457*
Orajel® **Brace-Aid Oral Anesthetic [OTC]** *see* benzocaine *on page 59*
Orajel® **Maximum Strength [OTC]** *see* benzocaine *on page 59*
Orajel® **Mouth-Aid [OTC]** *see* benzocaine *on page 59*
Orajel® **Perioseptic [OTC]** *see* carbamide peroxide *on page 90*
Oramorph SR™ **Oral** *see* morphine sulfate *on page 356*
Orap™ *see* pimozide *on page 418*
Orasept® **[OTC]** *see* benzocaine *on page 59*
Orasol® **[OTC]** *see* benzocaine *on page 59*
Orasone® *see* prednisone *on page 436*
Orazinc® **Oral [OTC]** *see* zinc sulfate *on page 561*
orciprenaline sulfate *see* metaproterenol *on page 332*
Ordrine AT® **Extended Release Capsule** *see* caramiphen and phenylpropanolamine *on page 88*
Oretic® *see* hydrochlorothiazide *on page 264*
Oreton® **Methyl** *see* methyltestosterone *on page 343*
Orexin® **[OTC]** *see* vitamin b complex *on page 553*
Organidin® **NR** *see* guaifenesin *on page 247*
Orgaran® *see* danaparoid *on page 148*
ORG NC 45 *see* vecuronium *on page 547*
Orimune® *see* poliovirus vaccine, live, trivalent, oral *on page 423*
Orinase® **Diagnostic Injection** *see* tolbutamide *on page 523*
Orinase® **Oral** *see* tolbutamide *on page 523*
ORLAAM® *see* levomethadyl acetate hydrochloride *on page 305*
Ormazine *see* chlorpromazine *on page 119*
Ornade® **Spansule**® *see* chlorpheniramine and phenylpropanolamine *on page 114*
Ornex® **No Drowsiness [OTC]** *see* acetaminophen and pseudoephedrine *on page 5*
Ornidyl® **Injection** *see* eflornithine *on page 191*

orphenadrine (or FEN a dreen)
Synonyms orphenadrine citrate
Brand Names Norflex™
(Continued)

orphenadrine *(Continued)*

Therapeutic Category Skeletal Muscle Relaxant
Use Treatment of muscle spasm associated with acute painful musculoskeletal conditions; supportive therapy in tetanus
Usual Dosage Adults:
Oral: 100 mg twice daily
I.M., I.V.: 60 mg every 12 hours
Dosage Forms
Injection, as citrate: 30 mg/mL (2 mL, 10 mL)
Tablet, as citrate: 100 mg
Sustained release: 100 mg

orphenadrine, aspirin and caffeine (or FEN a dreen, AS pir in, & KAF een)

Brand Names Norgesic™; Norgesic™ Forte
Therapeutic Category Analgesic, Non-narcotic; Skeletal Muscle Relaxant
Use Relief of discomfort associated with skeletal muscular conditions
Usual Dosage Oral: 1-2 tablets 3-4 times/day
Dosage Forms
Tablet: Orphenadrine citrate 25 mg, aspirin 385 mg, and caffeine 30 mg
Tablet (Norgesic® Forte): Orphenadrine citrate 50 mg, aspirin 770 mg, and caffeine 60 mg

orphenadrine citrate *see* orphenadrine *on previous page*

Ortho-Cept® *see* ethinyl estradiol and desogestrel *on page 207*

Orthoclone® OKT3 *see* muromonab-CD3 *on page 359*

Ortho-Cyclen® *see* ethinyl estradiol and norgestimate *on page 210*

Ortho-Dienestrol® Vaginal *see* dienestrol *on page 166*

Ortho-Est® Oral *see* estropipate *on page 206*

Ortho-Novum® 1/35 *see* ethinyl estradiol and norethindrone *on page 209*

Ortho-Novum® 1/50 *see* mestranol and norethindrone *on page 332*

Ortho-Novum® 7/7/7 *see* ethinyl estradiol and norethindrone *on page 209*

Ortho-Novum® 10/11 *see* ethinyl estradiol and norethindrone *on page 209*

Ortho Tri-Cyclen® *see* ethinyl estradiol and norgestimate *on page 210*

Or-Tyl® Injection *see* dicyclomine *on page 165*

Orudis® *see* ketoprofen *on page 297*

Orudis® KT [OTC] *see* ketoprofen *on page 297*

Oruvail® *see* ketoprofen *on page 297*

Os-Cal® 500 [OTC] *see* calcium carbonate *on page 82*

Osmitrol® Injection *see* mannitol *on page 321*

Osmoglyn® Ophthalmic *see* glycerin *on page 243*

Osmolite® HN [OTC] *see* enteral nutritional products *on page 194*

Osteocalcin® Injection *see* calcitonin *on page 81*

Otic-Care® Otic *see* neomycin, polymyxin b, and hydrocortisone *on page 369*

Otic Domeboro® *see* aluminum acetate and acetic acid *on page 20*

Otobiotic® Otic *see* polymyxin b and hydrocortisone *on page 424*

Otocalm® Ear *see* antipyrine and benzocaine *on page 38*

Otocort® Otic *see* neomycin, polymyxin b, and hydrocortisone *on page 369*

Otosporin® Otic *see* neomycin, polymyxin b, and hydrocortisone *on page 369*

Otrivin® Nasal [OTC] *see* xylometazoline *on page 558*

Ovcon® 35 *see* ethinyl estradiol and norethindrone *on page 209*

Ovcon® 50 *see* ethinyl estradiol and norethindrone *on page 209*

Ovide™ Topical *see* malathion *on page 320*

Ovral® *see* ethinyl estradiol and norgestrel *on page 210*

Ovrette® *see* norgestrel *on page 379*

oxacillin (oks a SIL in)

Synonyms methylphenyl isoxazolyl penicillin; oxacillin sodium; sodium oxacillin

Brand Names Bactocill®; Prostaphlin®

Therapeutic Category Penicillin

Use Treatment of bacterial infections such as osteomyelitis, septicemia, endocarditis, and CNS infections due to susceptible penicillinase-producing strains of *Staphylococcus*

Usual Dosage

Infants and Children:

I.M., I.V.: 150-200 mg/kg/day in divided doses every 6 hours; maximum dose: 12 g/day

Oral: 50-100 mg/kg/day divided every 6 hours

Adults:

Oral: 500-1000 mg every 4-6 hours for at least 5 days

I.M., I.V.: 250 mg to 2 g/dose every 4-6 hours

Dosage Forms

Capsule, as sodium: 250 mg, 500 mg

Powder:

For injection, as sodium: 250 mg, 500 mg, 1 g, 2 g, 4 g, 10 g

For oral solution, as sodium: 250 mg/5 mL (100 mL)

oxacillin sodium *see* oxacillin *on this page*

oxamniquine (oks AM ni kwin)

Brand Names Vansil™

Therapeutic Category Anthelmintic

Use Treat all stages of *Schistosoma mansoni* infection

Usual Dosage Oral:

Children <30 kg: 20 mg/kg in 2 divided doses of 10 mg/kg at 2- to 8-hour intervals

Adults: 12-15 mg/kg as a single dose

Dosage Forms Capsule: 250 mg

Oxandrin® *see* oxandrolone *on this page*

oxandrolone (oks AN droe lone)

Brand Names Oxandrin®

Therapeutic Category Androgen

Controlled Substance C-III

Use Treatment of catabolic or tissue-depleting processes

Usual Dosage Adults: Oral: 2.5 mg 2-4 times/day

Dosage Forms Tablet: 2.5 mg

oxaprozin (oks a PROE zin)

Brand Names Daypro™

Therapeutic Category Analgesic, Non-narcotic; Nonsteroidal Anti-Inflammatory Agent (NSAID)

Use Acute and long-term use in the management of signs and symptoms of osteoarthritis and rheumatoid arthritis

Usual Dosage Adults: Oral (individualize the dosage to the lowest effective dose to minimize adverse effects):

Osteoarthritis: 600-1200 mg once daily

(Continued)

oxaprozin *(Continued)*

Rheumatoid arthritis: 1200 mg once daily
Maximum dose: 1800 mg/day or 26 mg/kg (whichever is lower) in divided doses
Dosage Forms Tablet: 600 mg

oxazepam (oks A ze pam)

Brand Names Serax®
Therapeutic Category Anticonvulsant; Benzodiazepine
Controlled Substance C-IV
Use Treatment of anxiety and management of alcohol withdrawal; may also be used as an anticonvulsant in management of simple partial seizures
Usual Dosage Oral:
Children: 1 mg/kg/day has been administered
Adults:
Anxiety: 10-30 mg 3-4 times/day
Alcohol withdrawal: 15-30 mg 3-4 times/day
Hypnotic: 15-30 mg
Dosage Forms
Capsule: 10 mg, 15 mg, 30 mg
Tablet: 15 mg

oxiconazole (oks i KON a zole)

Synonyms oxiconazole nitrate
Brand Names Oxistat® Topical
Therapeutic Category Antifungal Agent
Use Treatment of tinea pedis, tinea cruris, and tinea corporis
Usual Dosage Topical: Apply once daily to affected areas for 2 weeks to 1 month
Dosage Forms
Cream, as nitrate: 1% (15 g, 30 g, 60 g)
Lotion, as nitrate: 1% (30 mL)

oxiconazole nitrate *see* oxiconazole *on this page*
oxilapine succinate *see* loxapine *on page 315*
Oxipor® VHC [OTC] *see* coal tar *on page 132*
Oxistat® Topical *see* oxiconazole *on this page*
oxpentifylline *see* pentoxifylline *on page 405*
Oxsoralen® *see* methoxsalen *on page 339*
Oxsoralen-Ultra® *see* methoxsalen *on page 339*

oxtriphylline (oks TRYE fi lin)

Synonyms choline theophyllinate
Therapeutic Category Theophylline Derivative
Use Bronchodilator in symptomatic treatment of asthma and reversible bronchospasm
Usual Dosage Oral:
Children:
1-9 years: 6.2 mg/kg/dose every 6 hours
9-16 years: 4.7 mg/kg/dose every 6 hours
Adults: 4.7 mg/kg every 8 hours; sustained release: administer every 12 hours
Dosage Forms
Elixir: 100 mg/5 mL (5 mL, 10 mL, 473 mL)
Syrup: 50 mg/5 mL (473 mL)
Tablet: 100 mg, 200 mg
Sustained release: 400 mg, 600 mg

Oxy-5® Advanced Formula for Sensitive Skin [OTC] *see* benzoyl peroxide *on page 61*

Oxy-5® Tinted [OTC] *see* benzoyl peroxide *on page 61*

Oxy-10® Advanced Formula for Sensitive Skin [OTC] *see* benzoyl peroxide *on page 61*

Oxy 10® Wash [OTC] *see* benzoyl peroxide *on page 61*

oxybutynin (oks i BYOO ti nin)
Synonyms oxybutynin chloride
Brand Names Ditropan®
Therapeutic Category Antispasmodic Agent, Urinary
Use Relief of bladder spasms associated with voiding in patients with uninhibited and reflex neurogenic bladder
Usual Dosage Oral:
Children:
1-5 years: 0.2 mg/kg/dose 2-4 times/day
>5 years: 5 mg twice daily, up to 5 mg 3 times/day
Adults: 5 mg 2-3 times/day up to 5 mg 4 times/day maximum
Dosage Forms
Syrup, as chloride: 5 mg/5 mL (473 mL)
Tablet, as chloride: 5 mg

oxybutynin chloride *see* oxybutynin *on this page*

Oxycel® *see* cellulose, oxidized *on page 102*

oxychlorosene (oks i KLOR oh seen)
Synonyms oxychlorosene sodium
Brand Names Clorpactin® WCS-90
Therapeutic Category Antibiotic, Topical
Use Treating localized infections
Usual Dosage Topical (0.1% to 0.5% solutions): Apply by irrigation, instillation, spray, soaks, or wet compresses
Dosage Forms Powder for solution, as sodium: 2 g, 5 g

oxychlorosene sodium *see* oxychlorosene *on this page*

oxycodone (oks i KOE done)
Synonyms dihydrohydroxycodeinone; oxycodone hydrochloride
Brand Names OxyContin®; OxyIR®; Roxicodone™
Therapeutic Category Analgesic, Narcotic
Controlled Substance C-II
Use Management of moderate to severe pain, normally used in combination with non-narcotic analgesics
Usual Dosage Oral:
Children:
6-12 years: 1.25 mg every 6 hours as needed
>12 years: 2.5 mg every 6 hours as needed
Adults: 5 mg every 6 hours as needed
Dosage Forms
Capsule, as hydrochloride, immediate release (OxyIR®): 5 mg
Liquid, oral, as hydrochloride: 5 mg/5 mL (500 mL)
Solution, oral concentrate, as hydrochloride: 20 mg/mL (30 mL)
Tablet, as hydrochloride: 5 mg
Controlled release (OxyContin®): 10 mg, 20 mg, 40 mg, 80 mg

oxycodone and acetaminophen (oks i KOE done & a seet a MIN oh fen)

Synonyms acetaminophen and oxycodone
Brand Names Percocet®; Roxicet® 5/500; Roxilox®; Tylox®
Therapeutic Category Analgesic, Narcotic
Controlled Substance C-II
Use Management of moderate to severe pain
Usual Dosage Oral (doses should be titrated to appropriate analgesic effects):
Children: Oxycodone: 0.05-0.15 mg/kg/dose to 5 mg/dose (maximum) every 4-6 hours as needed
Adults: 1-2 tablets every 4-6 hours as needed for pain
Maximum daily dose of acetaminophen: 8 g/day, in alcoholics: 4 g/day
Dosage Forms
Caplet: Oxycodone hydrochloride 5 mg and acetaminophen 500 mg
Capsule: Oxycodone hydrochloride 5 mg and acetaminophen 500 mg
Solution, oral: Oxycodone hydrochloride 5 mg and acetaminophen 325 mg per 5 mL (5 mL, 500 mL)
Tablet: Oxycodone hydrochloride 5 mg and acetaminophen 325 mg

oxycodone and aspirin (oks i KOE done & AS pir in)

Brand Names Codoxy®; Percodan®; Percodan®-Demi; Roxiprin®
Therapeutic Category Analgesic, Narcotic
Controlled Substance C-II
Use Relief of moderate to moderately severe pain
Usual Dosage Oral (based on oxycodone combined salts):
Children: 0.05-0.15 mg/kg/dose every 4-6 hours as needed; maximum: 5 mg/dose (1 tablet Percodan® or 2 tablets Percodan®-Demi/dose) **or**
Alternatively:
6-12 years: Percodan®-Demi: $1/4$ tablet every 6 hours as needed for pain
>12 years: $1/2$ tablet every 6 hours as needed for pain
Adults: Percodan®: 1 tablet every 6 hours as needed for pain or Percodan®-Demi: 1-2 tablets every 6 hours as needed for pain
Dosage Forms Tablet:
Percodan®: Oxycodone hydrochloride 4.5 mg, oxycodone terephthalate 0.38 mg, and aspirin 325 mg
Percodan®-Demi: Oxycodone hydrochloride 2.25 mg, oxycodone terephthalate 0.19 mg, and aspirin 325 mg

oxycodone hydrochloride see oxycodone on previous page

OxyContin® see oxycodone on previous page

OxyIR® see oxycodone on previous page

oxymetazoline (oks i met AZ oh leen)

Synonyms oxymetazoline hydrochloride
Brand Names Afrin® Children's Nose Drops [OTC]; Afrin® Sinus [OTC]; Allerest® 12 Hour Nasal Solution [OTC]; Chlorphed®-LA Nasal Solution [OTC]; Dristan® Long Lasting Nasal Solution [OTC]; Duramist® Plus [OTC]; Duration® Nasal Solution [OTC]; Neo-Synephrine® 12 Hour Nasal Solution [OTC]; Nōstrilla® [OTC]; NTZ® Long Acting Nasal Solution [OTC]; OcuClear® Ophthalmic [OTC]; Sinarest® 12 Hour Nasal Solution; Sinex® Long-Acting [OTC]; Twice-A-Day® Nasal [OTC]; Visine® L.R. Ophthalmic [OTC]; 4-Way® Long Acting Nasal Solution [OTC]
Therapeutic Category Adrenergic Agonist Agent
Use Symptomatic relief of nasal mucosal congestion associated with acute or chronic rhinitis, the common cold, sinusitis, hay fever, or other allergies
Usual Dosage
Intranasal:
Children 2-5 years: 0.025% solution: Instill 2-3 drops in each nostril twice daily

Children ≥6 years and Adults: 0.05% solution: Instill 2-3 drops or 2-3 sprays into each nostril twice daily

Ophthalmic: Adults: Instill 1-2 drops into affected eye(s) every 6 hours

Dosage Forms

Nasal solution, as hydrochloride:

Drops:

Afrin® Children's Nose Drops: 0.025% (20 mL)

Afrin®, NTZ® Long Acting Nasal Solution: 0.05% (15 mL, 20 mL)

Spray: Afrin® Sinus, Allerest® 12 Hours, Chlorphed®-LA, Dristan® Long Lasting, Duration®, 4-Way® Long Acting, Genasal®, Nasal Relief®, Neo-Synephrine® 12 Hour, Nōstrilla®, NTZ® Long Acting Nasal Solution, Sinex® Long-Acting, Twice-A-Day®: 0.05% (15 mL, 30 mL)

Ophthalmic solution, as hydrochloride (OcuClear®, Visine® L.R.): 0.025% (15 mL, 30 mL)

oxymetazoline hydrochloride *see* oxymetazoline *on previous page*

oxymetholone (oks i METH oh lone)

Brand Names Anadrol®

Therapeutic Category Anabolic Steroid

Controlled Substance C-III

Use Anemias caused by the administration of myelotoxic drugs

Usual Dosage Erythropoietic effects: 1-5 mg/kg/day in 1 daily dose; maximum: 100 mg/day

Dosage Forms Tablet: 50 mg

oxymorphone (oks i MOR fone)

Synonyms oxymorphone hydrochloride

Brand Names Numorphan®

Therapeutic Category Analgesic, Narcotic

Controlled Substance C-II

Use Management of moderate to severe pain and preoperatively as a sedative and a supplement to anesthesia

Usual Dosage Adults:

I.M., S.C.: Initial: 0.5 mg, then 1-1.5 mg every 4-6 hours as needed

I.V.: Initial: 0.5 mg

Rectal: 5 mg every 4-6 hours

Dosage Forms

Injection, as hydrochloride: 1 mg (1 mL); 1.5 mg/mL (1 mL, 10 mL)

Suppository, rectal, as hydrochloride: 5 mg

oxymorphone hydrochloride *see* oxymorphone *on this page*

oxyphenbutazone (oks i fen BYOO ta zone)

Therapeutic Category Analgesic, Non-narcotic; Nonsteroidal Anti-Inflammatory Agent (NSAID)

Use Management of inflammatory disorders, as an analgesic in the treatment of mild to moderate pain and as an antipyretic; I.V. form used as an alternate to surgery in management of patent ductus arteriosus in premature neonates; acute gouty arthritis

Usual Dosage Adults: Oral:

Rheumatoid arthritis: 100-200 mg 3-4 times/day until desired effect, then reduce dose to not exceeding 400 mg/day

Acute gouty arthritis: Initial: 400 mg then 100 mg every 4 hours until acute attack subsides

Dosage Forms Tablet: 100 mg

oxytetracycline (oks i tet ra SYE kleen)

Synonyms oxytetracycline hydrochloride
Brand Names Terramycin® I.M. Injection; Terramycin® Oral
Therapeutic Category Tetracycline Derivative
Use Treatment of susceptible bacterial infections; both gram-positive and gram-negative, as well as *Rickettsia* and *Mycoplasma* organisms
Usual Dosage
Oral:
Children: 40-50 mg/kg/day in divided doses every 6 hours (maximum: 2 g/24 hours)
Adults: 250-500 mg/dose every 6 hours
I.M.:
Children >8 years: 15-25 mg/kg/day (maximum: 250 mg/dose) in divided doses every 8-12 hours
Adults: 250-500 mg every 24 hours or 300 mg/day divided every 8-12 hours
Dosage Forms
Capsule, as hydrochloride: 250 mg
Injection, as hydrochloride, with lidocaine 2%: 5% [50 mg/mL] (2 mL, 10 mL); 12.5% [125 mg/mL] (2 mL)

oxytetracycline and hydrocortisone

(oks i tet ra SYE kleen & hye droe KOR ti sone)
Brand Names Terra-Cortril® Ophthalmic Suspension
Therapeutic Category Antibiotic/Corticosteroid, Ophthalmic
Use Treatment of susceptible ophthalmic bacterial infections with associated inflammation
Usual Dosage Ophthalmic: Adults: Instill 1-2 drops in eye(s) every 3-4 hours
Dosage Forms Suspension, ophthalmic: Oxytetracycline hydrochloride 0.5% and hydrocortisone 0.5% (5 mL)

oxytetracycline and polymyxin b

(oks i tet ra SYE kleen & pol i MIKS in bee)
Synonyms polymyxin b and oxytetracycline
Brand Names Terak® Ophthalmic Ointment; Terramycin® Ophthalmic Ointment; Terramycin® w/Polymyxin B Ophthalmic Ointment
Therapeutic Category Antibiotic, Ophthalmic
Use Treatment of superficial ocular infections involving the conjunctiva and/or cornea
Usual Dosage Ophthalmic: Apply ½" of ointment onto the lower lid of affected eye 2-4 times/day
Dosage Forms
Ointment, ophthalmic/otic: Oxytetracycline hydrochloride 5 mg and polymyxin B 10,000 units per g (3.5 g)
Tablet, vaginal: Oxytetracycline hydrochloride 100 mg and polymyxin B 100,000 units (10s)

oxytetracycline hydrochloride *see* oxytetracycline *on this page*

oxytocin (oks i TOE sin)

Synonyms pit
Brand Names Pitocin®; Syntocinon®
Therapeutic Category Oxytocic Agent
Use Induce labor at term; control postpartum bleeding; nasal preparation used to promote milk letdown in lactating females
Usual Dosage Adults:
Induction of labor: I.V.: 0.001-0.002 unit/minute; increase by 0.001-0.002 units every 15-30 minutes until contraction pattern has been established
Postpartum bleeding: I.V.: 0.001-0.002 unit/minute as needed

Promotion of milk letdown: Intranasal: 1 spray or 3 drops in one or both nostrils 2-3 minutes before breast feeding

Dosage Forms
Injection: 10 units/mL (1 mL, 10 mL)
Solution, nasal: 40 units/mL (2 mL, 5 mL)

Oyst-Cal 500 [OTC] *see* calcium carbonate *on page 82*

Oystercal® 500 *see* calcium carbonate *on page 82*

P-071 *see* cetirizine *on page 105*

paclitaxel (PAK li taks el)
Brand Names Taxol®
Therapeutic Category Antineoplastic Agent
Use Treatment of metastatic carcinoma of the ovary after failure of first-line or subsequent chemotherapy; treatment for AIDS-related Kaposi's sarcoma
Usual Dosage Adults: I.V.: 135 mg/m² over 24 hours every 3 weeks
Dosage Forms Injection: 6 mg/mL (5 mL, 16.7 mL)

Palmitate-A® 5000 [OTC] *see* vitamin a *on page 552*

PALS® [OTC] *see* chlorophyll *on page 110*

2-pam *see* pralidoxime *on page 432*

Pamelor® *see* nortriptyline *on page 379*

pamidronate (pa mi DROE nate)
Synonyms pamidronate disodium
Brand Names Aredia™
Therapeutic Category Bisphosphonate Derivative
Use Symptomatic treatment of Paget's disease; hypercalcemia associated with malignancy
Usual Dosage Drug must be diluted properly before administration and infused slowly (at least over 2 hours)

Adults: I.V.:
Moderate cancer-related hypercalcemia (12-13 mg/dL): 60-90 mg administered as a slow infusion over 2-24 hours
Severe cancer-related hypercalcemia (>13.5 mg/dL): 90 mg as a slow infusion over 2-24 hours
A period of 7 days should elapse before the use of second course; repeat infusions every 2-3 weeks have been suggested, however, could be administered every 2-3 months according to the degree and of severity of hypercalcemia and/or the type of malignancy
Paget's disease: 60 mg as a single 2- to 24-hour infusion
Dosage Forms Powder for injection, lyophilized, as disodium: 30 mg, 60 mg, 90 mg

pamidronate disodium *see* pamidronate *on this page*

Pamine® *see* methscopolamine *on page 340*

Panadol® [OTC] *see* acetaminophen *on page 3*

Panasal® 5/500 *see* hydrocodone and aspirin *on page 266*

Pancrease® *see* pancrelipase *on next page*

Pancrease® MT 4 *see* pancrelipase *on next page*

Pancrease® MT 10 *see* pancrelipase *on next page*

Pancrease® MT 16 *see* pancrelipase *on next page*

Pancrease® MT 20 *see* pancrelipase *on next page*

pancreatin (PAN kree a tin)

Brand Names Creon®; Digepepsin®; Donnazyme®; Hi-Vegi-Lip®
Therapeutic Category Enzyme
Use Replacement therapy in symptomatic treatment of malabsorption syndrome caused by pancreatic insufficiency
Usual Dosage Enteric coated microspheres: The following dosage recommendations are only an approximation for initial dosages. The actual dosage will depend on the digestive requirements of the individual patient.

Oral:
Children:
<1 year: 2000 units of lipase with meals/feedings
1-6 years: 4000-8000 units of lipase with meals and 4,000 units with snacks
7-12 years: 4000-12,000 units of lipase with meals and snacks
Adults: 4000-16,000 units of lipase with meals and with snacks

Dosage Forms
Capsule, enteric coated microspheres (Creon®): Lipase 8000 units, amylase 30,000 units, protease 13,000 units and pancreatin 300 mg
Tablet:
Digepepsin®: Pancreatin 300 mg, pepsin 250 mg, and bile salts 150 mg
Donnazyme®: Lipase 1000 units, amylase 12,500 units, protease 12,500 units and pancreatin 500 mg
Hi-Vegi-Lip®: Lipase 4800 units, amylase 60,000 units, protease 60,000 units and pancreatin 2400 mg

pancrelipase (pan kre LI pase)

Synonyms lipancreatin; lipase, protease, and amylase
Brand Names Cotazym®; Cotazym-S®; Creon® 10; Creon® 20; Ilozyme®; Ku-Zyme® HP; Pancrease®; Pancrease® MT 4; Pancrease® MT 10; Pancrease® MT 16; Pancrease® MT 20; Protilase®; Ultrase® MT12; Ultrase® MT20; Viokase®; Zymase®
Therapeutic Category Enzyme
Use Replacement therapy in symptomatic treatment of malabsorption syndrome caused by pancreatic insufficiency
Usual Dosage Oral:
Powder: Actual dose depends on the digestive requirements of the patient
Children <1 year: Start with 1/8 teaspoonful with feedings
Enteric coated microspheres and microtablets: The following dosage recommendations are only an approximation for initial dosages. The actual dosage will depend on the digestive requirements of the individual patient.
Children:
<1 year: 2000 units of lipase with meals/feedings
1-6 years: 4000-8000 units of lipase with meals and 4000 units with snacks
7-12 years: 4000-12,000 units of lipase with meals and snacks
Adults: 4000-16,000 units of lipase with meals and with snacks

Dosage Forms
Capsule:
Cotazym®: Lipase 8000 units, protease 30,000 units, amylase 30,000 units
Ku-Zyme® HP: Lipase 8000 units, protease 30,000 units, amylase 30,000 units
Ultrase® MT12: Lipase 12,000 units, protease 39,000 units, amylase 39,000 units
Ultrase® MT20: Lipase 20,000 units, protease 65,000 units, amylase 65,000 units
Enteric coated microspheres (Pancrease®): Lipase 4000 units, protease 25,000 units, amylase 20,000 units
Enteric coated microtablets:
Pancrease® MT 4: Lipase 4500 units, protease 12,000 units, amylase 12,000 units
Pancrease® MT 10: Lipase 10,000 units, protease 30,000 units, amylase 30,000 units
Pancrease® MT 16: Lipase 16,000 units, protease 48,000 units, amylase 48,000 units
Pancrease® MT 20: Lipase 20,000 units, protease 44,000 units, amylase 56,000 units

Enteric coated spheres:
Cotazym-S®: Lipase 5000 units, protease 20,000 units, amylase 20,000 units
Pancrelipase, Protilase®: Lipase 4000 units, protease 25,000 units, amylase 20,000 units
Zymase®: Lipase 12,000 units, protease 24,000 units, amylase 24,000 units
Delayed release:
Creon 10®: Lipase 10,000 units, protease 37,500 units, amylase 33,200 units
Creon 20®: Lipase 20,000 units, protease 75,000 units, amylase 66,400 units
Powder (Viokase®): Lipase 16,800 units, protease 70,000 units, amylase 70,000 units per 0.7 g
Tablet:
Ilozyme®: Lipase 11,000 units, protease 30,000 units, amylase 30,000 units
Viokase®: Lipase 8000 units, protease 30,000 units, amylase 30,000 units

pancuronium (pan kyoo ROE nee um)
Synonyms pancuronium bromide
Brand Names Pavulon®
Therapeutic Category Skeletal Muscle Relaxant
Use Produces skeletal muscle relaxation during surgery after induction of general anesthesia, increases pulmonary compliance during assisted mechanical respiration, facilitates endotracheal intubation
Usual Dosage Infants >1 month, Children, and Adults: I.V.: 0.04-0.1 mg/kg; maintenance dose: 0.02-0.1 mg/kg/dose every 30-60 minutes as needed
Dosage Forms Injection, as bromide: 1 mg/mL (10 mL); 2 mg/mL (2 mL, 5 mL)

pancuronium bromide *see* pancuronium *on this page*

Pandel® *see* hydrocortisone *on page 268*

Panhematin® *see* hemin *on page 257*

PanOxyl®-AQ *see* benzoyl peroxide *on page 61*

PanOxyl® Bar [OTC] *see* benzoyl peroxide *on page 61*

Panscol® [OTC] *see* salicylic acid *on page 472*

Panthoderm® Cream [OTC] *see* dexpanthenol *on page 158*

Pantopon® *see* opium alkaloids *on page 384*

pantothenic acid (pan toe THEN ik AS id)
Synonyms calcium pantothenate; vitamin b_5
Therapeutic Category Vitamin, Water Soluble
Use Pantothenic acid deficiency
Usual Dosage Adults: Oral: Recommended daily dose: 4-7 mg/day
Dosage Forms Tablet: 25 mg, 50 mg, 100 mg, 218 mg, 250 mg, 500 mg, 545 mg, 1000 mg

pantothenyl alcohol *see* dexpanthenol *on page 158*

papaverine (pa PAV er een)
Synonyms papaverine hydrochloride
Brand Names Genabid®; Pavabid®; Pavatine®
Therapeutic Category Vasodilator
Use Relief of peripheral and cerebral ischemia associated with arterial spasm

Investigational use: Prophylaxis of migraine headache
Usual Dosage Adults:
Oral: 100-300 mg 3-5 times/day
Oral, sustained release: 150-300 mg every 12 hours
Dosage Forms
Capsule, sustained release, as hydrochloride: 150 mg
(Continued)

papaverine *(Continued)*
Tablet, as hydrochloride: 30 mg, 60 mg, 100 mg, 150 mg, 200 mg, 300 mg
Timed release: 200 mg

papaverine hydrochloride *see* papaverine *on previous page*

para-aminosalicylate sodium *see* aminosalicylate sodium *on page 26*

parabromdylamine *see* brompheniramine *on page 73*

paracetaldehyde *see* paraldehyde *on this page*

paracetamol *see* acetaminophen *on page 3*

parachlorometaxylenol (PAIR a klor oh met a ZYE le nol)
Synonyms pcmx
Brand Names Metasep® [OTC]
Therapeutic Category Antiseborrheic Agent, Topical
Use Aid in relief of dandruff and associated conditions
Usual Dosage Massage to a foamy lather, allow to remain on hair for 5 minutes, rinse thoroughly and repeat
Dosage Forms Shampoo: 2% with isopropyl alcohol 9%

Paraflex® *see* chlorzoxazone *on page 120*

Parafon Forte™ DSC *see* chlorzoxazone *on page 120*

Paral® *see* paraldehyde *on this page*

paraldehyde (par AL de hyde)
Synonyms paracetaldehyde
Brand Names Paral®
Therapeutic Category Anticonvulsant
Controlled Substance C-IV
Use Treatment of status epilepticus and tetanus-induced seizures; has been used as a sedative/hypnotic and in the treatment of alcohol withdrawal symptoms
Usual Dosage Dilute in milk or iced fruit juice to mask taste and odor
Oral, rectal:
  Children: 0.15-0.3 mL/kg
  Adults:
    Hypnotic: 10-30 mL
    Sedative: 5-10 mL
  Rectal: Mix paraldehyde 2:1 with oil (cottonseed or olive)
Dosage Forms Liquid, oral or rectal: 1 g/mL (30 mL)

paramethasone acetate (par a METH a sone AS e tate)
Brand Names Haldrone®; Stemex®
Therapeutic Category Adrenal Corticosteroid
Use Treatment of variety of diseases including those of hematologic, allergic, inflammatory, neoplastic, and autoimmune in origin
Usual Dosage Oral: 2-24 mg/day
Dosage Forms Tablet: 1 mg

Paraplatin® *see* carboplatin *on page 92*

Parathar™ Injection *see* teriparatide *on page 506*

Par Decon® *see* chlorpheniramine, phenyltoloxamine, phenylpropanolamine, and phenylephrine *on page 117*

Paredrine® *see* hydroxyamphetamine *on page 273*

paregoric (par e GOR ik)
Synonyms camphorated tincture of opium
Therapeutic Category Analgesic, Narcotic
Controlled Substance C-III
Use Treatment of diarrhea or relief of pain; neonatal abstinence syndrome (neonatal opiate withdrawal)
Usual Dosage Oral:
Neonatal opiate withdrawal: 3-6 drops every 3-6 hours as needed, or initially 0.2 mL every 3 hours; increase dosage by approximately 0.05 mL every 3 hours until withdrawal symptoms are controlled; it is rare to exceed 0.7 mL/dose. Stabilize withdrawal symptoms for 3-5 days, then gradually decrease dosage over a 2- to 4-week period.
Children: 0.25-0.5 mL/kg 1-4 times/day
Adults: 5-10 mL 1-4 times/day
Dosage Forms Liquid: 2 mg morphine equivalent/5 mL [equivalent to 20 mg opium powder] (5 mL, 60 mL, 473 mL, 4000 mL)

Paremyd® Ophthalmic see hydroxyamphetamine and tropicamide on page 273

Parepectolin® see kaolin and pectin with opium on page 295

pargyline and methyclothiazide see methyclothiazide and pargyline on page 340

Parlodel® see bromocriptine on page 72

Parnate® see tranylcypromine on page 527

paromomycin (par oh moe MYE sin)
Synonyms paromomycin sulfate
Brand Names Humatin®
Therapeutic Category Amebicide
Use Treatment of acute and chronic intestinal amebiasis due to susceptible *Entamoeba histolytica* (not effective in the treatment of extraintestinal amebiasis); tapeworm infestations; adjunctive management of hepatic coma; treatment of cryptosporidial diarrhea
Usual Dosage Oral:
Intestinal amebiasis: Children and Adults: 25-35 mg/kg/day in 3 divided doses for 5-10 days
Tapeworm (fish, dog, bovine, porcine):
 Children: 11 mg/kg every 15 minutes for 4 doses
 Adults: 1 g every 15 minutes for 4 doses
Hepatic coma: Adults: 4 g/day in 2-4 divided doses for 5-6 days
Dwarf tapeworm: Children and Adults: 45 mg/kg/dose every day for 5-7 days
Dosage Forms Capsule, as sulfate: 250 mg

paromomycin sulfate see paromomycin on this page

paroxetine (pa ROKS e teen)
Brand Names Paxil™
Therapeutic Category Antidepressant, Selective Serotonin Reuptake Inhibitor
Use Treatment of depression, obsessive compulsive disorder (OCD) and panic disorder (PD)
Usual Dosage Adults: Oral: 20 mg once daily, preferably in the morning
Dosage Forms Tablet: 10 mg, 20 mg, 30 mg, 40 mg

Partuss® LA see guaifenesin and phenylpropanolamine on page 249

PAS see aminosalicylate sodium on page 26

Patanol® see olopatadine on page 383

Pathilon® see tridihexethyl on page 531

Pathocil® see dicloxacillin on page 165

Pavabid® *see* papaverine *on page 395*

Pavatine® *see* papaverine *on page 395*

Pavulon® *see* pancuronium *on page 395*

Paxil™ *see* paroxetine *on previous page*

Paxipam® *see* halazepam *on page 254*

PBZ® *see* tripelennamine *on page 535*

PBZ-SR® *see* tripelennamine *on page 535*

PCE® **Oral** *see* erythromycin *on page 199*

pcmx *see* parachlorometaxylenol *on page 396*

pectin and kaolin *see* kaolin and pectin *on page 295*

Pedameth® *see* methionine *on page 337*

Pedia Care® **Oral** *see* pseudoephedrine *on page 449*

Pediacof® *see* chlorpheniramine, phenylephrine, and codeine *on page 115*

Pediaflor® *see* fluoride *on page 228*

Pedialyte® **[OTC]** *see* enteral nutritional products *on page 194*

Pediapred® **Oral** *see* prednisolone *on page 434*

Pediatric Triban® *see* trimethobenzamide *on page 534*

Pediazole® *see* erythromycin and sulfisoxazole *on page 200*

Pedi-Boro® **[OTC]** *see* aluminum acetate and calcium acetate *on page 20*

Pedi-Cort V® **Creme** *see* clioquinol and hydrocortisone *on page 128*

Pediotic® **Otic** *see* neomycin, polymyxin b, and hydrocortisone *on page 369*

Pedi-Pro Topical [OTC] *see* undecylenic acid and derivatives *on page 541*

Pedituss® *see* chlorpheniramine, phenylephrine, and codeine *on page 115*

PedTE-PAK-4® *see* trace metals *on page 525*

Pedtrace-4® *see* trace metals *on page 525*

PedvaxHIB™ *see* haemophilus b conjugate vaccine *on page 254*

pegademase (bovine) (peg A de mase BOE vine)
Brand Names Adagen™
Therapeutic Category Enzyme
Use Enzyme replacement therapy for adenosine deaminase (ADA) deficiency in patients with severe combined immunodeficiency disease (SCID) who can not benefit from bone marrow transplant
Usual Dosage Children: I.M.: Dose administered every 7 days, 10 units/kg the first dose, 15 units/kg the second dose, and 20 units/kg the third; maintenance dose: 20 units/kg/week is recommended depending on patient's ADA level
Dosage Forms Injection: 250 units/mL (1.5 mL)

Peganone® *see* ethotoin *on page 211*

pegaspargase (peg AS par jase)
Synonyms peg-l-asparaginase
Brand Names Oncaspar®
Therapeutic Category Antineoplastic Agent
Use Induction treatment of acute lymphoblastic leukemia in combination with other chemotherapeutic agents in patients who have developed hypersensitivity to native forms of L-asparaginase derived from *E. coli* and/or *Erwinia chrysanthemia*, treatment of lymphoma

Usual Dosage **Refer to individual protocols**; I.M. administration may decrease the risk of anaphylaxis; dose must be individualized based upon clinical response and tolerance of the patient.

I.M., I.V.: 2000 units/m^2 every 14 days

Dosage Forms Injection, preservative free: 750 units/mL

peg-es *see* polyethylene glycol-electrolyte solution *on page 423*

peg-l-asparaginase *see* pegaspargase *on previous page*

pemoline (PEM oh leen)

Synonyms phenylisohydantoin; pio

Brand Names Cylert®

Therapeutic Category Central Nervous System Stimulant, Nonamphetamine

Controlled Substance C-IV

Use Treatment of attention deficit disorder with hyperactivity (ADDH); narcolepsy

Usual Dosage Oral:

Children: <6 years: Not recommended.

Children ≥6 years and Adults: Initial: 37.5 mg administered once daily in the morning, increase by 18.75 mg/day at weekly intervals; effective dose range: 56.25-75 mg/day; maximum: 112.5 mg/day; dosage range: 0.5-3 mg/kg/24 hours

Dosage Forms

Tablet: 18.75 mg, 37.5 mg, 75 mg

Chewable: 37.5 mg

penbutolol (pen BYOO toe lole)

Synonyms penbutolol sulfate

Brand Names Levatol®

Therapeutic Category Beta-Adrenergic Blocker

Use Treatment of mild to moderate arterial hypertension

Usual Dosage Adults: Oral: Initial: 20 mg once daily, full effect of a 20 or 40 mg dose is seen by the end of a 2-week period, doses of 40-80 mg have been tolerated but have shown little additional antihypertensive effects

Dosage Forms Tablet, as sulfate: 20 mg

penbutolol sulfate *see* penbutolol *on this page*

penciclovir (pen SYE kloe veer)

Brand Names Denavir®

Therapeutic Category Antiviral Agent

Use Antiviral cream for the treatment of recurrent herpes labialis (cold sores) in adults

Usual Dosage Apply cream at the first sign or symptom of cold sore (eg, tingling, swelling); apply every 2 hours during waking hours for 4 days

Dosage Forms Cream: 1% [10 mg/g] (2 g)

Penecort® *see* hydrocortisone *on page 268*

Penetrex™ *see* enoxacin *on page 194*

penicillamine (pen i SIL a meen)

Synonyms d-3-mercaptovaline; β,β-dimethylcysteine; d-penicillamine

Brand Names Cuprimine®; Depen®

Therapeutic Category Chelating Agent

Use Treatment of Wilson's disease, cystinuria, adjunct in the treatment of severe rheumatoid arthritis; lead poisoning, primary biliary cirrhosis

(Continued)

penicillamine (Continued)

Usual Dosage Oral:

Rheumatoid arthritis:

Children: Initial: 3 mg/kg/day (≤250 mg/day) for 3 months, then 6 mg/kg/day (≤500 mg/day) in divided doses twice daily for 3 months to a maximum of 10 mg/kg/day in 3-4 divided doses

Adults: 125-250 mg/day, may increase dose at 1- to 3-month intervals up to 1-1.5 g/day

Wilson's disease (doses titrated to maintain urinary copper excretion >1 mg/day):

Infants <6 months: 250 mg/dose once daily

Children <12 years: 250 mg/dose 2-3 times/day

Adults: 250 mg 4 times/day

Cystinuria:

Children: 30 mg/kg/day in 4 divided doses

Adults: 1-4 g/day in divided doses every 6 hours

Lead poisoning (continue until blood lead level is <60 mcg/dL):

Children: 25-40 mg/kg/day in 3 divided doses

Adults: 250 mg/dose every 8-12 hours

Primary biliary cirrhosis: 250 mg/day to start, increase by 250 mg every 2 weeks up to a maintenance dose of 1 g/day, usually administered 250 mg 4 times/day

Arsenic poisoning: Children: 100 mg/kg/day in divided doses every 6 hours for 5 days; maximum: 1 g/day

Dosage Forms

Capsule: 125 mg, 250 mg

Tablet: 250 mg

penicillin g benzathine (pen i SIL in jee BENZ a theen)

Synonyms benzathine benzylpenicillin; benzathine penicillin g; benzylpenicillin benzathine

Brand Names Bicillin® L-A; Permapen®

Therapeutic Category Penicillin

Use Active against most gram-positive organisms and some spirochetes; used only for the treatment of mild to moderately severe infections (ie, *Streptococcus* pharyngitis) caused by organisms susceptible to low concentrations of penicillin G, or for prophylaxis of infections caused by these organisms such as rheumatic fever prophylaxis

Usual Dosage I.M.: Administer undiluted injection, very slowly released from site of injection, providing uniform levels over 2-4 weeks; higher doses result in more sustained rather than higher levels. Use a penicillin g benzathine-penicillin g procaine combination to achieve early peak levels in acute infections

Infants and Children:

Group A streptococcal upper respiratory infection: 25,000 units/kg as a single dose; maximum: 1.2 million units

Prophylaxis of recurrent rheumatic fever: 25,000 units/kg every 3-4 weeks; maximum: 1.2 million units/dose

Early syphilis: 50,000 units/kg as a single injection; maximum: 2.4 million units

Syphilis of more than 1-year duration: 50,000 units/kg every week for 3 doses; maximum: 2.4 million units/dose

Adults:

Group A streptococcal upper respiratory infection: 1.2 million units as a single dose

Prophylaxis of recurrent rheumatic fever: 1.2 million units every 3-4 weeks or 600,000 units twice monthly; a single dose of 600,000 to 1,2000,000 units is effective in the prevention of rheumatic fever secondary to streptococcal pharyngitis

Early syphilis: 2.4 million units as a single dose

Syphilis of more than 1-year duration: 2.4 million units once weekly for 3 doses

Dosage Forms Injection: 300,000 units/mL (10 mL); 600,000 units/mL (1 mL, 2 mL, 4 mL)

penicillin g benzathine and procaine combined
(pen i SIL in jee BENZ a theen & PROE kane KOM bined)

Synonyms penicillin g procaine and benzathine combined

Brand Names Bicillin® C-R 900/300 Injection; Bicillin® C-R Injection

Therapeutic Category Penicillin

Use Active against most gram-positive organisms, mostly streptococcal and pneumococcal

Usual Dosage I.M.:
Children:
<30 lb: 600,000 units in a single dose
30-60 lb: 900,000 units to 1.2 million units in a single dose
Children >60 lb and Adults: 2.4 million units in a single dose

Dosage Forms
Injection:
300,000 units [150,000 units each of penicillin g benzathine and penicillin g procaine] (10 mL)
600,000 units [300,000 units each penicillin g benzathine and penicillin g procaine] (1 mL)
1,200,000 units [600,000 units each penicillin g benzathine and penicillin g procaine] (2 mL)
2,400,000 units [1,200,000 units each penicillin g benzathine and penicillin g procaine] (4 mL)
Injection: Penicillin g benzathine 900,000 units and penicillin g procaine 300,000 units per dose (2 mL)

penicillin g, parenteral, aqueous
(pen i SIL in jee, pa REN ter al, AYE kwee us)

Synonyms benzylpenicillin potassium; benzylpenicillin sodium; crystalline penicillin; penicillin g potassium; penicillin g sodium

Brand Names Pfizerpen®

Therapeutic Category Penicillin

Use Active against most gram-positive organisms except *Staphylococcus aureus*; some gram-negative such as *Neisseria gonorrhoeae* and some anaerobes and spirochetes; although ceftriaxone is now the drug of choice for lyme disease and gonorrhea

Usual Dosage I.M., I.V.:
Infants and Children (sodium salt is preferred in children): 100,000-250,000 units/kg/day in divided doses every 4 hours; maximum: 4.8 million units/24 hours
Severe infections: Up to 400,000 units/kg/day in divided doses every 4 hours; maximum dose: 24 million units/day
Adults: 2-24 million units/day in divided doses every 4 hours

Dosage Forms
Injection, as sodium: 5 million units
Injection:
Frozen premixed, as potassium: 1 million units, 2 million units, 3 million units
Powder, as potassium: 1 million units, 5 million units, 10 million units, 20 million units

penicillin g potassium *see* penicillin g, parenteral, aqueous *on this page*

penicillin g procaine (pen i SIL in jee PROE kane)

Synonyms appg; aqueous procaine penicillin g; procaine benzylpenicillin; procaine penicillin g

Brand Names Crysticillin® A.S.; Wycillin®

Therapeutic Category Penicillin

Use Moderately severe infections due to *Neisseria gonorrhoeae*, *Treponema pallidum*, and other penicillin G-sensitive microorganisms that are susceptible to low but prolonged serum penicillin concentrations
(Continued)

penicillin g procaine *(Continued)*

Usual Dosage I.M.:

Newborns: 50,000 units/kg/day administered every day (avoid using in this age group since sterile abscesses and procaine toxicity occur more frequently with neonates than older patients)

Children: 25,000-50,000 units/kg/day in divided doses 1-2 times/day; not to exceed 4.8 million units/24 hours

Gonorrhea: 100,000 units/kg one time (in 2 injection sites) along with probenecid 25 mg/kg (maximum: 1 g) orally 30 minutes prior to procaine penicillin

Adults: 0.6-4.8 million units/day in divided doses 1-2 times/day

Uncomplicated gonorrhea: 1 g probenecid orally, then 4.8 million units procaine penicillin divided into 2 injection sites 30 minutes later. When used in conjunction with an aminoglycoside for the treatment of endocarditis caused by susceptible *S. viridans*: 1.2 million units every 6 hours for 2-4 weeks

Dosage Forms Injection, suspension: 300,000 units/mL (10 mL); 500,000 units/mL (1.2 mL); 600,000 units/mL (1 mL, 2 mL, 4 mL)

penicillin g procaine and benzathine combined *see* penicillin g benzathine and procaine combined *on previous page*

penicillin g sodium *see* penicillin g, parenteral, aqueous *on previous page*

penicillin v potassium *(pen i SIL in vee poe TASS ee um)*

Synonyms pen vk; phenoxymethyl penicillin

Brand Names Beepen-VK®; Betapen®-VK; Pen.Vee® K; Robicillin® VK; Veetids®

Therapeutic Category Penicillin

Use Treatment of mild to moderately severe susceptible bacterial infections involving the upper respiratory tract, skin, and urinary tract; prophylaxis of pneumococcal infections and rheumatic fever

Usual Dosage Oral:

Systemic infections:

Children <12 years: 25-50 mg/kg/day in divided doses every 6-8 hours; maximum dose: 3 g/day

Children >12 years and Adults: 125-500 mg every 6-8 hours

Prophylaxis of pneumococcal infections:

Children <5 years: 125 mg twice daily

Children ≥5 years: 250 mg twice daily

Prophylaxis of recurrent rheumatic fever:

Children <5 years: 125 mg

Children ≥5 years and Adults: 250 mg twice daily

Dosage Forms

Powder for oral solution: 125 mg/5 mL (3 mL, 100 mL, 150 mL, 200 mL); 250 mg/5 mL (100 mL, 150 mL, 200 mL)

Tablet: 125 mg, 250 mg, 500 mg

penicilloyl-polylysine *see* benzylpenicilloyl-polylysine *on page 63*

Pentacarinat® Injection *see* pentamidine *on next page*

pentaerythritol tetranitrate *(pen ta er ITH ri tole te tra NYE trate)*

Synonyms petn

Brand Names Duotrate®; Peritrate®; Peritrate® SA

Therapeutic Category Vasodilator

Use Prophylactic long-term management of angina pectoris

Usual Dosage Adults: Oral: 10-20 mg 4 times/day (160 mg/day) up to 40 mg 4 times/day before or after meals and at bedtime; administer sustained release preparation every 12 hours; maximum daily dose: 240 mg

Dosage Forms

Capsule: sustained release: 15 mg, 30 mg

Tablet: 10 mg, 20 mg, 40 mg
Sustained release: 80 mg

pentagastrin (pen ta GAS trin)
Brand Names Peptavlon®
Therapeutic Category Diagnostic Agent
Use Evaluate gastric acid secretory function in pernicious anemia, gastric carcinoma; in suspected duodenal ulcer or Zollinger-Ellison tumor
Usual Dosage Adults: S.C.: 6 mcg/kg
Dosage Forms Injection: 0.25 mg/mL (2 mL)

Pentam-300® Injection see pentamidine on this page

pentamidine (pen TAM i deen)
Synonyms pentamidine isethionate
Brand Names NebuPent™ Inhalation; Pentacarinat® Injection; Pentam-300® Injection
Therapeutic Category Antiprotozoal
Use Treatment and prevention of pneumonia caused by *Pneumocystis carinii* in patients who cannot tolerate co-trimoxazole or who fail to respond to this drug; treatment of African trypanosomiasis; treatment of visceral leishmaniasis caused by *L. donovani*
Usual Dosage
Children:
Treatment: I.M., I.V. (I.V. preferred): 4 mg/kg/day once daily for 14-21 days
Prevention:
I.M., I.V.: 4 mg/kg monthly or biweekly
Inhalation (aerosolized pentamidine in children ≥5 years): 300 mg/dose administered every 3 weeks or monthly via Respirgard® II inhaler (8 mg/kg dose has also been used in children <5 years)
Treatment of trypanosomiasis: I.V.: 4 mg/kg/day once daily for 10 days
Adults:
Treatment: I.M., I.V. (I.V. preferred): 4 mg/kg/day once daily for 14 days
Prevention: Inhalation: 300 mg every 4 weeks via Respirgard® II nebulizer
Dosage Forms
Inhalation, as isethionate: 300 mg
Powder for injection, as isethionate, lyophilized: 300 mg

pentamidine isethionate see pentamidine on this page
Pentasa® Oral see mesalamine on page 331
Pentaspan® see pentastarch on this page

pentastarch (PEN ta starch)
Brand Names Pentaspan®
Therapeutic Category Blood Modifiers
Use Adjunct in leukapheresis to improve the harvesting and increase the yield of leukocytes by centrifugal means
Usual Dosage 250-700 mL to which citrate anticoagulant has been added is administered by adding to the input line of the centrifugation apparatus at a ratio of 1:8-1:13 to venous whole blood
Dosage Forms Injection, in NS: 10%

pentazocine (pen TAZ oh seen)
Synonyms pentazocine hydrochloride; pentazocine lactate
Brand Names Talwin®; Talwin® NX
Therapeutic Category Analgesic, Narcotic
Controlled Substance C-IV
Use Relief of moderate to severe pain; a sedative prior to surgery; supplement to surgical anesthesia
(Continued)

403

pentazocine *(Continued)*

Usual Dosage
Children: I.M., S.C.:
5-8 years: 15 mg
8-14 years: 30 mg
Children >12 years and Adults: Oral: 50 mg every 3-4 hours; may increase to 100 mg/dose if needed, but should not exceed 600 mg/day
Adults:
I.M., S.C.: 30-60 mg every 3-4 hours, not to exceed total daily dose of 360 mg
I.V.: 30 mg every 3-4 hours
Dosage Forms
Injection, as lactate: 30 mg/mL (1 mL, 1.5 mL, 2 mL, 10 mL)
Tablet: Pentazocine hydrochloride 50 mg and naloxone hydrochloride 0.5 mg

pentazocine compound (pen TAZ oh seen KOM pownd)
Brand Names Talacen®; Talwin® Compound
Therapeutic Category Analgesic, Narcotic
Use Relief of moderate to severe pain; has also been used as a sedative prior to surgery and as a supplement to surgical anesthesia
Usual Dosage Adults: Oral: 2 tablets 3-4 times/day
Dosage Forms Tablet:
Talacen®: Pentazocine hydrochloride 25 mg and acetaminophen 650 mg
Talwin® Compound: Pentazocine hydrochloride 12.5 mg and aspirin 325 mg

pentazocine hydrochloride *see* pentazocine *on previous page*

pentazocine lactate *see* pentazocine *on previous page*

Penthrane® *see* methoxyflurane *on page 339*

pentobarbital (pen toe BAR bi tal)
Synonyms pentobarbital sodium
Brand Names Nembutal®
Therapeutic Category Barbiturate
Controlled Substance C-II
Use Short-term treatment of insomnia; preoperative sedation; high-dose barbiturate coma for treatment of increased intracranial pressure or status epilepticus unresponsive to other therapy
Usual Dosage
Children:
Sedative: Oral: 2-6 mg/kg/day divided in 3 doses; maximum: 100 mg/day
Hypnotic: I.M.: 2-6 mg/kg; maximum: 100 mg/dose
Rectal:
2 months to 1 year (10-20 lb): 30 mg
1-4 years (20-40 lb): 30-60 mg
5-12 years (40-80 lb): 60 mg
12-14 years (80-110 lb): 60-120 mg **or**
<4 years: 3-6 mg/kg/dose
>4 years: 1.5-3 mg/kg/dose
Preoperative/preprocedure sedation: ≥6 months:
Oral, I.M., rectal: 2-6 mg/kg; maximum: 100 mg/dose
I.V.: 1-3 mg/kg to a maximum of 100 mg until asleep
Children 5-12 years: Conscious sedation prior to a procedure: I.V.: 2 mg/kg 5-10 minutes before procedures, may repeat one time
Adolescents: Conscious sedation: Oral, I.V.: 100 mg prior to a procedure

Children and Adults: Barbiturate coma in head injury patients: I.V.: Loading dose: 5-10 mg/kg administered slowly over 1-2 hours; monitor blood pressure and respiratory rate; Maintenance infusion: Initial: 1 mg/kg/hour; may increase to 2-3 mg/kg/hour; maintain burst suppression on EEG

Adults:
Hypnotic:
Oral: 100-200 mg at bedtime or 20 mg 3-4 times/day for daytime sedation
I.M.: 150-200 mg
I.V.: Initial: 100 mg, may repeat every 1-3 minutes up to 200-500 mg total dose
Rectal: 120-200 mg at bedtime
Preoperative sedation: I.M.: 150-200 mg
Dosage Forms
Capsule, as sodium (C-II): 50 mg, 100 mg
Elixir (C-II): 18.2 mg/5 mL (473 mL, 4000 mL)
Injection, as sodium (C-II): 50 mg/mL (1 mL, 2 mL, 20 mL, 50 mL)
Suppository, rectal (C-III): 30 mg, 60 mg, 120 mg, 200 mg

pentobarbital sodium *see* pentobarbital *on previous page*

pentosan polysulfate sodium (PEN toe san pol i SUL fate SOW dee um)
Synonyms PPS
Brand Names Elmiron®
Therapeutic Category Analgesic, Urinary
Use Bladder pain relief or discomfort associated with interstitial cystitis
Usual Dosage Adults: Oral: 100 mg capsule 3 times/day; take with water at least 1 hour before meals or 2 hours after meals
Dosage Forms Capsule: 100 mg

pentostatin (PEN toe stat in)
Synonyms dcf; 2'-deoxycoformycin
Brand Names Nipent™
Therapeutic Category Antineoplastic Agent
Use Treatment of adult patients with alpha-interferon-refractory hairy cell leukemia; significant antitumor activity in various lymphoid neoplasms has been demonstrated; pentostatin also is known as 2'-deoxycoformycin; it is a purine analogue capable of inhibiting adenosine deaminase
Usual Dosage Refractory hairy cell leukemia: Adults: I.V.: 4 mg/m^2 every other week
Dosage Forms Powder for injection: 10 mg/vial

Pentothal® Sodium *see* thiopental *on page 515*

pentoxifylline (pen toks I fi leen)
Synonyms oxpentifylline
Brand Names Trental®
Therapeutic Category Blood Viscosity Reducer Agent
Use Symptomatic management of peripheral vascular disease, mainly intermittent claudication

Investigational use: AIDS patients with increased tumor necrosis factor, cerebrovascular accidents, cerebrovascular diseases, new onset type I diabetes mellitus, diabetic atherosclerosis, diabetic neuropathy, gangrene, cutaneous polyarteritis nodosa, hemodialysis shunt thrombosis, cerebral malaria, septic shock, sepsis in premature neonates, sickle cell syndromes, vasculitis, Kawasaki disease, Raynaud's syndrome, cystic fibrosis, and persistent pulmonary hypertension of the newborn (case report)
Usual Dosage Adults: Oral: 400 mg 3 times/day with meals; may reduce to 400 mg twice daily if GI or CNS side effects occur
Dosage Forms Tablet, controlled release: 400 mg

Pentrax® [OTC] *see* coal tar *on page 132*
Pen.Vee® K *see* penicillin v potassium *on page 402*
pen vk *see* penicillin v potassium *on page 402*
Pepcid® *see* famotidine *on page 216*

Pepcid® AC Acid Controller [OTC] *see* famotidine *on page 216*

Peptavlon® *see* pentagastrin *on page 403*

Pepto-Bismol® [OTC] *see* bismuth subsalicylate *on page 68*

Pepto® Diarrhea Control [OTC] *see* loperamide *on page 313*

Perchloracap® *see* radiological/contrast media (ionic) *on page 457*

Percocet® *see* oxycodone and acetaminophen *on page 390*

Percodan® *see* oxycodone and aspirin *on page 390*

Percodan®-Demi *see* oxycodone and aspirin *on page 390*

Percogesic® [OTC] *see* acetaminophen and phenyltoloxamine *on page 5*

Perdiem® Plain [OTC] *see* psyllium *on page 451*

Perfectoderm® Gel [OTC] *see* benzoyl peroxide *on page 61*

pergolide (PER go lide)

Synonyms pergolide mesylate
Brand Names Permax®
Therapeutic Category Anti-Parkinson's Agent; Dopaminergic Agent (Antiparkinson's); Ergot Alkaloid
Use Adjunctive treatment to levodopa/carbidopa in the management of Parkinson's Disease
Usual Dosage Adults: Oral: Start with 0.05 mg/day for 2 days, then increase dosage by 0.1 or 0.15 mg/day every 3 days over next 12 days, increase dose by 0.25 mg/day every 3 days until optimal therapeutic dose is achieved
Dosage Forms Tablet, as mesylate: 0.05 mg, 0.25 mg, 1 mg

pergolide mesylate *see* pergolide *on this page*

Pergonal® *see* menotropins *on page 328*

Periactin® *see* cyproheptadine *on page 145*

Peri-Colace® [OTC] *see* docusate and casanthranol *on page 180*

Peridex® Oral Rinse *see* chlorhexidine gluconate *on page 109*

perindopril erbumine (per IN doe pril er BYOO meen)

Brand Names Aceon®
Therapeutic Category Miscellaneous Product
Use Treatment of hypertension
Usual Dosage Adults: Oral: 4 mg once daily; usual range: 4-8 mg/day, maximum of 16 mg/day
Dosage Forms Tablet: 2 mg, 4 mg, 8 mg

PerioGard® *see* chlorhexidine gluconate *on page 109*

Peritrate® *see* pentaerythritol tetranitrate *on page 402*

Peritrate® SA *see* pentaerythritol tetranitrate *on page 402*

Permapen® *see* penicillin g benzathine *on page 400*

Permax® *see* pergolide *on this page*

permethrin (per METH rin)

Brand Names Elimite™ Cream; Nix™ Creme Rinse
Therapeutic Category Scabicides/Pediculicides
Use Single application treatment of infestation with *Pediculus humanus capitis* (head louse) and its nits, or *Sarcoptes scabiei* (scabies)
Usual Dosage
Head lice: Children >2 months and Adults: Topical: After hair has been washed with shampoo, rinsed with water and towel dried, apply a sufficient volume to saturate the

hair and scalp. Leave on hair for 10 minutes before rinsing off with water; remove remaining nits.
Scabies: Apply cream from head to toe; leave on for 8-14 hours before washing off with water
Dosage Forms
Cream: 5% (60 g)
Creme rinse: 1% (60 mL with comb)

Permitil® Oral *see* fluphenazine *on page 230*

Pernox® [OTC] *see* sulfur and salicylic acid *on page 499*

Peroxin A5® *see* benzoyl peroxide *on page 61*

Peroxin A10® *see* benzoyl peroxide *on page 61*

perphenazine (per FEN a zeen)
Brand Names Trilafon®
Therapeutic Category Phenothiazine Derivative
Use Symptomatic management of psychotic disorders, as well as severe nausea and vomiting
Usual Dosage
Children:
Psychoses: Oral:
1-6 years: 4-6 mg/day in divided doses
6-12 years: 6 mg/day in divided doses
>12 years: 4-16 mg 2-4 times/day
I.M.: 5 mg every 6 hours
Nausea/vomiting: I.M.: 5 mg every 6 hours
Adults:
Psychoses:
Oral: 4-16 mg 2-4 times/day not to exceed 64 mg/day
I.M.: 5 mg every 6 hours up to 15 mg/day in ambulatory patients and 30 mg/day in hospitalized patients
Nausea/vomiting:
Oral: 8-16 mg/day in divided doses up to 24 mg/day
I.M.: 5-10 mg every 6 hours as necessary up to 15 mg/day in ambulatory patients and 30 mg/day in hospitalized patients
I.V. (severe): 1 mg at 1- to 2-minute intervals up to a total of 5 mg
Dosage Forms
Concentrate, oral: 16 mg/5 mL (118 mL)
Injection: 5 mg/mL (1 mL)
Tablet: 2 mg, 4 mg, 8 mg, 16 mg

perphenazine and amitriptyline *see* amitriptyline and perphenazine *on page 27*

Persa-Gel® *see* benzoyl peroxide *on page 61*

Persantine® *see* dipyridamole *on page 177*

Pertofrane® *see* desipramine *on page 154*

Pertussin® CS [OTC] *see* dextromethorphan *on page 160*

Pertussin® ES [OTC] *see* dextromethorphan *on page 160*

pethidine hydrochloride *see* meperidine *on page 328*

petn *see* pentaerythritol tetranitrate *on page 402*

pfa *see* foscarnet *on page 234*

Pfizerpen® *see* penicillin g, parenteral, aqueous *on page 401*

pge$_1$ *see* alprostadil *on page 18*

pge$_2$ *see* dinoprostone *on page 172*

pgf₂ₐ *see* dinoprost tromethamine *on page 172*

Phanatuss® Cough Syrup [OTC] *see* guaifenesin and dextromethorphan *on page 248*

Pharmaflur® *see* fluoride *on page 228*

Phazyme® [OTC] *see* simethicone *on page 480*

Phenadex® Senior [OTC] *see* guaifenesin and dextromethorphan *on page 248*

Phenahist-TR® *see* chlorpheniramine, phenylephrine, phenylpropanolamine, and belladonna alkaloids *on page 116*

Phenameth® DM *see* promethazine and dextromethorphan *on page 442*

phenantoin *see* mephenytoin *on page 329*

Phenaphen® With Codeine *see* acetaminophen and codeine *on page 3*

Phenazine® *see* promethazine *on page 441*

phenazopyridine (fen az oh PEER i deen)

Synonyms phenazopyridine hydrochloride; phenylazo diamino pyridine hydrochloride
Brand Names Azo-Standard® [OTC]; Baridium® [OTC]; Prodium® [OTC]; Pyridiate®; Pyridium®; Urodine®; Urogesic®
Therapeutic Category Analgesic, Urinary
Use Symptomatic relief of urinary burning, itching, frequency and urgency in association with urinary tract infection, or following urologic procedures
Usual Dosage Oral:
Children 6-12 years: 12 mg/kg/day in 3 divided doses administered after meals for 2 days
Adults: 100-200 mg 3-4 times/day for 2 days
Dosage Forms Tablet, as hydrochloride:
Azo-Standard®, Prodium®: 95 mg
Baridium®, Geridium®, Pyridiate®, Pyridium®, Urodine®, Urogesic®: 100 mg
Geridium®, Phenazodine®, Pyridium®, Urodine®: 200 mg

phenazopyridine hydrochloride *see* phenazopyridine *on this page*

Phenchlor® S.H.A. *see* chlorpheniramine, phenylephrine, phenylpropanolamine, and belladonna alkaloids *on page 116*

Phendry® Oral [OTC] *see* diphenhydramine *on page 173*

phenelzine (FEN el zeen)

Synonyms phenelzine sulfate
Brand Names Nardil®
Therapeutic Category Antidepressant, Monoamine Oxidase Inhibitor
Use Symptomatic treatment of atypical, nonendogenous or neurotic depression
Usual Dosage Adults: Oral: 15 mg 3 times/day; may increase to 60-90 mg/day during early phase of treatment, then reduce to dose for maintenance therapy slowly after maximum benefit is obtained; takes 2-4 weeks for a significant response to occur
Dosage Forms Tablet, as sulfate: 15 mg

phenelzine sulfate *see* phenelzine *on this page*

Phenerbel-S® *see* belladonna, phenobarbital, and ergotamine tartrate *on page 57*

Phenergan® *see* promethazine *on page 441*

Phenergan® VC Syrup *see* promethazine and phenylephrine *on page 442*

Phenergan® VC With Codeine *see* promethazine, phenylephrine, and codeine *on page 443*

Phenergan® With Codeine *see* promethazine and codeine *on page 442*

Phenergan® **with Dextromethorphan** *see* promethazine and dextromethorphan
on page 442

Phenhist® **Expectorant** *see* guaifenesin, pseudoephedrine, and codeine *on*
page 251

phenindamine (fen IN dah meen)
Synonyms phenindamine tartrate
Brand Names Nolahist® [OTC]
Therapeutic Category Antihistamine
Use Treatment of perennial and seasonal allergic rhinitis and chronic urticaria
Usual Dosage Oral:
  Children <6 years: As directed by physician
  Children 6 to <12 years: 12.5 mg every 4-6 hours, up to 75 mg/24 hours
  Adults: 25 mg every 4-6 hours, up to 150 mg/24 hours
Dosage Forms Tablet, as tartrate: 25 mg

phenindamine tartrate *see* phenindamine *on this page*
pheniramine and naphazoline *see* naphazoline and pheniramine *on page 365*

pheniramine, phenylpropanolamine, and pyrilamine
(fen EER a meen, fen il proe pa NOLE a meen, & peer IL a meen)
Brand Names Triaminic® Oral Infant Drops
Therapeutic Category Antihistamine/Decongestant Combination
Use Symptomatic relief of nasal congestion and postnasal drip as well as allergic rhinitis
Usual Dosage Infants <1 year: Drops: 0.05 mL/kg/dose 4 times/day
Dosage Forms Drops: Pheniramine maleate 10 mg, phenylpropanolamine hydrochloride
20 mg, and pyrilamine maleate 10 mg per mL (15 mL)

phenobarbital (fee noe BAR bi tal)
Synonyms phenobarbital sodium; phenobarbitone; phenylethylmalonylurea
Brand Names Barbita®; Luminal®; Solfoton®
Therapeutic Category Anticonvulsant; Barbiturate
Controlled Substance C-IV
Use Management of generalized tonic-clonic (grand mal) and partial seizures; neonatal
  seizures; febrile seizures in children; sedation; may also be used for prevention and
  treatment of neonatal hyperbilirubinemia and lowering of bilirubin in chronic cholestasis
Usual Dosage
Children:
  Sedation: Oral: 2 mg/kg 3 times/day
  Hypnotic: I.M., I.V., S.C.: 3-5 mg/kg at bedtime
  Hyperbilirubinemia: <12 years: Oral: 3-8 mg/kg/day in 2-3 divided doses; doses up to
    12 mg/kg/day have been used
  Preoperative sedation: Oral, I.M., I.V.: 1-3 mg/kg 1-1.5 hours before procedure

Anticonvulsant: Status epilepticus: **Loading dose:** I.V.:
  Infants, Children and Adults: 15-18 mg/kg in a single or divided dose; usual maximum
    loading dose: 20 mg/kg; in select patients may administer additional 5 mg/kg/dose
    every 15-30 minutes until seizure is controlled or a total dose of 30 mg/kg is reached
Anticonvulsant maintenance dose: Oral, I.V.:
  Infants: 5-6 mg/kg/day in 1-2 divided doses
  Children:
    1-5 years: 6-8 mg/kg/day in 1-2 divided doses
    5-12 years: 4-6 mg/kg/day in 1-2 divided doses
  Children >12 years and Adults: 1-3 mg/kg/day in divided doses

Adults:
  Sedation: Oral, I.M.: 30-120 mg/day in 2-3 divided doses
  Hypnotic: Oral, I.M., I.V., S.C.: 100-320 mg at bedtime
  Hyperbilirubinemia: Oral: 90-180 mg/day in 2-3 divided doses
(Continued)

phenobarbital *(Continued)*
Preoperative sedation: I.M.: 100-200 mg 1-1½ hours before procedure
Dosage Forms
Capsule: 16 mg
Elixir: 15 mg/5 mL (5 mL, 10 mL, 20 mL); 20 mg/5 mL (3.75 mL, 5 mL, 7.5 mL, 120 mL, 473 mL, 946 mL, 4000 mL)
Injection, as sodium: 30 mg/mL (1 mL); 60 mg/mL (1 mL); 65 mg/mL (1 mL); 130 mg/mL (1 mL)
Powder for injection: 120 mg
Tablet: 8 mg, 15 mg, 16 mg, 30 mg, 32 mg, 60 mg, 65 mg, 100 mg

phenobarbital sodium *see* phenobarbital *on previous page*
phenobarbitone *see* phenobarbital *on previous page*

phenol (FEE nol)
Synonyms carbolic acid
Brand Names Baker's P&S Topical [OTC]; Cēpastat® [OTC]; Chloraseptic® Oral [OTC]; Ulcerease® [OTC]
Therapeutic Category Pharmaceutical Aid
Use Relief of sore throat pain, mouth, gum, and throat irritations
Usual Dosage Oral: Allow to dissolve slowly in mouth; may be repeated every 2 hours as needed
Dosage Forms
Liquid:
  Oral, sugar free (Ulcerease®): 6% with glycerin (180 mL)
  Topical (Baker's P&S): 1% with sodium chloride, liquid paraffin oil and water (120 mL, 240 mL)
Lozenge:
  Cēpastat®: 1.45% with menthol and eucalyptus oil
  Cēpastat® Cherry: 0.72% with menthol and eucalyptus oil
  Chloraseptic®: 32.5 mg total phenol, sugar, corn syrup
Mouthwash (Chloraseptic®): 1.4% with thymol, sodium borate, menthol, and glycerin (180 mL)
Solution (Liquified Phenol): 88% [880 mg/mL]
Aqueous: 6% [60 mg/mL]

phenol red *see* phenolsulfonphthalein *on this page*

phenolsulfonphthalein (fee nol sul fon THAY leen)
Synonyms phenol red; psp
Therapeutic Category Diagnostic Agent
Use Evaluation of renal blood flow to aid in the determination of renal function
Usual Dosage I.M., I.V.: 6 mg
Dosage Forms Injection: 6 mg/mL (1 mL)

Phenoxine® [OTC] *see* phenylpropanolamine *on page 413*

phenoxybenzamine (fen oks ee BEN za meen)
Synonyms phenoxybenzamine hydrochloride
Brand Names Dibenzyline®
Therapeutic Category Alpha-Adrenergic Blocking Agent
Use Symptomatic management of hypertension and sweating in patients with pheochromocytoma
Usual Dosage Oral:
  Children: Initial: 0.2 mg/kg (maximum: 10 mg) once daily, increase by 0.2 mg/kg increments; usual maintenance dose: 0.4-1.2 mg/kg/day every 6-8 hours, maximum single dose: 10 mg

Adults: 10-40 mg every 8-12 hours
Dosage Forms Capsule, as hydrochloride: 10 mg

phenoxybenzamine hydrochloride *see* phenoxybenzamine *on previous page*

phenoxymethyl penicillin *see* penicillin v potassium *on page 402*

phensuximide (fen SUKS i mide)
Brand Names Milontin®
Therapeutic Category Anticonvulsant
Use Control of absence (petit mal) seizures
Usual Dosage Children and Adults: Oral: 0.5-1 g 2-3 times/day
Dosage Forms Capsule: 500 mg

phentolamine (fen TOLE a meen)
Synonyms phentolamine mesylate
Brand Names Regitine®
Therapeutic Category Alpha-Adrenergic Blocking Agent; Diagnostic Agent
Use Diagnosis of pheochromocytoma; treatment of hypertension associated with pheo-chromocytoma or other causes of excess sympathomimetic amines; local treatment of dermal necrosis after extravasation of drugs with alpha-adrenergic effects (dobutamine, dopamine, epinephrine, metaraminol, norepinephrine, phenylephrine)
Usual Dosage
Treatment of extravasation: Infiltrate area S.C. with small amount of solution made by diluting 5-10 mg in 10 mL 0.9% NaCl within 12 hours of extravasation; for children use 0.1-0.2 mg/kg up to a maximum of 10 mg

Children: I.M., I.V.:
Diagnosis of pheochromocytoma: 0.05-0.1 mg/kg/dose, maximum single dose: 5 mg
Hypertension: 0.05-0.1 mg/kg/dose administered 1-2 hours before procedure; repeat as needed until hypertension is controlled; maximum single dose: 5 mg
Adults: I.M., I.V.:
Diagnosis of pheochromocytoma: 5 mg
Hypertension: 5 mg administered 1-2 hours before procedure
Dosage Forms Injection, as mesylate: 5 mg/mL (1 mL)

phentolamine mesylate *see* phentolamine *on this page*

phenylalanine mustard *see* melphalan *on page 327*

phenylazo diamino pyridine hydrochloride *see* phenazopyridine *on page 408*

Phenyldrine® [OTC] *see* phenylpropanolamine *on page 413*

phenylephrine (fen il EF rin)
Synonyms phenylephrine hydrochloride
Brand Names AK-Dilate® Ophthalmic Solution; AK-Nefrin® Ophthalmic Solution; Alco-nefrin® Nasal Solution [OTC]; I-Phrine® Ophthalmic Solution; Mydfrin® Ophthalmic Solu-tion; Neo-Synephrine® Nasal Solution [OTC]; Neo-Synephrine® Ophthalmic Solution; Nostril® Nasal Solution [OTC]; Prefrin™ Ophthalmic Solution; Relief® Ophthalmic Solu-tion; Rhinall® Nasal Solution [OTC]; Sinarest® Nasal Solution [OTC]; St. Joseph® Measured Dose Nasal Solution [OTC]; Vicks Sinex® Nasal Solution [OTC]
Therapeutic Category Adrenergic Agonist Agent
Use Treatment of hypotension and vascular failure in shock; supraventricular tachy-cardia; as a vasoconstrictor in regional analgesia; symptomatic relief of nasal and nasopharyngeal mucosal congestion; as a mydriatic in ophthalmic procedures and treatment of wide-angle glaucoma
Usual Dosage
Ophthalmic procedures:
Infants <1 year: Instill 1 drop of 2.5% 15-30 minutes before procedures
(Continued)

phenylephrine *(Continued)*

Children and Adults: Instill 1 drop of 2.5% or 10% solution, may repeat in 10-60 minutes as needed

Nasal decongestant:

Children:

2-6 years: Instill 1 drop every 2-4 hours of 0.125% solution as needed

6-12 years: Instill 1-2 sprays or instill 1-2 drops every 4 hours of 0.25% solution as needed

Children >12 years and Adults: Instill 1-2 sprays or instill 1-2 drops every 4 hours of 0.25% to 0.5% solution as needed; 1% solution may be used in adult in cases of extreme nasal congestion; do not use nasal solutions more than 3 days

Hypotension/shock:

Children:

I.M., S.C.: 0.1 mg/kg/dose every 1-2 hours as needed (maximum: 5 mg)

I.V. bolus: 5-20 mcg/kg/dose every 10-15 minutes as needed

I.V. infusion: 0.1-0.5 mcg/kg/minute; the concentration and rate of infusion can be calculated using the following formulas: Dilute 0.6 mg x weight (kg) to 100 mL; then the dose in mcg/kg/minute = 0.1 x the infusion rate in mL/hour

Adults:

I.M., S.C.: 2-5 mg/dose every 1-2 hours as needed (initial dose should not exceed 5 mg)

I.V. bolus: 0.1-0.5 mg/dose every 10-15 minutes as needed (initial dose should not exceed 0.5 mg)

I.V. infusion: 10 mg in 250 mL D_5W or NS (1:25,000 dilution) (40 mcg/mL); start at 100-180 mcg/minute (2-5 mL/minute; 50-90 drops/minute) initially. When blood pressure is stabilized, maintenance rate: 40-60 mcg/minute (20-30 drops/minute)

Paroxysmal supraventricular tachycardia: I.V.:

Children: 5-10 mcg/kg/dose over 20-30 seconds

Adults: 0.25-0.5 mg/dose over 20-30 seconds

Dosage Forms

Injection, as hydrochloride (Neo-Synephrine®): 1% [10 mg/mL] (1 mL)

Nasal solution, as hydrochloride:

Drops:

Neo-Synephrine®: 0.125% (15 mL)

Alconefrin® 12: 0.16% (30 mL)

Alconefrin® 25, Neo-Synephrine®, Children's Nostril®, Rhinall®: 0.25% (15 mL, 30 mL, 40 mL)

Alconefrin®, Neo-Synephrine®: 0.5% (15 mL, 30 mL)

Spray:

Alconefrin® 25, Neo-Synephrine®, Rhinall®: 0.25% (15 mL, 30 mL, 40 mL)

Neo-Synephrine®, Nostril®, Sinex®: 0.5% (15 mL, 30 mL)

Neo-Synephrine®: 1% (15 mL)

Ophthalmic solution, as hydrochloride:

AK-Nefrin®, Prefrin™ Liquifilm®, Relief®: 0.12% (0.3 mL, 15 mL, 20 mL)

AK-Dilate®, Mydfrin®, Neo-Synephrine®, Phenoptic®: 2.5% (2 mL, 3 mL, 5 mL, 15 mL)

AK-Dilate®, Neo-Synephrine®, Neo-Synephrine® Viscous: 10% (1 mL, 2 mL, 5 mL, 15 mL)

phenylephrine and chlorpheniramine *see* chlorpheniramine and phenylephrine on page 113

phenylephrine and cyclopentolate *see* cyclopentolate and phenylephrine on page 143

phenylephrine and guaifenesin *see* guaifenesin and phenylephrine on page 249

phenylephrine and scopolamine *(fen il EF rin & skoe POL a meen)*

Synonyms scopolamine and phenylephrine

Brand Names Murocoll-2® Ophthalmic

Therapeutic Category Anticholinergic/Adrenergic Agonist
Use Mydriasis, cycloplegia and to break posterior synechiae in iritis
Usual Dosage Ophthalmic: Instill 1-2 drops into eye(s); repeat in 5 minutes
Dosage Forms Solution, ophthalmic: Phenylephrine hydrochloride 10% and scopolamine hydrobromide 0.3% (7.5 mL)

phenylephrine and zinc sulfate (fen il EF rin & zingk SUL fate)
Brand Names Zincfrin® Ophthalmic [OTC]
Therapeutic Category Adrenergic Agonist Agent
Use Soothe, moisturize, and remove redness due to minor eye irritation
Usual Dosage Ophthalmic: Instill 1-2 drops in eye(s) 2-4 times/day as needed
Dosage Forms Solution, ophthalmic: Phenylephrine hydrochloride 0.12% and zinc sulfate 0.25% (15 mL)

phenylephrine, chlorpheniramine, phenylpropanolamine, and belladonna alkaloids see chlorpheniramine, phenylephrine, phenylpropanolamine, and belladonna alkaloids on page 116

phenylephrine hydrochloride see phenylephrine on page 411

phenylethylmalonylurea see phenobarbital on page 409

Phenylfenesin® L.A. see guaifenesin and phenylpropanolamine on page 249

phenylisohydantoin see pemoline on page 399

phenylpropanolamine (fen il proe pa NOLE a meen)
Synonyms dl-norephedrine hydrochloride; phenylpropanolamine hydrochloride; ppa
Brand Names Acutrim® 16 Hours [OTC]; Acutrim® II, Maximum Strength [OTC]; Acutrim® Late Day [OTC]; Control® [OTC]; Dexatrim® Pre-Meal [OTC]; Maximum Strength Dex-A-Diet® [OTC]; Maximum Strength Dexatrim® [OTC]; Phenoxine® [OTC]; Phenyldrine® [OTC]; Prolamine® [OTC]; Propagest® [OTC]; Rhindecon®; Unitrol® [OTC]
Therapeutic Category Adrenergic Agonist Agent
Use Anorexiant and nasal decongestant
Usual Dosage Oral:
Children: Decongestant:
2-6 years: 6.25 mg every 4 hours
6-12 years: 12.5 mg every 4 hours not to exceed 75 mg/day
Adults:
Decongestant: 25 mg every 4 hours or 50 mg every 8 hours, not to exceed 150 mg/day
Anorexic: 25 mg 3 times/day 30 minutes before meals or 75 mg (timed release) once daily in the morning
Precision release: 75 mg after breakfast
Dosage Forms
Capsule, as hydrochloride: 37.5 mg
Timed release: 25 mg, 75 mg
Tablet, as hydrochloride: 25 mg, 50 mg
Precision release: 75 mg
Timed release: 75 mg

phenylpropanolamine and brompheniramine see brompheniramine and phenylpropanolamine on page 73

phenylpropanolamine and caramiphen see caramiphen and phenylpropanolamine on page 88

phenylpropanolamine and chlorpheniramine see chlorpheniramine and phenylpropanolamine on page 114

phenylpropanolamine and guaifenesin see guaifenesin and phenylpropanolamine on page 249

phenylpropanolamine and hydrocodone *see* hydrocodone and phenylpropanolamine *on page 267*

**phenylpropanolamine, chlorpheniramine, phenylephrine, and belladonna
alkaloids** *see* chlorpheniramine, phenylephrine, phenylpropanolamine, and belladonna alkaloids *on page 116*

phenylpropanolamine hydrochloride *see* phenylpropanolamine *on previous page*

phenyltoloxamine, phenylpropanolamine, and acetaminophen

(fen il tol OKS a meen, fen il proe pa NOLE a meen, & a seet a MIN oh fen)

Brand Names Sinubid®

Therapeutic Category Antihistamine/Decongestant/Analgesic

Use Intermittent symptomatic treatment of nasal congestion in sinus or other frontal
headache; allergic rhinitis, vasomotor rhinitis, coryza; facial pain and pressure of acute
and chronic sinusitis

Usual Dosage Oral:

Children 6-12 years: $^1/_2$ tablet every 12 hours (twice daily)

Adults: 1 tablet every 12 hours (twice daily)

Dosage Forms Tablet: Phenyltoloxamine citrate 22 mg, phenylpropanolamine hydrochloride 25 mg, and acetaminophen 325 mg

phenyltoloxamine, phenylpropanolamine, pyrilamine, and pheniramine

(fen il tol OKS a meen, fen il proe pa NOLE a meen, peer IL a meen, & fen IR a
meen)

Brand Names Poly-Histine-D® Capsule

Therapeutic Category Cold Preparation

Usual Dosage Adults: Oral: 1 capsule every 8-12 hours

Dosage Forms Capsule: Phenyltoloxamine citrate 16 mg, phenylpropanolamine hydrochloride 50 mg, pyrilamine maleate 16 mg, and pheniramine maleate 16 mg

phenytoin (FEN i toyn)

Synonyms diphenylhydantoin; DPH; phenytoin sodium; phenytoin sodium, extended;
phenytoin sodium, prompt

Brand Names Dilantin®

Therapeutic Category Antiarrhythmic Agent, Class I-B; Hydantoin

Use Management of generalized tonic-clonic (grand mal), simple partial and complex
partial seizures; prevention of seizures following head trauma/neurosurgery; ventricular
arrhythmias, including those associated with digitalis intoxication, prolonged Q-T
interval and surgical repair of congenital heart diseases in children; epidermolysis
bullosa

Usual Dosage

Status epilepticus: I.V.:

Infants and Children: Loading dose: 15-18 mg/kg in a single or divided dose; maintenance, anticonvulsant: Initial: 5 mg/kg/day in 2 divided doses, usual doses:

6 months to 3 years: 8-10 mg/kg/day

4-6 years: 7.5-9 mg/kg/day

7-9 years: 7-8 mg/kg/day

10-16 years: 6-7 mg/kg/day, some patients may require every 8 hours dosing

Adults: Loading dose: 15-18 mg/kg in a single or divided dose; maintenance, anticonvulsant: usual: 300 mg/day or 5-6 mg/kg/day in 3 divided doses or 1-2 divided doses
using extended release

Anticonvulsant: Children and Adults: Oral: Loading dose: 15-20 mg/kg; based on phenytoin serum concentrations and recent dosing history; administer oral loading dose in 3
divided doses administered every 2-4 hours to decrease GI adverse effects and to
ensure complete oral absorption; maintenance dose: same as I.V.

Arrhythmias:
Children and Adults: Loading dose: I.V.: 1.25 mg/kg IVP every 5 minutes may repeat up to total loading dose: 15 mg/kg
Children: Maintenance dose: Oral, I.V.: 5-10 mg/kg/day in 2 divided doses
Adults: Maintenance dose: Oral: 250 mg 4 times/day for 1 day, 250 mg twice daily for 2 days, then maintenance at 300-400 mg/day in divided doses 1-4 times/day

Dosage Forms
Capsule, as sodium:
Extended: 30 mg, 100 mg
Prompt: 30 mg, 100 mg
Injection, as sodium: 50 mg/mL (2 mL, 5 mL)
Suspension, oral: 30 mg/5 mL (5 mL, 240 mL); 125 mg/5 mL (5 mL, 240 mL)
Tablet, chewable: 50 mg

phenytoin sodium *see* phenytoin *on previous page*

phenytoin sodium, extended *see* phenytoin *on previous page*

phenytoin sodium, prompt *see* phenytoin *on previous page*

Pherazine® VC w/ Codeine *see* promethazine, phenylephrine, and codeine *on page 443*

Pherazine® w/DM *see* promethazine and dextromethorphan *on page 442*

Pherazine® With Codeine *see* promethazine and codeine *on page 442*

Phicon® [OTC] *see* pramoxine *on page 432*

Phillips'® LaxCaps® [OTC] *see* docusate and phenolphthalein *on page 180*

Phillips'® Milk of Magnesia [OTC] *see* magnesium hydroxide *on page 319*

pHisoHex® *see* hexachlorophene *on page 260*

Phos-Flur® *see* fluoride *on page 228*

PhosLo® *see* calcium acetate *on page 82*

phosphate, potassium *see* potassium phosphate *on page 430*

Phospholine Iodide® Ophthalmic *see* echothiophate iodide *on page 189*

phosphonoformic acid *see* foscarnet *on page 234*

phosphorated carbohydrate solution
(FOS for ate ed kar boe HYE drate soe LOO shun)
Synonyms dextrose, levulose and phosphoric acid; levulose, dextrose and phosphoric acid; phosphoric acid, levulose and dextrose
Brand Names Emecheck® [OTC]; Emetrol® [OTC]; Naus-A-Way® [OTC]; Nausetrol® [OTC]
Therapeutic Category Antiemetic
Use Relief of nausea associated with upset stomach that occurs with intestinal flu, pregnancy, food indiscretions, and emotional upsets
Usual Dosage Oral:
Morning sickness: 15-30 mL on arising; repeat every 3 hours or when nausea threatens
Motion sickness and vomiting due to drug therapy: 5 mL doses for young children; 15 mL doses for older children and adults
Regurgitation in infants: 5 or 10 mL, 10-15 minutes before each feeding; in refractory cases: 10-15 mL, 30 minutes before each feeding
Vomiting due to psychogenic factors:
Children: 5-10 mL; repeat dose every 15 minutes until distress subsides; do not take for more than 1 hour
Adults: 15-30 mL; repeat dose every 15 minutes until distress subsides; do not take for more than 1 hour
Dosage Forms Liquid, oral: Fructose, dextrose, and orthophosphoric acid (120 mL, 480 mL, 4000 mL)

415

phosphoric acid, levulose and dextrose *see* phosphorated carbohydrate solution *on previous page*

Photofrin® *see* porfimer *on page 425*

Phrenilin® *see* butalbital compound and acetaminophen *on page 78*

Phrenilin Forte® *see* butalbital compound and acetaminophen *on page 78*

***p*-hydroxyampicillin** *see* amoxicillin *on page 30*

Phyllocontin® *see* aminophylline *on page 25*

phylloquinone *see* phytonadione *on this page*

physostigmine (fye zoe STIG meen)

Synonyms eserine salicylate; physostigmine salicylate; physostigmine sulfate
Brand Names Antilirium®
Therapeutic Category Cholinesterase Inhibitor
Use Reverse toxic CNS and cardiac effects caused by anticholinergics and tricyclic antidepressants; ophthalmic solution is used to treat open-angle glaucoma
Usual Dosage
Children: Reserve for life-threatening situations only: I.V.: 0.01-0.03 mg/kg/dose; may repeat after 15-20 minutes to a maximum total dose of 2 mg
Adults:
I.M., I.V., S.C.: 0.5-2 mg to start, repeat every 20 minutes until response occurs or adverse effect occurs
I.M., I.V. to reverse the anticholinergic effects of atropine or scopolamine administered as preanesthetic medications: Administer twice the dose, on a weight basis of the anticholinergic drug
Ophthalmic: 1-2 drops of 0.25% or 0.5% solution every 4-8 hours (up to 4 times/day); the ointment can be instilled at night
Dosage Forms
Injection, as salicylate: 1 mg/mL (2 mL)
Ointment, ophthalmic, as sulfate: 0.25% (3.5 g, 3.7 g)

physostigmine salicylate *see* physostigmine *on this page*

physostigmine sulfate *see* physostigmine *on this page*

phytomenadione *see* phytonadione *on this page*

phytonadione (fye toe na DYE one)

Synonyms methylphytyl napthoquinone; phylloquinone; phytomenadione; vitamin k_1
Brand Names AquaMEPHYTON® Injection; Konakion® Injection; Mephyton® Oral
Therapeutic Category Vitamin, Fat Soluble
Use Prevention and treatment of hypoprothrombinemia caused by vitamin K deficiency or anticoagulant-induced hypoprothrombinemia; hemorrhagic disease of the newborn
Usual Dosage I.V. route should be restricted for emergency use only
Hemorrhagic disease of the newborn:
Prophylaxis: I.M., S.C.: 0.5-1 mg within 1 hour of birth
Treatment: I.M., S.C.: 1-2 mg/dose/day
Oral anticoagulant overdose:
Infants: I.M., I.V., S.C.: 1-2 mg/dose every 4-8 hours
Children and Adults: Oral, I.M., I.V., S.C.: 2.5-10 mg/dose; rarely up to 25-50 mg has been used; may repeat in 6-8 hours if administered by I.M., I.V., S.C. route; may repeat 12-48 hours after oral route
Vitamin K deficiency: Due to drugs, malabsorption or decreased synthesis of vitamin K
Infants and Children:
Oral: 2.5-5 mg/24 hours
I.M., I.V.: 1-2 mg/dose as a single dose
Adults:
Oral: 5-25 mg/24 hours

I.M., I.V.: 10 mg
Minimum daily requirement: Not well established
Infants: 1-5 mcg/kg/day
Adults: 0.03 mcg/kg/day

Dosage Forms
Injection:
Aqueous colloidal: 2 mg/mL (0.5 mL); 10 mg/mL (1 mL, 2.5 mL, 5 mL)
Aqueous (I.M. only): 2 mg/mL (0.5 mL); 10 mg/mL (1 mL)
Tablet: 5 mg

Pilagan® Ophthalmic *see pilocarpine on this page*

Pilocar® Ophthalmic *see pilocarpine on this page*

pilocarpine (pye loe KAR peen)

Synonyms pilocarpine hydrochloride; pilocarpine nitrate
Brand Names Adsorbocarpine® Ophthalmic; Akarpine® Ophthalmic; Isopto® Carpine Ophthalmic; Ocusert Pilo-20® Ophthalmic; Ocusert Pilo-40® Ophthalmic; Pilagan® Ophthalmic; Pilocar® Ophthalmic; Pilopine HS® Ophthalmic; Piloptic® Ophthalmic; Pilostat® Ophthalmic; Salagen® Oral
Therapeutic Category Cholinergic Agent
Use
Ophthalmic: Management of chronic simple glaucoma, chronic and acute angle-closure glaucoma; counter effects of cycloplegics
Oral: Symptomatic treatment of xerostomia caused by salivary gland hypofunction resulting from radiotherapy for cancer of the head and neck
Usual Dosage Adults:
Oral: 5 mg 3 times/day, titration up to 10 mg 3 times/day may be considered for patients who have not responded adequately
Ophthalmic:
Nitrate solution: Shake well before using; instill 1-2 drops 2-4 times/day
Hydrochloride solution:
Instill 1-2 drops up to 6 times/day; adjust the concentration and frequency as required to control elevated intraocular pressure
To counteract the mydriatic effects of sympathomimetic agents: Instill 1 drop of a 1% solution in the affected eye
Gel: Instill 0.5" ribbon into lower conjunctival sac once daily at bedtime
Ocular systems: Systems are labeled in terms of mean rate of release of pilocarpine over 7 days; begin with 20 mcg/hour at night and adjust based on response
Dosage Forms
Gel, ophthalmic, as hydrochloride (Pilopine HS®): 4% (3.5 g)
Ocular therapeutic system (Ocusert® Pilo): Releases 20 or 40 mcg per hour for 1 week (8s)
Solution, ophthalmic:
As hydrochloride (Adsorbocarpine®, Akarpine®, Isopto® Carpine, Pilagan®, Pilocar®, Piloptic®, Pilostat®): 0.25% (15 mL); 0.5% (15 mL, 30 mL); 1% (1 mL, 2 mL, 15 mL, 30 mL); 2% (1 mL, 2 mL, 15 mL, 30 mL); 3% (15 mL, 30 mL); 4% (1 mL, 2 mL, 15 mL, 30 mL); 5% (15 mL); 6% (15 mL, 30 mL); 8% (2 mL); 10% (15 mL)
As nitrate (Pilagan®): 1% (15 mL); 2% (15 mL); 4% (15 mL)
Tablet, as hydrochloride: 5 mg

pilocarpine and epinephrine (pye loe KAR peen & ep i NEF rin)

Brand Names E-Pilo-x® Ophthalmic; P$_x$E$_x$® Ophthalmic
Therapeutic Category Cholinergic Agent
Use Treatment of glaucoma; counter effect of cycloplegics
Usual Dosage Ophthalmic: Instill 1-2 drops up to 6 times/day
Dosage Forms Solution, ophthalmic: Epinephrine bitartrate 1% and pilocarpine hydrochloride 1%, 2%, 4%, 6% (15 mL)

pilocarpine hydrochloride *see* pilocarpine *on previous page*
pilocarpine nitrate *see* pilocarpine *on previous page*
Pilopine HS® Ophthalmic *see* pilocarpine *on previous page*
Piloptic® Ophthalmic *see* pilocarpine *on previous page*
Pilostat® Ophthalmic *see* pilocarpine *on previous page*
Pima® *see* potassium iodide *on page 430*
pimaricin *see* natamycin *on page 366*

pimozide (PI moe zide)
Brand Names Orap™
Therapeutic Category Neuroleptic Agent
Use Suppression of severe motor and phonic tics in patients with Tourette's disorder
Usual Dosage Children >12 years and Adults: Oral: Initial: 1-2 mg/day, then increase dosage as needed every other day; range is usually 7-16 mg/day, maximum dose: 20 mg/day or 0.3 mg/kg/day should not be exceeded
Dosage Forms Tablet: 2 mg

pindolol (PIN doe lole)
Brand Names Visken®
Therapeutic Category Beta-Adrenergic Blocker
Use Management of hypertension
Usual Dosage Oral: 5 mg twice daily
Dosage Forms Tablet: 5 mg, 10 mg

Pin-Rid® [OTC] *see* pyrantel pamoate *on page 451*
Pin-X® [OTC] *see* pyrantel pamoate *on page 451*
pio *see* pemoline *on page 399*

pipecuronium (pi pe kur OH nee um)
Synonyms pipecuronium bromide
Brand Names Arduan®
Therapeutic Category Skeletal Muscle Relaxant
Use Adjunct to general anesthesia, to provide skeletal muscle relaxation during surgery and to provide skeletal muscle relaxation for endotracheal intubation; recommended only for procedures anticipated to last 90 minutes or longer
Usual Dosage I.V.:
Children:
3 months to 1 year: Adult dosage
1-14 years: May be less sensitive to effects
Adults: Dose is individualized based on ideal body weight, ranges are 85-100 mcg/kg initially to a maintenance dose of 5-25 mcg/kg
Dosage Forms Injection, as bromide: 10 mg (10 mL)

pipecuronium bromide *see* pipecuronium *on this page*

piperacillin (pi PER a sil in)
Synonyms piperacillin sodium
Brand Names Pipracil®
Therapeutic Category Penicillin
Use Treatment of serious infections caused by susceptible strains of gram-positive, gram-negative, and anaerobic bacilli; mixed aerobic-anaerobic bacterial infections or empiric antibiotic therapy in granulocytopenic patients. Its primary use is in the treatment of serious carbenicillin-resistant or ticarcillin-resistant *Pseudomonas aeruginosa* infections susceptible to piperacillin.

Usual Dosage
Infants and Children: I.M., I.V.: 200-300 mg/kg/day in divided doses every 4-6 hours; maximum dose: 24 g/day
Higher doses have been used in cystic fibrosis: 350-500 mg/kg/day in divided doses every 4 hours
Adults:
I.M.: 2-3 g/dose every 6-12 hours I.M.; maximum 24 g/24 hours
I.V.: 3-4 g/dose every 4-6 hours; maximum 24 g/24 hours
Dosage Forms Powder for injection, as sodium: 2 g, 3 g, 4 g, 40 g

piperacillin and tazobactam sodium
(pi PER a sil in & ta zoe BAK tam SOW dee um)
Brand Names Zosyn™
Therapeutic Category Penicillin
Use Treatment of infections caused by piperacillin-resistant, beta-lactamase producing strains that are piperacillin/tazobactam susceptible involving the lower respiratory tract, urinary tract, skin and skin structures, gynecologic, intra-abdominal, and septicemia. Tazobactam expands activity of piperacillin to include beta-lactamase producing strains of S. aureus, H. influenzae, B. fragilis, Klebsiella, E. coli, and Acinetobacter.
Usual Dosage Adults: I.V.: 3.375 g (3 g piperacillin/0.375 g tazobactam) every 6 hours
Dosage Forms Injection: Piperacillin sodium 2 g and tazobactam sodium 0.25 g; piperacillin sodium 3 g and tazobactam sodium 0.375 g; piperacillin sodium 4 g and tazobactam sodium 0.5 g (vials at an 8:1 ratio of piperacillin sodium to tazobactam sodium)

piperacillin sodium see piperacillin on previous page

piperazine (PI per a zeen)
Synonyms piperazine citrate
Brand Names Vermizine®
Therapeutic Category Anthelmintic
Use Treatment of pinworm (Enterobius vermicularis) and roundworm (Ascaris lumbricoides) infections; used as an alternative to first-line agents mebendazole or pyrantel pamoate for the treatment of these infections
Usual Dosage Oral:
Pinworms:
Children and Adults: 65 mg/kg/day as a single daily dose for 7 days, in severe infections, repeat course after a 1-week interval; not to exceed 2.5 g/day
Roundworms:
Children: 75 mg/kg/day as a single daily dose for 2 days; maximum: 3.5 g/day;
Adults: 3.5 g/day for 2 days (in severe infections, repeat course, after a 1-week interval)
Dosage Forms
Syrup, as citrate: 500 mg/5 mL (473 mL, 4000 mL)
Tablet, as citrate: 250 mg

piperazine citrate see piperazine on this page
piperazine estrone sulfate see estropipate on page 206

pipobroman (pi poe BROE man)
Therapeutic Category Antineoplastic Agent
Use Treat polycythemia vera; chronic myelocytic leukemia
Usual Dosage Children >15 years and Adults: Oral:
Polycythemia: 1 mg/kg/day for 30 days; may increase to 1.5-3 mg/kg until hematocrit reduced to 50% to 55%; maintenance: 0.1-0.2 mg/kg/day
Myelocytic leukemia: 1.5-2.5 mg/kg/day until WBC drops to 10,000 mm^3 then start maintenance 7-175 mg/day; stop if WBC falls below 3000/mm^3 or platelets fall below 150,000/mm^3
(Continued)

419

pipobroman *(Continued)*
Dosage Forms Tablet: 25 mg

Pipracil® *see* piperacillin *on page 418*

pirbuterol (peer BYOO ter ole)
Synonyms pirbuterol acetate
Brand Names Maxair™ Inhalation Aerosol
Therapeutic Category Adrenergic Agonist Agent
Use Prevention and treatment of reversible bronchospasm including asthma
Usual Dosage Children >12 years and Adults: 2 inhalations every 4-6 hours for prevention; two inhalations at an interval of at least 1-3 minutes, followed by a third inhalation in treatment of bronchospasm, not to exceed 12 inhalations/day
Dosage Forms Aerosol, oral, as acetate: 0.2 mg per actuation (25.6 g)

pirbuterol acetate *see* pirbuterol *on this page*

piroxicam (peer OKS i kam)
Brand Names Feldene®
Therapeutic Category Analgesic, Non-narcotic; Nonsteroidal Anti-Inflammatory Agent (NSAID)
Use Management of inflammatory disorders; symptomatic treatment of acute and chronic rheumatoid arthritis, osteoarthritis, and ankylosing spondylitis; also used to treat sunburn; dysmenorrhea
Usual Dosage Oral:
Children: 0.2-0.3 mg/kg/day once daily; maximum dose: 15 mg/day
Adults: 10-20 mg/day once daily; although associated with increases in GI adverse effects, doses >20 mg/day have been used (ie, 30-40 mg/day)

Therapeutic efficacy of the drug should not be assessed for at least 2 weeks after initiation of therapy or adjustment of dosage
Dosage Forms Capsule: 10 mg, 20 mg

***p*-isobutylhydratropic acid** *see* ibuprofen *on page 278*

pit *see* oxytocin *on page 392*

Pitocin® *see* oxytocin *on page 392*

Pitressin® **Injection** *see* vasopressin *on page 547*

pit vipers antivenin *see* antivenin (*Crotalidae*) polyvalent *on page 38*

pix carbonis *see* coal tar *on page 132*

Placidyl® *see* ethchlorvynol *on page 207*

plague vaccine (plaig vak SEEN)
Therapeutic Category Vaccine, Inactivated Bacteria
Use Vaccination of persons at high risk exposure to plaque
Usual Dosage Three I.M. doses: First dose 1 mL, second dose (0.2 mL) 1 month later, third dose (0.2 mL) 5 months after the second dose; booster doses (0.2 mL) at 1- to 2-year intervals if exposure continues
Dosage Forms Injection: 2 mL, 20 mL

plantago seed *see* psyllium *on page 451*

plantain seed *see* psyllium *on page 451*

Plaquenil® *see* hydroxychloroquine *on page 273*

Plasbumin® *see* albumin *on page 13*

Plasmanate® *see* plasma protein fraction *on next page*

Plasma-Plex® *see* plasma protein fraction *on next page*

plasma protein fraction (PLAS mah PROE teen FRAK shun)
Brand Names Plasmanate®; Plasma-Plex®; Plasmatein®; Protenate®
Therapeutic Category Blood Product Derivative
Use Plasma volume expansion and maintenance of cardiac output in the treatment of certain types of shock or impending shock
Usual Dosage I.V.: 250-1500 mL/day
Dosage Forms Injection: 5% (50 mL, 250 mL, 500 mL)

Plasmatein® see plasma protein fraction on this page

Platinol® see cisplatin on page 125

Platinol®-AQ see cisplatin on page 125

Plendil® see felodipine on page 218

plicamycin (plye kay MYE sin)
Synonyms mithramycin
Brand Names Mithracin®
Therapeutic Category Antidote; Antineoplastic Agent
Use Malignant testicular tumors; treatment of hypercalcemia and hypercalciuria of malignancy not responsive to conventional treatment; chronic myelogenous leukemia in blast phase; Paget's disease
Usual Dosage Refer to individual protocols. Adults: I.V. (dose based on ideal body weight):
Testicular cancer: 25-50 mcg/kg/day or every other day for 5-10 days
Blastic chronic granulocytic leukemia: 25 mcg/kg over 2-4 hours every other day for 3 weeks
Paget's disease: 15 mcg/kg/day once daily for 10 days
Hypercalcemia:
25 mcg/kg single dose which may be repeated in 48 hours if no response occurs
OR 25 mcg/kg/day for 3-4 days
OR 25-50 mcg/kg/dose every other day for 3-8 doses
Dosage Forms Powder for injection: 2.5 mg

pneumococcal polysaccharide vaccine see pneumococcal vaccine on this page

pneumococcal vaccine (noo moe KOK al vak SEEN)
Synonyms pneumococcal polysaccharide vaccine
Brand Names Pneumovax® 23; Pnu-Imune® 23
Therapeutic Category Vaccine, Inactivated Bacteria
Use Immunity to pneumococcal lobar pneumonia and bacteremia in individuals ≥2 years of age who are at high risk of morbidity and mortality from pneumococcal infection
Usual Dosage Children >2 years and Adults: I.M., S.C.: 0.5 mL
Revaccination should be considered if ≥6 years since initial vaccination; revaccination is recommended in patients who received 14-valent pneumococcal vaccine and are at highest risk (asplenic) for fatal infection, or at ≥6 years in patients with nephrotic syndrome, renal failure, or transplant recipients, or 3-5 years in children with nephrotic syndrome, asplenia or sickle cell disease
Dosage Forms Injection: 25 mcg each of 23 polysaccharide isolates/0.5 mL dose (0.5 mL, 1 mL, 5 mL)

Pneumomist® see guaifenesin on page 247

Pneumovax® 23 see pneumococcal vaccine on this page

Pnu-Imune® 23 see pneumococcal vaccine on this page

Pod-Ben-25® see podophyllum resin on next page

Podocon-25® see podophyllum resin on next page

podofilox (po do FIL oks)
Brand Names Condylox®
Therapeutic Category Keratolytic Agent
Use Treatment of external genital warts
Usual Dosage Adults: Topical: Apply twice daily (morning and evening) for 3 consecutive days, then withhold use for 4 consecutive days; repeat this cycle may be repeated up to 4 times until there is no visible wart tissue
Dosage Forms Solution, topical: 0.5% (3.5 mL)

Podofin® *see* podophyllum resin *on this page*

podophyllin and salicylic acid (po DOF fil um & sal i SIL ik AS id)
Synonyms salicylic acid and podophyllin
Brand Names Verrex-C&M®
Therapeutic Category Keratolytic Agent
Use Topical treatment of benign growths including external genital and perianal warts, papillomas, fibroids
Usual Dosage Topical: Apply daily with applicator, allow to dry; remove necrotic tissue before each application
Dosage Forms Solution, topical: Podophyllum 10% and salicylic acid 30% with penederm 0.5% (7.5 mL)

podophyllum resin (po DOF fil um REZ in)
Synonyms mandrake; may apple
Brand Names Pod-Ben-25®; Podocon-25®; Podofin®
Therapeutic Category Keratolytic Agent
Use Topical treatment of benign growths including external genital and perianal warts (condylomata acuminata), papillomas, fibroids
Usual Dosage Topical:
Children and Adults: 10% to 25% solution in compound benzoin tincture; apply drug to dry surface, use 1 drop at a time allowing drying between drops until area is covered; total volume should be limited to <0.5 mL per treatment session

Condylomata acuminatum: 25% solution is applied daily; use a 10% solution when applied to or near mucous membranes
Verrucae: 25% solution is applied 3-5 times/day directly to the wart
Dosage Forms Liquid, topical: 25% in benzoin tincture (5 mL, 7.5 mL, 30 mL)

Point-Two® *see* fluoride *on page 228*

Poladex® *see* dexchlorpheniramine *on page 158*

Polaramine® *see* dexchlorpheniramine *on page 158*

poliomyelitis vaccine *see* poliovirus vaccine, inactivated *on this page*

poliovirus vaccine, inactivated
(POE lee oh VYE rus vak SEEN, in ak ti VAY ted)
Synonyms ipv; poliomyelitis vaccine; Salk vaccine
Brand Names IPOL™
Therapeutic Category Vaccine, Live Virus and Inactivated Virus
Use Active immunization for the prevention of poliomyelitis
Usual Dosage
S.C.: 3 doses of 0.5 mL; the first 2 doses should be administered at an interval of 8 weeks; the third dose should be administered at least 6 and preferably 12 months after the second dose
Booster dose: All children who have received the 3 dose primary series in infancy and early childhood should receive a booster dose of 0.5 mL before entering school. However, if the third dose of the primary series is administered on or after the fourth birthday, a fourth (booster) dose is not required at school entry.

Dosage Forms Injection, Suspension: Three types of poliovirus (Types 1, 2, and 3) grown in monkey kidney cell cultures (0.5 mL)

poliovirus vaccine, live, trivalent, oral
(POE lee oh VYE rus vak SEEN, live, try VAY lent, OR al)
Synonyms opv; Sabin vaccine; topv
Brand Names Orimune®
Therapeutic Category Vaccine, Live Virus
Use Poliovirus immunization
Usual Dosage Oral:
Infants: 0.5 mL dose at age 2 months, 4 months, and 18 months; optional dose may be administered at 6 months in areas where poliomyelitis is endemic
Older Children, Adolescents and Adults: Two 0.5 mL doses 8 weeks apart; third dose of 0.5 mL 6-12 months after second dose; a reinforcing dose of 0.5 mL should be administered before entry to school, in children who received the third primary dose before their fourth birthday
Dosage Forms Solution, oral: Mixture of type 1, 2, and 3 viruses in monkey kidney tissue (0.5 mL)

Polocaine® *see* mepivacaine *on page 329*

Polycillin® *see* ampicillin *on page 33*

Polycillin-N® *see* ampicillin *on page 33*

Polycillin-PRB® *see* ampicillin and probenecid *on page 33*

Polycitra® *see* sodium citrate and potassium citrate mixture *on page 485*

Polycitra®-K *see* potassium citrate and citric acid *on page 429*

Polycose® [OTC] *see* enteral nutritional products *on page 194*

Polycose® [OTC] *see* glucose polymers *on page 242*

Polydine® [OTC] *see* povidone-iodine *on page 431*

polyestradiol (pol i es tra DYE ole)
Synonyms polyestradiol phosphate
Therapeutic Category Estrogen Derivative
Use Palliative treatment of advanced, inoperable carcinoma of the prostate
Usual Dosage Adults: I.M.: 40 mg every 2-4 weeks or less frequently
Dosage Forms Powder for injection, as phosphate: 40 mg

polyestradiol phosphate *see* polyestradiol *on this page*

polyethylene glycol-electrolyte solution
(pol i ETH i leen GLY kol ee LEK troe lite soe LOO shun)
Synonyms electrolyte lavage solution; peg-es
Brand Names Colovage®; CoLyte®; GoLYTELY®; NuLytely®; OCL®
Therapeutic Category Laxative
Use For bowel cleansing prior to GI examination
Usual Dosage The recommended dose for adults is 4 L of solution prior to gastrointestinal examination, as ingestion of this dose produces a satisfactory preparation in >95% of patients. The solution is usually administered orally, but may be administered via nasogastric tube to patients who are unwilling or unable to drink the solution.
Children: Oral: 25-40 mL/kg/hour for 4-10 hours
Adults:
Oral: At a rate of 240 mL (8 oz) every 10 minutes, until 4 liters are consumed or the rectal effluent is clear; rapid drinking of each portion is preferred to drinking small amounts continuously
Nasogastric tube: At the rate of 20-30 mL/minute (1.2-1.8 L/hour); the first bowel movement should occur approximately one hour after the start of administration
(Continued)

polyethylene glycol-electrolyte solution *(Continued)*

Dosage Forms Powder, for oral solution: PEG 3350 236 g, sodium sulfate 22.74 g, sodium bicarbonate 6.74 g, sodium chloride 5.86 g and potassium chloride 2.97 g (2000 mL, 4000 mL, 4800 mL, 6000 mL)

Polygam® *see* immune globulin, intravenous *on page 281*

Polygam® **S/D** *see* immune globulin, intravenous *on page 281*

Poly-Histine CS® *see* brompheniramine, phenylpropanolamine, and codeine *on page 74*

Poly-Histine-D® **Capsule** *see* phenyltoloxamine, phenylpropanolamine, pyrilamine, and pheniramine *on page 414*

Polymox® *see* amoxicillin *on page 30*

polymyxin b and hydrocortisone
(pol i MIKS in bee & hye droe KOR ti sone)
Brand Names Otobiotic® Otic
Therapeutic Category Antibiotic/Corticosteroid, Otic
Use Treatment of superficial bacterial infections of external ear canal
Usual Dosage Otic: Instill 4 drops 3-4 times/day
Dosage Forms Solution, otic: Polymyxin B sulfate 10,000 units and hydrocortisone 0.5% [5 mg/mL] per mL (10 mL, 15 mL)

polymyxin b and neomycin *see* neomycin and polymyxin b *on page 368*

polymyxin b and oxytetracycline *see* oxytetracycline and polymyxin b *on page 392*

polymyxin b and trimethoprim *see* trimethoprim and polymyxin b *on page 534*

Poly-Pred® **Ophthalmic Suspension** *see* neomycin, polymyxin b, and prednisolone *on page 370*

polysaccharide-iron complex (pol i SAK a ride-EYE ern KOM pleks)
Brand Names Hytinic® [OTC]; Niferex® [OTC]; Nu-Iron® [OTC]
Therapeutic Category Electrolyte Supplement
Use Prevention and treatment of iron deficiency anemias
Usual Dosage Oral:
  Children: 3 mg/kg 3 times/day
  Adults: 200 mg 3-4 times/day
Dosage Forms
  Capsule: Elemental iron 150 mg
  Elixir: Elemental iron 100 mg/5 mL (240 mL)
  Tablet: Elemental iron 50 mg

Polysporin® **Ophthalmic** *see* bacitracin and polymyxin b *on page 53*

Polysporin® **Topical** *see* bacitracin and polymyxin b *on page 53*

Polytar® **[OTC]** *see* coal tar *on page 132*

polythiazide (pol i THYE a zide)
Brand Names Renese®
Therapeutic Category Diuretic, Thiazide
Use Adjunctive therapy in treatment of edema and hypertension
Usual Dosage Adults: Oral: 1-4 mg/day
Dosage Forms Tablet: 1 mg, 2 mg, 4 mg

Polytrim® **Ophthalmic** *see* trimethoprim and polymyxin b *on page 534*

Poly-Vi-Flor® *see* vitamin, multiple (pediatric) *on page 554*

polyvinyl alcohol *see* artificial tears *on page 42*

Poly-Vi-Sol® [OTC] *see* vitamin, multiple (pediatric) *on page 554*

Ponstel® *see* mefenamic acid *on page 326*

Pontocaine® *see* tetracaine *on page 509*

Pontocaine® With Dextrose Injection *see* tetracaine and dextrose *on page 509*

Porcelana® [OTC] *see* hydroquinone *on page 272*

Porcelana® Sunscreen [OTC] *see* hydroquinone *on page 272*

porfimer (POR fi mer)
Synonyms porfimer sodium
Brand Names Photofrin®
Therapeutic Category Antineoplastic Agent
Use Esophageal cancer: Photodynamic therapy (PDT) with porfimer for palliation of patients with completely obstructing esophageal cancer, or of patients with partially obstructing esophageal cancer who cannot be satisfactorily treated with Nd:YAG laser therapy
Usual Dosage I.V. (refer to individual protocols):
Children: Safety and efficacy have not been established
Adults: I.V.: 2 mg/kg over 3-5 minutes
Photodynamic therapy is a two-stage process requiring administration of both drug and light. The first stage of PDT is the I.V. injection of porfimer. Illumination with laser light 40-50 hours following the injection with porfimer constitutes the second stage of therapy. A second laser light application may be administered 90-120 hours after injection, preceded by gentle debridement of residual tumor.
Patients may receive a second course of PDT a minimum of 30 days after the initial therapy; up to three courses of PDT (each separated by a minimum of 30 days) can be given. Before each course of treatment, evaluate patients for the presence of a tracheoesophageal or bronchoesophageal fistula.
Dosage Forms Powder for injection, as sodium: 75 mg

porfimer sodium *see* porfimer *on this page*

Pork NPH Iletin® II *see* insulin preparations *on page 284*

Pork Regular Iletin® II *see* insulin preparations *on page 284*

Portagen® [OTC] *see* enteral nutritional products *on page 194*

Porton Asparaginase *see* erwinia asparaginase *on page 199*

Posicor® *see* mibefradil *on page 348*

Posture® [OTC] *see* calcium phosphate, dibasic *on page 86*

Potasalan® *see* potassium chloride *on page 427*

potassium acetate (poe TASS ee um AS e tate)
Therapeutic Category Electrolyte Supplement
Use Potassium deficiency, treatment of hypokalemia, correction of metabolic acidosis through conversion of acetate to bicarbonate
Usual Dosage I.V. infusion:
Children: Not to exceed 3 mEq/kg/day
Adults: Up to 150 mEq/day administered at a rate up to 20 mEq/hour; maximum concentration: 40 mEq/L
Dosage Forms Injection: 2 mEq/mL (20 mL, 50 mL, 100 mL); 4 mEq/mL (50 mL)

potassium acetate, potassium bicarbonate, and potassium citrate

(poe TASS ee um AS e tate, poe TASS ee um bye KAR bun ate, & poe TASS ee um SIT rate)

Brand Names Tri-K®

Therapeutic Category Electrolyte Supplement

Use Treatment or prevention of hypokalemia

Usual Dosage Oral:

Children: 1-4 mEq/kg/24 hours in divided doses as required to maintain normal serum potassium

Adults:

Prevention: 16-24 mEq/day in 2-4 divided doses

Treatment: 40-100 mEq/day in 2-4 divided doses

Dosage Forms Solution, oral: 45 mEq/15 mL from potassium acetate 1500 mg, potassium bicarbonate 1500 mg, and potassium citrate 1500 mg per 15 mL

potassium acid phosphate (poe TASS ee um AS id FOS fate)

Brand Names K-Phos® Original

Therapeutic Category Urinary Acidifying Agent

Use Acidify the urine and lower urinary calcium concentration; reduces odor and rash caused by ammoniacal urine

Usual Dosage Adults: Oral: 1000 mg dissolved in 6-8 oz of water 4 times/day with meals and at bedtime

Dosage Forms Tablet, sodium free: 500 mg [potassium 3.67 mEq]

potassium bicarbonate (poe TASS ee um bye KAR bun ate)

Brand Names K+ Care® Effervescent; K-Electrolyte® Effervescent; K-Gen® Effervescent; K-Lyte® Effervescent

Therapeutic Category Electrolyte Supplement

Use Potassium deficiency, hypokalemia

Usual Dosage Oral:

Normal daily requirements:

Children: 2-3 mEq/kg/day

Adults: 40-80 mEq/day

Prevention during diuretic therapy:

Children: 1-2 mEq/kg/day in 1-2 divided doses

Adults: 20-40 mEq/day in 1-2 divided doses

Treatment of hypokalemia: Children: 1-2 mEq/kg initially, then as needed based on frequently obtained lab values. If deficits are severe or ongoing losses are great, I.V. route should be considered.

Treatment of hypokalemia: Adults:

Potassium >2.5 mEq/L: 60-80 mEq/day plus additional amounts if needed

Potassium <2.5 mEq/L: Up to 40-60 mEq initial dose, followed by further doses based on lab values; deficits at a plasma level of 2 mEq/L may be as high as 400-800 mEq of potassium

Dosage Forms

Tablet for oral solution, effervescent: 6.5 mEq, 25 mEq

K+ Care® Effervescent; K-Electrolyte® Effervescent; K-Gen® Effervescent; K-Ide®; K-Lyte® Effervescent: 25 mEq

potassium bicarbonate and potassium chloride, effervescent

(poe TASS ee um bye KAR bun ate & poe TASS ee um KLOR ide, ef er VES ent)

Brand Names Klorvess® Effervescent; K/Lyte/CL®

Therapeutic Category Electrolyte Supplement

Use Treatment or prevention of hypokalemia

Usual Dosage Oral:
Children: 1-4 mEq/kg/24 hours in divided doses as required to maintain normal serum potassium
Adults:
Prevention: 16-24 mEq/day in 2-4 divided doses
Treatment: 40-100 mEq/day in 2-4 divided doses
Dosage Forms
Granules for oral solution, effervescent (Klorvess®): 20 mEq per packet
Tablet for oral solution, effervescent
Klorvess®: 20 mEq per packet
K/Lyte/CL®: 25 mEq, 50 mEq per packet

potassium bicarbonate and potassium citrate, effervescent

(poe TASS ee um bye KAR bun ate & poe TASS ee um SIT rate, ef er VES ent)
Synonyms potassium citrate and potassium bicarbonate, effervescent
Brand Names Effer-K™; K-Ide®; Klor-con®/EF; K-Lyte®; K-Vescent®
Therapeutic Category Electrolyte Supplement
Use Treatment or prevention of hypokalemia
Usual Dosage Oral:
Children: 1-4 mEq/kg/24 hours as required to maintain normal serum potassium
Adults:
Prevention: 16-24 mEq/day in 2-4 divided doses
Treatment: 40-100 mEq/day in 2-4 divided doses
Dosage Forms
Capsule, extended release: 8 mEq, 10 mEq
Powder for oral solution: 15 mEq/packet; 20 mEq/packet; 25 mEq/packet
Tablet, effervescent: 25 mEq, 50 mEq

potassium bicarbonate, potassium chloride, and potassium citrate

(poe TASS ee um bye KAR bun ate, poe TASS ee um KLOR ide & poe TASS ee um SIT rate)
Brand Names Kaochlor-Eff®
Therapeutic Category Electrolyte Supplement
Use Treatment or prevention of hypokalemia
Usual Dosage Oral:
Children: 1-4 mEq/kg/24 hours in divided doses as required to maintain normal serum potassium
Adults:
Prevention: 16-24 mEq/day in 2-4 divided doses
Treatment: 40-100 mEq/day in 2-4 divided doses
Dosage Forms Tablet for oral solution: 20 mEq from potassium bicarbonate 1 g, potassium chloride 600 mg, and potassium citrate 220 mg

potassium chloride (poe TASS ee um KLOR ide)
Synonyms KCl
Brand Names Cena-K®; Gen-K®; K+ 10®; Kaochlor®; Kaochlor® SF; Kaon-Cl®; Kaon-Cl-10®; Kay Ciel®; K+ Care®; K-Dur® 10; K-Dur® 20; K-Lease®; K-Lor™; Klor-Con®; Klor-Con® 8; Klor-Con® 10; Klor-Con/25®; Klorvess®; Klotrix®; K-Lyte®/Cl; K-Norm®; K-Tab®; Micro-K® 10; Micro-K Extencaps®; Micro-K® LS; Potasalan®; Rum-K®; Slow-K®; Ten-K®
Therapeutic Category Electrolyte Supplement
Use Potassium deficiency, treatment or prevention of hypokalemia
Usual Dosage I.V. doses should be incorporated into the patient's maintenance I.V. fluids, intermittent I.V. potassium administration should be reserved for severe depletion situations in patients undergoing EKG monitoring.

Normal daily requirement: Oral, I.V.:
Newborns: 2-6 mEq/kg/day
(Continued)

427

potassium chloride *(Continued)*

Children: 2-3 mEq/kg/day
Adults: 40-80 mEq/day

Prevention during diuretic therapy: Oral:
Children: 1-2 mEq/kg/day in 1-2 divided doses
Adults: 20-40 mEq/day in 1-2 divided doses
Treatment: Oral, I.V.:
Children: 2-3 mEq/kg/day
Adults: 40-100 mEq/day
I.V. intermittent infusion:
Children: Dose should not exceed 0.5 mEq/kg/hour, not to exceed 20 mEq/hour
Adults: 10-20 mEq/hour, not to exceed 40 mEq/hour and 150 mEq/day

Dosage Forms
Capsule, controlled release (microcapsulated): 600 mg [8 mEq]; 750 mg [10 mEq]
Micro-K® Extencaps®: 600 mg [8 mEq]
K-Lease®, K-Norm®, Micro-K® 10: 750 mg [10 mEq]
Crystals for oral suspension, extended release (Micro-K® LS®): 20 mEq per packet
Liquid: 10% [20 mEq/15 mL] (480 mL, 4000 mL); 20% [40 mEq/15 mL] (480 mL, 4000 mL)
Cena-K®, Kaochlor®, Kaochlor® SF, Kay Ciel®, Klorvess®, Potasalan®: 10% [20 mEq/15 mL] (480 mL, 4000 mL)
Rum-K®: 15% [30 mEq/15 mL] (480 mL, 4000 mL)
Cena-K®, Kaon-Cl® 20%: 20% [40 mEq/15 mL]
Powder: 20 mEq per packet (30s, 100s)
K+ Care®, K-Lor™: 15 mEq per packet (30s, 100s)
Gen-K®, Kay Ciel®, K+ Care®, K-Lor™, Klor-Con®: 20 mEq per packet (30s, 100s)
K+ Care®, Klor-Con/25®: 25 mEq per packet (30s, 100s)
K-Lyte/Cl®: 25 mEq per dose (30s)
Infusion, concentrate: 0.1 mEq/mL, 0.2 mEq/mL, 0.3 mEq/mL, 0.4 mEq/mL
Injection, concentrate: 1.5 mEq/mL, 2 mEq/mL, 3 mEq/mL
Tablet, controlled release (microencapsulated)
K-Dur® 10, Ten-K®: 750 mg [10 mEq]
K-Dur® 20: 1500 mg [20 mEq]
Tablet, controlled release (wax matrix): 600 mg [8 mEq]; 750 mg [10 mEq]
Kaon-Cl®: 500 mg [6.7 mEq]
Klor-Con® 8, Slow-K®: 600 mg [8 mEq]
K+ 10®, Kaon-Cl-10®, Klor-Con® 10, Klotrix®, K-Tab®: 750 mg [10 mEq]

potassium chloride and potassium gluconate

(poe TASS ee um KLOR ide & poe TASS ee um GLOO coe nate)
Brand Names Kolyum®
Therapeutic Category Electrolyte Supplement
Use Treatment or prevention of hypokalemia
Usual Dosage Oral:
Children: 1-4 mEq/kg/24 hours in divided doses as required to maintain normal serum potassium
Adults:
Prevention: 16-24 mEq/day in 2-4 divided doses
Treatment: 40-100 mEq/day in 2-4 divided doses
Dosage Forms Solution, oral: Potassium 20 mEq/15 mL

potassium citrate (poe TASS ee um SIT rate)

Brand Names Urocit®-K
Therapeutic Category Alkalinizing Agent
Use Prevention of uric acid nephrolithiasis; prevention of calcium renal stones in patients with hypocitraturia; urinary alkalinizer when sodium citrate is contraindicated
Usual Dosage Adults: Oral: 10-20 mEq 3 times/day with meals up to 100 mEq/day

Dosage Forms Tablet: 540 mg [5 mEq], 1080 mg [10 mEq]

potassium citrate and citric acid
(poe TASS ee um SIT rate & SI trik AS id)

Brand Names Polycitra®-K

Therapeutic Category Alkalinizing Agent

Use Treatment of metabolic acidosis; alkalinizing agent in conditions where long-term maintenance of an alkaline urine is desirable

Usual Dosage Oral:
Mild to moderate hypocitraturia: 10 mEq 3 times/day with meals
Severe hypocitraturia: Initial: 20 mEq 3 times/day or 15 mEq 4 times/day with meals or within 30 minutes after meals; do not exceed 100 mEq/day

Dosage Forms
Crystals for reconstitution: Potassium citrate 3300 mg and citric acid 1002 mg per packet
Solution, oral: Potassium citrate 1100 mg and citric acid 334 mg per 5 mL

potassium citrate and potassium bicarbonate, effervescent *see* potassium bicarbonate and potassium citrate, effervescent *on page 427*

potassium citrate and potassium gluconate
(poe TASS ee um SIT rate & poe TASS ee um GLOO coe nate)

Brand Names Twin-K®

Therapeutic Category Electrolyte Supplement

Use Treatment or prevention of hypokalemia

Usual Dosage Oral:
Children: 1-4 mEq/kg/24 hours in divided doses as required to maintain normal serum potassium
Adults:
Prevention: 16-24 mEq/day in 2-4 divided doses
Treatment: 40-100 mEq/day in 2-4 divided doses

Dosage Forms Solution, oral: 20 mEq/5 mL from potassium citrate 170 mg and potassium gluconate 170 mg per 5 mL

potassium gluconate (poe TASS ee um GLOO coe nate)

Brand Names Kaon®; K-G®

Therapeutic Category Electrolyte Supplement

Use Treatment or prevention of hypokalemia

Usual Dosage Oral:
Normal daily requirement:
Children: 2-3 mEq/kg/day
Adults: 40-80 mEq/day

Prevention during diuretic therapy:
Children: 1-2 mEq/kg/day in 1-2 divided doses
Adults: 20-40 mEq/day in 1-2 divided doses
Treatment of hypokalemia:
Children: 2-3 mEq/kg/day in 2-4 divided doses
Adults: 40-100 mEq/day in 2-4 divided doses

Dosage Forms
Elixir: 20 mEq/15 mL
K-G®, Kaon®, Kaylixir®: 20 mEq/15 mL
Tablet:
Glu-K®: 2 mEq
Kaon®: 5 mEq

potassium iodide (poe TASS ee um EYE oh dide)

Synonyms KI; Lugol's solution; strong iodine solution
Brand Names Pima®; SSKI®; Thyro-Block®
Therapeutic Category Antithyroid Agent; Expectorant
Use Facilitate bronchial drainage and cough; to reduce thyroid vascularity prior to thyroid-ectomy and management of thyrotoxic crisis; block thyroidal uptake of radioactive isotopes of iodine in a radiation emergency
Usual Dosage Oral:
Adults RDA: 130 mcg

Expectorant:
Children: 60-250 mg every 6-8 hours; maximum single dose: 500 mg
Adults: 300-1000 mg 2-3 times/day, may increase to 1-1.5 g 3 times/day
Preoperative thyroidectomy: Children and Adults: 50-250 mg 3 times/day (2-6 drops strong iodine solution); administer for 10 days before surgery
Thyrotoxic crisis:
Infants <1 year: $\frac{1}{2}$ adult dosage
Children and Adults: 300 mg = 6 drops SSKI® every 8 hours
Graves' disease in neonates: 1 drop of Lugol's solution every 8 hours
Sporotrichosis:
Initial:
Preschool: 50 mg/dose 3 times/day
Children: 250 mg/dose 3 times/day
Adults: 500 mg/dose 3 times/day
Oral increase 50 mg/dose daily
Maximum dose:
Preschool: 500 mg/dose 3 times/day
Children and Adults: 1-2 g/dose 3 times/day
Continue treatment for 4-6 weeks after lesions have completely healed
Dosage Forms
Solution, oral:
SSKI®: 1 g/mL (30 mL, 240 mL, 473 mL)
Lugol's solution, strong iodine: 100 mg/mL with iodine 50 mg/mL (120 mL)
Syrup: 325 mg/5 mL
Tablet: 130 mg

potassium phosphate (poe TASS ee um FOS fate)

Synonyms phosphate, potassium
Brand Names Neutra-Phos®-K
Therapeutic Category Electrolyte Supplement
Use Treatment and prevention of hypophosphatemia
Usual Dosage I.V. doses should be incorporated into the patient's maintenance I.V. fluids; intermittent I.V. infusion should be reserved for severe depletion situations and requires continuous cardiac monitoring. It is difficult to determine total body phosphorus deficit, the following dosages are empiric guidelines: **Note:** Doses listed as mmol of **phosphate**:

Replacement intermittent infusion: I.V.:
Children:
Low dose: 0.08 mmol/kg over 6 hours; use if recent losses and uncomplicated
Intermediate dose: 0.16-0.24 mmol/kg over 4-6 hours; use if serum phosphorus level 0.5-1 mg/dL
High dose: 0.36 mmol/kg over 6 hours; use if serum phosphorus <0.5 mg/dL
Adults: Varying dosages: 0.15-0.3 mmol/kg/dose over 12 hours; may repeat as needed to achieve desired serum level **or**
15 mmol/dose over 2 hours; use if serum phosphorus <2 mg/dL **or**
Low dose: 0.16 mmol/kg over 4-6 hours; use if serum phosphorus level 2.3-3 mg/dL
Intermediate dose: 0.32 mmol/kg over 4-6 hours; use if serum phosphorus level 1.6-2.2 mg/dL

High dose: 0.64 mmol/kg over 8-12 hours; use if serum phosphorus <1.5 mg/dL
Maintenance:
Children: 0.5-1.5 mmol/kg/24 hours I.V. or 2-3 mmol/kg/24 hours orally in divided doses
Adults: 50-70 mmol/24 hours I.V. or 50-150 mmol/24 hours orally in divided doses

Dosage Forms
Capsule: Neutra-Phos®-K: Phosphorus 250 mg [8 mmol] and potassium 556 mg [14.25 mEq] per capsule
Injection: Potassium phosphate monobasic anhydrous 224 mg and potassium phosphate dibasic anhydrous 236 mg per mL; [phosphorus 3 mmol and potassium 4.4 mEq per mL] (15 mL)
Powder: Neutra-Phos®-K: Phosphorus 250 mg [8 mmol] and potassium 556 mg [14.25 mEq] per packet

potassium phosphate and sodium phosphate
(poe TASS ee um FOS fate & SOW dee um FOS fate)
Synonyms sodium phosphate and potassium phosphate
Brand Names K-Phos® Neutral; Neutra-Phos®; Uro-KP-Neutral®
Therapeutic Category Electrolyte Supplement
Use Treatment of conditions associated with excessive renal phosphate loss or inadequate GI absorption of phosphate
Usual Dosage All dosage forms to be mixed in 6-8 oz of water prior to administration

Children: 2-3 mmol phosphate/kg/24 hours administered 4 times/day
Adults: 100-150 mmol phosphate/24 hours in divided doses after meals and at bedtime; 1-8 tablets or capsules/day, administered 4 times/day
Dosage Forms
Powder, concentrate: Phosphate 8 mmol, sodium 7.125 mEq, and potassium 7.125 mEq per 75 mL when reconstituted
Tablet: Phosphate 8 mmol, sodium 13 mEq, and potassium 1.1 mEq (114 mg of phosphorus)

povidone-iodine (POE vi done EYE oh dyne)
Brand Names ACU-dyne® [OTC]; Aerodine® [OTC]; Betadine® [OTC]; Betadine® 5% Sterile Ophthalmic Prep Solution; Betagen [OTC]; Biodine [OTC]; Efodine® [OTC]; Iodex® [OTC]; Iodex-p® [OTC]; Mallisol® [OTC]; Massengill® Medicated Douche w/ Ceptcin [OTC]; Minidyne® [OTC]; Operand® [OTC]; Polydine® [OTC]; Summer's Eve® Medicated Douche [OTC]; Yeast-Gard® Medicated Douche
Therapeutic Category Antibacterial, Topical
Use External antiseptic with broad microbicidal spectrum against bacteria, fungi, viruses, protozoa, and yeasts
Usual Dosage Apply as needed for treatment and prevention of susceptible microbial infections
Dosage Forms
Aerosol: 5% (90 mL)
Cleanser, topical: 7.5% (30 mL, 120 mL)
Concentrate:
Whirlpool: 10% (3840 mL)
Perineal wash: 10% (240 mL)
Douche: 10% [0.3% when reconstituted]
Foam, topical: 10% (250 g)
Gel, vaginal: 10% (3 oz)
Mouthwash: 0.5% (180 mL)
Ointment, topical: 10% (0.9 g foil packet, 0.94 g, 28 g, 480 g)
Pads, antiseptic gauze: 10% (3" x 9", 5" x 9")
Scrub, surgical: 7.5% (480 mL, 946 mL)
Shampoo: 7.5% (120 mL)
Solution:
Ophthalmic, sterile prep: 5% (50 mL)
(Continued)

povidone-iodine *(Continued)*
Swab aid: 10% (100s)
Swabsticks, 4": 10%
Topical: 10% (240 mL, 480 mL, 946 mL)
Suppository, vaginal: 10%

ppa *see* phenylpropanolamine *on page 413*

ppd *see* tuberculin tests *on page 539*

ppl *see* benzylpenicilloyl-polylysine *on page 63*

PPS *see* pentosan polysulfate sodium *on page 405*

pralidoxime (pra li DOKS eem)
Synonyms 2-pam; pralidoxime chloride; 2-pyridine aldoxime methochloride
Brand Names Protopam®
Therapeutic Category Antidote
Use Reverse muscle paralysis associated with toxic exposure to organophosphate anticholinesterase pesticides and chemicals; control of overdosage by anticholinesterase drugs used to treat myasthenia gravis
Usual Dosage Poisoning: I.V.:
Children: 20-50 mg/kg/dose; repeat in 1-2 hours if muscle weakness has not been relieved, then at 10- to 12-hour intervals if cholinergic signs recur
Adults: 1-2 g; repeat in 1-2 hours if muscle weakness has not been relieved, then at 10- to 12-hour intervals if cholinergic signs recur
Dosage Forms
Injection: 20 mL vial containing 1 g each pralidoxime chloride with one 20 mL ampul diluent, disposable syringe, needle, and alcohol swab
Injection, as chloride: 300 mg/mL (2 mL)
Tablet, as chloride: 500 mg

pralidoxime chloride *see* pralidoxime *on this page*

PrameGel® [OTC] *see* pramoxine *on this page*

Pramet® FA *see* vitamin, multiple (prenatal) *on page 554*

Pramilet® FA *see* vitamin, multiple (prenatal) *on page 554*

pramipexole (pram i PREKS ole)
Brand Names Mirapex®
Therapeutic Category Ectoparasiticide and Ovicide
Use Treatment of the signs and symptoms of idiopathic Parkinson's Disease
Usual Dosage Adults: Oral: Initial: 0.375 mg/day given in 3 divided doses, increase gradually by 0.125 mg/dose every 5-7 days; range: 1.5-4.5 mg/day
Dosage Forms Tablet: 0.125 mg, 0.25 mg, 1 mg, 1.5 mg

Pramosone® *see* pramoxine and hydrocortisone *on next page*

pramoxine (pra MOKS een)
Synonyms pramoxine hydrochloride
Brand Names Anusol® Ointment [OTC]; Fleet® Pain Relief [OTC]; Itch-X® [OTC]; Phicon® [OTC]; PrameGel® [OTC]; Prax® [OTC]; ProctoFoam® NS [OTC]; Tronolane® [OTC]
Therapeutic Category Local Anesthetic
Use Temporary relief of pain and itching associated with anogenital pruritus or irritation; dermatosis, minor burns or hemorrhoids
Usual Dosage Apply as directed, usually every 3-4 hours
Dosage Forms
Aerosol foam, as hydrochloride (ProctoFoam® NS): 1% (15 g)

Cream, as hydrochloride:
Prax®: 1% (30 g, 113.4 g, 454 g)
Tronolane®: 1% (30 g, 60 g)
Tronothane® HCl: 1% (28.4 g)
Gel, topical, as hydrochloride:
Itch-X®: 1% (35.4 g)
PrameGel®: 1% (118 g)
Lotion, as hydrochloride (Prax®): 1% (15 mL, 120 mL, 240 mL)
Ointment, as hydrochloride (Anusol®): 1% (30 g)
Pads, as hydrochloride (Fleet® Pain Relief): 1% (100s)
Spray, as hydrochloride (Itch-X®): 1% (60 mL)

pramoxine and hydrocortisone (pra MOKS een & hye droe KOR ti sone)
Synonyms hydrocortisone and pramoxine
Brand Names Enzone®; Pramosone®; Proctofoam®-HC; Zone-A Forte®
Therapeutic Category Anesthetic/Corticosteroid
Use Treatment of severe anorectal or perianal inflammation
Usual Dosage Apply to affected areas 3-4 times/day
Dosage Forms
Cream, topical: Pramoxine hydrochloride 1% and hydrocortisone acetate 0.5% (30 g); pramoxine hydrochloride 1% and hydrocortisone acetate 1%
Foam, rectal: Pramoxine hydrochloride 1% and hydrocortisone acetate 1% (10 g)
Lotion, topical: Pramoxine hydrochloride 1% and hydrocortisone 0.25%; pramoxine hydrochloride 1% and hydrocortisone 2.5%; pramoxine hydrochloride 2.5% and hydrocortisone 1% (37.5 mL, 120 mL, 240 mL)

pramoxine hydrochloride *see* pramoxine *on previous page*
Pravachol® *see* pravastatin *on this page*

pravastatin (PRA va stat in)
Synonyms pravastatin sodium
Brand Names Pravachol®
Therapeutic Category HMG-CoA Reductase Inhibitor
Use Adjunct to diet for the reduction of elevated total and LDL-cholesterol levels in patients with hypercholesterolemia (Type IIa and IIb)
Usual Dosage Adults: Oral: 10-20 mg once daily at bedtime
Dosage Forms Tablet, as sodium: 10 mg, 20 mg, 40 mg

pravastatin sodium *see* pravastatin *on this page*
Prax® [OTC] *see* pramoxine *on previous page*

praziquantel (pray zi KWON tel)
Brand Names Biltricide®
Therapeutic Category Anthelmintic
Use Treatment of all stages of schistosomiasis caused by *Schistosoma* species pathogenic to humans; also active in the treatment of clonorchiasis, opisthorchiasis, cysticercosis, and many intestinal tapeworm infections and trematode
Usual Dosage Children and Adults: Oral:
Schistosomiasis: 20 mg/kg/dose 2-3 times/day for 1 day at 4- to 6-hour intervals
Flukes: 25 mg/kg/dose every 8 hours for 1-2 days
Cysticercosis: 50 mg/kg/day divided every 8 hours for 14 days
Tapeworms: 10-20 mg/kg as a single dose (25 mg/kg for *H. nana*)
Dosage Forms Tablet, tri-scored: 600 mg

prazosin (PRA zoe sin)
Synonyms furazosin; prazosin hydrochloride
Brand Names Minipress®
(Continued)

prazosin *(Continued)*

Therapeutic Category Alpha-Adrenergic Blocking Agent
Use Hypertension, severe congestive heart failure (in conjunction with diuretics and cardiac glycosides)
Unlabeled use: Symptoms of benign prostatic hyperplasia
Usual Dosage Oral:
Children: Initial: 5 mcg/kg/dose (to assess hypotensive effects); usual dosing interval every 6 hours; increase dosage gradually up to maintenance of 25-150 mcg/kg/day divided every 6 hours
Adults: Initial: 1 mg/dose 2-3 times/day; usual maintenance dose: 3-15 mg/day in divided doses 2-4 times/day; maximum daily dose: 20 mg
Dosage Forms Capsule, as hydrochloride: 1 mg, 2 mg, 5 mg

prazosin and polythiazide *(PRA zoe sin & pol i THYE a zide)*

Brand Names Minizide®
Therapeutic Category Antihypertensive, Combination
Use Management of mild to moderate hypertension
Usual Dosage Adults: Oral: 1 capsule 2-3 times/day
Dosage Forms Capsule:
1: Prazosin 1 mg and polythiazide 0.5 mg
2: Prazosin 2 mg and polythiazide 0.5 mg
5: Prazosin 5 mg and polythiazide 0.5 mg

prazosin hydrochloride *see prazosin on previous page*

Precose® *see acarbose on page 2*

Predalone Injection *see prednisolone on this page*

Predcor-TBA® Injection *see prednisolone on this page*

Pred Forte® Ophthalmic *see prednisolone on this page*

Pred-G® Ophthalmic *see prednisolone and gentamicin on next page*

Pred Mild® Ophthalmic *see prednisolone on this page*

prednicarbate *(PRED ni kar bate)*

Brand Names Dermatop®
Therapeutic Category Corticosteroid, Topical
Use Relief of the inflammatory and pruritic manifestations of corticosteroid-responsive dermatoses
Usual Dosage Adults: Topical: Apply a thin film to affected area twice daily
Dosage Forms Cream: 0.1% (15 g, 60 g)

Prednicen-M® *see prednisone on page 436*

prednisolone *(pred NIS oh lone)*

Synonyms deltahydrocortisone; metacortandralone prednisolone acetate; prednisolone sodium phosphate; prednisolone tebutate
Brand Names AK-Pred® Ophthalmic; Articulose-50® Injection; Delta-Cortef® Oral; Econopred® Ophthalmic; Econopred® Plus Ophthalmic; Hydeltrasol® Injection; Inflamase® Forte Ophthalmic; Inflamase® Mild Ophthalmic; Key-Pred® Injection; Key-Pred-SP® Injection; Pediapred® Oral; Predalone Injection; Predcor-TBA® Injection; Pred Forte® Ophthalmic; Pred Mild® Ophthalmic; Prednisol® TBA Injection; Prelone® Oral
Therapeutic Category Adrenal Corticosteroid
Use Treatment of endocrine disorders, rheumatic disorders, collagen diseases, dermatologic diseases, allergic states, ophthalmic diseases, respiratory diseases, hematologic disorders, neoplastic diseases, edematous states, and gastrointestinal diseases

Ophthalmic: Treatment of palpebral and bulbar conjunctivitis; corneal injury from chemical, radiation, thermal burns, or foreign body penetration

Usual Dosage Dose depends upon condition being treated and response of patient; dosage for infants and children should be based on severity of the disease and response of the patient rather than on strict adherence to dosage indicated by age, weight, or body surface area. Consider alternate day therapy for long-term therapy. Discontinuation of long-term therapy requires gradual withdrawal by tapering the dose.

Children:
Acute asthma:
Oral: 1-2 mg/kg/day in divided doses 1-2 times/day for 3-5 days
I.V.: 2-4 mg/kg/day divided 3-4 times/day
Anti-inflammatory or immunosuppressive dose: Oral, I.V.: 0.1-2 mg/kg/day in divided doses 1-4 times/day
Nephrotic syndrome: Oral: Initial: 2 mg/kg/day (maximum: 80 mg/day) in divided doses 3-4 times/day until urine is protein free for 5 days (maximum: 28 days); if proteinuria persists, use 4 mg/kg/dose every other day for an additional 28 days (maximum: 120 mg/day); maintenance: 2 mg/kg/dose every other day for 28 days (maximum: 80 mg/dose); then taper over 4-6 weeks
Adults:
Oral, I.V.: 5-60 mg/day
Ophthalmic suspension: 1-2 drops into conjunctival sac every hour during day, every 2 hours at night until favorable response is obtained, then use 1 drop every 4 hours

Dosage Forms
Injection:
As acetate (for I.M., intralesional, intra-articular, or soft tissue administration only): 25 mg/mL (10 mL, 30 mL); 50 mg/mL (30 mL)
As sodium phosphate (for I.M., I.V., intra-articular, intralesional, or soft tissue administration): 20 mg/mL (2 mL, 5 mL, 10 mL)
As tebutate (for intra-articular, intralesional, soft tissue administration only): 20 mg/mL (1 mL, 5 mL, 10 mL)
Liquid, oral, as sodium phosphate: 5 mg/5 mL (120 mL)
Solution, ophthalmic, as sodium phosphate: 0.125% (5 mL, 10 mL, 15 mL); 1% (5 mL, 10 mL, 15 mL)
Suspension, ophthalmic, as acetate: 0.12% (5 mL, 10 mL); 0.125% (5 mL, 10 mL, 15 mL); 1% (1 mL, 5 mL, 10 mL, 15 mL)
Syrup: 15 mg/5 mL (240 mL)
Tablet: 5 mg

prednisolone acetate and sodium sulfacetamide *see* sulfacetamide sodium and prednisolone *on page 497*

prednisolone and gentamicin (pred NIS oh lone & jen ta MYE sin)

Synonyms gentamicin and prednisolone
Brand Names Pred-G® Ophthalmic
Therapeutic Category Antibiotic/Corticosteroid, Ophthalmic
Use Treatment of steroid responsive inflammatory conditions and superficial ocular infections due to strains of microorganisms susceptible to gentamicin such as *Staphylococcus*, *E. coli*, *H. influenzae*, *Klebsiella*, *Neisseria*, *Pseudomonas*, *Proteus*, and *Serratia* species
Usual Dosage Children and Adults: Ophthalmic: 1 drop 2-4 times/day; during the initial 24-48 hours, the dosing frequency may be increased if necessary
Dosage Forms
Ointment, ophthalmic: Prednisolone acetate 0.6% and gentamicin sulfate 0.3% (3.5 g)
Suspension, ophthalmic: Prednisolone acetate 1% and gentamicin sulfate 0.3% (2 mL, 5 mL, 10 mL)

prednisolone sodium phosphate *see* prednisolone *on previous page*

prednisolone tebutate *see* prednisolone *on previous page*

Prednisol® TBA Injection *see* prednisolone *on previous page*

prednisone (PRED ni sone)

Synonyms deltacortisone; deltadehydrocortisone

Brand Names Deltasone®; Liquid Pred®; Meticorten®; Orasone®; Prednicen-M®; Sterapred®

Therapeutic Category Adrenal Corticosteroid

Use Management of adrenocortical insufficiency; used for its anti-inflammatory or immunosuppressant effects

Usual Dosage Dose depends upon condition being treated and response of patient; dosage for infants and children should be based on severity of the disease and response of the patient rather than on strict adherence to dosage indicated by age, weight, or body surface area. Consider alternate day therapy for long-term therapy. Discontinuation of long-term therapy requires gradual withdrawal by tapering the dose.

Children: Oral: 0.05-2 mg/kg/day (anti-inflammatory or immunosuppressive dose) divided 1-4 times/day

Acute asthma: Oral: 1-2 mg/kg/day in divided doses 1-2 times/day for 3-5 days

Nephrotic syndrome: Oral: Initial: 2 mg/kg/day (maximum: of 80 mg/day) in divided doses 3-4 times/day until urine is protein free for 5 days (maximum: 28 days); if proteinuria persists, use 4 mg/kg/dose every other day (maximum: 120 mg/day) for an additional 28 days; maintenance: 2 mg/kg/dose every other day for 28 days (maximum: 80 mg/day); then taper over 4-6 weeks

Children and Adults: Physiologic replacement: 4-5 mg/m^2/day

Adults: Oral: 5-60 mg/day in divided doses 1-4 times/day

Dosage Forms

Solution:

Concentrate: 5 mg/mL (5 mL, 30 mL)

Oral: 5 mg/5 mL (10 mL, 20 mL, 500 mL)

Syrup: 5 mg/5 mL (120 mL, 240 mL)

Tablet: 1 mg, 2.5 mg, 5 mg, 10 mg, 20 mg, 50 mg

Prefrin™ Ophthalmic Solution *see* phenylephrine *on page 411*

Pregestimil® [OTC] *see* enteral nutritional products *on page 194*

pregnenedione *see* progesterone *on page 440*

Pregnyl® *see* chorionic gonadotropin *on page 122*

Prelone® Oral *see* prednisolone *on page 434*

Premarin® *see* estrogens, conjugated *on page 205*

Premarin® With Methyltestosterone *see* estrogens and methyltestosterone *on page 204*

Premphase™ *see* estrogens and medroxyprogesterone *on page 204*

Prempro™ *see* estrogens and medroxyprogesterone *on page 204*

prenatal vitamins *see* vitamin, multiple (prenatal) *on page 554*

Prenavite® [OTC] *see* vitamin, multiple (prenatal) *on page 554*

Prepcat® *see* radiological/contrast media (ionic) *on page 457*

Pre-Pen® *see* benzylpenicilloyl-polylysine *on page 63*

Prepidil® Vaginal Gel *see* dinoprostone *on page 172*

Prescription Strength Desenex® [OTC] *see* miconazole *on page 348*

PreSun® 29 [OTC] *see* methoxycinnamate and oxybenzone *on page 339*

Pretz® [OTC] *see* sodium chloride *on page 483*

Pretz-D® [OTC] *see* ephedrine *on page 194*

Prevacid® *see* lansoprazole *on page 302*

Prevalite® *see* cholestyramine resin *on page 121*

PreviDent® *see* fluoride *on page 228*

prilocaine (PRIL oh kane)
Brand Names Citanest® Forte; Citanest® Plain
Therapeutic Category Local Anesthetic
Use In dentistry for infiltration anesthesia and for nerve block anesthesia
Usual Dosage Dose varies with procedure, desired depth, and duration of anesthesia, desired muscle relaxation, vascularity of tissues, physical condition, and age of patient
Dosage Forms
Injection:
Citanest® Plain: 4% (1.8 mL)
Citanest® Forte: 4% with epinephrine bitartrate 1:200,000 (1.8 mL)

Prilosec™ *see* omeprazole *on page 383*

primaclone *see* primidone *on this page*

Primacor® *see* milrinone *on page 351*

primaquine and chloroquine *see* chloroquine and primaquine *on page 110*

primaquine phosphate (PRIM a kween FOS fate)
Synonyms prymaccone
Therapeutic Category Aminoquinoline (Antimalarial)
Use In conjunction with a blood schizonticidal agent to provide radical cure of *P. vivax* or *P. ovale* malaria after a clinical attack has been confirmed by blood smear or serologic titer; prevention of relapse of *P. ovale* or *P. vivax* malaria; malaria postexposure prophylaxis
Usual Dosage Oral:
Children: 0.3 mg base/kg/day once daily for 14 days not to exceed 15 mg/day or 0.9 mg base/kg once weekly for 8 weeks not to exceed 45 mg base/week
Adults: 15 mg/day (base) once daily for 14 days or 45 mg base once weekly for 8 weeks
Dosage Forms Tablet: 26.3 mg [15 mg base]

Primatene® **Mist [OTC]** *see* epinephrine *on page 195*

Primaxin® *see* imipenem and cilastatin *on page 280*

primidone (PRI mi done)
Synonyms desoxyphenobarbital; primaclone
Brand Names Mysoline®
Therapeutic Category Anticonvulsant; Barbiturate
Use Management of generalized tonic-clonic (grand mal), complex partial and simple partial (focal) seizures
Usual Dosage Oral:
Children: 0.3 mg base/kg/day once daily for 14 days (not to exceed 15 mg/day) or 0.9 mg base/kg once weekly for 8 weeks not to exceed 45 mg base/week
Adults: 15 mg/day (base) once daily for 14 days or 45 mg base once weekly for 8 weeks
Dosage Forms
Suspension, oral: 250 mg/5 mL (240 mL)
Tablet: 50 mg, 250 mg

Principen® *see* ampicillin *on page 33*

Prinivil® *see* lisinopril *on page 311*

Prinzide® *see* lisinopril and hydrochlorothiazide *on page 311*

Priscoline® *see* tolazoline *on page 523*

Privine® **Nasal [OTC]** *see* naphazoline *on page 364*

ProAmatine™ *see* midodrine *on page 350*

Probampacin® *see* ampicillin and probenecid *on page 33*

Pro-Banthine® *see* propantheline *on page 444*

probenecid (proe BEN e sid)
Therapeutic Category Uricosuric Agent
Use Prevention of gouty arthritis; hyperuricemia; prolong serum levels of penicillin/cephalosporin
Usual Dosage Oral:
Children:
<2 years: Not recommended
2-14 years: Prolong penicillin serum levels: 25 mg/kg starting dose, then 40 mg/kg/day administered 4 times/day
Gonorrhea: <45 kg: 25 mg/kg x 1 (maximum: 1 g/dose) 30 minutes before penicillin, ampicillin or amoxicillin
Adults:
Hyperuricemia with gout: 250 mg twice daily for one week; increase to 500 mg 2 times/day; may increase by 500 mg/month, if needed, to maximum of 2-3 g/day (dosages may be decreased by 500 mg every 6 months if serum urate concentrations are controlled)
Prolong penicillin serum levels: 500 mg 4 times/day
Gonorrhea: 1 g 30 minutes before penicillin, ampicillin or amoxicillin
Dosage Forms Tablet: 500 mg

probenecid and colchicine *see* colchicine and probenecid *on page 135*

procainamide (proe kane A mide)
Synonyms procainamide hydrochloride; procaine amide hydrochloride
Brand Names Procanbid®; Pronestyl®
Therapeutic Category Antiarrhythmic Agent, Class I-A
Use Ventricular tachycardia, premature ventricular contractions, paroxysmal atrial tachycardia, and atrial fibrillation; to prevent recurrence of ventricular tachycardia, paroxysmal supraventricular tachycardia, atrial fibrillation or flutter
Usual Dosage Must be titrated to patient's response
Children:
Oral: 15-50 mg/kg/24 hours divided every 3-6 hours; maximum 4 g/24 hours
I.M.: 20-30 mg/kg/24 hours divided every 4-6 hours in divided doses; maximum 4 g/24 hours
I.V.: Load: 3-6 mg/kg/dose over 5 minutes not to exceed 100 mg/dose; may repeat every 5-10 minutes to maximum of 15 mg/kg/load; maintenance as continuous I.V. infusion: 20-80 mcg/kg/minute; maximum: 2 g/24 hours
Adults:
Oral: 250-500 mg/dose every 3-6 hours or 500 mg to 1 g every 6 hours sustained release; usual dose: 50 mg/kg/24 hours or 2-4 g/24 hours
I.V.: Load: 50-100 mg/dose, repeated every 5-10 minutes until patient controlled; or load with 15-18 mg/kg, maximum loading dose: 1-1.5 g; maintenance: 2-6 mg/minute continuous I.V. infusion, usual maintenance: 3-4 mg/minute
Dosage Forms
Capsule, as hydrochloride: 250 mg, 375 mg, 500 mg
Injection, as hydrochloride: 100 mg/mL (10 mL); 500 mg/mL (2 mL)
Tablet, as hydrochloride: 250 mg, 375 mg, 500 mg
Sustained release: 250 mg, 500 mg, 750 mg, 1000 mg
Sustained release (Procanbid®): 500 mg, 1000 mg

procainamide hydrochloride *see* procainamide *on this page*

procaine (PROE kane)
Synonyms procaine hydrochloride
Brand Names Novocain® Injection
Therapeutic Category Local Anesthetic
Use Produce spinal anesthesia and epidural and peripheral nerve block by injection and infiltration methods

Usual Dosage Dose varies with procedure, desired depth, and duration of anesthesia, desired muscle relaxation, vascularity of tissues, physical condition, and age of patient
Dosage Forms Injection, as hydrochloride: 1% [10 mg/mL] (2 mL, 6 mL, 30 mL, 100 mL); 2% [20 mg/mL] (30 mL, 100 mL); 10% (2 mL)

procaine amide hydrochloride *see* procainamide *on previous page*

procaine benzylpenicillin *see* penicillin g procaine *on page 401*

procaine hydrochloride *see* procaine *on previous page*

procaine penicillin g *see* penicillin g procaine *on page 401*

Pro-Cal-Sof® [OTC] *see* docusate *on page 179*

Procanbid® *see* procainamide *on previous page*

procarbazine (proe KAR ba zeen)
Synonyms ibenzmethyzin; mih; n-methylhydrazine; procarbazine hydrochloride
Brand Names Matulane®
Therapeutic Category Antineoplastic Agent
Use Treatment of Hodgkin's disease, non-Hodgkin's lymphoma, brain tumor, bronchogenic carcinoma
Usual Dosage Refer to individual protocols. Oral:
Children: 50-100 mg/m^2/day once daily; doses as high as 100-200 mg/m^2/day once daily have been used for neuroblastoma and medulloblastoma
Adults: Initial: 2-4 mg/kg/day in single or divided doses for 7 days then increase dose to 4-6 mg/kg/day until response is obtained or leukocyte count decreased <4000/mm^3 or the platelet count decreased <100,000/mm^3; maintenance: 1-2 mg/kg/day
Dose reductions are necessary in patients with reduced renal function, reduced hepatic function, and/or bone marrow disorders
Dosage Forms Capsule, as hydrochloride: 50 mg

procarbazine hydrochloride *see* procarbazine *on this page*

Procardia® *see* nifedipine *on page 374*

Procardia XL® *see* nifedipine *on page 374*

procetofene *see* fenofibrate *on page 218*

prochlorperazine (proe klor PER a zeen)
Synonyms prochlorperazine edisylate; prochlorperazine maleate
Brand Names Compazine®
Therapeutic Category Phenothiazine Derivative
Use Management of nausea and vomiting; acute and chronic psychosis
Usual Dosage
Children: Oral, rectal:
>10 kg: 0.4 mg/kg/24 hours in 3-4 divided doses; **or**
9-14 kg: 2.5 mg every 12-24 hours as needed; maximum: 7.5 mg/day
14-18 kg: 2.5 mg every 8-12 hours as needed; maximum: 10 mg/day
18-39 kg: 2.5 mg every 8 hours or 5 mg every 12 hours as needed; maximum: 15 mg/day
I.M.: 0.1-0.15 mg/kg/dose; usual: 0.13 mg/kg/dose; change to oral as soon as possible
I.V.: Not recommended
Adults:
Oral: 5-10 mg 3-4 times/day; usual maximum: 40 mg/day; doses up to 150 mg/day may be required in some patients
I.M.: 5-10 mg every 3-4 hours; usual maximum: 40 mg/day; doses up to 10-20 mg every 4-6 hours may be required in some patients
I.V.: 2.5-10 mg; maximum 10 mg/dose or 40 mg/day; may repeat dose every 3-4 hours as needed
Rectal: 25 mg twice daily
(Continued)

prochlorperazine *(Continued)*

Dosage Forms
Capsule, sustained action, as maleate: 10 mg, 15 mg, 30 mg
Injection, as edisylate: 5 mg/mL (2 mL, 10 mL)
Suppository, rectal: 2.5 mg, 5 mg, 25 mg (12/box)
Syrup, as edisylate: 5 mg/5 mL (120 mL)
Tablet, as maleate: 5 mg, 10 mg, 25 mg

prochlorperazine edisylate *see* prochlorperazine *on previous page*

prochlorperazine maleate *see* prochlorperazine *on previous page*

Procort® [OTC] *see* hydrocortisone *on page 268*

Procrit® *see* epoetin alfa *on page 197*

Proctocort™ *see* hydrocortisone *on page 268*

proctofene *see* fenofibrate *on page 218*

Proctofoam®-HC *see* pramoxine and hydrocortisone *on page 433*

ProctoFoam® NS [OTC] *see* pramoxine *on page 432*

procyclidine (proe SYE kli deen)

Synonyms procyclidine hydrochloride
Brand Names Kemadrin®
Therapeutic Category Anticholinergic Agent; Anti-Parkinson's Agent
Use Relief of symptoms of Parkinsonian syndrome and drug-induced extrapyramidal symptoms
Usual Dosage Adults: Oral: 2-2.5 mg 3 times/day after meals; if tolerated, gradually increase dose to 4-5 mg 3 times/day
Dosage Forms Tablet, as hydrochloride: 5 mg

procyclidine hydrochloride *see* procyclidine *on this page*

Prodium® [OTC] *see* phenazopyridine *on page 408*

Profasi® HP *see* chorionic gonadotropin *on page 122*

Profenal® Ophthalmic *see* suprofen *on page 501*

Profen II® *see* guaifenesin and phenylpropanolamine *on page 249*

Profen II DM® *see* guaifenesin, phenylpropanolamine, and dextromethorphan *on page 251*

Profen LA® *see* guaifenesin and phenylpropanolamine *on page 249*

Profilate® OSD *see* antihemophilic factor (human) *on page 37*

Profilate® SD *see* antihemophilic factor (human) *on page 37*

Profilnine® Heat-Treated *see* factor ix complex (human) *on page 215*

Progestasert® *see* progesterone *on this page*

progesterone (proe JES ter one)

Synonyms pregnenedione; progestin
Brand Names Crinone®; Progestasert®
Therapeutic Category Progestin
Use
Gel: Progesterone supplementation or replacement as part of an assisted reproductive technology treatment for infertile women with progesterone deficiency
Reservoir: Endometrial carcinoma or renal carcinoma as well as secondary amenorrhea or abnormal uterine bleeding due to hormonal imbalance
Usual Dosage Adults:
Amenorrhea: I.M.: 5-10 mg/day for 6-8 consecutive days
Functional uterine bleeding: I.M.: 5-10 mg/day for 6 doses

Contraception: Female: Intrauterine device: Insert a single system into the uterine cavity; contraceptive effectiveness is retained for 1 year and system must be replaced 1 year after insertion

Dosage Forms
Gel, single use: 8% (90 mg applicator)
Intrauterine system, reservoir: 38 mg in silicone fluid

progestin *see* progesterone *on previous page*

Proglycem® Oral *see* diazoxide *on page 163*

Prograf® *see* tacrolimus *on page 502*

ProHIBiT® *see* haemophilus b conjugate vaccine *on page 254*

Prolamine® [OTC] *see* phenylpropanolamine *on page 413*

Prolastin® Injection *see* alpha$_1$-proteinase inhibitor *on page 18*

Proleukin® *see* aldesleukin *on page 15*

Prolixin Decanoate® Injection *see* fluphenazine *on page 230*

Prolixin Enanthate® Injection *see* fluphenazine *on page 230*

Prolixin® Injection *see* fluphenazine *on page 230*

Prolixin® Oral *see* fluphenazine *on page 230*

Proloprim® *see* trimethoprim *on page 534*

promazine (PROE ma zeen)

Synonyms promazine hydrochloride
Brand Names Sparine®
Therapeutic Category Phenothiazine Derivative
Use Treatment of psychoses
Usual Dosage Oral, I.M.:
  Children >12 years: Antipsychotic: 10-25 mg every 4-6 hours
  Adults:
    Psychosis: 10-200 mg every 4-6 hours not to exceed 1000 mg/day
    Antiemetic: 25-50 mg every 4-6 hours as needed
Dosage Forms
  Injection, as hydrochloride: 25 mg/mL (10 mL); 50 mg/mL (1 mL, 2 mL, 10 mL)
  Tablet, as hydrochloride: 25 mg, 50 mg, 100 mg

promazine hydrochloride *see* promazine *on this page*

Prometa® *see* metaproterenol *on page 332*

promethazine (proe METH a zeen)

Synonyms promethazine hydrochloride
Brand Names Anergan®; Phenazine®; Phenergan®; Prorex®
Therapeutic Category Antiemetic; Phenothiazine Derivative
Use Symptomatic treatment of various allergic conditions and motion sickness; sedative and an antiemetic
Usual Dosage
  Children:
    Antihistamine: Oral: 0.1 mg/kg/dose every 6 hours during the day and 0.5 mg/kg/dose at bedtime as needed
    Antiemetic: Oral, I.M., I.V., rectal: 0.25-1 mg/kg 4-6 times/day as needed
    Motion sickness: Oral: 0.5 mg/kg 30 minutes to 1 hour before departure, then every 12 hours as needed
    Sedation: Oral, I.M., I.V., rectal: 0.5-1 mg/kg/dose every 6 hours as needed
  Adults:
    Antihistamine:
      Oral: 25 mg at bedtime or 12.5 mg 3 times/day
(Continued)

promethazine *(Continued)*

I.M., I.V., rectal: 25 mg, may repeat in 2 hours
Antiemetic: Oral, I.M., I.V., rectal: 12.5-25 mg every 4 hours as needed
Motion sickness: Oral: 25 mg 30 minutes to 1 hour before departure, then every 12 hours as needed
Sedation: Oral, I.M., I.V., rectal: 25-50 mg/dose

Dosage Forms
Injection, as hydrochloride: 25 mg/mL (1 mL, 10 mL); 50 mg/mL (1 mL, 10 mL)
Suppository, rectal, as hydrochloride: 12.5 mg, 25 mg, 50 mg
Syrup, as hydrochloride: 6.25 mg/5 mL (5 mL, 120 mL, 240 mL, 480 mL, 4000 mL); 25 mg/5 mL (120 mL, 480 mL, 4000 mL)
Tablet, as hydrochloride: 12.5 mg, 25 mg, 50 mg

promethazine and codeine (proe METH a zeen & KOE deen)

Brand Names Phenergan® With Codeine; Pherazine® With Codeine; Prothazine-DC®
Therapeutic Category Antihistamine/Antitussive
Controlled Substance C-V
Use Temporary relief of coughs and upper respiratory symptoms associated with allergy or the common cold
Usual Dosage Oral (in terms of codeine):
Children: 1-1.5 mg/kg/day every 4 hours as needed; maximum: 30 mg/day **or**
2-6 years: 1.25-2.5 mL every 4-6 hours or 2.5-5 mg/dose every 4-6 hours as needed; maximum: 30 mg codeine/day
6-12 years: 2.5-5 mL every 4-6 hours as needed or 5-10 mg/dose every 4-6 hours as needed; maximum: 60 mg codeine/day
Adults: 10-20 mg/dose every 4-6 hours as needed; maximum: 120 mg codeine/day; or 5-10 mL every 4-6 hours as needed
Dosage Forms Syrup: Promethazine hydrochloride 6.25 mg and codeine phosphate 10 mg per 5 mL (120 mL, 180 mL, 473 mL)

promethazine and dextromethorphan

(proe METH a zeen & deks troe meth OR fan)
Brand Names Phenameth® DM; Phenergan® with Dextromethorphan; Pherazine® w/DM
Therapeutic Category Antihistamine/Antitussive
Use Temporary relief of coughs and upper respiratory symptoms associated with allergy or the common cold
Usual Dosage Oral:
Children:
2-6 years: 1.25-2.5 mL every 4-6 hours up to 10 mL in 24 hours
6-12 years: 2.5-5 mL every 4-6 hours up to 20 mL in 24 hours
Adults: 5 mL every 4-6 hours up to 30 mL in 24 hours
Dosage Forms Syrup: Promethazine hydrochloride 6.25 mg and dextromethorphan hydrobromide 15 mg per 5 mL with alcohol 7% (120 mL, 480 mL, 4000 mL)

promethazine and phenylephrine (proe METH a zeen & fen il EF rin)

Brand Names Phenergan® VC Syrup; Promethazine VC Plain Syrup; Promethazine VC Syrup; Prometh VC Plain Liquid
Therapeutic Category Antihistamine/Decongestant Combination
Use Temporary relief of upper respiratory symptoms associated with allergy or the common cold
Usual Dosage Oral:
Children:
2-6 years: 1.25 mL every 4-6 hours, not to exceed 7.5 mL in 24 hours
6-12 years: 2.5 mL every 4-6 hours, not to exceed 15 mL in 24 hours
Children >12 years and Adults: 5 mL every 4-6 hours, not to exceed 30 mL in 24 hours
Dosage Forms Liquid: Promethazine hydrochloride 6.25 mg and phenylephrine hydrochloride 5 mg per 5 mL

promethazine hydrochloride *see* promethazine *on page 441*

promethazine, phenylephrine, and codeine
(proe METH a zeen, fen il EF rin, & KOE deen)

Brand Names Phenergan® VC With Codeine; Pherazine® VC w/ Codeine; Promethist® with Codeine; Prometh® VC with Codeine

Therapeutic Category Antihistamine/Decongestant/Antitussive

Controlled Substance C-V

Use Temporary relief of coughs and upper respiratory symptoms including nasal congestion

Usual Dosage Oral:

Children (expressed in terms of codeine dosage): 1-1.5 mg/kg/day every 4 hours, maximum: 30 mg/day **or**

<2 years: Not recommended

2 to 6 years:

Weight 25 lb: 1.25-2.5 mL every 4-6 hours, not to exceed 6 mL/24 hours

Weight 30 lb: 1.25-2.5 mL every 4-6 hours, not to exceed 7 mL/24 hours

Weight 35 lb: 1.25-2.5 mL every 4-6 hours, not to exceed 8 mL/24 hours

Weight 40 lb: 1.25-2.5 mL every 4-6 hours, not to exceed 9 mL/24 hours

6 to <12 years: 2.5-5 mL every 4-6 hours, not to exceed 15 mL/24 hours

Adults: 5 mL every 4-6 hours, not to exceed 30 mL/24 hours

Dosage Forms Liquid: Promethazine hydrochloride 6.25 mg, phenylephrine hydrochloride 5 mg, and codeine phosphate 10 mg per 5 mL with alcohol 7% (120 mL, 240 mL, 480 mL, 4000 mL)

Promethazine VC Plain Syrup *see* promethazine and phenylephrine *on previous page*

Promethazine VC Syrup *see* promethazine and phenylephrine *on previous page*

Promethist® with Codeine *see* promethazine, phenylephrine, and codeine *on this page*

Prometh VC Plain Liquid *see* promethazine and phenylephrine *on previous page*

Prometh® VC with Codeine *see* promethazine, phenylephrine, and codeine *on this page*

Promit® *see* dextran 1 *on page 159*

Pronestyl® *see* procainamide *on page 438*

Pronto® Shampoo [OTC] *see* pyrethrins *on page 452*

Propac™ [OTC] *see* enteral nutritional products *on page 194*

Propacet® *see* propoxyphene and acetaminophen *on page 445*

propafenone (proe pa FEEN one)

Synonyms propafenone hydrochloride

Brand Names Rythmol®

Therapeutic Category Antiarrhythmic Agent, Class I-C

Use Life-threatening ventricular arrhythmias; an oral sodium channel blocker similar to encainide and flecainide; in clinical trials was used effectively to treat atrial flutter, atrial fibrillation and other arrhythmias, but are not labeled indications; can worsen or even cause new ventricular arrhythmias (proarrhythmic effect)

Usual Dosage Adults: Oral: 150 mg every 8 hours, up to 300 mg every 8 hours

Dosage Forms Tablet, as hydrochloride: 150 mg, 225 mg, 300 mg

propafenone hydrochloride *see* propafenone *on this page*

Propagest® [OTC] *see* phenylpropanolamine *on page 413*

propantheline (proe PAN the leen)
Synonyms propantheline bromide
Brand Names Pro-Banthine®
Therapeutic Category Anticholinergic Agent
Use Adjunctive treatment of peptic ulcer, irritable bowel syndrome, pancreatitis, ureteral and urinary bladder spasm; to reduce duodenal motility during diagnostic radiologic procedures
Usual Dosage Oral:
Antisecretory:
Children: 1-2 mg/kg/day in 3-4 divided doses
Elderly patients: 7.5 mg 3 times/day before meals and at bedtime
Antispasmodic:
Children: 2-3 mg/kg/day in divided doses every 4-6 hours and at bedtime
Adults: 15 mg 3 times/day before meals or food and 30 mg at bedtime
Dosage Forms Tablet, as bromide: 7.5 mg, 15 mg

propantheline bromide *see* propantheline *on this page*

proparacaine (proe PAR a kane)
Synonyms proparacaine hydrochloride; proxymetacaine
Brand Names AK-Taine®; Alcaine®; I-Paracaine®; Ophthetic®
Therapeutic Category Local Anesthetic
Use Local anesthesia for tonometry, gonioscopy; suture removal from cornea; removal of corneal foreign body; cataract extraction, glaucoma surgery; short operative procedure involving the cornea and conjunctiva
Usual Dosage Children and Adults:
Ophthalmic surgery: Instill 1 drop of 0.5% solution in eye every 5-10 minutes for 5-7 doses
Tonometry, gonioscopy, suture removal: Instill 1-2 drops 0.5% solution in eye just prior to procedure
Dosage Forms Ophthalmic, solution, as hydrochloride: 0.5% (2 mL, 15 mL)

proparacaine and fluorescein (proe PAR a kane & FLURE e seen)
Brand Names Fluoracaine® Ophthalmic
Therapeutic Category Diagnostic Agent; Local Anesthetic
Use Anesthesia for tonometry, gonioscopy; suture removal from cornea; removal of corneal foreign body; cataract extraction, glaucoma surgery
Usual Dosage
Tonometry, gonioscopy, suture removal: Adults: Instill 1-2 drops 0.5% solution in eye just prior to procedure
Ophthalmic surgery: Children and Adults: Instill 1 drop of 0.5% solution in eye every 5-10 minutes for 5-7 doses
Dosage Forms Solution: Proparacaine hydrochloride 0.5% and fluorescein sodium 0.25% (2 mL, 5 mL)

proparacaine hydrochloride *see* proparacaine *on this page*

Propine® Ophthalmic *see* dipivefrin *on page 176*

propiomazine (proe pee OH ma zeen)
Synonyms propiomazine hydrochloride
Brand Names Largon® Injection
Therapeutic Category Phenothiazine Derivative
Use Relief of restlessness, nausea and apprehension before and during surgery or during labor
Usual Dosage I.M., I.V.:
Children: 0.55-1.1 mg/kg
Adults: 10-40 mg prior to procedure, additional may be repeated at 3-hour intervals

Dosage Forms Injection, as hydrochloride: 20 mg/mL (1 mL)

propiomazine hydrochloride *see* propiomazine *on previous page*

Proplex® SX-T *see* factor ix complex (human) *on page 215*

Proplex® T *see* factor ix complex (human) *on page 215*

propofol (PROE po fole)

Brand Names Diprivan® Injection

Therapeutic Category General Anesthetic

Use Induction or maintenance of anesthesia; sedation

Usual Dosage Dosage must be individualized and titrated to the desired clinical effect; however, as a general guideline:

No pediatric dose has been established

Induction: I.V.:

Adults ≤55 years, and/or ASA I or II patients: 2-2.5 mg/kg of body weight (approximately 40 mg every 10 seconds until onset of induction)

Elderly, debilitated, hypovolemic, and/or ASA III or IV patients: 1-1.5 mg/kg of body weight (approximately 20 mg every 10 seconds until onset of induction)

Maintenance: I.V. infusion:

Adults ≤55 years, and/or ASA I or II patients: 0.1-0.2 mg/kg of body weight/minute (6-12 mg/kg of body weight/hour)

Elderly, debilitated, hypovolemic, and/or ASA III or IV patients: 0.05-0.1 mg/kg of body weight/minute (3-6 mg/kg of body weight/hour)

I.V. intermittent: 25-50 mg increments, as needed

Dosage Forms Injection: 10 mg/mL (20 mL, 50 mL, 100 mL)

propoxyphene (proe POKS i feen)

Synonyms dextropropoxyphene; propoxyphene hydrochloride; propoxyphene napsylate

Brand Names Darvon®; Darvon-N®; Dolene®

Therapeutic Category Analgesic, Narcotic

Controlled Substance C-IV

Use Management of mild to moderate pain

Usual Dosage Adults: Oral:

Hydrochloride: 65 mg every 3-4 hours as needed for pain; maximum: 390 mg/day

Napsylate: 100 mg every 4 hours as needed for pain; maximum: 600 mg/day

Dosage Forms

Capsule, as hydrochloride: 65 mg

Tablet, as napsylate: 100 mg

propoxyphene and acetaminophen

(proe POKS i feen & a seet a MIN oh fen)

Synonyms propoxyphene hydrochloride and acetaminophen; propoxyphene napsylate and acetaminophen

Brand Names Darvocet-N®; Darvocet-N® 100; Propacet®; Wygesic®

Therapeutic Category Analgesic, Narcotic

Controlled Substance C-IV

Use Management of mild to moderate pain

Usual Dosage Adults: Oral:

Darvocet-N®: 1-2 tablets every 4 hours as needed; maximum: 600 mg propoxyphene napsylate/day

Darvocet-N® 100: 1 tablet every 4 hours as needed; maximum: 600 mg propoxyphene napsylate/day

Dosage Forms Tablet:

Darvocet-N®: Propoxyphene napsylate 50 mg and acetaminophen 325 mg

Darvocet-N® 100: Propoxyphene napsylate 100 mg and acetaminophen 650 mg

(Continued)

propoxyphene and acetaminophen *(Continued)*

Genagesic®, Wygesic®: Propoxyphene hydrochloride 65 mg and acetaminophen 650 mg

propoxyphene and aspirin (proe POKS i feen & AS pir in)

Synonyms propoxyphene hydrochloride and aspirin; propoxyphene napsylate and aspirin

Brand Names Bexophene®; Darvon® Compound-65 Pulvules®

Therapeutic Category Analgesic, Narcotic

Controlled Substance C-IV

Use Management of mild to moderate pain

Usual Dosage Oral: 1-2 capsules every 4 hours as needed

Dosage Forms

Capsule: Propoxyphene hydrochloride 65 mg and aspirin 389 mg with caffeine 32.4 mg

Tablet (Darvon-N® with A.S.A.): Propoxyphene napsylate 100 mg and aspirin 325 mg

propoxyphene hydrochloride *see* propoxyphene *on previous page*

propoxyphene hydrochloride and acetaminophen *see* propoxyphene and acetaminophen *on previous page*

propoxyphene hydrochloride and aspirin *see* propoxyphene and aspirin *on this page*

propoxyphene napsylate *see* propoxyphene *on previous page*

propoxyphene napsylate and acetaminophen *see* propoxyphene and acetaminophen *on previous page*

propoxyphene napsylate and aspirin *see* propoxyphene and aspirin *on this page*

propranolol (proe PRAN oh lole)

Synonyms propranolol hydrochloride

Brand Names Betachron E-R® Capsule; Inderal®; Inderal® LA

Therapeutic Category Antiarrhythmic Agent, Class II; Beta-Adrenergic Blocker

Use Management of hypertension, angina pectoris, pheochromocytoma, essential tremor, tetralogy of Fallot cyanotic spells, and arrhythmias (such as atrial fibrillation and flutter, A-V nodal re-entrant tachycardias, and catecholamine-induced arrhythmias); prevention of myocardial infarction, migraine headache; symptomatic treatment of hypertrophic subaortic stenosis; short-term adjunctive therapy of thyrotoxicosis

Usual Dosage

Tachyarrhythmias:

Oral:

Children: Initial: 0.5-1 mg/kg/day in divided doses every 6-8 hours; titrate dosage upward every 3-7 days; usual dose: 2-4 mg/kg/day; higher doses may be needed; do not exceed 16 mg/kg/day or 60 mg/day

Adults: 10-80 mg/dose every 6-8 hours

I.V.:

Children: 0.01-0.1 mg/kg slow IVP over 10 minutes; maximum dose: 1 mg

Adults: 1 mg/dose slow IVP; repeat every 5 minutes up to a total of 5 mg

Hypertension: Oral:

Children: Initial: 0.5-1 mg/kg/day in divided doses every 6-12 hours; increase gradually every 3-7 days; maximum: 2 mg/kg/24 hours

Adults: Initial: 40 mg twice daily or 60-80 mg once daily as sustained release capsules; increase dosage every 3-7 days; usual dose: ≤320 mg divided in 2-3 doses/day or once daily as sustained release; maximum daily dose: 640 mg

Migraine headache prophylaxis: Oral:

Children: 0.6-1.5 mg/kg/day **or**

≤35 kg: 10-20 mg 3 times/day

>35 kg: 20-40 mg 3 times/day

Adults: Initial: 80 mg/day divided every 6-8 hours; increase by 20-40 mg/dose every 3-4 weeks to a maximum of 160-240 mg/day administered in divided doses every 6-8 hours; if satisfactory response not achieved within 6 weeks of starting therapy, drug should be withdrawn gradually over several weeks

Tetralogy spells: Children: Oral: 1-2 mg/kg/day every 6 hours as needed, may increase by 1 mg/kg/day to a maximum of 5 mg/kg/day, or if refractory may increase slowly to a maximum of 10-15 mg/kg/day

Thyrotoxicosis:

Adolescents and Adults: Oral: 10-40 mg/dose every 6 hours

Adults: I.V.: 1-3 mg/dose slow IVP as a single dose

Adults: Oral:

Angina: 80-320 mg/day in doses divided 2-4 times/day or 80-160 mg of sustained release once daily

Pheochromocytoma: 30-60 mg/day in divided doses

Myocardial infarction prophylaxis: 180-240 mg/day in 3-4 divided doses

Hypertrophic subaortic stenosis: 20-40 mg 3-4 times/day

Essential tremor: 40 mg twice daily initially; maintenance doses: usually 120-320 mg/day

Dosage Forms

Capsule, as hydrochloride, sustained action: 60 mg, 80 mg, 120 mg, 160 mg

Injection, as hydrochloride: 1 mg/mL (1 mL)

Solution, oral:

As hydrochloride (strawberry-mint flavor): 4 mg/mL (5 mL, 500 mL); 8 mg/mL (5 mL, 500 mL)

Concentrate, as hydrochloride: 80 mg/mL (30 mL)

Tablet, as hydrochloride: 10 mg, 20 mg, 40 mg, 60 mg, 80 mg, 90 mg

propranolol and hydrochlorothiazide
(proe PRAN oh lole & hye droe klor oh THYE a zide)

Brand Names Inderide®

Therapeutic Category Antihypertensive, Combination

Use Management of hypertension

Usual Dosage Dose is individualized

Dosage Forms

Capsule, long acting (Inderide® LA):

80/50 Propranolol hydrochloride 80 mg and hydrochlorothiazide 50 mg

120/50 Propranolol hydrochloride 120 mg and hydrochlorothiazide 50 mg

160/50 Propranolol hydrochloride 160 mg and hydrochlorothiazide 50 mg

Tablet (Inderide®):

40/25 Propranolol hydrochloride 40 mg and hydrochlorothiazide 25 mg

80/25 Propranolol hydrochloride 80 mg and hydrochlorothiazide 25 mg

propranolol hydrochloride *see* propranolol *on previous page*

Propulsid® *see* cisapride *on page 124*

propylene glycol and salicylic acid *see* salicylic acid and propylene glycol *on page 472*

propylhexedrine (proe pil HEKS e dreen)
Brand Names Benzedrex® [OTC]

Therapeutic Category Adrenergic Agonist Agent

Use Topical nasal decongestant

Usual Dosage Inhale through each nostril while blocking the other

Dosage Forms Inhaler: 250 mg

2-propylpentanoic acid *see* valproic acid and derivatives *on page 544*

propylthiouracil (proe pil thye oh YOOR a sil)
Synonyms ptu
Therapeutic Category Antithyroid Agent
Use Palliative treatment of hyperthyroidism, adjunct to ameliorate hyperthyroidism in preparation for surgical treatment or radioactive iodine therapy, management of thyrotoxic crisis
Usual Dosage Oral:
Children: Initial: 5-7 mg/kg/day in divided doses every 8 hours or
6-10 years: 50-150 mg/day
>10 years: 150-300 mg/day
Maintenance: $1/3$ to $2/3$ of the initial dose in divided doses every 8-12 hours
Adults: Initial: 300-450 mg/day in divided doses every 8 hours; maintenance: 100-150 mg/day in divided doses every 8-12 hours
Dosage Forms Tablet: 50 mg

2-propylvaleric acid *see* valproic acid and derivatives *on page 544*

Prorex® *see* promethazine *on page 441*

Proscar® *see* finasteride *on page 223*

Pro-Sof® Plus [OTC] *see* docusate and casanthranol *on page 180*

ProSom™ *see* estazolam *on page 202*

prostaglandin e₁ *see* alprostadil *on page 18*

prostaglandin e₂ *see* dinoprostone *on page 172*

prostaglandin f₂ alpha *see* dinoprost tromethamine *on page 172*

Prostaphlin® *see* oxacillin *on page 387*

ProStep® Patch *see* nicotine *on page 373*

Prostigmin® *see* neostigmine *on page 370*

Prostin/15M® *see* carboprost tromethamine *on page 92*

Prostin E₂® Vaginal Suppository *see* dinoprostone *on page 172*

Prostin F₂ Alpha® *see* dinoprost tromethamine *on page 172*

Prostin VR Pediatric® Injection *see* alprostadil *on page 18*

protamine sulfate (PROE ta meen SUL fate)
Therapeutic Category Antidote
Use Treatment of heparin overdosage; neutralize heparin during surgery or dialysis procedures
Usual Dosage Children and Adults: I.V.: 1 mg of protamine neutralizes 90 USP units of heparin (lung) and 115 USP units of heparin (intestinal); heparin neutralization occurs within 5 minutes following I.V. injection; administer 1 mg for each 100 units of heparin administered in preceding 3-4 hours up to a maximum dose of 50 mg
Dosage Forms Injection: 10 mg/mL (5 mL, 10 mL, 25 mL)

Protenate® *see* plasma protein fraction *on page 421*

Prothazine-DC® *see* promethazine and codeine *on page 442*

Protilase® *see* pancrelipase *on page 394*

protirelin (proe TYE re lin)
Synonyms lopremone
Brand Names Relefact® TRH Injection; Thypinone® Injection
Therapeutic Category Diagnostic Agent
Use Adjunct in the diagnostic assessment of thyroid function, and an adjunct to other diagnostic procedures in assessment of patients with pituitary or hypothalamic dysfunction; also causes release of prolactin from the pituitary and is used to detect defective control of prolactin secretion.

Usual Dosage I.V.:
Children: 7 mcg/kg to a maximum dose of 500 mcg
Adults: 500 mcg (range: 200-500 mcg)
Dosage Forms Injection: 500 mcg/mL (1 mL)

Protopam® *see* pralidoxime *on page 432*

Protostat® **Oral** *see* metronidazole *on page 346*

protriptyline (proe TRIP ti leen)
Synonyms protriptyline hydrochloride
Brand Names Vivactil®
Therapeutic Category Antidepressant, Tricyclic (Secondary Amine)
Use Treatment of various forms of depression, often in conjunction with psychotherapy
Usual Dosage Oral:
Adolescents: 15-20 mg/day
Adults: 15-60 mg in 3-4 divided doses
Elderly: 15-20 mg/day
Dosage Forms Tablet, as hydrochloride: 5 mg, 10 mg

protriptyline hydrochloride *see* protriptyline *on this page*

Protropin® **Injection** *see* human growth hormone *on page 262*

Provatene® **[OTC]** *see* beta-carotene *on page 64*

Proventil® *see* albuterol *on page 14*

Proventil® **HFA** *see* albuterol *on page 14*

Provera® **Oral** *see* medroxyprogesterone acetate *on page 326*

Provocholine® *see* methacholine *on page 334*

Proxigel® **Oral [OTC]** *see* carbamide peroxide *on page 90*

proxymetacaine *see* proparacaine *on page 444*

Prozac® *see* fluoxetine *on page 229*

prp-d *see haemophilus* b conjugate vaccine *on page 254*

prymaccone *see* primaquine phosphate *on page 437*

Pseudo-Car® **DM** *see* carbinoxamine, pseudoephedrine, and dextromethorphan *on page 91*

pseudoephedrine (soo doe e FED rin)
Synonyms *d*-isoephedrine hydrochloride; pseudoephedrine hydrochloride; pseudoephedrine sulfate
Brand Names Actifed® Allergy Tablet (Day) [OTC]; Afrin® Tablet [OTC]; Cenafed® [OTC]; Children's Silfedrine® [OTC]; Decofed® Syrup [OTC]; Drixoral® Non-Drowsy [OTC]; Efidac/24® [OTC]; Pedia Care® Oral; Sudafed® [OTC]; Sudafed® 12 Hour [OTC]; Triaminic® AM Decongestant Formula [OTC]
Therapeutic Category Adrenergic Agonist Agent
Use Temporary symptomatic relief of nasal congestion due to common cold, upper respiratory allergies, and sinusitis; also promotes nasal or sinus drainage
Usual Dosage Oral:
Children:
<2 years: 4 mg/kg/day in divided doses every 6 hours
2-5 years: 15 mg every 6 hours; maximum: 60 mg/24 hours
6-12 years: 30 mg every 6 hours; maximum: 120 mg/24 hours
Adults: 60 mg every 6 hours; maximum: 240 mg/24 hours
Dosage Forms
Capsule: 60 mg
Timed release, as hydrochloride: 120 mg
Drops, oral, as hydrochloride: 7.5 mg/0.8 mL (15 mL)
(Continued)

pseudoephedrine *(Continued)*
Liquid, as hydrochloride: 15 mg/5 mL (120 mL); 30 mg/5 mL (120 mL, 240 mL, 473 mL)
Syrup, as hydrochloride: 15 mg/5 mL (118 mL)
Tablet:
As hydrochloride: 30 mg, 60 mg
Timed release, as hydrochloride: 120 mg
Extended release, as sulfate: 120 mg, 240 mg

pseudoephedrine, acetaminophen, and dextromethorphan *see* acetaminophen, dextromethorphan, and pseudoephedrine *on page 6*

pseudoephedrine and acetaminophen *see* acetaminophen and pseudoephedrine *on page 5*

pseudoephedrine and acrivastine *see* acrivastine and pseudoephedrine *on page 9*

pseudoephedrine and azatadine *see* azatadine and pseudoephedrine *on page 50*

pseudoephedrine and chlorpheniramine *see* chlorpheniramine and pseudoephedrine *on page 114*

pseudoephedrine and dexbrompheniramine *see* dexbrompheniramine and pseudoephedrine *on page 157*

pseudoephedrine and dextromethorphan
(soo doe e FED rin & deks troe meth OR fan)
Brand Names Drixoral® Cough & Congestion Liquid Caps [OTC]; Vicks® 44D Cough & Head Congestion; Vicks® 44 Non-Drowsy Cold & Cough Liqui-Caps [OTC]
Therapeutic Category Antitussive/Decongestant
Use Temporary symptomatic relief of nasal congestion due to common cold, upper respiratory allergies, and sinusitis; also promotes nasal or sinus drainage; symptomatic relief of coughs caused by minor viral upper respiratory tract infections or inhaled irritants; most effective for a chronic nonproductive cough
Usual Dosage Adults: Oral: 1 capsule every 6 hours
Dosage Forms
Capsule: Pseudoephedrine hydrochloride 60 mg and dextromethorphan hydrobromide 30 mg
Liquid: Pseudoephedrine hydrochloride 20 mg and dextromethorphan hydrobromide 10 mg per 5 mL

pseudoephedrine and guaifenesin *see* guaifenesin and pseudoephedrine *on page 250*

pseudoephedrine and ibuprofen
(soo doe e FED rin & eye byoo PROE fen)
Brand Names Advil® Cold & Sinus Caplets [OTC]; Dimetapp® Sinus Caplets [OTC]; Dristan® Sinus Caplets [OTC]; Motrin® IB Sinus [OTC]; Sine-Aid® IB [OTC]
Therapeutic Category Decongestant/Analgesic
Use Temporary symptomatic relief of nasal congestion due to common cold, upper respiratory allergies, and sinusitis; also promotes nasal or sinus drainage; sinus headaches and pains
Usual Dosage Adults: Oral: 1-2 caplets every 4-6 hours
Dosage Forms Caplet: Pseudoephedrine hydrochloride 30 mg and ibuprofen 200 mg

pseudoephedrine and triprolidine *see* triprolidine and pseudoephedrine *on page 536*

pseudoephedrine, dextromethorphan, and acetaminophen *see* acetaminophen, dextromethorphan, and pseudoephedrine *on page 6*

pseudoephedrine, dextromethorphan, and guaifenesin *see* guaifenesin, pseudoephedrine, and dextromethorphan *on page 252*

pseudoephedrine hydrochloride *see* pseudoephedrine *on page 449*

pseudoephedrine sulfate *see* pseudoephedrine *on page 449*

Pseudo-Gest Plus® Tablet [OTC] *see* chlorpheniramine and pseudoephedrine *on page 114*

pseudomonic acid a *see* mupirocin *on page 358*

Psor-a-set® Soap [OTC] *see* salicylic acid *on page 472*

Psorcon™ *see* diflorasone *on page 167*

psoriGel® [OTC] *see* coal tar *on page 132*

psp *see* phenolsulfonphthalein *on page 410*

P&S® Shampoo [OTC] *see* salicylic acid *on page 472*

psyllium (SIL i yum)
Synonyms plantago seed; plantain seed
Brand Names Effer-Syllium® [OTC]; Fiberall® Powder [OTC]; Fiberall® Wafer [OTC]; Hydrocil® [OTC]; Konsyl® [OTC]; Konsyl-D® [OTC]; Metamucil® [OTC]; Metamucil® Instant Mix [OTC]; Modane® Bulk [OTC]; Perdiem® Plain [OTC]; Reguloid® [OTC]; Serutan® [OTC]; Syllact® [OTC]; V-Lax® [OTC]
Therapeutic Category Laxative
Use Treatment of chronic atonic or spastic constipation and in constipation associated with rectal disorders; management of irritable bowel syndrome
Usual Dosage Oral:
Children 6-11 years: 1/2 to 1 rounded teaspoonful 1-3 times/day
Adults: 1-2 rounded teaspoonfuls or 1-2 packets 1-4 times/day
Dosage Forms
Granules: 4.03 g per rounded teaspoon (100 g, 250 g); 2.5 g per rounded teaspoon
Powder: Psyllium 50% and dextrose 50% (6.5 g, 325 g, 420 g, 480 g, 500 g)
Effervescent: 3 g/dose (270 g, 480 g); 3.4 g/dose (single-dose packets)
Psyllium hydrophilic: 3.4 g per rounded teaspoon (210 g, 300 g, 420 g, 630 g)
Squares, chewable: 1.7 g, 3.4 g
Wafers: 3.4 g

P.T.E.-4® *see* trace metals *on page 525*

P.T.E.-5® *see* trace metals *on page 525*

pteroylglutamic acid *see* folic acid *on page 233*

ptu *see* propylthiouracil *on page 448*

Pulmicort® Turbuhaler® *see* budesonide *on page 75*

Pulmozyme® *see* dornase alfa *on page 181*

Puralube® Tears Solution [OTC] *see* artificial tears *on page 42*

Purge® [OTC] *see* castor oil *on page 95*

Puri-Clens™ [OTC] *see* methylbenzethonium chloride *on page 341*

purified protein derivative *see* tuberculin tests *on page 539*

Purinethol® *see* mercaptopurine *on page 330*

P-V-Tussin® *see* hydrocodone, phenylephrine, pyrilamine, phenindamine, chlorpheniramine, and ammonium chloride *on page 268*

P$_x$E$_x$® Ophthalmic *see* pilocarpine and epinephrine *on page 417*

pyrantel pamoate (pi RAN tel PAM oh ate)
Brand Names Antiminth® [OTC]; Pin-Rid® [OTC]; Pin-X® [OTC]; Reese's® Pinworm Medicine [OTC]
(Continued)

451

pyrantel pamoate *(Continued)*
Therapeutic Category Anthelmintic
Use Roundworm (*Ascaris lumbricoides*), pinworm (*Enterobius vermicularis*), and hookworm (*Ancylostoma duodenale* and *Necator americanus*) infestations, and trichostrongyliasis
Usual Dosage Children and Adults: Oral:
Roundworm, pinworm, or trichostrongyliasis: 11 mg/kg administered as a single dose; maximum dose is 1 g; dosage should be repeated in 2 weeks for pinworm infection
Hookworm: 11 mg/kg/day once daily for 3 days
Dosage Forms
Capsule: 180 mg
Liquid: 50 mg/mL (30 mL); 144 mg/mL (30 mL)
Suspension, oral (caramel-currant flavor): 50 mg/mL (60 mL)

pyrazinamide (peer a ZIN a mide)
Synonyms pyrazinoic acid amide
Therapeutic Category Antitubercular Agent
Use In combination with other antituberculosis agents in the treatment of *Mycobacterium tuberculosis* infection (especially useful in disseminated and meningeal tuberculosis); CDC currently recommends a 3 or 4 multidrug regimen which includes pyrazinamide, rifampin, INH, and at times ethambutol or streptomycin for the treatment of tuberculosis
Usual Dosage Oral:
Children: 15-30 mg/kg/day in divided doses every 12-24 hours; daily dose not to exceed 2 g
Adults: 15-30 mg/kg/day in 3-4 divided doses; maximum daily dose: 2 g/day
Dosage Forms Tablet: 500 mg

pyrazinoic acid amide *see* pyrazinamide *on this page*

pyrethrins (pye RE thrins)
Brand Names A-200™ Shampoo [OTC]; Barc™ Liquid [OTC]; End Lice® Liquid [OTC]; Lice-Enz® Shampoo [OTC]; Pronto® Shampoo [OTC]; Pyrinex® Pediculicide Shampoo [OTC]; Pyrinyl II® Liquid [OTC]; Pyrinyl Plus® Shampoo [OTC]; R & C® Shampoo [OTC]; RID® Shampoo [OTC]; Tisit® Blue Gel [OTC]; Tisit® Liquid [OTC]; Tisit® Shampoo [OTC]; Triple X® Liquid [OTC]
Therapeutic Category Scabicides/Pediculicides
Use Treatment of *Pediculus humanus* infestations
Usual Dosage Application of pyrethrins: Topical:
Apply enough solution to completely wet infested area, including hair
Allow to remain on area for 10 minutes
Wash and rinse with large amounts of warm water
Use fine-toothed comb to remove lice and eggs from hair
Shampoo hair to restore body and luster
Treatment may be repeated if necessary once in a 24-hours period
Repeat treatment in 7-10 days to kill newly hatched lice
Dosage Forms
Gel, topical: 0.3% (30 g, 480 g)
Liquid, topical: 0.18% (60 mL); 0.2% (60 mL, 120 mL); 0.3% (60 mL, 120 mL, 240 mL)
Shampoo: 0.3% (60 mL, 118 mL); 0.33% (60 mL, 120 mL)

Pyridiate® *see* phenazopyridine *on page 408*
2-pyridine aldoxime methochloride *see* pralidoxime *on page 432*
Pyridium® *see* phenazopyridine *on page 408*

pyridostigmine (peer id oh STIG meen)
Synonyms pyridostigmine bromide
Brand Names Mestinon® Injection; Mestinon® Oral; Regonol® Injection

Therapeutic Category Cholinergic Agent

Use Symptomatic treatment of myasthenia gravis by improving muscle strength; reversal of effects of nondepolarizing neuromuscular blocking agents

Usual Dosage Normally, sustained release dosage form is used at bedtime for patients who complain of morning weakness

Myasthenia gravis:
Oral:
Children: 7 mg/kg/day in 5-6 divided doses
Adults: Initial: 60 mg 3 times/day with maintenance dose ranging from 60 mg to 1.5 g/day; sustained release formulation should be dosed at least every 6 hours (usually 12-24 hours)
I.M., I.V.:
Children: 0.05-0.15 mg/kg/dose (maximum single dose: 10 mg)
Adults: 2 mg every 2-3 hours or 1/30th of oral dose
Reversal of nondepolarizing neuromuscular blocker: I.M., I.V.:
Children: 0.1-0.25 mg/kg/dose preceded by atropine
Adults: 10-20 mg preceded by atropine

Dosage Forms
Injection, as bromide: 5 mg/mL (2 mL, 5 mL)
Syrup, as bromide (raspberry flavor): 60 mg/5 mL (480 mL)
Tablet, as bromide: 60 mg
Sustained release: 180 mg

pyridostigmine bromide *see* pyridostigmine *on previous page*

pyridoxine (peer i DOKS een)

Synonyms pyridoxine hydrochloride; vitamin b_6
Brand Names Nestrex®
Therapeutic Category Vitamin, Water Soluble
Use Prevent and treat vitamin B_6 deficiency, pyridoxine-dependent seizures in infants, treatment of drug-induced deficiency (eg, isoniazid or hydralazine)
Usual Dosage
Pyridoxine-dependent Infants:
Oral: 2-100 mg/day
I.M., I.V.: 10-100 mg
Dietary deficiency: Oral:
Children: 5-10 mg/24 hours for 3 weeks
Adults: 10-20 mg/day for 3 weeks
Drug induced neuritis (eg, isoniazid, hydralazine, penicillamine, cycloserine): Oral treatment:
Children: 10-50 mg/24 hours; prophylaxis: 1-2 mg/kg/24 hours
Adults: 100-200 mg/24 hours; prophylaxis: 10-100 mg/24 hours

For the treatment of seizures and/or coma from acute isoniazid toxicity, a dose of pyridoxine hydrochloride equal to the amount of INH ingested can be administered I.M./I.V. in divided doses together with other anticonvulsants

Dosage Forms
Injection, as hydrochloride: 100 mg/mL (10 mL, 30 mL)
Tablet, as hydrochloride: 25 mg, 50 mg, 100 mg
Extended release: 100 mg

pyridoxine hydrochloride *see* pyridoxine *on this page*

pyrimethamine (peer i METH a meen)

Brand Names Daraprim®
Therapeutic Category Folic Acid Antagonist (Antimalarial)
Use Prophylaxis of malaria due to susceptible strains of plasmodia; used in conjunction with quinine and sulfadoxine for the treatment of uncomplicated attacks of chloroquine-resistant *P. falciparum* malaria; used in conjunction with fast-acting schizonticide to
(Continued)

pyrimethamine *(Continued)*

initiate transmission control and suppression cure; synergistic combination with sulfadiazine in treatment of toxoplasmosis

Usual Dosage Oral:

Malaria chemoprophylaxis:

Children: 0.5 mg/kg once weekly; not to exceed 25 mg/dose **or**

Children:

<4 years: 6.25 mg once weekly

4-10 years: 12.5 mg once weekly

Children >10 years and Adults: 25 mg once weekly

Dosage should be continued for all age groups for at least 6-10 weeks after leaving endemic areas

Chloroquine-resistant *P. falciparum* malaria (when used in conjunction with quinine and sulfadiazine):

Children:

<10 kg: 6.25 mg/day once daily for 3 days

10-20 kg: 12.5 mg/day once daily for 3 days

20-40 kg: 25 mg/day once daily for 3 days

Adults: 25 mg twice daily for 3 days

Toxoplasmosis (with sulfadiazine or trisulfapyrimidines):

Children: 1 mg/kg/day divided into 2 equal daily doses; decrease dose after 2-4 days by 50%, continue for about 1 month; used with 100 mg sulfadiazine/kg/day divided every 6 hours; **or** 2 mg/kg/day divided every 12 hours for 3 days followed by 1 mg/kg/day once daily for 4 weeks

Adults: 50-75 mg/day together with 1-4 g of a sulfonamide for 1-3 weeks depending on patient's tolerance and response

Dosage Forms Tablet: 25 mg

Pyrinex® **Pediculicide Shampoo [OTC]** *see* pyrethrins *on page 452*

Pyrinyl II® **Liquid [OTC]** *see* pyrethrins *on page 452*

Pyrinyl Plus® **Shampoo [OTC]** *see* pyrethrins *on page 452*

pyrithione zinc *(peer i THYE one zingk)*

Brand Names DHS Zinc® [OTC]; Head & Shoulders® [OTC]; Theraplex Z® [OTC]; Zincon® Shampoo [OTC]; ZNP® Bar [OTC]

Therapeutic Category Antiseborrheic Agent, Topical

Use Relieves the itching, irritation and scalp flaking associated with dandruff and/or seborrheal dermatitis of the scalp

Usual Dosage Topical: Shampoo hair twice weekly, wet hair, apply to scalp and massage vigorously, rinse and repeat

Dosage Forms

Bar: 2% (119 g)

Shampoo: 1% (120 mL); 2% (120 mL, 180 mL, 240 mL, 360 mL)

quazepam *(KWAY ze pam)*

Brand Names Doral®

Therapeutic Category Benzodiazepine

Controlled Substance C-IV

Use Short-term treatment of insomnia

Usual Dosage Adults: Oral: Initial: 15 mg at bedtime, in some patients the dose may be reduced to 7.5 mg after a few nights

Dosage Forms Tablet: 7.5 mg, 15 mg

Quelicin® **Injection** *see* succinylcholine *on page 494*

Questran® *see* cholestyramine resin *on page 121*

Questran® **Light** *see* cholestyramine resin *on page 121*

quetiapine (kwe TYE a peen)
Synonyms quetiapine fumarate
Brand Names Seroquel®
Therapeutic Category Antipsychotic Agent
Use Management of psychotic disorders; this antipsychotic drug belongs to a new chemical class, the dibenzothiazepine derivatives
Usual Dosage Adults: Oral: 25-100 mg 2-3 times daily
Dosage Forms Tablet: 25 mg, 100 mg, 200 mg

quetiapine fumarate *see* quetiapine *on this page*

Quibron® *see* theophylline and guaifenesin *on page 512*

Quibron®-T *see* theophylline *on page 511*

Quibron®-T/SR *see* theophylline *on page 511*

Quinaglute® Dura-Tabs® *see* quinidine *on this page*

Quinalan® *see* quinidine *on this page*

quinalbarbitone sodium *see* secobarbital *on page 475*

quinapril (KWIN a pril)
Synonyms quinapril hydrochloride
Brand Names Accupril®
Therapeutic Category Angiotensin-Converting Enzyme (ACE) Inhibitors
Use Treatment of hypertension, either alone or in combination with other antihypertensive agents
Usual Dosage Adults: Oral: Initial: 10 mg once daily, adjust according to blood pressure response at peak and trough blood levels; in general, the normal dosage range is 40-80 mg/day
Dosage Forms Tablet, as hydrochloride: 5 mg, 10 mg, 20 mg, 40 mg

quinapril hydrochloride *see* quinapril *on this page*

quinethazone (kwin ETH a zone)
Brand Names Hydromox®
Therapeutic Category Diuretic, Thiazide
Use Adjunctive therapy in treatment of edema and hypertension
Usual Dosage Adults: Oral: 50-100 mg once daily up to a maximum of 200 mg daily
Dosage Forms Tablet: 50 mg

Quinidex® Extentabs® *see* quinidine *on this page*

quinidine (KWIN i deen)
Synonyms quinidine gluconate; quinidine polygalacturonate; quinidine sulfate
Brand Names Cardioquin®; Quinaglute® Dura-Tabs®; Quinalan®; Quinidex® Extentabs®; Quinora®
Therapeutic Category Antiarrhythmic Agent, Class I-A
Use Prophylaxis after cardioversion of atrial fibrillation and/or flutter to maintain normal sinus rhythm; also used to prevent reoccurrence of paroxysmal supraventricular tachycardia, paroxysmal A-V junctional rhythm, paroxysmal ventricular tachycardia, paroxysmal atrial fibrillation, and atrial or ventricular premature contractions; also has activity against *Plasmodium falciparum* malaria
Usual Dosage Note: Dosage expressed in terms of the salt: 267 mg of quinidine gluconate = 275 mg of quinidine polygalacturonate = 200 mg of quinidine sulfate

Children: Test dose for idiosyncratic reaction (sulfate, oral or gluconate, I.M.): 2 mg/kg or 60 mg/m^2
(Continued)

quinidine *(Continued)*

Oral (quinidine sulfate): 15-60 mg/kg/day in 4-5 divided doses or 6 mg/kg every 4-6 hours (AMA 1991); usual 30 mg/kg/day or 900 mg/m^2/day administered in 5 daily doses

I.V. **not** recommended (quinidine gluconate): 2-10 mg/kg/dose every 3-6 hours as needed

Adults: Test dose: 200 mg administered several hours before full dosage (to determine possibility of idiosyncratic reaction)

Oral (sulfate): 100-600 mg/dose every 4-6 hours; begin at 200 mg/dose and titrate to desired effect

Oral (gluconate): 324-972 mg every 8-12 hours

Oral (polygalacturonate): 275 mg every 8-12 hours

I.M.: 400 mg/dose every 4-6 hours

I.V.: 200-400 mg/dose diluted and administered at a rate ≤10 mg/minute

Dosage Forms

Injection, as gluconate: 80 mg/mL (10 mL)

Tablet:

As polygalacturonate: 275 mg

As sulfate: 200 mg, 300 mg

Sustained action, as sulfate: 300 mg

Sustained release, as gluconate: 324 mg

quinidine gluconate *see* quinidine *on previous page*

quinidine polygalacturonate *see* quinidine *on previous page*

quinidine sulfate *see* quinidine *on previous page*

quinine *(KWYE nine)*

Synonyms quinine sulfate

Brand Names Formula Q®

Therapeutic Category Antimalarial Agent; Skeletal Muscle Relaxant

Use Suppression or treatment of chloroquine-resistant *P. falciparum* malaria (inactive against sporozoites, pre-erythrocytic or exoerythrocytic forms of plasmodia); treatment of *Babesia microti* infection; prevention and treatment of nocturnal recumbency leg muscle cramps

Usual Dosage Oral (parenteral dosage form may be obtained from Centers for Disease Control if needed):

Children: Chloroquine-resistant malaria and babesiosis: 25 mg/kg/day in divided doses every 8 hours for 7 days; maximum: 650 mg/dose

Adults:

Chloroquine-resistant malaria: 650 mg every 8 hours for 7 days in conjunction with another agent

Babesiosis: 650 mg every 6-8 hours for 7 days

Leg cramps: 200-300 mg at bedtime

Dosage Forms

Capsule, as sulfate: 64.8 mg, 65 mg, 200 mg, 300 mg, 325 mg

Tablet, as sulfate: 162.5 mg, 260 mg

quinine sulfate *see* quinine *on this page*

quinol *see* hydroquinone *on page 272*

Quinora® *see* quinidine *on previous page*

Quinsana Plus® **[OTC]** *see* tolnaftate *on page 523*

QYS® *see* hydroxyzine *on page 275*

rabies immune globulin (human)
(RAY beez i MYUN GLOB yoo lin, HYU man)
Synonyms rig
Brand Names Hyperab®; Imogam®
Therapeutic Category Immune Globulin
Use Passive immunity to rabies for postexposure prophylaxis of individuals exposed to the virus
Usual Dosage Children and Adults: I.M.: 20 units/kg in a single dose (RIG should always be administered in conjunction with rabies vaccine (HDCV)) (Infiltrate 1/2 of the dose locally around the wound; administer the remainder I.M.)
Dosage Forms Injection: 150 units/mL (2 mL, 10 mL)

rabies virus vaccine (RAY beez VYE rus vak SEEN)
Synonyms hdcv; hdrs
Brand Names Imovax® Rabies I.D. Vaccine; Imovax® Rabies Vaccine
Therapeutic Category Vaccine, Inactivated Virus
Use Pre-exposure rabies immunization for high risk persons; postexposure antirabies immunization along with local treatment and immune globulin
Usual Dosage
Pre-exposure prophylaxis: Two 1 mL doses I.M. or I.D. 1 week apart, third dose 3 weeks after second. If exposure continues, booster doses can be administered every 2 years, or an antibody titer determined and a booster dose administered if the titer is inadequate.

Postexposure prophylaxis: All postexposure treatment should begin with immediate cleansing of the wound with soap and water. Persons not previously immunized as above: Rabies immune globulin 20 units/kg body weight, half infiltrated at bite site if possible, remainder I.M.; and 5 doses of rabies vaccine, 1 mL I.M., one each on days 0, 3, 7, 14, 28.

Persons who have previously received postexposure prophylaxis with rabies vaccine, received a recommended I.M. or I.D. pre-exposure series of rabies vaccine or have a previously documented rabies antibody titer considered adequate: Two doses of rabies vaccine, 1 mL I.M., one each on days 0 and 3
Dosage Forms Injection:
I.M. (HDCV): Rabies antigen 2.5 units/mL (1 mL)
Intradermal: Rabies antigen 0.25 units/mL (1 mL)

radiological/contrast media (ionic)
Brand Names Anatrast®; Angio Conray®; Angiovist®; Baricon®; Barobag®; Baro-CAT®; Baroflave®; Barosperse®; Bar-Test®; Bilopaque®; Cholebrine®; Cholografin® Meglumine; Conray®; Cystografin®; Dionosil Oily®; Enecat®; Entrobar®; Epi-C®; Ethiodol®; Flo-Coat®; Gastrografin®; HD 85®; HD 200 Plus®; Hexabrix™; Hypaque-Cysto®; Hypaque® Meglumine; Hypaque® Sodium; Liquid Barosperse®; Liquipake®; Lymphazurin®; Magnevist®; MD-Gastroview®; Oragrafin® Calcium; Oragrafin® Sodium; Perchloracap®; Prepcat®; Reno-M-30®; Reno-M-60®; Reno-M-Dip®; Renovue®-65; Renovue®-DIP; Sinografin®; Telepaque®; Tomocat®; Tonopaque®; Urovist Cysto®; Urovist® Meglumine; Urovist® Sodium 300; Vascoray®
Therapeutic Category Radiopaque Agents
Dosage Forms
Oral cholecystographic agents:
Iocetamic acid: Tablet (Cholebrine®): 750 mg
Iopanoic acid: Tablet (Telepaque®): 500 mg
Ipodate calcium: Granules for oral suspension (Oragrafin® Calcium): 3 g
Ipodate sodium: Capsule (Bilivist®, Oragrafin® Sodium): 500 mg
Tyropanoate sodium: Capsule (Bilopaque®): 750 mg

GI contrast agents: Barium sulfate:
Paste (Anatrast®): 100% (500 g)
(Continued)

457

radiological/contrast media (ionic) *(Continued)*

Powder:
Baroflave®: 100%
Baricon®, HD 200 Plus®: 98%
Barosperse®, Tonopaque®: 95%
Suspension:
Baro-CAT®, Prepcat®: 1.5%
Enecat®, Tomocat®: 5%
Entrobar®: 50%
Liquid Barasperse®: 60%
HD 85®: 85%
Barobag®: 97%
Flo-Coat®, Liquipake®: 100%
Epi-C®: 150%
Tablet (Bar-Test®): 650 mg

Parenteral agents: Injection:
Diatrizoate meglumine:
Hypaque® Meglumine
Reno-M-DIP®
Urovist® Meglumine
Angiovist® 282
Hypaque® Meglumine
Reno-M-60®
Diatrizoate sodium:
Hypaque® Sodium
Hypaque® Sodium
Urovist® Sodium 300
Gadopentetate dimeglumine: Magnevist®
Iodamide meglumine:
Renovue®-DIP
Renovue®-65
Iodipamide meglumine: Cholografin® meglumine
Iothalamate meglumine:
Conray® 30
Conray® 43
Conray®
Iothalamate sodium:
Angio Conray®
Conray® 325
Conray® 400
Diatrizoate meglumine and diatrizoate sodium:
Angiovist® 292
Angiovist® 370
Hypaque-76®
Hypaque-M®, 75%
Hypaque-M®, 90%
MD-60®
MD-76®
Renografin-60®
Renografin-76®
Renovist® II
Renovist®
Iothalamate meglumine and iothalamate sodium:
Vascoray®
Hexabrix™

Miscellaneous agents: (**NOT** for intravascular use, for instillation into various cavities)
Diatrizoate meglumine: Urogenital solution, sterile:
Crystografin®

Crystografin® Dilute
Hypaque-Cysto®
Reno-M-30®
Urovist Cysto®
Diatrizoate meglumine and diatrizoate sodium: Solution, oral or rectal:
Gastrografin®
MD-Gastroview®
Diatrizoate sodium:
Solution, oral or rectal (Hypaque® sodium oral)
Solution, urogenital (Hypaque® sodium 20%)
Iothalamate meglumine: Solution, urogenital:
Cysto-Conray®
Cysto-Conray® II

Diatrizoate meglumine and iodipamide meglumine:
Injection, urogenital for intrauterine instillation (Sinografin®)
Ethiodized oil: Injection (Ethiodol®)
Propyliodone: Suspension (Dionosil Oily®)
Isosulfan blue: Injection (Lymphazurin® 1%)
Potassium perchlorate: Capsule (Perchloracap®): 200 mg

radiological/contrast media (non-ionic)

Brand Names Amnipaque®; Isovue®; Omnipaque®; Optiray®
Therapeutic Category Radiopaque Agents
Dosage Forms
Parenteral agents: Injection:
Iohexol: Omnipaque®: 140 mg/mL; 180 mg/mL; 210 mg/mL; 240 mg/mL; 300 mg/mL; 350 mg/mL
Iopamidol:
Isovue-128®
Isovue-200®
Isovue-M 200®
Isovue-300®
Isovue-M 300®
Isovue-370®
Ioversol:
Optiray® 160
Optiray® 240
Optiray® 320
Metrizamide: Amnipaque®

ramipril (ra MI pril)
Brand Names Altace™
Therapeutic Category Angiotensin-Converting Enzyme (ACE) Inhibitors
Use Treatment of hypertension, alone or in combination with thiazide diuretics; congestive heart failure immediately after myocardial infarction
Usual Dosage Adults: Oral: 2.5-5 mg once daily
Dosage Forms Capsule: 1.25 mg, 2.5 mg, 5 mg, 10 mg

Ramses® [OTC] *see* nonoxynol 9 *on page 377*

ranitidine bismuth citrate (ra NI ti deen BIZ muth SIT rate)
Synonyms RBC
Brand Names Tritec®
Therapeutic Category Gastrointestinal Agent, Gastric or Duodenal Ulcer Treatment
Use In combination with clarithromycin for the treatment of active duodenal ulcer associated with *H. pylori* infection; not to be used alone for the treatment of active duodenal ulcer
(Continued)

ranitidine bismuth citrate *(Continued)*

Usual Dosage Adults: Oral: 400 mg twice daily for 4 weeks (28 days) in conjunction with clarithromycin 500 mg 3 times/day for first 2 weeks
Dosage Forms Tablet: 400 mg

ranitidine hydrochloride (ra NI ti deen hye droe KLOR ide)

Brand Names Zantac®; Zantac® 75 [OTC]
Therapeutic Category Histamine H₂ Antagonist
Use Short-term treatment of active duodenal ulcers and benign gastric ulcers; long-term prophylaxis of duodenal ulcer and gastric hypersecretory states; gastroesophageal reflux (GER)
Usual Dosage
Children:
Oral: 1.5-2 mg/kg/dose every 12 hours
I.M., I.V.: 0.75-1.5 mg/kg/dose every 6-8 hours, maximum daily dose: 400 mg
Continuous infusion: 0.1-0.25 mg/kg/hour (preferred for stress ulcer prophylaxis in patients with concurrent maintenance I.V.s or TPNs)
Adults:
Short-term treatment of ulceration: 150 mg/dose twice daily or 300 mg at bedtime
Prophylaxis of recurrent duodenal ulcer: 150 mg at bedtime
Gastric hypersecretory conditions: Oral: 150 mg twice daily, up to 6 g/day
I.M., I.V.: 50 mg/dose every 6-8 hours (dose not to exceed 400 mg/day)
Dosage Forms
Capsule (GELdose™): 150 mg, 300 mg
Granules, effervescent (EFFERdose™): 150 mg
Infusion, preservative free, in NaCl 0.45%: 1 mg/mL (50 mL)
Injection: 25 mg/mL (2 mL, 10 mL, 40 mL)
Syrup (peppermint flavor): 15 mg/mL (473 mL)
Tablet: 75 mg [OTC]; 150 mg, 300 mg
Effervescent (EFFERdose™): 150 mg

Raudixin® *see* rauwolfia serpentina *on this page*
Rauverid® *see* rauwolfia serpentina *on this page*

rauwolfia serpentina (rah WOOL fee a ser pen TEEN ah)

Synonyms whole root rauwolfia
Brand Names Raudixin®; Rauverid®; Wolfina®
Therapeutic Category Rauwolfia Alkaloid
Use Mild essential hypertension; relief of agitated psychotic states
Usual Dosage Adults: Oral: 200-400 mg/day in 2 divided doses
Dosage Forms Tablet: 50 mg, 100 mg

RBC *see* ranitidine bismuth citrate *on previous page*
R & C® **Shampoo [OTC]** *see* pyrethrins *on page 452*
Rea-Lo® **[OTC]** *see* urea *on page 542*
recombinant human deoxyribonuclease *see* dornase alfa *on page 181*
Recombinate® *see* antihemophilic factor (recombinant) *on page 37*
Recombivax HB® *see* hepatitis b vaccine *on page 259*
Redutemp® **[OTC]** *see* acetaminophen *on page 3*
Reese's® **Pinworm Medicine [OTC]** *see* pyrantel pamoate *on page 451*
Refresh® **Ophthalmic Solution [OTC]** *see* artificial tears *on page 42*
Refresh® **Plus Ophthalmic Solution [OTC]** *see* artificial tears *on page 42*
Regitine® *see* phentolamine *on page 411*
Reglan® *see* metoclopramide *on page 344*

Regonol® **Injection** *see* pyridostigmine *on page 452*

Regulace® **[OTC]** *see* docusate and casanthranol *on page 180*

Regular (Concentrated) Iletin® II U-500 *see* insulin preparations *on page 284*

Regular Iletin® I *see* insulin preparations *on page 284*

Regular Insulin *see* insulin preparations *on page 284*

Regular Purified Pork Insulin *see* insulin preparations *on page 284*

Regular Strength Bayer® Enteric 500 Aspirin [OTC] *see* aspirin *on page 44*

Regulax SS® [OTC] *see* docusate *on page 179*

Reguloid® [OTC] *see* psyllium *on page 451*

Relafen® *see* nabumetone *on page 360*

Relefact® TRH Injection *see* protirelin *on page 448*

Relief® Ophthalmic Solution *see* phenylephrine *on page 411*

Remeron® *see* mirtazapine *on page 352*

remifentanil (rem i FEN ta nil)
Brand Names Ultiva®
Therapeutic Category Analgesic, Narcotic
Use Analgesic for use during general anesthesia for continued analgesia
Usual Dosage Adults: I.V. continuous infusion:
During induction: 0.5-1 mcg/kg/minute
During maintenance:
With nitrous oxide (66%): 0.4 mcg/kg/minute (range: 0.1-2 mcg/kg/min)
With isoflurane: 0.25 mcg/kg/minute (range: 0.05-2 mcg/kg/min)
With propofol: 0.25 mcg/kg/minute (range: 0.05-2 mcg/kg/min)
Continuation as an analgesic in immediate postoperative period: 0.1 mcg/kg/minute (range: 0.025-0.2 mcg/kg/min)
Dosage Forms Powder for injection, lyophilized: 1 mg/3 mL vial, 2 mg/5 mL vial, 5 mg/10 mL vial

Renacidin® *see* citric acid bladder mixture *on page 125*

Renese® *see* polythiazide *on page 424*

Reno-M-30® *see* radiological/contrast media (ionic) *on page 457*

Reno-M-60® *see* radiological/contrast media (ionic) *on page 457*

Reno-M-Dip® *see* radiological/contrast media (ionic) *on page 457*

Renoquid® *see* sulfacytine *on page 497*

Renormax® *see* spirapril *on page 491*

Renovue®-65 *see* radiological/contrast media (ionic) *on page 457*

Renovue®-DIP *see* radiological/contrast media (ionic) *on page 457*

Rentamine® *see* chlorpheniramine, ephedrine, phenylephrine, and carbetapentane *on page 115*

ReoPro™ *see* abciximab *on page 2*

Repan® *see* butalbital compound and acetaminophen *on page 78*

Reposans-10® Oral *see* chlordiazepoxide *on page 109*

Repronex® *see* menotropins *on page 328*

Requip™ *see* ropinirole *on page 469*

Resaid® *see* chlorpheniramine and phenylpropanolamine *on page 114*

Rescaps-D® S.R. Capsule *see* caramiphen and phenylpropanolamine *on page 88*

Rescon Liquid [OTC] *see* chlorpheniramine and phenylpropanolamine *on page 114*

Rescriptor™ *see* delavirdine *on page 152*

Resectisol® Irrigation Solution *see* mannitol *on page 321*

reserpine (re SER peen)
Brand Names Serpalan®
Therapeutic Category Rauwolfia Alkaloid
Use Management of mild to moderate hypertension
Usual Dosage Adults: Oral: 0.1-0.5 mg/day in 1-2 doses
Dosage Forms Tablet: 0.1 mg, 0.25 mg

reserpine and chlorothiazide *see* chlorothiazide and reserpine *on page 112*

reserpine and hydrochlorothiazide *see* hydrochlorothiazide and reserpine *on page 265*

Respa-1st® *see* guaifenesin and pseudoephedrine *on page 250*

Respa-DM® *see* guaifenesin and dextromethorphan *on page 248*

Respa-GF® *see* guaifenesin *on page 247*

Respaire®-60 SR *see* guaifenesin and pseudoephedrine *on page 250*

Respaire®-120 SR *see* guaifenesin and pseudoephedrine *on page 250*

Respbid® *see* theophylline *on page 511*

RespiGam® *see* respiratory syncytial virus immune globulin (intravenous) *on this page*

respiratory syncytial virus immune globulin (intravenous)
(RES peer rah tor ee sin SISH al VYE rus i MYUN GLOB yoo lin in tra VEE nus)
Synonyms rsv-igiv
Brand Names RespiGam®
Therapeutic Category Immune Globulin
Use Prevention of serious lower respiratory infection caused by respiratory syncytial virus (RSV) in children <24 months of age with bronchopulmonary dysplasia (BPD) or a history of premature birth (≤35 weeks gestation)
Usual Dosage I.V.: 750 mg/kg/month according to the following infusion schedule: 1.5 mL/kg/hour for 15 minutes, then at 3 mL/kg/hour for the next 15 minutes if the clinical condition does not contraindicate a higher rate, and finally, administer at 6 mL/kg/hour until completion of dose
Dosage Forms Injection: 2500 mg RSV immunoglobulin/50 mL vial

Restoril® *see* temazepam *on page 504*

Retavase® *see* reteplase *on this page*

reteplase (RE ta plase)
Brand Names Retavase®
Therapeutic Category Thrombolytic Agent
Use Management of acute myocardial infarction
Usual Dosage Adults: I.V.: Given as two (2) bolus doses of 10 units each over a period of 2 minutes (second dose given 30 minutes after the initiation of the first dose)
Dosage Forms Powder for injection, lyophilized: 10.8 units [reteplase 18.8 mg]

Retin-A™ Micro Topical *see* tretinoin (topical) *on page 528*

Retin-A™ Topical *see* tretinoin (topical) *on page 528*

retinoic acid *see* tretinoin (topical) *on page 528*

Retrovir® *see* zidovudine *on page 559*

Reversol® Injection *see* edrophonium *on page 190*

Revex® *see* nalmefene *on page 363*

Rēv-Eyes™ *see* dapiprazole *on page 149*

ReVia® *see* naltrexone *on page 363*

Rezulin® *see* troglitazone *on page 537*

R-Gel® **[OTC]** *see* capsaicin *on page 87*

R-Gene® *see* arginine *on page 41*

rgm-csf *see* sargramostim *on page 474*

Rheaban® **[OTC]** *see* attapulgite *on page 48*

Rheomacrodex® *see* dextran *on page 159*

Rheumatrex® *see* methotrexate *on page 338*

Rhinall® **Nasal Solution [OTC]** *see* phenylephrine *on page 411*

Rhinatate® **Tablet** *see* chlorpheniramine, pyrilamine, and phenylephrine *on page 118*

Rhindecon® *see* phenylpropanolamine *on page 413*

Rhinocort® *see* budesonide *on page 75*

Rhinosyn-DMX® **[OTC]** *see* guaifenesin and dextromethorphan *on page 248*

Rhinosyn® **Liquid [OTC]** *see* chlorpheniramine and pseudoephedrine *on page 114*

Rhinosyn-PD® **Liquid [OTC]** *see* chlorpheniramine and pseudoephedrine *on page 114*

Rhinosyn-X® **Liquid [OTC]** *see* guaifenesin, pseudoephedrine, and dextromethorphan *on page 252*

$Rh_o(D)$ immune globulin (ar aych oh (dee) i MYUN GLOB yoo lin)

Brand Names Gamulin® Rh; HypRho®-D; HypRho®-D Mini-Dose; MICRhoGAM™; Mini-Gamulin® Rh; RhoGAM™

Therapeutic Category Immune Globulin

Use Prevent isoimmunization in Rh-negative individuals exposed to Rh-positive blood during delivery of an Rh-positive infant, as a result of an abortion, following amniocentesis or abdominal trauma, or following a transfusion accident; to prevent hemolytic disease of the newborn if there is a subsequent pregnancy with an Rh-positive fetus

Usual Dosage Adults: I.M.:

Obstetrical usage: 1 vial (300 mcg) prevents maternal sensitization if fetal packed red blood cell volume that has entered the circulation is <15 mL; if it is more, administer additional vials. The number of vials = RBC volume of the calculated fetomaternal hemorrhage divided by 15 mL

Postpartum prophylaxis: 300 mcg within 72 hours of delivery

Antepartum prophylaxis: 300 mcg at approximately 26-28 weeks gestation; followed by 300 mcg within 72 hours of delivery if infant is Rh-positive

Following miscarriage, abortion, or termination of ectopic pregnancy at up to 13 weeks of gestation: 50 mcg ideally within 3 hours, but may be administered up to 72 hours after; if pregnancy has been terminated at 13 or more weeks of gestation, administer 300 mcg

Dosage Forms

Injection: Each package contains one single dose 300 mcg of Rh_o (D) immune globulin

Injection, microdose: Each package contains one single dose of microdose, 50 mcg of Rh_o (D) immune globulin

$rh_o(D)$ immune globulin (intravenous-human)

(ar aych oh (dee) i MYUN GLOB yoo lin, eye vee, HYU man)

Synonyms RhoIGIV

Brand Names WinRho SD®

Therapeutic Category Immune Globulin

(Continued)

rh₀(D) immune globulin (intravenous-human) *(Continued)*

Use

Prevention of Rh isoimmunization in nonsensitized Rho(D) antigen-negative women within 7 hours after spontaneous or induced abortion, amniocentesis, chorionic vilus sampling, ruptured tubal pregnancy, abdominal trauma, transplacental hemorrhage, or in the normal course of pregnancy unless the blood type of the fetus or father is known to be Rho(D) antigen-negative

Suppression of Rh isoimmunization in Rho(D) antigen-negative female children and female adults in their childbearing years transfused with Rho(D) antigen-positive RBCs or blood components containing Rho(D) antigen-positive RBCs

Treatment of immune thrombocytopenic purpura (ITP) innon-spenectomized Rho(D) antigen-positive patients

Usual Dosage

Prevention of Rh isoimmunization: I.V.: 1500 units (300 mcg) at 28 weeks gestation or immediately after amniocentesis if <34 weeks gestation or after chorionic vilus sampling; repeat this dose every 12 weeks during the pregnancy, 600 units (120 mcg) at delivery (within 72 hours) and after invasive intrauterine procedures such as abortion, amniocentesis, or any other manipulation if at >34 weeks gestation. **Note:** If the Rh status of the baby is not known at 72 hours, administer Rho(D) immune globulin to the mother at 72 hours after delivery. If >72 hours have elapsed, do not withhold Rho(D) immune globulin, but administer as soon as possible, up to 28 days after delivery.

I.M.: Reconstitute vial with 1.25 mL and administer as above

Transfusion: Administer within 72 hours after exposure for treatment of incompatible blood transfusions or massive fetal hemorrhage as follows:

I.V.: 3000 units (600 mcg) every 8 hours until the total dose is administered (45 units [9 mcg] of Rh+ blood/mL blood; 90 units [18 mcg] Rh+ red cells/mL cells)

I.M.: 6000 units [1200 mcg] every 12 hours until the total dose is administered (60 units [12 mcg] of Rh+ blood/mL blood; 120 units [24 mcg] Rh+ red cells/mL cells)

Treatment of ITP: I.V.: Initial: 25-50 mcg/kg depending on the patient's Hg concentration; maintenance: 25-60 mcg/kg depending on the clinical response

Dosage Forms Injection: 600 units [120 mcg], 1500 units [300 mcg]

RhoGAM™ *see* Rh₀(D) immune globulin *on previous page*

RhoIGIV *see* rh₀(D) immune globulin (intravenous-human) *on previous page*

rhuepo-α *see* epoetin alfa *on page 197*

Rhulicaine® **[OTC]** *see* benzocaine *on page 59*

ribavirin (rye ba VYE rin)

Synonyms rtca; tribavirin

Brand Names Virazole® Aerosol

Therapeutic Category Antiviral Agent

Use Treatment of patients with respiratory syncytial virus (RSV) infections; specially indicated for treatment of severe lower respiratory tract RSV infections in patients with an underlying compromising condition (prematurity, bronchopulmonary dysplasia and other chronic lung conditions, congenital heart disease, immunodeficiency, immunosuppression), and recent transplant recipients; may also be used in other viral infections including influenza A and B and adenovirus

Usual Dosage Infants, Children, and Adults: Aerosol inhalation:

Use with Viratek® small particle aerosol generator (SPAG-2) at a concentration of 20 mg/mL (6 g reconstituted with 300 mL of sterile water without preservatives)

Aerosol only: 12-18 hours/day for 3 days, up to 7 days in length

Dosage Forms Powder for aerosol: 6 g (100 mL)

riboflavin (RYE boe flay vin)

Synonyms lactoflavin; vitamin b$_2$; vitamin g
Brand Names Riobin®
Therapeutic Category Vitamin, Water Soluble
Use Prevent riboflavin deficiency and treat ariboflavinosis
Usual Dosage Oral:
  Riboflavin deficiency:
    Children: 2.5-10 mg/day in divided doses
    Adults: 5-30 mg/day in divided doses
    Required daily allowance: Adults:
    Male: 1.4-4.8 mg
    Female: 1.2-1.3 mg
Dosage Forms Tablet: 25 mg, 50 mg, 100 mg

Rid-A-Pain® [OTC] *see* benzocaine *on page 59*

Ridaura® *see* auranofin *on page 48*

Ridenol® [OTC] *see* acetaminophen *on page 3*

RID® Shampoo [OTC] *see* pyrethrins *on page 452*

rifabutin (rif a BYOO tin)

Synonyms ansamycin
Brand Names Mycobutin®
Therapeutic Category Antibiotic, Miscellaneous
Use Prevention of disseminated *Mycobacterium avium* complex (MAC) in patients with advanced HIV infection; utilized in multiple drug regimens for treatment of MAC
Usual Dosage Oral:
  Children: Efficacy and safety of rifabutin have not been established in children; a limited number of HIV-positive children with MAC (n=22) have been given rifabutin for MAC prophylaxis; doses of 5 mg/kg/day have been useful
  Adults: 300 mg once daily; for patients who experience gastrointestinal upset, rifabutin can be administered 150 mg twice daily with food
Dosage Forms Capsule: 150 mg

Rifadin® Injection *see* rifampin *on this page*

Rifadin® Oral *see* rifampin *on this page*

Rifamate® *see* rifampin and isoniazid *on next page*

rifampicin *see* rifampin *on this page*

rifampin (RIF am pin)

Synonyms rifampicin
Brand Names Rifadin® Injection; Rifadin® Oral; Rimactane® Oral
Therapeutic Category Antibiotic, Miscellaneous
Use Used in combination with other antitubercular drugs for the treatment of active tuberculosis; eliminate meningococci from asymptomatic carriers; prophylaxis in contacts of patients with *Haemophilus influenzae* type B infection; used in combination with other anti-infectives in the treatment of staphylococcal infections
Usual Dosage I.V. infusion dose is the same as for the oral route
  Tuberculosis: Oral:
    Children: 10-20 mg/kg/day in divided doses every 12-24 hours
    Adults: 10 mg/kg/day; maximum: 600 mg/day
  American Thoracic Society and CDC currently recommend twice weekly therapy as part of a short-course regimen which follows 1-2 months of daily treatment of uncomplicated pulmonary tuberculosis in the compliant patient
    Children: 10-20 mg/kg/dose (up to 600 mg) twice weekly under supervision to ensure compliance
    Adults: 10 mg/kg (up to 600 mg) twice weekly
(Continued)

rifampin *(Continued)*

H. influenza prophylaxis:
Infants and Children: 20 mg/kg/day every 24 hours for 4 days
Adults: 600 mg every 24 hours for 4 days
Meningococcal prophylaxis:
<1 month: 10 mg/kg/day in divided doses every 12 hours
Infants and Children: 20 mg/kg/day in divided doses every 12 hours for 2 days
Adults: 600 mg every 12 hours for 2 days
Nasal carriers of *Staphylococcus aureus*: Adults: 600 mg/day for 5-10 days in combination with other antibiotics
Dosage Forms
Capsule: 150 mg, 300 mg
Powder for injection: 600 mg (contains a sulfite)

rifampin and isoniazid (RIF am pin & eye soe NYE a zid)

Brand Names Rifamate®
Therapeutic Category Antibiotic, Miscellaneous
Use Management of active tuberculosis; see individual monographs for additional information
Usual Dosage Oral: 2 capsules/day
Dosage Forms Capsule: Rifampin 300 mg and isoniazid 150 mg

rifampin, isoniazid, and pyrazinamide

(RIF am pin , eye soe NYE a zid, & peer a ZIN a mide)
Brand Names Rifater®
Therapeutic Category Antibiotic, Miscellaneous
Use Management of active tuberculosis
Usual Dosage Adults: Oral: Patients weighing:
≤44 kg: 4 tablets
45-54 kg: 5 tablets
≥55 kg: 6 tablets
Doses should be administered in a single daily dose
Dosage Forms Tablet: Rifampin 120 mg, isoniazid 50 mg, and pyrazinamide 300 mg

Rifater® *see* rifampin, isoniazid, and pyrazinamide *on this page*

rIFN-A *see* interferon alfa-2a *on page 285*

rig *see* rabies immune globulin (human) *on page 457*

Rilutek® *see* riluzole *on this page*

riluzole (RIL yoo zole)

Synonyms 2-amino-6-trifluoromethoxy-benzothiazole; RP54274
Brand Names Rilutek®
Therapeutic Category Miscellaneous Product
Use Treatment of amyotrophic lateral sclerosis (ALS), also known as Lou Gehrig's disease
Usual Dosage Adults: Oral: 50 mg twice daily
Dosage Forms Tablet: 50 mg

Rimactane® Oral *see* rifampin *on previous page*

rimantadine (ri MAN ta deen)

Synonyms rimantadine hydrochloride
Brand Names Flumadine®
Therapeutic Category Antiviral Agent
Use Prophylaxis (adults and children) and treatment (adults) of influenza A viral infection

Usual Dosage Oral:
Prophylaxis:
Children (<10 years of age): 5 mg/kg administered once daily
Children (>10 years of age) and Adults: 100 mg twice daily
Treatment: Adults: 100 mg twice daily
In patients with severe hepatic dysfunction or renal function, and in geriatric nursing home patients, the dosage should be reduced to 100 mg/day
Dosage Forms
Syrup, as hydrochloride: 50 mg/5 mL (60 mL, 240 mL, 480 mL)
Tablet, as hydrochloride: 100 mg

rimantadine hydrochloride *see* rimantadine *on previous page*

rimexolone (ri MEKS oh lone)
Brand Names Vexol® Ophthalmic Suspension
Therapeutic Category Adrenal Corticosteroid
Use Treatment of inflammation after ocular surgery and the treatment of anterior uveitis
Usual Dosage Children >2 years and Adults: Ophthalmic: Instill 1-2 drops into conjunctival sac every hour during day, every 2 hours at night until favorable response is obtained, then use 1 drop every 4 hours; for mild to moderate inflammation, instill 1-2 drops into conjunctival sac 2-4 times/day
Dosage Forms Suspension, ophthalmic: 1% (5 mL, 10 mL)

Rimso®-50 *see* dimethyl sulfoxide *on page 172*
Riobin® *see* riboflavin *on page 465*
Riopan® [OTC] *see* magaldrate *on page 317*
Riopan Plus® [OTC] *see* magaldrate and simethicone *on page 317*
Risperdal® *see* risperidone *on this page*

risperidone (ris PER i done)
Brand Names Risperdal®
Therapeutic Category Antipsychotic Agent, Benzisoxazole
Use Management of psychotic disorders (eg, schizophrenia)
Usual Dosage Oral: Recommended starting dose: 1 mg twice daily; slowly increase to the optimum range of 4-8 mg/day; daily dosages >10 mg does not appear to confer any additional benefit, and the incidence of extrapyramidal reactions is higher than with lower doses
Dosage Forms
Solution, oral: 1 mg/mL
Tablet: 1 mg, 2 mg, 3 mg, 4 mg

Ritalin® *see* methylphenidate *on page 342*
Ritalin-SR® *see* methylphenidate *on page 342*

ritodrine (RI toe dreen)
Synonyms ritodrine hydrochloride
Brand Names Yutopar®
Therapeutic Category Adrenergic Agonist Agent
Use Inhibit uterine contraction in preterm labor
Usual Dosage Adults:
Oral: Start 30 minutes before stopping I.V. infusion; 10 mg every 2 hours for 24 hours, then 10-20 mg every 4-6 hours up to 120 mg/day. Continue treatment as long as it is desirable to prolong pregnancy.
I.V.: 50-100 mcg/minute; increase by 50 mcg/minute every 10 minutes; continue for 12 hours after contractions have stopped
(Continued)

ritodrine *(Continued)*
Dosage Forms
Infusion, in D_5W: 0.3 mL (500 mL)
Injection, as hydrochloride: 10 mg/mL (5 mL); 15 mg/mL (10 mL)

ritodrine hydrochloride *see* ritodrine *on previous page*

ritonavir (rye TON a veer)
Brand Names Norvir®
Therapeutic Category Antiviral Agent
Use Treatment of HIV, especially advanced cases; usually is used as part of triple or double therapy with other nucleoside and protease inhibitors
Usual Dosage Adults: Oral: 600 mg twice daily with meals
Dosage Forms
Capsule: 100 mg
Solution: 80 mg/mL (240 mL)

rLFN-α2 *see* interferon alfa-2b *on page 286*

rlfn-b *see* interferon beta-1b *on page 286*

RMS® Rectal *see* morphine sulfate *on page 356*

Robafen® AC *see* guaifenesin and codeine *on page 247*

Robafen® CF [OTC] *see* guaifenesin, phenylpropanolamine, and dextromethorphan *on page 251*

Robafen DM® [OTC] *see* guaifenesin and dextromethorphan *on page 248*

Robaxin® *see* methocarbamol *on page 337*

Robaxisal® *see* methocarbamol and aspirin *on page 337*

Robicillin® VK *see* penicillin v potassium *on page 402*

Robinul® *see* glycopyrrolate *on page 244*

Robinul® Forte *see* glycopyrrolate *on page 244*

Robitussin® [OTC] *see* guaifenesin *on page 247*

Robitussin® A-C *see* guaifenesin and codeine *on page 247*

Robitussin-CF® [OTC] *see* guaifenesin, phenylpropanolamine, and dextromethorphan *on page 251*

Robitussin® Cough Calmers [OTC] *see* dextromethorphan *on page 160*

Robitussin®-DAC *see* guaifenesin, pseudoephedrine, and codeine *on page 251*

Robitussin®-DM [OTC] *see* guaifenesin and dextromethorphan *on page 248*

Robitussin-PE® [OTC] *see* guaifenesin and pseudoephedrine *on page 250*

Robitussin® Pediatric [OTC] *see* dextromethorphan *on page 160*

Robitussin® Severe Congestion Liqui-Gels [OTC] *see* guaifenesin and pseudoephedrine *on page 250*

Rocaltrol® *see* calcitriol *on page 81*

Rocephin® *see* ceftriaxone *on page 101*

rocky mountain spotted fever vaccine
(ROK ee MOUN ten SPOT ted FEE ver vak SEEN)
Therapeutic Category Vaccine, Live Bacteria
Dosage Forms Injection: 3 mL

rocuronium (roe kyoor OH nee um)
Synonyms rocuronium bromide
Brand Names Zemuron®

Therapeutic Category Skeletal Muscle Relaxant

Use Produces skeletal muscle relaxation during surgery after induction of general anesthesia, increases pulmonary compliance during assisted mechanical respiration, facilitates endotracheal intubation

Usual Dosage

Children:

Initial: 0.6 mg/kg under halothane anesthesia produce excellent to good intubating conditions within 1 minute and will provide a median time of 41 minutes of clinical relaxation in children 3 months to 1 year of age, and 27 minutes in children 1-12 years

Maintenance: 0.075-0.125 mg/kg administered upon return of T_1 to 25% of control provides clinical relaxation for 7-10 minutes

Adults:

Tracheal intubation: I.V.:

Initial: 0.6 mg/kg is expected to provide approximately 31 minutes of clinical relaxation under opioid/nitrous oxide/oxygen anesthesia with neuromuscular block sufficient for intubation attained in 1-2 minutes; lower doses (0.45 mg/kg) may be used to provide 22 minutes of clinical relaxation with median time to neuromuscular block of 1-3 minutes; maximum blockade is achieved in <4 minutes

Maximum: 0.9-1.2 mg/kg may be administered during surgery under opioid/nitrous oxide/oxygen anesthesia without adverse cardiovascular effects and is expected to provide 58-67 minutes of clinical relaxation; neuromuscular blockade sufficient for intubation is achieved in <2 minutes with maximum blockade in <3 minutes

Maintenance: 0.1, 0.15, and 0.2 mg/kg administered at 25% recovery of control T_1 (defined as 3 twitches of train-of-four) provides a median of 12, 17, and 24 minutes of clinical duration under anesthesia

Rapid sequence intubation: 0.6-1.2 mg/kg in appropriately premedicated and anesthetized patients with excellent or good intubating conditions within 2 minutes

Continuous infusion: Initial: 0.01-0.012 mg/kg/minute only after early evidence of spontaneous recovery of neuromuscular function is evident

Dosage Forms Injection, as bromide: 10 mg/mL

rocuronium bromide *see rocuronium on previous page*

Roferon-A® *see interferon alfa-2a on page 285*

Rogaine® **for Men [OTC]** *see minoxidil on page 352*

Rogaine® **for Women [OTC]** *see minoxidil on page 352*

Rolaids® **[OTC]** *see dihydroxyaluminum sodium carbonate on page 170*

Rolaids® **Calcium Rich [OTC]** *see calcium carbonate on page 82*

Rolatuss® **Plain Liquid** *see chlorpheniramine and phenylephrine on page 113*

Romazicon™ *see flumazenil on page 226*

Rondamine-DM® **Drops** *see carbinoxamine, pseudoephedrine, and dextromethorphan on page 91*

Rondec®**-DM** *see carbinoxamine, pseudoephedrine, and dextromethorphan on page 91*

Rondec® **Drops** *see carbinoxamine and pseudoephedrine on page 91*

Rondec® **Filmtab**® *see carbinoxamine and pseudoephedrine on page 91*

Rondec® **Syrup** *see carbinoxamine and pseudoephedrine on page 91*

Rondec-TR® *see carbinoxamine and pseudoephedrine on page 91*

ropinirole (roe pin' i role)

Synonyms ropinirole hydrochloride

Brand Names Requip™

Therapeutic Category Anti-Parkinson's Agent

(Continued)

ropinirole *(Continued)*

Use Treatment of idiopathic Parkinson's disease; in patients with early Parkinson's disease who were not receiving concomitant levodopa therapy as well as in patients with advanced disease on concomitant levodopa

Usual Dosage Adults: Oral: The dosage should be increased to achieve a maximum therapeutic effect, balanced against the principal side effects of nausea, dizziness, somnolence and dyskinesia

Recommended starting dose is 0.25 mg three times/day; based on individual patient response, the dosage should be titrated with weekly increments as described below:
Week 1 = 0.25 mg 3 times/day Total daily dose= 0.75 mg
Week 2 = 0.5 mg 3 times/day Total daily dose= 1.5 mg
Week 3 = 0.75 mg 3 times/day Total daily dose= 2.25 mg
Week 4 = 1 mg 3 times/day Total daily dose= 3 mg

After week 4, if necessary, daily dosage may be increased by 1.5 mg per day on a weekly basis up to a dose of 9 mg/day, and then by up to 3 mg/day weekly to a total of 24 mg/day

Dosage Forms Tablet: 0.25 mg, 0.5 mg, 1 mg, 2 mg, 5 mg

ropinirole hydrochloride *see* ropinirole *on previous page*

ropivacaine (roe PIV a kane)

Synonyms ropivacaine hydrochloride
Brand Names Naropin™
Therapeutic Category Local Anesthetic
Use Production of local or regional anesthesia for surgery, postoperative pain management and obstetrical procedures by infiltration anesthesia and nerve block anesthesia
Usual Dosage Administer the smallest dose and concentration required to produce the desired result
Dosage Forms
Infusion, as hydrochloride: 2 mg/mL (100 mL, 200 mL)
Injection, as hydrochloride (single dose): 2 mg/mL (20 mL); 5 mg/mL (30 mL); 7.5 mg/mL (10 mL, 20 mL); 10 mg/mL (10 mL, 20 mL)

ropivacaine hydrochloride *see* ropivacaine *on this page*

Rowasa® Rectal *see* mesalamine *on page 331*

Roxanol™ Oral *see* morphine sulfate *on page 356*

Roxanol Rescudose® *see* morphine sulfate *on page 356*

Roxanol SR™ Oral *see* morphine sulfate *on page 356*

Roxicet® 5/500 *see* oxycodone and acetaminophen *on page 390*

Roxicodone™ *see* oxycodone *on page 389*

Roxilox® *see* oxycodone and acetaminophen *on page 390*

Roxiprin® *see* oxycodone and aspirin *on page 390*

RP54274 *see* riluzole *on page 466*

rsv-igiv *see* respiratory syncytial virus immune globulin (intravenous) *on page 462*

R-Tannamine® Tablet *see* chlorpheniramine, pyrilamine, and phenylephrine *on page 118*

R-Tannate® Tablet *see* chlorpheniramine, pyrilamine, and phenylephrine *on page 118*

rtca *see* ribavirin *on page 464*

rubella and measles vaccines, combined *see* measles and rubella vaccines, combined *on page 323*

rubella and mumps vaccines, combined
(rue BEL a & mumpz vak SEENS, kom BINED)
Brand Names Biavax® II
Therapeutic Category Vaccine, Live Virus
Use Promote active immunity to rubella and mumps by inducing production of antibodies
Usual Dosage Children >12 months and Adults: 1 vial in outer aspect of the upper arm
Dosage Forms Injection (mixture of 2 viruses):
  1. Wistar RA 27/3 strain of rubella virus
  2. Jeryl Lynn (B level) mumps strain grown cell cultures of chick embryo

rubella virus vaccine, live (rue BEL a VYE rus vak SEEN, live)
Synonyms german measles vaccine
Brand Names Meruvax® II
Therapeutic Category Vaccine, Live Virus
Use Provide vaccine-induced immunity to rubella
Usual Dosage S.C.: 1000 $TCID_{50}$ of rubella
Dosage Forms Injection, single dose: 1000 $TCID_{50}$ (Wistar RA 27/3 Strain)

rubeola vaccine *see* measles virus vaccine, live *on page 323*

Rubex® *see* doxorubicin *on page 183*

rubidomycin hydrochloride *see* daunorubicin hydrochloride *on page 150*

Rum-K® *see* potassium chloride *on page 427*

Ru-Tuss® *see* chlorpheniramine, phenylephrine, phenylpropanolamine, and belladonna alkaloids *on page 116*

Ru-Tuss® DE *see* guaifenesin and pseudoephedrine *on page 250*

Ru-Tuss® Expectorant [OTC] *see* guaifenesin, pseudoephedrine, and dextromethorphan *on page 252*

Ru-Tuss® Liquid *see* chlorpheniramine and phenylephrine *on page 113*

Ru-Vert-M® *see* meclizine *on page 324*

Rymed® *see* guaifenesin and pseudoephedrine *on page 250*

Rymed-TR® *see* guaifenesin and phenylpropanolamine *on page 249*

Ryna-C® Liquid *see* chlorpheniramine, pseudoephedrine, and codeine *on page 118*

Ryna-CX® *see* guaifenesin, pseudoephedrine, and codeine *on page 251*

Ryna® Liquid [OTC] *see* chlorpheniramine and pseudoephedrine *on page 114*

Rynatan® Pediatric Suspension *see* chlorpheniramine, pyrilamine, and phenylephrine *on page 118*

Rynatan® Tablet *see* chlorpheniramine, pyrilamine, and phenylephrine *on page 118*

Rynatuss® Pediatric Suspension *see* chlorpheniramine, ephedrine, phenylephrine, and carbetapentane *on page 115*

Rythmol® *see* propafenone *on page 443*

Sabin vaccine *see* poliovirus vaccine, live, trivalent, oral *on page 423*

Safe Tussin® 30 [OTC] *see* guaifenesin and dextromethorphan *on page 248*

Sal-Acid® Plaster [OTC] *see* salicylic acid *on next page*

Salactic® Film [OTC] *see* salicylic acid *on next page*

Salagen® Oral *see* pilocarpine *on page 417*

salbutamol *see* albuterol *on page 14*

Saleto-200® [OTC] *see* ibuprofen *on page 278*

Saleto-400® *see* ibuprofen *on page 278*

Saleto-600® *see* ibuprofen *on page 278*

Saleto-800® *see* ibuprofen *on page 278*

Salflex® *see* salsalate *on next page*

Salgesic® *see* salsalate *on next page*

salicylazosulfapyridine *see* sulfasalazine *on page 498*

salicylic acid (sal i SIL ik AS id)

Brand Names Clear Away® Disc [OTC]; Compound W® [OTC]; Dr Scholl's® Disk [OTC]; Dr Scholl's® Wart Remover [OTC]; DuoFilm® [OTC]; DuoPlant® Gel [OTC]; Freezone® Solution [OTC]; Gordofilm® Liquid; Mediplast® Plaster [OTC]; Mosco® Liquid [OTC]; Occlusal-HP Liquid; Off-Ezy® Wart Remover [OTC]; Panscol® [OTC]; Psor-a-set® Soap [OTC]; P&S® Shampoo [OTC]; Sal-Acid® Plaster [OTC]; Salactic® Film [OTC]; Sal-Plant® Gel [OTC]; Trans-Ver-Sal® AdultPatch [OTC]; Trans-Ver-Sal® PediaPatch [OTC]; Trans-Ver-Sal® PlantarPatch [OTC]; Wart-Off® [OTC]

Therapeutic Category Keratolytic Agent

Use Topically for its keratolytic effect in controlling seborrheic dermatitis or psoriasis of body and scalp, dandruff, and other scaling dermatoses; to remove warts, corns, calluses; also used in the treatment of acne

Usual Dosage

Shampoo: Apply to scalp and allow to remain for a few minutes, then rinse, initially use every day or every other day; 2 treatments/week are usually sufficient to maintain control

Topical: Apply to affected area and place under occlusion at night; hydrate skin for at least 5 minutes before use

Dosage Forms

Cream: 2% (30 g)

Disk: 40%

Gel: 5% (60 g); 6% (30 g); 17% (7.5 g)

Liquid: 13.6% (9.3 mL); 17% (9.3 mL, 13.5 mL, 15 mL); 16.7% (15 mL)

Lotion: 3% (120 mL)

Ointment: 3% (90 g)

Patch, transdermal: 15% (20 mm); 40% (20 mm)

Plaster: 40%

Soap: 2% (97.5 g)

Strip: 40%

salicylic acid and benzoic acid *see* benzoic acid and salicylic acid *on page 61*

salicylic acid and lactic acid (sal i SIL ik AS id & LAK tik AS id)

Synonyms lactic acid and salicylic acid

Brand Names Duofilm® Solution

Therapeutic Category Keratolytic Agent

Use Treatment of benign epithelial tumors such as warts

Usual Dosage Topical: Apply a thin layer directly to wart once daily (may be useful to apply at bedtime and wash off in morning)

Dosage Forms Solution, topical: Salicylic acid 16.7% and lactic acid 16.7% in flexible collodion (15 mL)

salicylic acid and podophyllin *see* podophyllin and salicylic acid *on page 422*

salicylic acid and propylene glycol

(sal i SIL ik AS id & PROE pi leen GLYE cole)

Synonyms propylene glycol and salicylic acid

Brand Names Keralyt® Gel

Therapeutic Category Keratolytic Agent

Use Removal of excessive keratin in hyperkeratotic skin disorders, including various ichthyosis, keratosis palmaris and plantaris and psoriasis; may be used to remove excessive keratin in dorsal and plantar hyperkeratotic lesions

Usual Dosage Topical: Apply to area at night after soaking region for at least 5 minutes to hydrate area, and place under occlusion; medication is washed off in morning

Dosage Forms Gel, topical: Salicylic acid 6% and propylene glycol 60% in ethyl alcohol 19.4% with hydroxypropyl methylcellulose and water (30 g)

salicylic acid and sulfur *see* sulfur and salicylic acid *on page 499*

SalineX® [OTC] *see* sodium chloride *on page 483*

Salivart® Solution [OTC] *see* saliva substitute *on this page*

saliva substitute (sa LYE va SUB stee tute)

Brand Names Entertainer's Secret® Spray [OTC]; Moi-Stir® Solution [OTC]; Moi-Stir® Swabsticks [OTC]; Mouthkote® Solution [OTC]; Optimoist® Solution [OTC]; Salivart® Solution [OTC]; Salix® Lozenge [OTC]

Therapeutic Category Gastrointestinal Agent, Miscellaneous

Use Relief of dry mouth and throat in xerostomia

Usual Dosage Use as needed

Dosage Forms
Lozenge: 100s
Solution: 60 mL, 75 mL, 120 mL, 180 mL, 240 mL
Swabstix: 3s

Salix® Lozenge [OTC] *see* saliva substitute *on this page*

Salk vaccine *see* poliovirus vaccine, inactivated *on page 422*

salmeterol (sal ME te role)

Synonyms salmeterol xinafoate

Brand Names Serevent®

Therapeutic Category Adrenergic Agonist Agent

Use Maintenance treatment of asthma; prevention of bronchospasm in patients >12 years of age with reversible obstructive airway disease, including patients with symptoms of nocturnal asthma who require regular treatment with inhaled, short-acting beta$_2$ agonists; prevention of exercise-induced bronchospasm

Usual Dosage
Inhalation: 42 mcg (2 puffs) twice daily (12 hours apart) for maintenance and prevention of symptoms of asthma
Prevention of exercise-induced asthma: 42 mcg (2 puffs) 30-60 minutes prior to exercise; additional doses should not be used for 12 hours

Dosage Forms Aerosol, oral, as xinafoate: 21 mcg/spray [60 inhalations] (6.5 g), [120 inhalations] (13 g)

salmeterol xinafoate *see* salmeterol *on this page*

Salmonine® Injection *see* calcitonin *on page 81*

Sal-Plant® Gel [OTC] *see* salicylic acid *on previous page*

salsalate (SAL sa late)

Synonyms disalicylic acid

Brand Names Argesic®-SA; Artha-G®; Disalcid®; Marthritic®; Mono-Gesic®; Salflex®; Salgesic®; Salsitab®

Therapeutic Category Analgesic, Non-narcotic; Antipyretic; Nonsteroidal Anti-Inflammatory Agent (NSAID)

Use Treatment of minor pain or fever; rheumatoid arthritis, osteoarthritis, and related inflammatory conditions

Usual Dosage Adults: Oral: 1 g 2-4 times/day

(Continued)

salsalate *(Continued)*
Dosage Forms
Capsule: 500 mg
Tablet: 500 mg, 750 mg

Salsitab® *see* salsalate *on previous page*

salt *see* sodium chloride *on page 483*

Saluron® *see* hydroflumethiazide *on page 271*

Salutensin® *see* hydroflumethiazide and reserpine *on page 271*

Sandimmune® **Injection** *see* cyclosporine *on page 145*

Sandimmune® **Oral** *see* cyclosporine *on page 145*

Sandoglobulin® *see* immune globulin, intravenous *on page 281*

Sandostatin® *see* octreotide acetate *on page 382*

Sani-Supp® **Suppository [OTC]** *see* glycerin *on page 243*

Sanorex® *see* mazindol *on page 323*

Sansert® *see* methysergide *on page 344*

Santyl® *see* collagenase *on page 136*

saquinavir (sa KWIN a veer)
Synonyms saquinavir mesylate
Brand Names Invirase®
Therapeutic Category Antiviral Agent
Use Treatment of advanced HIV infection, used in combination with older nucleoside analog medications
Usual Dosage Adults: Oral: 200 mg 3 times/day within 2 hours after a full meal
Dosage Forms Capsule, as mesylate: 200 mg

saquinavir mesylate *see* saquinavir *on this page*

sargramostim (sar GRAM oh stim)
Synonyms gm-csf; granulocyte-macrophage colony stimulating factor; rgm-csf
Brand Names Leukine™
Therapeutic Category Colony Stimulating Factor
Use Myeloid reconstitution after autologous bone marrow transplantation; to accelerate myeloid recovery in patients with non-Hodgkin's lymphoma, Hodgkin's lymphoma, and acute lymphoblastic leukemia undergoing autologous BMT; following induction chemotherapy in patients with acute myelogenous leukemia to shorten time to neutrophil recovery
Usual Dosage
Children and Adults (may also administer S.C.):
Bone marrow transplant: I.V.: 250 mcg/m^2/day over at least 2 hours to begin 2-4 hours after the marrow infusion on day 0 of autologous bone marrow transplant or not <24 hours after chemotherapy or 12 hours after last dose of radiotherapy. If significant adverse effects or "first dose" reaction is seen at this dose, discontinue the drug until toxicity resolves, then restart at a reduced dose of 125 mcg/m^2/day
Cancer chemotherapy recovery: I.V.: 3-15 mcg/kg/day over at least 2 hours for 14-21 days; maximum daily dose is 15 mcg/kg/day due to dose-related adverse effects
Discontinue therapy if the ANC count is >20,000/mm^3.

Excessive blood counts return to normal or baseline levels within 3-7 days following cessation of therapy.

Length of therapy: Bone marrow transplant patients: GM-CSF should be administered daily for up to 30 days or until the ANC has reached 1000/mm^3 for 3 consecutive days following the expected chemotherapy-induced neutrophil-nadir.

Dosage Forms Injection: 250 mcg, 500 mcg

Sarna [OTC] *see* camphor, menthol, and phenol *on page 87*

SAStid® Plain Therapeutic Shampoo and Acne Wash [OTC] *see* sulfur and salicylic acid *on page 499*

Scabene® *see* lindane *on page 309*

Scalpicin® *see* hydrocortisone *on page 268*

Scleromate™ *see* morrhuate sodium *on page 357*

Scopace® Tablet *see* scopolamine *on this page*

scopolamine (skoe POL a meen)

Synonyms hyoscine
Brand Names Isopto® Hyoscine Ophthalmic; Scopace® Tablet; Transderm Scop® Patch
Therapeutic Category Anticholinergic Agent
Use Preoperative medication to produce amnesia and decrease salivary and respiratory secretions; to produce cycloplegia and mydriasis; treatment of iridocyclitis; prevention of motion sickness
Usual Dosage
Preoperatively:
Children: I.M., S.C.: 6 mcg/kg/dose (maximum: 0.3 mg/dose) or 0.2 mg/m² may be repeated every 6-8 hours **or** alternatively:
4-7 months: 0.1 mg
7 months to 3 years: 0.15 mg
3-8 years: 0.2 mg
8-12 years: 0.3 mg
Adults: I.M., I.V., S.C.: 0.3-0.65 mg; may be repeated every 4-6 hours
Motion sickness: Transdermal: Children >12 years and Adults: Apply 1 disc behind the ear at least 4 hours prior to exposure and every 3 days as needed
Ophthalmic:
Refraction:
Children: Instill 1 drop of 0.25% to eye(s) twice daily for 2 days before procedure
Adults: Instill 1-2 drops of 0.25% to eye(s) 1 hour before procedure
Iridocyclitis:
Children: Instill 1 drop of 0.25% to eye(s) up to 3 times/day
Adults: Instill 1-2 drops of 0.25% to eye(s) up to 4 times/day
Dosage Forms
Disc, transdermal: 1.5 mg/disc (4's)
Injection, as hydrobromide: 0.3 mg/mL (1 mL); 0.4 mg/mL (0.5 mL, 1 mL); 0.86 mg/mL (0.5 mL); 1 mg/mL (1 mL)
Solution, ophthalmic, as hydrobromide: 0.25% (5 mL, 15 mL)
Tablet: 0.4 mg

scopolamine and phenylephrine *see* phenylephrine and scopolamine *on page 412*

Scot-Tussin® [OTC] *see* guaifenesin *on page 247*

Scot-Tussin DM® Cough Chasers [OTC] *see* dextromethorphan *on page 160*

Scot-Tussin® Senior Clear [OTC] *see* guaifenesin and dextromethorphan *on page 248*

SeaMist® [OTC] *see* sodium chloride *on page 483*

Sebizon® Topical Lotion *see* sulfacetamide sodium *on page 496*

secobarbital (see koe BAR bi tal)

Synonyms quinalbarbitone sodium; secobarbital sodium
Brand Names Seconal™ Injection
Therapeutic Category Barbiturate
(Continued)

secobarbital *(Continued)*

Controlled Substance C-II
Use Short-term treatment of insomnia and as preanesthetic agent
Usual Dosage Hypnotic:
  Children: I.M.: 3-5 mg/kg/dose; maximum: 100 mg/dose
  Adults:
    I.M.: 100-200 mg/dose
    I.V.: 50-250 mg/dose
Dosage Forms Injection, as sodium: 50 mg/mL (2 mL)

secobarbital and amobarbital *see* amobarbital and secobarbital *on page 29*

secobarbital sodium *see* secobarbital *on previous page*

Seconal™ Injection *see* secobarbital *on previous page*

Secran® *see* vitamin, multiple (prenatal) *on page 554*

secretin (SEE kre tin)

Brand Names Secretin-Ferring Powder
Therapeutic Category Diagnostic Agent
Use Diagnosis of Zollinger-Ellison syndrome, chronic pancreatic dysfunction, and some hepatobiliary diseases such as obstructive jaundice resulting from cancer or stones in the biliary tract
Usual Dosage I.V.:
  Pancreatic function: 1 CU/kg slow I.V. injection over 1 minute
  Zollinger-Ellison: 2 CU/kg slow I.V. injection over 1 minute
Dosage Forms Powder for injection: 75 units (10 mL)

Secretin-Ferring Powder *see* secretin *on this page*

Sectral® *see* acebutolol *on page 2*

Sedapap-10® *see* butalbital compound and acetaminophen *on page 78*

Seldane® *see* terfenadine *on page 506*

Seldane-D® *see* terfenadine and pseudoephedrine *on page 506*

selegiline (seh LEDGE ah leen)

Synonyms deprenyl; l-deprenyl; selegiline hydrochloride
Brand Names Eldepryl®
Therapeutic Category Anti-Parkinson's Agent; Dopaminergic Agent (Antiparkinson's)
Use Adjunct in the management of Parkinsonian patients in which levodopa/carbidopa therapy is deteriorating
  Unlabeled uses: Early Parkinson's disease, Alzheimer's disease
Usual Dosage Adults: Oral: 5 mg twice daily
Dosage Forms
  Capsule, as hydrochloride (Eldepryl®): 5 mg
  Tablet: 5 mg

selegiline hydrochloride *see* selegiline *on this page*

selenium sulfide (se LEE nee um SUL fide)

Brand Names Exsel®; Head & Shoulders® Intensive Treatment [OTC]; Selsun®; Selsun Blue® [OTC]; Selsun Gold® for Women [OTC]
Therapeutic Category Antiseborrheic Agent, Topical
Use Treat itching and flaking of the scalp associated with dandruff; to control scalp seborrheic dermatitis; treatment of tinea versicolor

Usual Dosage Topical:

Dandruff, seborrhea: Massage 5-10 mL into wet scalp, leave on scalp 2-3 minutes, rinse thoroughly and repeat application; shampoo twice weekly for 2 weeks initially, then use once every 1-4 weeks as indicated depending upon control

Tinea versicolor: Apply the 2.5% lotion to affected area and lather with small amounts of water; leave on skin for 10 minutes, then rinse thoroughly; apply every day for 7 days

Dosage Forms Shampoo: 1% (120 mL, 210 mL, 240 mL, 330 mL); 2.5% (120 mL)

Sele-Pak® *see* trace metals *on page 525*

Selepen® *see* trace metals *on page 525*

Selsun® *see* selenium sulfide *on previous page*

Selsun Blue® [OTC] *see* selenium sulfide *on previous page*

Selsun Gold® for Women [OTC] *see* selenium sulfide *on previous page*

Semicid® [OTC] *see* nonoxynol 9 *on page 377*

Semprex-D® *see* acrivastine and pseudoephedrine *on page 9*

Senexon® [OTC] *see* senna *on this page*

senna (SEN na)

Brand Names Black Draught® [OTC]; Senexon® [OTC]; Senna-Gen® [OTC]; Senokot® [OTC]; Senolax® [OTC]; X-Prep® Liquid [OTC]

Therapeutic Category Laxative

Use Short-term treatment of constipation; evacuate the colon for bowel or rectal examinations

Usual Dosage

Children:

Oral:

>6 years: 10-20 mg/kg/dose at bedtime; maximum daily dose: 872 mg

6-12 years, >27 kg: 1 tablet at bedtime, up to 4 tablets/day **or** ½ teaspoonful of granules (326 mg/tsp) at bedtime (up to 2 teaspoonfuls/day)

Liquid:

2-5 years: 5-10 mL at bedtime

6-15 years: 10-15 mL at bedtime

Suppository: ½ at bedtime

Syrup:

1 month to 1 year: 1.25-2.5 mL at bedtime up to 5 mL/day

1-5 years: 2.5-5 mL at bedtime up to 10 mL/day

5-10 years: 5-10 mL at bedtime up to 20 mL/day

Adults:

Granules (326 mg/teaspoon): 1 teaspoonful at bedtime, not to exceed 2 teaspoonfuls twice daily

Liquid: 15-30 mL with meals and at bedtime

Suppository: 1 at bedtime, may repeat once in 2 hours

Syrup: 2-3 teaspoonfuls at bedtime, not to exceed 30 mL/day

Tablet: 187 mg: 2 tablets at bedtime, not to exceed 8 tablets/day

Tablet: 374 mg: 1 at bedtime, up to 4/day; 600 mg: 2 tablets at bedtime, up to 3 tablets/day

Dosage Forms

Granules: 326 mg/teaspoonful

Liquid: 7% [70 mg/mL] (130 mL, 360 mL); 6.5% [65 mg/mL] (75 mL, 150 mL)

Suppository, rectal: 652 mg

Syrup: 218 mg/5 mL (60 mL, 240 mL)

Tablet: 187 mg, 217 mg, 600 mg

Senna-Gen® [OTC] *see* senna *on this page*

Senokot® [OTC] *see* senna *on this page*

Senolax® [OTC] *see* senna *on this page*

Sensorcaine® *see* bupivacaine *on page 76*

Sensorcaine®**-MPF** *see* bupivacaine *on page 76*

Septa® **Topical Ointment [OTC]** *see* bacitracin, neomycin, and polymyxin b *on page 53*

Septisol® *see* hexachlorophene *on page 260*

Septra® *see* co-trimoxazole *on page 140*

Septra® **DS** *see* co-trimoxazole *on page 140*

Ser-Ap-Es® *see* hydralazine, hydrochlorothiazide, and reserpine *on page 264*

Serax® *see* oxazepam *on page 388*

Serentil® *see* mesoridazine *on page 332*

Serevent® *see* salmeterol *on page 473*

sermorelin acetate (ser moe REL in AS e tate)
Brand Names Geref® Injection
Therapeutic Category Diagnostic Agent
Use Evaluate ability of the somatotroph of the pituitary gland to secrete growth hormone
Usual Dosage I.V. (in a single dose in the morning following an overnight fast):
   Children or subjects <50 kg: Draw venous blood samples for GH determinations 15 minutes before and immediately prior to administration, then administer 1 mcg/kg followed by a 3 mL normal saline flush, draw blood samples again for GH determinations
   Adults or subjects >50 kg: Determine the number of ampules needed based on a dose of 1 mcg/kg, draw venous blood samples for GH determinations 15 minutes before and immediately prior to administration, then administer 1 mcg/kg followed by a 3 mL normal saline flush, draw blood samples again for GH determinations
Dosage Forms Powder for injection, lyophilized: 50 mcg

Seromycin® **Pulvules**® *see* cycloserine *on page 144*

Serophene® *see* clomiphene *on page 129*

Seroquel® *see* quetiapine *on page 455*

Serostim® **Injection** *see* human growth hormone *on page 262*

Serpalan® *see* reserpine *on page 462*

sertraline (SER tra leen)
Synonyms sertraline hydrochloride
Brand Names Zoloft™
Therapeutic Category Antidepressant, Selective Serotonin Reuptake Inhibitor
Use Treatment of major depression; also being studied for use in obesity and obsessive-compulsive disorder
Usual Dosage Oral: Initial: 50 mg/day as a single dose, dosage may be increased at intervals of at least 1 week to a maximum recommended dosage of 200 mg/day
Dosage Forms Tablet, as hydrochloride: 25 mg, 50 mg, 100 mg

sertraline hydrochloride *see* sertraline *on this page*

Serutan® **[OTC]** *see* psyllium *on page 451*

Serzone® *see* nefazodone *on page 367*

sevoflurane (see voe FLOO rane)
Brand Names Ultane®
Therapeutic Category General Anesthetic
Use General induction and maintenance of anesthesia (inhalation)
Usual Dosage Surgical levels of anesthesia can usually be obtained with concentrations of 0.5% to 3%

Dosage Forms Liquid for inhalation: 250 mL

Shur-Seal® [OTC] *see* nonoxynol 9 *on page 377*

Silace-C® [OTC] *see* docusate and casanthranol *on page 180*

Siladryl® Oral [OTC] *see* diphenhydramine *on page 173*

Silafed® Syrup [OTC] *see* triprolidine and pseudoephedrine *on page 536*

Silaminic® Cold Syrup [OTC] *see* chlorpheniramine and phenylpropanolamine *on page 114*

Silaminic® Expectorant [OTC] *see* guaifenesin and phenylpropanolamine *on page 249*

Sildicon-E® [OTC] *see* guaifenesin and phenylpropanolamine *on page 249*

Silphen® Cough [OTC] *see* diphenhydramine *on page 173*

Silphen DM® [OTC] *see* dextromethorphan *on page 160*

Siltussin® [OTC] *see* guaifenesin *on page 247*

Siltussin-CF® [OTC] *see* guaifenesin, phenylpropanolamine, and dextromethorphan *on page 251*

Siltussin DM® [OTC] *see* guaifenesin and dextromethorphan *on page 248*

Silvadene® *see* silver sulfadiazine *on this page*

silver nitrate (SIL ver NYE trate)
Synonyms AgNO₃
Brand Names Dey-Drop® Ophthalmic Solution
Therapeutic Category Topical Skin Product
Use Prevention of gonococcal ophthalmia neonatorum; cauterization of wounds and sluggish ulcers, removal of granulation tissue and warts
Usual Dosage
Neonates: Ophthalmic: Instill 2 drops immediately after birth into conjunctival sac of each eye as a single dose; do not irrigate eyes following instillation of eye drops
Children and Adults:
Sticks: Apply to mucous membranes and other moist skin surfaces only on area to be treated 2-3 times/week for 2-3 weeks
Topical solution: Apply a cotton applicator dipped in solution on the affected area 2-3 times/week for 2-3 weeks
Dosage Forms
Applicator, topical: 75% with potassium nitrate 25% (6")
Ointment, topical: 10% (30 g)
Solution:
Ophthalmic: 1% (wax ampuls)
Topical: 10% (30 mL); 25% (30 mL); 50% (30 mL)

silver protein, mild (SIL ver PRO teen mild)
Therapeutic Category Antibiotic, Topical
Use Stain and coagulate mucus in eye surgery which is then removed by irrigation; eye infections
Usual Dosage
Preop in eye surgery: Place 2-3 drops into eye(s), then rinse out with sterile irrigating solution
Eye infections: 1-3 drops into the affected eye(s) every 3-4 hours for several days
Dosage Forms Solution, ophthalmic: 20% (15 mL, 30 mL)

silver sulfadiazine (SIL ver sul fa DYE a zeen)
Brand Names Silvadene®; SSD® AF; SSD® Cream; Thermazene®
Therapeutic Category Antibacterial, Topical
Use Adjunct in the prevention and treatment of infection in second and third degree burns
(Continued)

479

silver sulfadiazine *(Continued)*

Usual Dosage Children and Adults: Topical: Apply once or twice daily with a sterile gloved hand; apply to a thickness of 1/16"; burned area should be covered with cream at all times

Dosage Forms Cream, topical: 1% [10 mg/g] (20 g, 50 g, 100 g, 400 g, 1000 g)

simethicone (sye METH i kone)

Synonyms activated dimethicone; activated methylpolysiloxane

Brand Names Degas® [OTC]; Flatulex® [OTC]; Gas Relief®; Gas-X® [OTC]; Maalox Anti-Gas® [OTC]; Mylanta Gas® [OTC]; Mylicon® [OTC]; Phazyme® [OTC]

Therapeutic Category Antiflatulent

Use Relieve flatulence, functional gastric bloating, and postoperative gas pains

Usual Dosage Oral:

Infants: 20 mg 4 times/day

Children <12 years: 40 mg 4 times/day

Children >12 years and Adults: 40-120 mg after meals and at bedtime as needed, not to exceed 500 mg/day

Dosage Forms

Capsule: 125 mg

Drops, oral: 40 mg/0.6 mL (30 mL)

Tablet: 50 mg, 60 mg, 95 mg

Chewable: 40 mg, 80 mg, 125 mg

simethicone and calcium carbonate *see* calcium carbonate and simethicone *on page 83*

simethicone and magaldrate *see* magaldrate and simethicone *on page 317*

Simron® [OTC] *see* ferrous gluconate *on page 220*

simvastatin (SIM va stat in)

Brand Names Zocor®

Therapeutic Category HMG-CoA Reductase Inhibitor

Use Adjunct to dietary therapy to decrease elevated serum total and LDL cholesterol concentrations in primary hypercholesterolemia

Usual Dosage Adults: Oral: Start with 5-10 mg/day as a single bedtime dose; starting dose of 5 mg/day should be considered for patients with LDL-C of ≤190 mg/dL and for the elderly; patients with LDL-C levels >190 mg/dL should be started on 10 mg/day; adjustments of dosage should be made at intervals of 4 weeks or more; maximum recommended dose: 40 mg/day

Dosage Forms Tablet: 5 mg, 10 mg, 20 mg, 40 mg

Sinarest® 12 Hour Nasal Solution *see* oxymetazoline *on page 390*

Sinarest® Nasal Solution [OTC] *see* phenylephrine *on page 411*

Sinarest®, No Drowsiness [OTC] *see* acetaminophen and pseudoephedrine *on page 5*

sincalide (SIN ka lide)

Synonyms c8-cck; op-cck

Brand Names Kinevac®

Therapeutic Category Diagnostic Agent

Use Postevacuation cholecystography; gallbladder bile sampling; stimulate pancreatic secretion for analysis

Usual Dosage Adults: I.V.:

Contraction of gallbladder: 0.02 mcg/kg over 30 seconds to 1 minute, may repeat in 15 minutes a 0.04 mcg/kg dose

Pancreatic function: 0.02 mcg/kg over 30 minutes

Dosage Forms Injection: 5 mcg

Sine-Aid® IB [OTC] *see* pseudoephedrine and ibuprofen *on page 450*

Sine-Aid®, Maximum Strength [OTC] *see* acetaminophen and pseudoephedrine *on page 5*

Sinemet® *see* levodopa and carbidopa *on page 305*

Sine-Off® Maximum Strength No Drowsiness Formula [OTC] *see* acetaminophen and pseudoephedrine *on page 5*

Sinequan® Oral *see* doxepin *on page 183*

Sinex® Long-Acting [OTC] *see* oxymetazoline *on page 390*

Sinografin® *see* radiological/contrast media (ionic) *on page 457*

Sinubid® *see* phenyltoloxamine, phenylpropanolamine, and acetaminophen *on page 414*

Sinufed® Timecelles® *see* guaifenesin and pseudoephedrine *on page 250*

Sinumist®-SR Capsulets® *see* guaifenesin *on page 247*

Sinupan® *see* guaifenesin and phenylephrine *on page 249*

Sinus Excedrin® Extra Strength [OTC] *see* acetaminophen and pseudoephedrine *on page 5*

Sinus-Relief® [OTC] *see* acetaminophen and pseudoephedrine *on page 5*

Sinutab® Tablets [OTC] *see* acetaminophen, chlorpheniramine, and pseudoephedrine *on page 5*

Sinutab® Without Drowsiness [OTC] *see* acetaminophen and pseudoephedrine *on page 5*

sk *see* streptokinase *on page 492*

Skelaxin® *see* metaxalone *on page 333*

Skelid® *see* tiludronate *on page 519*

SKF 104864 *see* topotecan *on page 524*

skin test antigens, multiple (skin test AN tee gens, MUL ti pul)

Brand Names Multitest CMI®

Therapeutic Category Diagnostic Agent

Use Detection of nonresponsiveness to antigens by means of delayed hypersensitivity skin testing

Usual Dosage Select only test sites that permit sufficient surface area and subcutaneous tissue to allow adequate penetration of all 8 points, avoid hairy areas

Press loaded unit into the skin with sufficient pressure to puncture the skin and allow adequate penetration of all points, maintain firm contact for at least five seconds, during application the device should not be "rocked" back and forth and side to side without removing any of the test heads from the skin sites

If adequate pressure is applied it will be possible to observe:

1. The puncture marks of the nine tines on each of the eight test heads
2. An imprint of the circular platform surrounding each test head
3. Residual antigen and glycerin at each of the eight sites

If any of the above three criteria are not fully followed, the test results may not be reliable

Reading should be done in good light, read the test sites at both 24 and 48 hours, the largest reaction recorded from the two readings at each test site should be used; if two readings are not possible, a single 48 hour is recommended

A positive reaction from any of the seven delayed hypersensitivity skin test antigens is **induration of ≥2 mm** providing there is no induration at the negative control site; the size of the induration reactions with this test may be smaller than those obtained with other intradermal procedures

Dosage Forms Individual carton containing one preloaded skin test antigen for cellular hypersensitivity

Sleep-eze 3® Oral [OTC] *see* diphenhydramine *on page 173*

Sleepinal® [OTC] *see* diphenhydramine *on page 173*

Sleepwell 2-nite® [OTC] *see* diphenhydramine *on page 173*

Slim-Mint® [OTC] *see* benzocaine *on page 59*

Slo-bid™ *see* theophylline *on page 511*

Slo-Niacin® [OTC] *see* niacin *on page 372*

Slo-Phyllin® *see* theophylline *on page 511*

Slo-Phyllin GG® *see* theophylline and guaifenesin *on page 512*

Slow FE® [OTC] *see* ferrous sulfate *on page 221*

Slow-K® *see* potassium chloride *on page 427*

Slow-Mag® [OTC] *see* magnesium chloride *on page 318*

smelling salts *see* ammonia spirit, aromatic *on page 28*

smx-tmp *see* co-trimoxazole *on page 140*

snake (pit vipers) antivenin *see* antivenin (*Crotalidae*) polyvalent *on page 38*

Snaplets-EX® [OTC] *see* guaifenesin and phenylpropanolamine *on page 249*

Snooze Fast® [OTC] *see* diphenhydramine *on page 173*

sodium 2-mercaptoethane sulfonate *see* mesna *on page 331*

sodium acetate (SOW dee um AS e tate)
Therapeutic Category Alkalinizing Agent; Electrolyte Supplement
Use Sodium salt replacement; correction of acidosis through conversion of acetate to bicarbonate
Usual Dosage Sodium acetate is metabolized to bicarbonate on an equimolar basis outside the liver; administer in large volume I.V. fluids as a sodium source. Refer to sodium bicarbonate monograph.

Maintenance electrolyte requirements of sodium in parenteral nutrition solutions:
Daily requirements: 3-4 mEq/kg/24 hours or 25-40 mEq/1000 kcal/24 hours
Maximum: 100-150 mEq/24 hours
Dosage Forms Injection: 2 mEq/mL (20 mL, 50 mL); 4 mEq/mL (50 mL)

sodium acid carbonate *see* sodium bicarbonate *on next page*

sodium ascorbate (SOW dee um a SKOR bate)
Brand Names Cenolate®
Therapeutic Category Vitamin, Water Soluble
Use Prevention and treatment of scurvy and to acidify the urine; large doses may decrease the severity of "colds"
Usual Dosage Oral, I.V.:
Children:
Scurvy: 100-300 mg/day in divided doses for at least 2 weeks
Urinary acidification: 500 mg every 6-8 hours
Dietary supplement: 35-45 mg/day
Adults:
Scurvy: 100-250 mg 1-2 times/day for at least 2 weeks
Urinary acidification: 4-12 g/day in divided doses
Dietary supplement: 50-60 mg/day
Prevention and treatment of cold: 1-3 g/day
Dosage Forms
Crystals: 1020 mg per 1/4 teaspoonful [ascorbic acid 900 mg]
Injection: 250 mg/mL [ascorbic acid 222 mg/mL] (30 mL); 562.5 mg/mL [ascorbic acid 500 mg/mL] (1 mL, 2 mL)
Tablet: 585 mg [ascorbic acid 500 mg]

sodium benzoate and caffeine *see* caffeine and sodium benzoate *on page 80*

sodium bicarbonate (SOW dee um bye KAR bun ate)

Synonyms baking soda; NaHCO$_3$; sodium acid carbonate; sodium hydrogen carbonate
Brand Names Neut® Injection
Therapeutic Category Alkalinizing Agent; Antacid; Electrolyte Supplement
Use Management of metabolic acidosis; antacid; alkalinize urine; stabilization of acid base status in cardiac arrest, and treatment of life-threatening hyperkalemia
Usual Dosage
Cardiac arrest (patient should be adequately ventilated before administering NaHCO$_3$):
Infants: Use 1:1 dilution of 1 mEq/mL NaHCO$_3$ or use 0.5 mEq/mL NaHCO$_3$ at a dose of 1 mEq/kg slow IVP initially; may repeat with 0.5 mEq/kg in 10 minutes one time or as indicated by the patient's acid-base status. Rate of administration should not exceed 10 mEq/minute.
Children and Adults: IVP: 1 mEq/kg initially; may repeat with 0.5 mEq/kg in 10 minutes one time or as indicated by the patient's acid-base status

Metabolic acidosis: Dosage should be based on the following formula if blood gases and pH measurements are available:
Infants and Children: HCO$_3$-(mEq) = 0.3 x weight (kg) x base deficit (mEq/L) **or** HCO$_3$-(mEq) = 0.5 x weight (kg) x (24 - serum HCO$_3$-) (mEq/L)

Adults: HCO$_3$-(mEq) = 0.2 x weight (kg) x base deficit (mEq/L) **or** HCO$_3$-(mEq) = 0.5 x weight (kg) x (24 - serum HCO$_3$-) (mEq/L)
If acid-base status is not available: Dose for older Children and Adults: 2-5 mEq/kg I.V. infusion over 4-8 hours; subsequent doses should be based on patient's acid-base status

Chronic renal failure: Oral: Children: 1-3 mEq/kg/day

Renal tubular acidosis: Oral:
Distal:
Children: 2-3 mEq/kg/day
Adults: 1 mEq/kg/day
Proximal: Children: Initial: 5-10 mEq/kg/day; maintenance: Increase as required to maintain serum bicarbonate in the normal range

Urine alkalinization: Oral:
Children: 1-10 mEq (84-840 mg)/kg/day in divided doses; dose should be titrated to desired urinary pH
Adults: 48 mEq (4 g) initially, then 12-24 mEq (1-2 g) every 4 hours; dose should be titrated to desired urinary pH; doses up to 16 g/day have been used
Dosage Forms
Injection: 4% [40 mg/mL = 2.4 mEq/5 mL] (5 mL); 4.2% [42 mg/mL = 5 mEq/10 mL] (10 mL); 7.5% [75 mg/mL = 8.92 mEq/10 mL] (10 mL, 50 mL); 8.4% [84 mg/mL = 10 mEq/10 mL] (10 mL, 50 mL)
Powder: 120 g, 480 g
Tablet: 300 mg [3.6 mEq]; 325 mg [3.8 mEq]; 520 mg [6.3 mEq]; 600 mg [7.3 mEq]; 650 mg [7.6 mEq]

sodium cellulose phosphate *see* cellulose sodium phosphate *on page 102*

sodium chloride (SOW dee um KLOR ide)

Synonyms NaCl; normal saline; salt
Brand Names Adsorbonac® Ophthalmic [OTC]; Afrin® Saline Mist [OTC]; AK-NaCl® [OTC]; Ayr® Saline [OTC]; Breathe Free® [OTC]; Dristan® Saline Spray [OTC]; HuMist® Nasal Mist [OTC]; Muro 128® Ophthalmic [OTC]; Muroptic-5® [OTC]; NāSal™ [OTC]; Nasal Moist® [OTC]; Ocean Nasal Mist [OTC]; Pretz® [OTC]; SalineX® [OTC]; SeaMist® [OTC]
Therapeutic Category Electrolyte Supplement; Lubricant, Ocular
(Continued)

sodium chloride (Continued)

Use Prevention of muscle cramps and heat prostration; restoration of sodium ion in hyponatremia; restore moisture to nasal membranes; reduction of corneal edema

Usual Dosage

Newborn electrolyte requirement:

Premature: 2-8 mEq/kg/24 hours

Term:

0-48 hours: 0-2 mEq/kg/24 hours

>48 hours: 1-4 mEq/kg/24 hours

Children: I.V.: Hypertonic solutions (>0.9%) should only be used for the initial treatment of acute serious symptomatic hyponatremia; maintenance: 3-4 mEq/kg/day; maximum: 100-150 mEq/day; dosage varies widely depending on clinical condition

Replacement: Determined by laboratory determinations mEq

Sodium deficiency (mEq/kg) = [% dehydration (L/kg)/100 x 70 (mEq/L) = [0.6 (L/kg) x (140 - serum sodium) (mEq/L)]

Nasal: Use as often as needed

Adults:

GI irrigant: 1-3 L/day by intermittent irrigation

Heat cramps: Oral: 0.5-1 g with full glass of water, up to 4.8 g/day

Replacement I.V.: Determined by laboratory determinations mEq

Sodium deficiency (mEq/kg) = [% dehydration (L/kg)/100 x 70 (mEq/L)] + [0.6 (L/kg) x (140 - serum sodium) (mEq/L)]

To correct acute, serious hyponatremia: mEq sodium = (desired sodium (mEq/L) - actual sodium (mEq/L) x 0.6 x wt (kg)); for acute correction use 125 mEq/L as the desired serum sodium; acutely correct serum sodium in 5 mEq/L/dose increments; more gradual correction in increments of 10 mEq/L/day is indicated in the asymptomatic patient

Chloride maintenance electrolyte requirement in parenteral nutrition: 2-4 mEq/kg/24 hours or 25-40 mEq/1000 kcals/24 hours; maximum: 100-150 mEq/24 hours

Sodium maintenance electrolyte requirement in parenteral nutrition: 3-4 mEq/kg/24 hours or 25-40 mEq/1000 kcals/24 hours; maximum: 100-150 mEq/24 hours.

Nasal: Use as often as needed

Ophthalmic:

Ointment: Apply once daily or more often

Solution: Instill 1-2 drops into affected eye(s) every 3-4 hours

Abortifacient: 20% (250 mL) administered by transabdominal intra-amniotic instillation

Dosage Forms

Drops, nasal: 0.9% with dropper

Injection: 0.2% (3 mL); 0.45% (3 mL, 5 mL, 500 mL, 1000 mL); 0.9% (1 mL, 2 mL, 3 mL, 4 mL, 5 mL, 10 mL, 20 mL, 25 mL, 30 mL, 50 mL, 100 mL, 130 mL, 150 mL, 250 mL, 500 mL, 1000 mL); 3% (500 mL); 5% (500 mL); 20% (250 mL); 23.4% (30 mL, 100 mL)

Injection:

Admixtures: 50 mEq (20 mL); 100 mEq (40 mL); 625 mEq (250 mL)

Bacteriostatic: 0.9% (30 mL)

Concentrated: 14.6% (20 mL, 40 mL, 200 mL); 23.4% (10 mL, 20 mL, 30 mL)

Irrigation: 0.45% (500 mL, 1000 mL, 1500 mL); 0.9% (250 mL, 500 mL, 1000 mL, 1500 mL, 2000 mL, 3000 mL, 4000 mL)

Ointment, ophthalmic (Muro 128®): 5% (3.5 g)

Solution:

Irrigation: 0.9% (1000 mL, 2000 mL)

Nasal: 0.4% (15 mL, 50 mL); 0.6% (15 mL); 0.65% (20 mL, 45 mL, 50 mL)

Ophthalmic (Adsorbonac®): 2% (15 mL); 5% (15 mL, 30 mL)

Tablet: 650 mg, 1 g, 2.25 g

Enteric coated: 1 g

Slow release: 600 mg

sodium citrate and potassium citrate mixture
(SOW dee um SIT rate & poe TASS ee um SIT rate MIKS chur)
Brand Names Polycitra®
Therapeutic Category Alkalinizing Agent
Use Conditions where long-term maintenance of an alkaline urine is desirable as in control and dissolution of uric acid and cystine calculi of the urinary tract
Usual Dosage Oral:
Children: 5-15 mL diluted in water after meals and at bedtime
Adults: 15-30 mL diluted in water after meals and at bedtime
Dosage Forms Syrup: Sodium citrate 500 mg, potassium citrate 550 mg, with citric acid 334 mg per 5 mL [sodium 1 mEq, potassium 1 mEq, bicarbonate 2 mEq]

sodium edetate *see* edetate disodium *on page 190*

sodium ethacrynate *see* ethacrynic acid *on page 206*

sodium etidronate *see* etidronate disodium *on page 212*

sodium fluoride *see* fluoride *on page 228*

sodium hyaluronate (SOW dee um hye al yoor ON nate)
Synonyms hyaluronic acid
Brand Names AMO Vitrax®; Amvisc®; Amvisc® Plus; Healon®; Healon® GV
Therapeutic Category Ophthalmic Agent, Viscoelastic
Use Surgical aid in cataract extraction, intraocular implantation, corneal transplant, glaucoma filtration, and retinal attachment surgery
Usual Dosage Depends upon procedure (slowly introduce a sufficient quantity into eye)
Dosage Forms Injection, intraocular:
Healon®: 10 mg/mL (0.4 mL, 0.55 mL, 0.85 mL, 2 mL)
Amvisc®: 12 mg/mL (0.5 mL, 0.8 mL)
Healon® GV: 14 mg/mL (0.55 mL, 0.85 mL)
Amvisc® Plus: 16 mg/mL (0.5 mL, 8 mL)
AMO Vitrax®: 30 mg/mL (0.65 mL)

sodium hyaluronate-chrondroitin sulfate *see* chondroitin sulfate-sodium hyaluronate *on page 122*

sodium hydrogen carbonate *see* sodium bicarbonate *on page 483*

sodium hypochlorite solution
(SOW dee um hye poe KLOR ite soe LOO shun)
Synonyms Dakin's solution; modified Dakin's solution
Therapeutic Category Disinfectant
Use Treatment of athlete's foot (0.5%); wound irrigation (0.5%); to disinfect utensils and equipment (5%)
Usual Dosage Topical irrigation
Dosage Forms
Solution: 5% (4000 mL)
Modified Dakin's solution:
Full strength: 0.5% (1000 mL)
Half strength: 0.25% (1000 mL)
Quarter strength: 0.125% (1000 mL)

sodium lactate (SOW dee um LAK tate)
Therapeutic Category Alkalinizing Agent
Use Source of bicarbonate for prevention and treatment of mild to moderate metabolic acidosis
Usual Dosage Dosage depends on degree of acidosis
Dosage Forms Injection:
1.87 g/100 mL [sodium 16.7 mEq and lactate 16.7 mEq per 100 mL] (1000 mL)
(Continued)

sodium lactate *(Continued)*

560 mg/mL [sodium 5 mEq sodium and lactate 5 mEq per mL] (10 mL)

sodium *l*-triiodothyronine *see* liothyronine *on page 309*

sodium methicillin *see* methicillin *on page 336*

sodium nitroferricyanide *see* nitroprusside *on page 377*

sodium nitroprusside *see* nitroprusside *on page 377*

sodium oxacillin *see* oxacillin *on page 387*

sodium-pca and lactic acid *see* lactic acid and sodium-PCA *on page 299*

sodium phenylacetate and sodium benzoate

(SOW dee um fen il AS e tate & SOW dee um BENZ oh ate)

Brand Names Ucephan®

Therapeutic Category Ammonium Detoxicant

Use Adjunctive therapy to prevent/treat hyperammonemia in patients with urea cycle enzymopathy involving partial or complete deficiencies of carbamoyl-phosphate synthetase, ornithine transcarbamoylase or argininosuccinate synthetase

Usual Dosage Infants and Children: Oral: 2.5 mL (250 mg sodium benzoate and 250 mg sodium phenylacetate)/kg/day divided 3-6 times/day; total daily dose should not exceed 100 mL

Dosage Forms Solution: Sodium phenylacetate 100 mg and sodium benzoate 100 mg per mL (100 mL)

sodium phenylbutyrate (SOW dee um fen il BYOO ti rate)

Synonyms Ammonapse

Brand Names Buphenyl®

Therapeutic Category Miscellaneous Product

Use Adjunctive therapy in the chronic management of patients with urea cycle disorder involving deficiencies of carbamoylphosphate synthetase, ornithine transcarbamylase, or argininosuccinic acid synthetase

Usual Dosage

Powder: Patients weighing <20 kg: 450-600 mg/kg/day or 9.9-13 g/m^2/day, administered in equally divided amounts with each meal or feeding, 4-6 times/day; safety and efficacy of doses >20 g/day have not been established

Tablet: Children >20 kg and Adults: 450-600 mg/kg/day or 9.9-13 g/m^2/day, administered in equally divided amounts with each meal; safety and efficacy of doses >20 g/day have not been established

Dosage Forms

Powder: 3.2 g [sodium phenylbutyrate 3 g] per teaspoon (500 mL, 950 mL); 9.1 g [sodium phenylbutyrate 8.6 g] per **tablespoon** (500 mL, 950 mL)

Tablet: 500 mg

sodium phosphate (SOW dee um FOS fate)

Brand Names Fleet® Enema [OTC]; Fleet® Phospho®-Soda [OTC]

Therapeutic Category Electrolyte Supplement; Laxative

Use Source of phosphate in large volume I.V. fluids; short-term treatment of constipation (oral/rectal) and to evacuate the colon for rectal and bowel exams; treatment and prevention of hypophosphatemia

Usual Dosage

Normal requirements elemental phosphate: Oral:

0-6 months: 240 mg

6-12 months: 360 mg

1-10 years: 800 mg

>10 years: 1200 mg

Pregnancy lactation: Additional 400 mg/day

Treatment:

It is difficult to provide concrete guidelines for the treatment of severe hypophospha-temia because the extent of total body deficits and response to therapy are difficult to predict. Aggressive doses of phosphate may result in a transient serum elevation followed by redistribution into intracellular compartments or bone tissue. It is recommended that repletion of severe hypophosphatemia (<1 mg/dL in adults) be done I.V. because large doses of oral phosphate may cause diarrhea and intestinal absorption may be unreliable

Pediatric I.V. phosphate repletion:

Children: 0.25-0.5 mmol/kg **administer over 4-6 hours and repeat if symptomatic hypophosphatemia persists;** to assess the need for further phosphate administration: obtain serum inorganic phosphate after administration of the first dose and base further doses on serum levels and clinical status

Adult I.V. phosphate repletion:

Initial dose: 0.08 mmol/kg if recent uncomplicated hypophosphatemia

Initial dose: 0.16 mmol/kg if prolonged hypophosphatemia with presumed total body deficits; increase dose by 25% to 50% if patient symptomatic with severe hypophosphatemia

Severe hypophosphatemia:

High-dose = 0.36 mmol/kg over 6 hours; use if serum PO_4 <0.5 mg/dL

Adults: 0.15-0.3 mmol/kg/dose over 12 hours, may repeat as needed to achieve desired serum level

With orders for I.V. phosphate, there is considerable confusion associated with the use of millimoles (mmol) versus milliequivalents (mEq) to express the phosphate requirement. Because inorganic phosphate exists as monobasic and dibasic anions, with the mixture of valences is dependent on pH, ordering by mEq amounts is unreliable and may lead to large dosing errors. In addition, I.V. phosphate is available in the sodium and potassium salt; therefore, the content of these cations must be considered when ordering phosphate. The most reliable method of ordering I.V. phosphate is by millimoles, then specifying the potassium or sodium salt. For example, an order for 15 mmol of phosphate as potassium phosphate in one liter of normal saline would also provide 22 mEq of potassium.

Phosphate maintenance electrolyte requirement in parenteral nutrition: 2 mmol/kg/24 hours or 35 mmol/kcal/24 hours; Maximum: 15-30 mmol/24 hours

Maintenance:

Children: 0.5-1.5 mmol/kg/24 hours I.V. **or** 2-3 mmol/kg/24 hours orally in divided doses

Adults: 15-30 mmol/24 hours I.V. **or** 50-150 mmol/24 hours orally in divided doses

Laxative (Fleet®): Rectal:

Children 2-12 years: 67.5 mL (½ bottle) as a single dose, may repeat

Children ≥12 years and Adults: 133 mL enema as a single dose, may repeat

Laxative (Fleet® Phospho®-Soda): Oral:

Children:

5-9 years: 5 mL as a single dose

10-12 years: 10 mL as a single dose

Children ≥12 years and Adults: 20-30 mL as a single dose

Dosage Forms

Enema: Sodium phosphate 6 g and sodium biphosphate 16 g/100 mL (67.5 mL pediatric enema unit, 135 mL adult enema unit)

Injection: Phosphate 3 mmol and sodium 4 mEq per mL (5 mL, 10 mL, 15 mL, 30 mL, 50 mL)

Solution, oral: Sodium phosphate 18 g and sodium biphosphate 48 g/100 mL (45 mL, 90 mL, 273 mL)

See table on following page.

sodium phosphate and potassium phosphate *see* potassium phosphate and sodium phosphate *on page 431*

	Phosphate (mmol)	Sodium (mEq)	Potassium (mEq)
Oral			
Whole cow's milk	0.29/mL	0.025/mL	0.035/mL
Fleet® Phospho®-Soda	4.15/mL	4.8/mL	None
Intravenous			
Sodium phosphate	3/mL	4/mL	None

sodium polystyrene sulfonate
(SOW dee um pol ee STYE reen SUL fon ate)
Brand Names Kayexalate®; SPS®
Therapeutic Category Antidote
Use Treatment of hyperkalemia
Usual Dosage
Children:
Oral: 1 g/kg/dose every 6 hours
Rectal: 1 g/kg/dose every 2-6 hours (In small children and infants employ lower doses by using the practical exchange ratio of 1 mEq potassium/g of resin as the basis for calculation)
Adults:
Oral: 15 g (60 mL) 1-4 times/day
Rectal: 30-50 g every 6 hours
Dosage Forms Oral or rectal:
Powder for suspension: 454 g
Suspension: 1.25 g/5 mL with sorbitol 33% and alcohol 0.3% (60 mL, 120 mL, 200 mL, 500 mL)

sodium salicylate (SOW dee um sa LIS i late)
Brand Names Uracel®
Therapeutic Category Analgesic, Non-narcotic; Antipyretic
Use Treatment of minor pain or fever; arthritis
Usual Dosage Adults: Oral: 325-650 mg every 4 hours
Dosage Forms Tablet, enteric coated: 325 mg, 650 mg

Sodium Sulamyd® Ophthalmic see sulfacetamide sodium on page 496

sodium sulfacetamide see sulfacetamide sodium on page 496

sodium sulfacetamide and sulfur see sulfur and sulfacetamide sodium on page 500

sodium tetradecyl (SOW dee um tetra DEK il)
Synonyms sodium tetradecyl sulfate
Brand Names Sotradecol® Injection
Therapeutic Category Sclerosing Agent
Use Treatment of small, uncomplicated varicose veins of the lower extremities; endoscopic sclerotherapy in the management of bleeding esophageal varices
Usual Dosage I.V.: 0.5-2 mL of 1% (5-20 mg) for small veins; 0.5-2 mL of 3% (15-60 mg) for medium or large veins
Dosage Forms Injection, as sulfate: 1% [10 mg/mL] (2 mL); 3% [30 mg/mL] (2 mL)

sodium tetradecyl sulfate see sodium tetradecyl on this page

sodium thiosulfate (SOW dee um thye oh SUL fate)
Brand Names Tinver® Lotion
Therapeutic Category Antidote; Antifungal Agent

Use
Parenteral: Used alone or with sodium nitrite or amyl nitrite in cyanide poisoning or arsenic poisoning; reduce the risk of nephrotoxicity associated with cisplatin therapy; local infiltration (in diluted form) of selected chemotherapy extravasation
Topical: Treatment of tinea versicolor
Usual Dosage I.V.:
Cyanide and nitroprusside antidote:
Children <25 kg: 50 mg/kg after receiving 4.5-10 mg/kg sodium nitrite; a half dose of each may be repeated if necessary
Children >25 kg and Adults: 12.5 g after 300 mg of sodium nitrite; a half dose of each may be repeated if necessary
Cyanide poisoning: Dose should be based on determination as with nitrite, at rate of 2.5-5 mL/minute to maximum of 50 mL
Dosage Forms
Injection: 100 mg/mL (10 mL); 250 mg/mL (50 mL)
Lotion: 25% with salicylic acid 1% and isopropyl alcohol 10% (120 mL, 180 mL)

Solaquin® [OTC] *see* hydroquinone *on page 272*

Solaquin Forte® *see* hydroquinone *on page 272*

Solarcaine® [OTC] *see* benzocaine *on page 59*

Solarcaine® Aloe Extra Burn Relief [OTC] *see* lidocaine *on page 307*

Solatene® *see* beta-carotene *on page 64*

Solfoton® *see* phenobarbital *on page 409*

Solganal® *see* aurothioglucose *on page 49*

soluble fluorescein *see* fluorescein sodium *on page 227*

Solu-Cortef® *see* hydrocortisone *on page 268*

Solu-Medrol® Injection *see* methylprednisolone *on page 343*

Solurex® *see* dexamethasone *on page 156*

Solurex L.A.® *see* dexamethasone *on page 156*

Soma® *see* carisoprodol *on page 93*

Soma® Compound *see* carisoprodol and aspirin *on page 93*

Soma® Compound w/Codeine *see* carisoprodol, aspirin, and codeine *on page 93*

somatrem *see* human growth hormone *on page 262*

somatropin *see* human growth hormone *on page 262*

Sominex® Oral [OTC] *see* diphenhydramine *on page 173*

sorbitol (SOR bi tole)

Therapeutic Category Genitourinary Irrigant; Laxative
Use Humectant; sweetening agent; hyperosmotic laxative; facilitate the passage of sodium polystyrene sulfonate or a charcoal-toxin complex through the intestinal tract
Usual Dosage Hyperosmotic laxative (as single dose, at infrequent intervals):
Children 2-11 years:
Oral: 2 mL/kg (as 70% solution)
Rectal enema: 30-60 mL as 25% to 30% solution
Children >12 years and Adults:
Oral: 30-150 mL (as 70% solution)
Rectal enema: 120 mL as 25% to 30% solution
Adjunct to sodium polystyrene sulfonate: 15 mL as 70% solution orally until diarrhea occurs (10-20 mL/2 hours) or 20-100 mL as an oral vehicle for the sodium polystyrene sulfonate resin

When administered with charcoal: Oral:
Children: 4.3 mL/kg of 35% sorbitol with 1 g/kg of activated charcoal
(Continued)

ALPHABETICAL LISTING OF DRUGS

sorbitol *(Continued)*
Adults: 4.3 mL/kg of 70% sorbitol with 1 g/kg of activated charcoal
Dosage Forms
Solution: 70%
Solution, genitourinary irrigation: 3% (1500 mL, 3000 mL); 3.3% (2000 mL)

Sorbitrate® *see* isosorbide dinitrate *on page 292*

sotalol (SOE ta lole)
Synonyms sotalol hydrochloride
Brand Names Betapace®
Therapeutic Category Antiarrhythmic Agent, Class II; Antiarrhythmic Agent, Class III
Use Treatment of ventricular arrhythmias
Usual Dosage Adults: Oral: Initial: 80 mg twice daily; may be increased to 240-320 mg/day and up to 480-640 mg/day in patients with life-threatening refractory ventricular arrhythmias
Dosage Forms Tablet, as hydrochloride: 80 mg, 120 mg, 160 mg, 240 mg

sotalol hydrochloride *see* sotalol *on this page*

Sotradecol® Injection *see* sodium tetradecyl *on page 488*

Soyacal® *see* fat emulsion *on page 216*

Soyalac® [OTC] *see* enteral nutritional products *on page 194*

Span-FF® [OTC] *see* ferrous fumarate *on page 220*

sparfloxacin (spar FLOKS a sin)
Brand Names Zagam®
Therapeutic Category Quinolone
Use Treatment of adult patients with community acquired pneumonia caused by susceptible strains of *Chlamydia pneumoniae, Haemophilus influenzae, Haemophilus parainfluenzae, Moraxella catarrhalis, Mycoplasma pneumoniae*, or *Streptococcus pneumoniae* and acute bacterial exacerbations of acute bronchitis caused by susceptible strains of *Chlamydia pneumoniae, Enterobacter cloacae, Haemophilus influenzae, Haemophilus parainfluenzae, Klebsiella pneumoniae, Moraxella catarrhalis, Staphylococcus aureus*, or *Streptococcus pneumoniae*
Usual Dosage Adults: Oral: 400 mg on day 1, then 200 mg daily for the next 9 days (11 tablets total). In patients with creatinine clearance <50 mL/minute, administer 400 mg on day 1, then begin 200 mg every 48 hours on day 3 for a total of 9 days (6 tablets total).
Dosage Forms Tablet: 200 mg

Sparine® *see* promazine *on page 441*

Spasmolin® *see* hyoscyamine, atropine, scopolamine, and phenobarbital *on page 276*

Spec-T® [OTC] *see* benzocaine *on page 59*

Spectazole™ *see* econazole *on page 189*

spectinomycin (spek ti noe MYE sin)
Synonyms spectinomycin hydrochloride
Brand Names Trobicin®
Therapeutic Category Antibiotic, Miscellaneous
Use Treatment of uncomplicated gonorrhea (ineffective against syphilis)
Usual Dosage I.M.:
Children:
<45 kg: 40 mg/kg/dose 1 time
≥45 kg: See adult dose

Children >8 years who are allergic to penicillins/cephalosporins may be treated with oral tetracycline

Adults: 2 g deep I.M. or 4 g where antibiotic resistance is prevalent 1 time; 4 g (10 mL) dose should be administered as 2-5 mL injections

Dosage Forms Injection, as hydrochloride: 2 g, 4 g

spectinomycin hydrochloride *see* spectinomycin *on previous page*

Spectrobid® *see* bacampicillin *on page 52*

Spherulin® *see* coccidioidin skin test *on page 134*

spirapril (SPYE ra pril)

Brand Names Renormax®
Therapeutic Category Angiotensin-Converting Enzyme (ACE) Inhibitors
Use Management of mild to severe hypertension
Usual Dosage Adults: Oral: 12 mg/day in 1-2 divided doses
Dosage Forms Tablet: 3 mg, 6 mg, 12 mg, 24 mg

spironolactone (speer on oh LAK tone)

Brand Names Aldactone®
Therapeutic Category Diuretic, Potassium Sparing
Use Management of edema associated with excessive aldosterone excretion; hypertension; primary hyperaldosteronism; hypokalemia; treatment of hirsutism
Usual Dosage Oral:
  Children: 1.5-3.5 mg/kg/day in divided doses every 6-24 hours
  Diagnosis of primary aldosteronism: 125-375 mg/m^2/day in divided doses
  Vaso-occlusive disease: 7.5 mg/kg/day in divided doses twice daily (non-FDA approved dose)
  Adults:
  Edema, hypertension, hypokalemia: 25-200 mg/day in 1-2 divided doses
  Diagnosis of primary aldosteronism: 100-400 mg/day in 1-2 divided doses
Dosage Forms Tablet: 25 mg, 50 mg, 100 mg

spironolactone and hydrochlorothiazide *see* hydrochlorothiazide and spironolactone *on page 265*

Sporanox® *see* itraconazole *on page 293*

Sportscreme® **[OTC]** *see* triethanolamine salicylate *on page 532*

SPS® *see* sodium polystyrene sulfonate *on page 488*

S-P-T *see* thyroid *on page 518*

SRC® **Expectorant** *see* hydrocodone, pseudoephedrine, and guaifenesin *on page 268*

SSD® **AF** *see* silver sulfadiazine *on page 479*

SSD® **Cream** *see* silver sulfadiazine *on page 479*

SSKI® *see* potassium iodide *on page 430*

Stadol® *see* butorphanol *on page 79*

Stadol® **NS** *see* butorphanol *on page 79*

Stagesic® *see* hydrocodone and acetaminophen *on page 266*

Stahist® *see* chlorpheniramine, phenylephrine, phenylpropanolamine, and belladonna alkaloids *on page 116*

stannous fluoride *see* fluoride *on page 228*

stanozolol (stan OH zoe lole)

Brand Names Winstrol®
Therapeutic Category Anabolic Steroid
(Continued)

stanozolol *(Continued)*
Controlled Substance C-III
Use Prophylactic use against angioedema
Usual Dosage
Children: Acute attacks:
<6 years: 1 mg/day
6-12 years: 2 mg/day
Adults: Oral: Initial: 2 mg 3 times/day, may then reduce to a maintenance dose of 2 mg/day or 2 mg every other day after 1-3 months
Dosage Forms Tablet: 2 mg

Staphcillin® *see* methicillin *on page 336*

Staticin® **Topical** *see* erythromycin, topical *on page 201*

stavudine (STAV yoo deen)
Synonyms d4T
Brand Names Zerit®
Therapeutic Category Antiviral Agent
Use Treatment of advanced HIV infection in patients who experience intolerance, toxicity, resistance, or HIV disease progression with either zidovudine or didanosine therapy; active against most zidovudine-resistant strains; in adults, stavudine used alone in patients with 50-500 CD4 cells/mm^3 and at least 6 months previous treatment with zidovudine was more effective than continued zidovudine in preventing disease progression and death
Usual Dosage Oral:
Children 7 months to 15 years: 1-2 mg/kg/day divided twice daily
Adults: 0.5-1 mg/kg/day **or**
<60 kg: 30 mg every 12 hours
≥60 kg: 40 mg every 12 hours
If peripheral neuropathy or elevations in liver enzymes occur, stavudine should be discontinued; once adverse effects resolve, reinitiate therapy at a lower dose of 20 mg every 12 hours (for ≥60 kg patients) or 15 mg every 12 hours (for <60 kg patients)
Dosage Forms
Capsule: 15 mg, 20 mg, 30 mg, 40 mg
Powder for oral solution: 1 mg/mL (200 mL)

S-T Cort® *see* hydrocortisone *on page 268*

Stelazine® *see* trifluoperazine *on page 532*

Stemex® *see* paramethasone acetate *on page 396*

Sterapred® *see* prednisone *on page 436*

stilbestrol *see* diethylstilbestrol *on page 167*

Stilphostrol® *see* diethylstilbestrol *on page 167*

Stimate® **Nasal** *see* desmopressin acetate *on page 155*

St Joseph® **Adult Chewable Aspirin [OTC]** *see* aspirin *on page 44*

St. Joseph® **Cough Suppressant [OTC]** *see* dextromethorphan *on page 160*

St. Joseph® **Measured Dose Nasal Solution [OTC]** *see* phenylephrine *on page 411*

Stop® **[OTC]** *see* fluoride *on page 228*

Streptase® *see* streptokinase *on this page*

streptokinase (strep toe KYE nase)
Synonyms sk
Brand Names Kabikinase®; Streptase®
Therapeutic Category Thrombolytic Agent

Use Thrombolytic agent used in treatment of recent severe or massive deep vein thrombosis, pulmonary emboli, myocardial infarction, and occluded arteriovenous cannulas

Usual Dosage I.V.:

Children: Safety and efficacy not established; limited studies have used: 3500-4000 units/kg over 30 minutes followed by 1000-1500 units/kg/hour; clotted catheter: 25,000 units, clamp for 2 hours then aspirate contents and flush with normal saline

Adults (best results are realized if used within 5-6 hours of myocardial infarction; antibodies to streptokinase remain for 3-6 months after initial dose, use another thrombolytic enzyme, ie, urokinase, if thrombolytic therapy is indicated):

Guidelines for Acute Myocardial Infarction (AMI):

1.5 million units infused over 60 minutes. Monitor for the first few hours for signs of anaphylaxis or allergic reaction. **Infusion should be slowed if lowering of 25 mm Hg in blood pressure or terminated if asthmatic symptoms appear.** Begin heparin 5000-10,000 unit bolus followed by 1000 units/hour approximately 3-4 hours after completion of streptokinase infusion or when PTT is <100 seconds.

Guidelines for Acute Pulmonary Embolism (APE):

3 million unit dose; administer 250,000 units over 30 minutes followed by 100,000 units/hour for 24 hours. Monitor for the first few hours for signs of anaphylaxis or allergic reaction. **Infusion should be slowed if blood pressure is lowered by 25 mm Hg or if asthmatic symptoms appear.** Begin heparin 1000 units/hour approximately 3-4 hours after completion of streptokinase infusion or when PTT is <100 seconds.

Thromboses: 250,000 units to start, then 100,000 units/hour for 24-72 hours depending on location

Cannula occlusion: 250,000 units into cannula, clamp for 2 hours, then aspirate contents and flush with normal saline

Dosage Forms Powder for injection: 250,000 units (5 mL, 6.5 mL); 600,000 units (5 mL); 750,000 units (6 mL, 6.5 mL); 1,500,000 units (6.5 mL, 10 mL, 50 mL)

streptozocin (strep toe ZOE sin)

Brand Names Zanosar®

Therapeutic Category Antineoplastic Agent

Use Treat metastatic islet cell carcinoma of the pancreas, carcinoid tumor and syndrome, Hodgkin's disease, palliative treatment of colorectal cancer

Usual Dosage Children and Adults: I.V.: 500 mg/m^2 for 5 days every 6 weeks until optimal benefit or toxicity occurs; or may be administered in single dose 1000 mg/m^2 at weekly intervals for 2 doses, then increased to 1500 mg/m^2 weekly; the median total dose to onset of response is about 2000 mg/m^2 and the median total dose to maximum response is about 4000 mg/m^2

Dosage Forms Injection: 1 g

Stresstabs® 600 Advanced Formula Tablets [OTC] *see* vitamins, multiple (oral, adult) *on page 556*

Stromectol® *see* ivermectin *on page 293*

strong iodine solution *see* potassium iodide *on page 430*

strontium-89 (STRON shee um atey nine)

Synonyms strontium-89 chloride

Brand Names Metastron® Injection

Therapeutic Category Radiopharmaceutical

Use Relief of bone pain in patients with skeletal metastases

Usual Dosage Adults: I.V.: 148 megabecquerel (4 millicurie) administered by slow I.V. injection over 1-2 minutes or 1.5-2.2 megabecquerel (40-60 microcurie)/kg; repeated doses are generally not recommended at intervals <90 days

Dosage Forms Injection, as chloride: 10.9-22.6 mg/mL [148 megabecquerel, 4 millicurie] (10 mL)

strontium-89 chloride *see* strontium-89 *on this page*

Stuartnatal® 1+1 *see* vitamin, multiple (prenatal) *on page 554*

Stuart Prenatal® [OTC] *see* vitamin, multiple (prenatal) *on page 554*

Sublimaze® Injection *see* fentanyl *on page 219*

succimer (SUKS i mer)
Brand Names Chemet®
Therapeutic Category Chelating Agent
Use Treatment of lead poisoning in children with blood levels >45 mcg/dL. It is not indicated for prophylaxis of lead poisoning in a lead-containing environment.
Usual Dosage Children and Adults: Oral: 30 mg/kg/day in divided doses every 8 hours for an additional 5 days followed by 20 mg/kg/day for 14 days
Dosage Forms Capsule: 100 mg

succinylcholine (suks in il KOE leen)
Synonyms succinylcholine chloride; suxamethonium chloride
Brand Names Anectine® Chloride Injection; Anectine® Flo-Pack®; Quelicin® Injection
Therapeutic Category Skeletal Muscle Relaxant
Use Used to produce skeletal muscle relaxation in procedures of short duration such as endotracheal intubation or endoscopic exams
Usual Dosage I.M., I.V.:
  Children: 1-2 mg/kg
  Intermittent: Initial: 1 mg/kg/dose one time; maintenance: 0.3-0.6 mg/kg every 5-10 minutes as needed
  Adults: 0.6 mg/kg (range: 0.3-1.1 mg/kg) over 10-30 seconds, up to 150 mg total dose
  Maintenance: 0.04-0.07 mg/kg every 5-10 minutes as needed
  Continuous infusion: 2.5 mg/minute (or 0.5-10 mg/minute); dilute to concentration of 1-2 mg/mL in D_5W or NS

Note: Pretreatment with atropine may reduce occurrence of bradycardia
Dosage Forms
  Injection, as chloride: 20 mg/mL (10 mL); 50 mg/mL (10 mL); 100 mg/mL (5 mL, 10 mL, 20 mL)
  Powder for injection, as chloride: 100 mg, 500 mg, 1 g

succinylcholine chloride *see* succinylcholine *on this page*

sucralfate (soo KRAL fate)
Synonyms aluminum sucrose sulfate, basic
Brand Names Carafate®
Therapeutic Category Gastrointestinal Agent, Gastric or Duodenal Ulcer Treatment
Use Short-term management of duodenal ulcers; gastric ulcers; suspension may be used topically for treatment of stomatitis due to cancer chemotherapy or other causes of esophageal and gastric erosions
Usual Dosage
  Children: Dose not established, doses of 40-80 mg/kg/day divided every 6 hours have been used
  Stomatitis: Oral: 2.5-5 mL (1 g/15 mL suspension), swish and spit or swish and swallow 4 times/day
  Adults:
  Duodenal ulcer treatment: Oral: 1 g 4 times/day, 1 hour before meals or food and at bedtime for 4-8 weeks, or alternatively 2 g twice daily
  Duodenal ulcer maintenance therapy: Oral: 1 g twice daily
  Stomatitis: Oral: 1 g/15 mL suspension, swish and spit or swish and swallow 4 times/day
Dosage Forms
  Suspension, oral: 1 g/10 mL (420 mL)
  Tablet: 1 g

Sucrets® **[OTC]** *see* dyclonine *on page 188*

Sucrets® **Cough Calmers [OTC]** *see* dextromethorphan *on page 160*

Sucrets® **Sore Throat [OTC]** *see* hexylresorcinol *on page 260*

Sudafed® **[OTC]** *see* pseudoephedrine *on page 449*

Sudafed® **12 Hour [OTC]** *see* pseudoephedrine *on page 449*

Sudafed® **Cold & Cough Liquid Caps [OTC]** *see* guaifenesin, pseudoephedrine, and dextromethorphan *on page 252*

Sudafed Plus® **Liquid [OTC]** *see* chlorpheniramine and pseudoephedrine *on page 114*

Sudafed Plus® **Tablet [OTC]** *see* chlorpheniramine and pseudoephedrine *on page 114*

Sudafed® **Severe Cold [OTC]** *see* acetaminophen, dextromethorphan, and pseudoephedrine *on page 6*

Sufenta® **Injection** *see* sufentanil *on this page*

sufentanil (soo FEN ta nil)
Synonyms sufentanil citrate
Brand Names Sufenta® Injection
Therapeutic Category Analgesic, Narcotic; General Anesthetic
Controlled Substance C-II
Use Analgesia; analgesia adjunct; anesthetic agent
Usual Dosage I.V.:
Children <12 years: 10-25 mcg/kg with 100% O_2, maintenance: 25-50 mcg as needed (total dose of up to 1-2 mcg/kg)
Adults: Dose should be based on body weight. **Note:** In obese patients (ie, >20% above ideal body weight), use lean body weight to determine dosage
1-2 mcg/kg with N_2O/O_2 for endotracheal intubation; maintenance: 10-25 mcg as needed
2-8 mcg/kg with N_2O/O_2 more complicated major surgical procedures; maintenance: 10-50 mcg as needed
8-30 mcg/kg with 100% O_2 and muscle relaxant produces sleep; at doses of ≥8 mcg/kg maintains a deep level of anesthesia; maintenance: 10-50 mcg as needed
Dosage Forms Injection, as citrate: 50 mcg/mL (1 mL, 2 mL, 5 mL)

sufentanil citrate *see* sufentanil *on this page*

Sular™ *see* nisoldipine *on page 375*

sulbactam and ampicillin *see* ampicillin and sulbactam *on page 33*

sulconazole (sul KON a zole)
Synonyms sulconazole nitrate
Brand Names Exelderm® Topical
Therapeutic Category Antifungal Agent
Use Treatment of superficial fungal infections of the skin, including tinea cruris, tinea corporis, tinea versicolor and possibly tinea pedis
Usual Dosage Topical: Apply once or twice daily for 4-6 weeks
Dosage Forms
Cream, as nitrate: 1% (15 g, 30 g, 60 g)
Solution, as nitrate, topical: 1% (30 mL)

sulconazole nitrate *see* sulconazole *on this page*

Sulf-10® **Ophthalmic** *see* sulfacetamide sodium *on next page*

sulfabenzamide, sulfacetamide, and sulfathiazole
(sul fa BENZ a mide, sul fa SEE ta mide & sul fa THYE a zole)

Synonyms triple sulfa

Brand Names Femguard®; Gyne-Sulf®; Sulfa-Gyn®; Sulfa-Trip®; Sultrin™; Trysul®; V.V.S.®

Therapeutic Category Antibiotic, Vaginal

Use Treatment of *Haemophilus vaginalis* vaginitis

Usual Dosage Adults: Vaginal:
Cream: Insert one applicatorful in vagina twice daily for 4-6 days; dosage may then be decreased to 1/2 to 1/4 of an applicatorful twice daily
Tablet: Insert one intravaginally twice daily for 10 days

Dosage Forms
Cream, vaginal: Sulfabenzamide 3.7%, sulfacetamide 2.86%, and sulfathiazole 3.42% (78 g with applicator, 90 g, 120 g)
Tablet, vaginal: Sulfabenzamide 184 mg, sulfacetamide 143.75 mg, and sulfathiazole 172.5 mg (20 tablets/box with vaginal applicator)

sulfacetamide sodium (sul fa SEE ta mide SOW dee um)

Synonyms sodium sulfacetamide

Brand Names AK-Sulf® Ophthalmic; Bleph®-10 Ophthalmic; Cetamide® Ophthalmic; Isopto® Cetamide® Ophthalmic; Klaron® Lotion; Ocusulf-10® Ophthalmic; Sebizon® Topical Lotion; Sodium Sulamyd® Ophthalmic; Sulf-10® Ophthalmic

Therapeutic Category Antibiotic, Ophthalmic

Use Treatment and prophylaxis of conjunctivitis, corneal ulcers, and other superficial ocular infections due to susceptible organisms; adjunctive treatment with systemic sulfonamides for therapy of trachoma

Usual Dosage Children >2 months and Adults: Ophthalmic:
Ointment: Apply to lower conjunctival sac 1-4 times/day and at bedtime
Solution: 1-2 drops every 2-3 hours in the lower conjunctival sac during the waking hours and less frequently at night

Dosage Forms
Lotion: 10% (59 mL, 85 mL)
Ointment, ophthalmic: 10% (3.5 g)
Solution, ophthalmic: 10% (1 mL, 2 mL, 2.5 mL, 5 mL, 15 mL); 15% (5 mL, 15 mL); 30% (15 mL)

sulfacetamide sodium and fluorometholone
(sul fa SEE ta mide SOW dee um & flure oh METH oh lone)

Brand Names FML-S® Ophthalmic Suspension

Therapeutic Category Antibiotic/Corticosteroid, Ophthalmic

Use Steroid-responsive inflammatory ocular conditions where infection is present or there is a risk of infection

Usual Dosage Children >2 months and Adults: Ophthalmic: Instill 1-3 drops every 2-3 hours while awake

Dosage Forms Suspension, ophthalmic: Sulfacetamide sodium 10% and fluorometholone 0.1% (5 mL, 10 mL)

sulfacetamide sodium and phenylephrine
(sul fa SEE ta mide SOW dee um & fen il EF rin)

Brand Names Vasosulf® Ophthalmic

Therapeutic Category Antibiotic, Ophthalmic

Usual Dosage Ophthalmic: Instill 1-3 drops in lower conjunctival sac every 3-4 hours

Dosage Forms Solution, ophthalmic: Sulfacetamide sodium 15% and phenylephrine hydrochloride 0.125% (5 mL, 15 mL)

sulfacetamide sodium and prednisolone
(sul fa SEE ta mide SOW dee um & pred NIS oh lone)

Synonyms prednisolone acetate and sodium sulfacetamide

Brand Names AK-Cide® Ophthalmic; Blephamide® Ophthalmic; Cetapred® Ophthalmic; Isopto® Cetapred® Ophthalmic; Metimyd® Ophthalmic; Vasocidin® Ophthalmic

Therapeutic Category Antibiotic/Corticosteroid, Ophthalmic

Use Steroid-responsive inflammatory ocular conditions where infection is present or there is a risk of infection; ophthalmic suspension may be used as an otic preparation

Usual Dosage Children >2 and Adults: Ophthalmic:
Ointment: Apply to lower conjunctival sac 1-4 times/day
Solution: Instill 1-3 drops every 2-3 hours while awake

Dosage Forms
Ointment, ophthalmic:
AK-Cide®, Metimyd®, Vasocidin®: Sulfacetamide sodium 10% and prednisolone acetate 0.5% (3.5 g)
Blephamide®: Sulfacetamide sodium 10% and prednisolone acetate 0.2% (3.5 g)
Cetapred®: Sulfacetamide sodium 10% and prednisolone acetate 0.25% (3.5 g)
Suspension, ophthalmic: Sulfacetamide sodium 10% and prednisolone sodium phosphate 0.25% (5 mL)
Suspension, ophthalmic:
AK-Cide®, Metimyd®: Sulfacetamide sodium 10% and prednisolone acetate 0.5% (5 mL)
Blephamide®: Sulfacetamide sodium 10% and prednisolone acetate 0.2% (2.5 mL, 5 mL, 10 mL)
Isopto® Cetapred®: Sulfacetamide sodium 10% and prednisolone acetate 0.25% (5 mL, 15 mL)
Vasocidin®: Sulfacetamide sodium 10% and prednisolone sodium phosphate: 0.25% (5 mL, 10 mL)

Sulfacet-R® Topical *see* sulfur and sulfacetamide sodium *on page 500*

sulfacytine (sul fa SYE teen)
Brand Names Renoquid®
Therapeutic Category Sulfonamide
Use Treatment of urinary tract infections
Usual Dosage Adults: Oral: Initial: 500 mg, then 250 mg every 4 hours for 10 days
Dosage Forms Tablet: 250 mg

sulfadiazine (sul fa DYE a zeen)
Therapeutic Category Sulfonamide
Use Adjunctive treatment in toxoplasmosis; treatment of urinary tract infections and nocardiosis; rheumatic fever prophylaxis in penicillin-allergic patient; uncomplicated attack of malaria

Usual Dosage Oral:
Congenital toxoplasmosis:
Newborns and Children <2 months: 100 mg/kg/day divided every 6 hours in conjunction with pyrimethamine 1 mg/kg/day once daily and supplemental folinic acid 5 mg every 3 days for 6 months
Children >2 months: 25-50 mg/kg/dose 4 times/day
Toxoplasmosis:
Children: 120-150 mg/kg/day, maximum dose: 6 g/day; divided every 6 hours in conjunction with pyrimethamine 2 mg/kg/day divided every 12 hours for 3 days followed by 1 mg/kg/day once daily (maximum: 25 mg/day) with supplemental folinic acid
Adults: 2-8 g/day divided every 6 hours in conjunction with pyrimethamine 25 mg/day and with supplemental folinic acid

Dosage Forms Tablet: 500 mg

sulfadiazine, sulfamethazine, and sulfamerazine
(sul fa DYE a zeen sul fa METH a zeen & sul fa MER a zeen)
Synonyms multiple sulfonamides; trisulfapyrimidines
Therapeutic Category Sulfonamide
Use Treatment of toxoplasmosis
Usual Dosage Adults: Oral: 2-4 g to start, then 2-4 g/day in 3-6 divided doses
Dosage Forms Tablet: Sulfadiazine 167 mg, sulfamethazine 167 mg, and sulfamerazine 167 mg

Sulfa-Gyn® *see* sulfabenzamide, sulfacetamide, and sulfathiazole *on page 496*

Sulfalax® [OTC] *see* docusate *on page 179*

sulfamethoxazole (sul fa meth OKS a zole)
Brand Names Gantanol®; Urobak®
Therapeutic Category Sulfonamide
Use Treatment of urinary tract infections, nocardiosis, chlamydial infections, toxoplasmosis, acute otitis media, and acute exacerbations of chronic bronchitis due to susceptible organisms
Usual Dosage Oral:
Children >2 months: 50-60 mg/kg/day divided every 12 hours; maximum: 3 g/24 hours or 75 mg/kg/day
Adults: 2 g stat, 1 g 2-3 times/day; maximum: 3 g/24 hours
Dosage Forms
Suspension, oral (cherry flavor): 500 mg/5 mL (480 mL)
Tablet: 500 mg

sulfamethoxazole and phenazopyridine
(sul fa meth OKS a zole & fen az oh PEER i deen)
Therapeutic Category Sulfonamide
Use Treatment of urinary tract infections complicated with pain
Usual Dosage Oral: 4 tablets to start, then 2 tablets twice daily for up to 2 days, then switch to sulfamethoxazole only
Dosage Forms Tablet: Sulfamethoxazole 500 mg and phenazopyridine 100 mg

sulfamethoxazole and trimethoprim *see* co-trimoxazole *on page 140*

Sulfamylon® Topical *see* mafenide *on page 317*

sulfanilamide (sul fa NIL a mide)
Brand Names AVC™ Cream; AVC™ Suppository; Vagitrol®
Therapeutic Category Antifungal Agent
Use Treatment of vulvovaginitis caused by *Candida albicans*
Usual Dosage Vaginal: One applicatorful once or twice daily continued through 1 complete menstrual cycle
Dosage Forms
Cream, vaginal (AVC™, Vagitrol®): 15% [150 mg/g] (120 g with applicator)
Suppository, vaginal (AVC™): 1.05 g (16s)

sulfasalazine (sul fa SAL a zeen)
Synonyms salicylazosulfapyridine
Brand Names Azulfidine®; Azulfidine® EN-tabs®
Therapeutic Category 5-Aminosalicylic Acid Derivative
Use Management of ulcerative colitis; treatment of active Crohn's disease
Usual Dosage Oral:
Children >2 years:
Initial: 40-60 mg/kg/day divided every 4-6 hour

Maintenance dose: 20-30 mg/kg/day divided every 6 hours, up to a maximum of 2 g/day

Adults:

Initial: 3-4 g/day divided every 4-6 hours

Maintenance dose: 2 g/day divided every 6 hours

Dosage Forms

Suspension, oral: 250 mg/5 mL (473 mL)

Tablet: 500 mg

Enteric coated: 500 mg

Sulfatrim® *see* co-trimoxazole *on page 140*

Sulfa-Trip® *see* sulfabenzamide, sulfacetamide, and sulfathiazole *on page 496*

sulfinpyrazone (sul fin PEER a zone)

Brand Names Anturane®

Therapeutic Category Uricosuric Agent

Use Treatment of chronic gouty arthritis and intermittent gouty arthritis

Usual Dosage Oral: 200 mg twice daily

Dosage Forms

Capsule: 200 mg

Tablet: 100 mg

sulfisoxazole (sul fi SOKS a zole)

Synonyms sulfisoxazole acetyl; sulphafurazole

Brand Names Gantrisin®

Therapeutic Category Sulfonamide

Use Treatment of uncomplicated urinary tract infections, otitis media, *Chlamydia*; nocardiosis; treatment of acute pelvic inflammatory disease in prepubertal children

Usual Dosage

Children >2 months: Oral: 75 mg/kg stat, 120-150 mg/kg/day in divided doses every 4-6 hours; not to exceed 6 g/day

Pelvic inflammatory disease: 100 mg/kg/day in divided doses every 6 hours; used in combination with ceftriaxone

Chlamydia trachomatis: 100 mg/kg/day divided every 6 hours

Adults: Oral: 2-4 g stat, 4-8 g/day in divided doses every 4-6 hours

Dosage Forms

Suspension, oral, pediatric, as acetyl (raspberry flavor): 500 mg/5 mL (480 mL)

Tablet: 500 mg

sulfisoxazole acetyl *see* sulfisoxazole *on this page*

sulfisoxazole and erythromycin *see* erythromycin and sulfisoxazole *on page 200*

sulfisoxazole and phenazopyridine

(sul fi SOKS a zole & fen az oh PEER i deen)

Therapeutic Category Sulfonamide

Use Treatment of urinary tract infections and nocardiosis

Usual Dosage Oral: 4-6 tablets to start, then 2 tablets 4 times/day for 2 days, then continue with sulfisoxazole only

Dosage Forms Tablet: Sulfisoxazole 500 mg and phenazopyridine 50 mg

sulfur and salicylic acid (SUL fur & sal i SIL ik AS id)

Synonyms salicylic acid and sulfur

Brand Names Aveeno® Cleansing Bar [OTC]; Fostex® [OTC]; Pernox® [OTC]; SAStid® Plain Therapeutic Shampoo and Acne Wash [OTC]

Therapeutic Category Antiseborrheic Agent, Topical

Use Therapeutic shampoo for dandruff and seborrheal dermatitis; acne skin cleanser

(Continued)

sulfur and salicylic acid *(Continued)*

Usual Dosage Children and Adults: Topical:
Shampoo: Initial: Use daily or every other day; 1-2 treatments/week will usually maintain control
Soap: Use daily or every other day

Dosage Forms
Cake: Sulfur 2% and salicylic acid 2% (123 g)
Cleanser: Sulfur 2% and salicylic acid 1.5% (60 mL, 120 mL)
Shampoo: Micropulverized sulfur 2% and salicylic acid 2% (120 mL, 240 mL)
Soap: Micropulverized sulfur 2% and salicylic acid 2% (113 g)
Wash: Sulfur 1.6% and salicylic acid 1.6% (75 mL)

sulfur and sulfacetamide sodium

(SUL fur & sul fa SEE ta mide SOW dee um)
Synonyms sodium sulfacetamide and sulfur
Brand Names Novacet® Topical; Sulfacet-R® Topical
Therapeutic Category Antiseborrheic Agent, Topical
Use Aid in the treatment of acne vulgaris, acne rosacea and seborrheic dermatitis
Usual Dosage Topical: Apply in a thin film 1-3 times/day
Dosage Forms Lotion, topical: Sulfur colloid 5% and sulfacetamide sodium 10% (30 mL)

sulindac (sul IN dak)

Brand Names Clinoril®
Therapeutic Category Analgesic, Non-narcotic; Nonsteroidal Anti-Inflammatory Agent (NSAID)
Use Management of inflammatory disease, rheumatoid disorders; acute gouty arthritis
Usual Dosage Oral:
Children: Dose not established
Adults: 150-200 mg twice daily; not to exceed 400 mg/day
Dosage Forms Tablet: 150 mg, 200 mg

sulphafurazole *see* sulfisoxazole *on previous page*

Sultrin™ *see* sulfabenzamide, sulfacetamide, and sulfathiazole *on page 496*

Sumacal® **[OTC]** *see* glucose polymers *on page 242*

sumatriptan succinate (SOO ma trip tan SUKS i nate)

Brand Names Imitrex®
Therapeutic Category Antimigraine Agent
Use Acute treatment of migraine with or without aura
Unlabeled use: Cluster headaches
Usual Dosage Adults:
Oral: Maximum dose: 300 mg every 24 hours
S.C.: 6 mg; a second injection may be administered at least 1 hour after the initial dose, but not more than 2 injections in a 24-hour period
Dosage Forms
Injection: 12 mg/mL (0.5 mL, 2 mL)
Tablet: 25 mg, 50 mg

Summer's Eve® **Medicated Douche [OTC]** *see* povidone-iodine *on page 431*

Sumycin® **Oral** *see* tetracycline *on page 510*

sunscreen (paba-free) *see* methoxycinnamate and oxybenzone *on page 339*

SuperChar® **[OTC]** *see* charcoal *on page 105*

Supprelin™ **Injection** *see* histrelin *on page 261*

Suppress® **[OTC]** *see* dextromethorphan *on page 160*

Suprane® *see* desflurane *on page 154*

Suprax® *see* cefixime *on page 97*

suprofen (soo PROE fen)
Brand Names Profenal® Ophthalmic
Therapeutic Category Nonsteroidal Anti-Inflammatory Agent (NSAID)
Use Inhibition of intraoperative miosis
Usual Dosage Ophthalmic: On day of surgery, instill 2 drops in conjunctival sac at 3, 2, and 1 hour prior to surgery; or 2 drops in sac every 4 hours, while awake, the day preceding surgery
Dosage Forms Solution, ophthalmic: 1% (2.5 mL)

Surbex® **[OTC]** *see* vitamin b complex *on page 553*

Surbex-T® **Filmtabs**® **[OTC]** *see* vitamin b complex with vitamin c *on page 553*

Surbex® **with C Filmtabs**® **[OTC]** *see* vitamin b complex with vitamin c *on page 553*

Surfak® **[OTC]** *see* docusate *on page 179*

Surgicel® *see* cellulose, oxidized *on page 102*

Surmontil® *see* trimipramine *on page 535*

Survanta® *see* beractant *on page 63*

Sus-Phrine® *see* epinephrine *on page 195*

Sustaire® *see* theophylline *on page 511*

suxamethonium chloride *see* succinylcholine *on page 494*

Sween Cream® **[OTC]** *see* methylbenzethonium chloride *on page 341*

Swim-Ear® **Otic [OTC]** *see* boric acid *on page 70*

Syllact® **[OTC]** *see* psyllium *on page 451*

Symmetrel® *see* amantadine *on page 22*

Synacol® **CF [OTC]** *see* guaifenesin and dextromethorphan *on page 248*

Synacort® *see* hydrocortisone *on page 268*

synacthen *see* cosyntropin *on page 139*

Synalar® *see* fluocinolone *on page 226*

Synalar-HP® *see* fluocinolone *on page 226*

Synalgos®**-DC** *see* dihydrocodeine compound *on page 169*

Synarel® *see* nafarelin *on page 361*

Synemol® *see* fluocinolone *on page 226*

synthetic lung surfactant *see* colfosceril palmitate *on page 136*

Synthroid® *see* levothyroxine *on page 306*

Syntocinon® *see* oxytocin *on page 392*

Syprine® *see* trientine *on page 531*

Syracol-CF® **[OTC]** *see* guaifenesin and dextromethorphan *on page 248*

t₃/t₄ liotrix *see* liotrix *on page 310*

t₃ thyronine sodium *see* liothyronine *on page 309*

t₄ thyroxine sodium *see* levothyroxine *on page 306*

Tac™**-3** *see* triamcinolone *on page 528*

Tac™**-40** *see* triamcinolone *on page 528*

TACE® *see* chlorotrianisene *on page 112*

tacrine (TAK reen)
Synonyms tacrine hydrochloride; tetrahydroaminoacrine; tha
Brand Names Cognex®
Therapeutic Category Acetylcholinesterase Inhibitor
Use Treatment of Alzheimer's disease
Usual Dosage Adults: Oral: 40 mg/day
Dosage Forms Capsule, as hydrochloride: 10 mg, 20 mg, 30 mg, 40 mg

tacrine hydrochloride *see* tacrine *on this page*

tacrolimus (ta KROE li mus)
Synonyms FK506
Brand Names Prograf®
Therapeutic Category Immunosuppressant Agent
Use Potent immunosuppressive drug used in liver, kidney, heart, lung, or small bowel transplant recipients
Usual Dosage
Initial: I.V. continuous infusion: 0.1 mg/kg/day until the tolerance of oral intake
Oral: Usually 3-4 times the I.V. dose, or 0.3 mg/kg/day in divided doses every 12 hours
Dosage Forms
Capsule: 1 mg, 5 mg
Injection, with alcohol and surfactant: 5 mg/mL (1 mL)

Tagamet® *see* cimetidine *on page 123*

Tagamet® HB [OTC] *see* cimetidine *on page 123*

Talacen® *see* pentazocine compound *on page 404*

Talwin® *see* pentazocine *on page 403*

Talwin® Compound *see* pentazocine compound *on page 404*

Talwin® NX *see* pentazocine *on page 403*

Tambocor™ *see* flecainide *on page 223*

Tamine® [OTC] *see* brompheniramine and phenylpropanolamine *on page 73*

tamoxifen (ta MOKS i fen)
Synonyms tamoxifen citrate
Brand Names Nolvadex®
Therapeutic Category Antineoplastic Agent
Use Palliative or adjunctive treatment of advanced breast cancer in postmenopausal women
Usual Dosage Oral: 10-20 mg twice daily
Dosage Forms Tablet, as citrate: 10 mg, 20 mg

tamoxifen citrate *see* tamoxifen *on this page*

tamsulosin (tam SOO loe sin)
Synonyms tamsulosin hydrochloride
Brand Names Flomax™
Therapeutic Category Alpha-Adrenergic Blocking Agent
Use Treatment of sings and symptoms of benign prostatic hyperplasia (BPH)
Usual Dosage Oral: Adults: 0.4 mg once daily approximately 30 minutes after the same meal each day
Dosage Forms Capsule, as hydrochloride: 0.4 mg

tamsulosin hydrochloride *see* tamsulosin *on this page*

Tanac® [OTC] *see* benzocaine *on page 59*

Tanoral® **Tablet** *see* chlorpheniramine, pyrilamine, and phenylephrine *on page 118*

Tao® *see* troleandomycin *on page 537*

Tapazole® *see* methimazole *on page 336*

Tarka® *see* trandolapril and verapamil *on page 526*

tat *see* tetanus antitoxin *on page 508*

Tavist® *see* clemastine *on page 126*

Tavist®**-1 [OTC]** *see* clemastine *on page 126*

Tavist-D® *see* clemastine and phenylpropanolamine *on page 127*

Taxol® *see* paclitaxel *on page 393*

Taxotere® *see* docetaxel *on page 179*

tazarotene (taz AR oh teen)
   Brand Names Tazorac®
   Therapeutic Category Keratolytic Agent
   Use Topical treatment of facial acne fulgaris; topical treatment of stable plaque psoriasis of up to,20% body surface area involvement
   Dosage Forms Gel: 0.05% (30 g, 100 g); 0.1% (30 g, 100 g)

Tazicef® *see* ceftazidime *on page 100*

Tazidime® *see* ceftazidime *on page 100*

Tazorac® *see* tazarotene *on this page*

3TC *see* lamivudine *on page 301*

tcn *see* tetracycline *on page 510*

td *see* diphtheria and tetanus toxoid *on page 174*

Tear Drop® **Solution [OTC]** *see* artificial tears *on page 42*

TearGard® **Ophthalmic Solution [OTC]** *see* artificial tears *on page 42*

Teargen® **Ophthalmic Solution [OTC]** *see* artificial tears *on page 42*

Tearisol® **Solution [OTC]** *see* artificial tears *on page 42*

Tears Naturale® **Free Solution [OTC]** *see* artificial tears *on page 42*

Tears Naturale® **II Solution [OTC]** *see* artificial tears *on page 42*

Tears Naturale® **Solution [OTC]** *see* artificial tears *on page 42*

Tears Plus® **Solution [OTC]** *see* artificial tears *on page 42*

Tears Renewed® **Solution [OTC]** *see* artificial tears *on page 42*

Tebamide® *see* trimethobenzamide *on page 534*

Teczem® *see* enalapril and diltiazem *on page 192*

Tedral® *see* theophylline, ephedrine, and phenobarbital *on page 513*

Tegison® *see* etretinate *on page 214*

Tegopen® *see* cloxacillin *on page 132*

Tegretol® *see* carbamazepine *on page 89*

Tegretol-XR® *see* carbamazepine *on page 89*

Tegrin®**-HC [OTC]** *see* hydrocortisone *on page 268*

Telachlor® *see* chlorpheniramine *on page 113*

Teladar® *see* betamethasone *on page 64*

Teldrin® **[OTC]** *see* chlorpheniramine *on page 113*

Telepaque® *see* radiological/contrast media (ionic) *on page 457*

temazepam (te MAZ e pam)
Brand Names Restoril®
Therapeutic Category Benzodiazepine
Controlled Substance C-IV
Use Treatment of anxiety and as an adjunct in the treatment of depression; also may be used in the management of panic attacks; transient insomnia and sleep latency
Usual Dosage Adults: Oral: 15-30 mg at bedtime
Dosage Forms Capsule: 7.5 mg, 15 mg, 30 mg

Temazin® Cold Syrup [OTC] *see* chlorpheniramine and phenylpropanolamine *on page 114*

Temovate® *see* clobetasol *on page 128*

Tempra® [OTC] *see* acetaminophen *on page 3*

Tenex® *see* guanfacine *on page 253*

teniposide (ten i POE side)
Synonyms ept; vm-26
Brand Names Vumon Injection
Therapeutic Category Antineoplastic Agent
Use Treatment of Hodgkin's and non-Hodgkin's lymphomas, acute lymphocytic leukemia, bladder carcinoma and neuroblastoma
Usual Dosage I.V.:
Children: 130 mg/m^2/week, increasing to 150 mg/m^2 after 3 weeks and to 180 mg/m^2 after 6 weeks
Adults: 50-180 mg/m^2 once or twice weekly for 4-6 weeks
Dosage Forms Injection: 10 mg/mL (5 mL)

Ten-K® *see* potassium chloride *on page 427*

Tenoretic® *see* atenolol and chlorthalidone *on page 46*

Tenormin® *see* atenolol *on page 45*

Tensilon® Injection *see* edrophonium *on page 190*

Tenuate® *see* diethylpropion *on page 166*

Tenuate® Dospan® *see* diethylpropion *on page 166*

Terak® Ophthalmic Ointment *see* oxytetracycline and polymyxin b *on page 392*

Terazol® Vaginal *see* terconazole *on next page*

terazosin (ter AY zoe sin)
Brand Names Hytrin®
Therapeutic Category Alpha-Adrenergic Blocking Agent
Use Management of mild to moderate hypertension; considered a step 2 drug in stepped approach to hypertension; benign prostate hypertrophy
Usual Dosage Adults: Oral: 1 mg; slowly increase dose to achieve desired blood pressure, up to 20 mg/day
Dosage Forms
Capsule: 1 mg, 2 mg, 5 mg, 10 mg
Tablet: 1 mg, 2 mg, 5 mg, 10 mg

terbinafine, oral (TER bin a feen, OR al)
Brand Names Lamisil® Oral
Therapeutic Category Antifungal Agent
Use Treatment of onychomycosis infections of the toenail or fingernail
Usual Dosage Adults: Oral:
Fingernail onychomycosis: 250 mg once daily for 6 weeks

Toenail onychomycosis: 250 mg once daily for 12 weeks
Dosage Forms Tablet: 250 mg

terbinafine, topical (TER bin a feen, TOP i kal)
Brand Names Lamisil® Cream
Therapeutic Category Antifungal Agent
Use Topical antifungal for the treatment of tinea pedis (athlete's foot), tinea cruris (jock itch), and tinea corporis (ring worm)
Unlabeled use: Cutaneous candidiasis and pityriasis versicolor
Usual Dosage Adults: Topical:
Athlete's foot: Apply to affected area twice daily for at least 1 week, not to exceed 4 weeks
Ringworm and jock itch: Apply to affected area once or twice daily for at least 1 week, not to exceed 4 weeks
Dosage Forms Cream: 1% (15 g, 30 g)

terbutaline (ter BYOO ta leen)
Synonyms terbutaline sulfate
Brand Names Brethaire®; Brethine®; Bricanyl®
Therapeutic Category Adrenergic Agonist Agent
Use Bronchodilator in reversible airway obstruction and bronchial asthma
Usual Dosage
Children <12 years:
Oral: Initial: 0.05 mg/kg/dose 3 times/day, increased gradually as required; maximum: 0.15 mg/kg/dose 3-4 times/day or a total of 5 mg/24 hours
S.C.: 0.005-0.01 mg/kg/dose to a maximum of 0.3 mg/dose every 15-20 minutes for 3 doses
Inhalation nebulization dose: 0.06 mg/kg; maximum: 8 mg
Inhalation: 0.3 mg/kg/dose up to maximum of 10 mg/dose every 4-6 hours
Children >12 years and Adults:
Oral:
12-15 years: 2.5 mg every 6 hours 3 times/day; not to exceed 7.5 mg in 24 hours
>15 years: 5 mg/dose every 6 hours 3 times/day; if side effects occur, reduce dose to 2.5 mg every 6 hours; not to exceed 15 mg in 24 hours
S.C.: 0.25 mg/dose repeated in 15-30 minutes for one time only; a total dose of 0.5 mg should not be exceeded within a 4-hour period
Nebulization: 0.01-0.03 mL/kg (1 mg = 1 mL); minimum dose: 0.1 mL; maximum dose: 2.5 mL diluted with 1-2 mL normal saline
Inhalation: 2 inhalations every 4-6 hours; wait 1 minute between inhalations
Dosage Forms
Aerosol, oral, as sulfate: 0.2 mg/actuation (10.5 g)
Injection, as sulfate: 1 mg/mL (1 mL)
Tablet, as sulfate: 2.5 mg, 5 mg

terbutaline sulfate see terbutaline on this page

terconazole (ter KONE a zole)
Synonyms triaconazole
Brand Names Terazol® Vaginal
Therapeutic Category Antifungal Agent
Use Local treatment of vulvovaginal candidiasis
Usual Dosage Vaginal: 1 applicatorful in vagina at bedtime for 7 consecutive days
Dosage Forms
Cream, vaginal: 0.4% (45 g); 0.8% (20 g)
Suppository, vaginal: 80 mg (3s)

terfenadine (ter FEN a deen)
Brand Names Seldane®
Therapeutic Category Antihistamine
Use Perennial and seasonal allergic rhinitis and other allergic symptoms including urticaria
Usual Dosage Oral:
Children:
3-6 years: 15 mg twice daily
6-12 years: 30 mg twice daily
Children >12 years and Adults: 60 mg twice daily
Dosage Forms Tablet: 60 mg

terfenadine and pseudoephedrine (ter FEN a deen & soo doe e FED rin)
Brand Names Seldane-D®
Therapeutic Category Antihistamine/Decongestant Combination
Use Perennial and seasonal allergic rhinitis and other allergic symptoms including urticaria; has drying effect in patients with asthma
Usual Dosage Adults: Oral: 1 tablet every morning and at bedtime
Dosage Forms Tablet: Terfenadine 60 mg and pseudoephedrine hydrochloride 120 mg

teriparatide (ter i PAR a tide)
Brand Names Parathar™ Injection
Therapeutic Category Diagnostic Agent
Use Diagnosis of hypocalcemia in either hypoparathyroidism or pseudohypoparathyroidism
Usual Dosage I.V.:
Children ≥3 years: 3 units/kg up to 200 units
Adults: 200 units over 10 minutes
Dosage Forms Powder for injection: 200 units hPTH activity (10 mL)

terpin hydrate (TER pin HYE drate)
Therapeutic Category Expectorant
Use Symptomatic relief of cough
Usual Dosage Adults: Oral: 5-10 mL every 4-6 hours as needed
Dosage Forms Elixir: 85 mg/5 mL (120 mL)

terpin hydrate and codeine (TER pin HYE drate & KOE deen)
Synonyms eth and c
Therapeutic Category Antitussive/Expectorant
Controlled Substance C-V
Use Symptomatic relief of cough
Usual Dosage Based on codeine content: Oral:
Children (not recommended): 1-1.5 mg/kg/24 hours divided every 4 hours; maximum: 30 mg/24 hours
2-6 years: 1.25-2.5 mL every 4-6 hours as needed
6-12 years: 2.5-5 mL every 4-6 hours as needed
Adults: 10-20 mg/dose every 4-6 hours as needed
Dosage Forms Elixir: Terpin hydrate 85 mg and codeine 10 mg per 5 mL with alcohol 42.5%

Terra-Cortril® Ophthalmic Suspension *see* oxytetracycline and hydrocortisone *on page 392*

Terramycin® I.M. Injection *see* oxytetracycline *on page 392*

Terramycin® Ophthalmic Ointment *see* oxytetracycline and polymyxin b *on page 392*

Terramycin® Oral *see* oxytetracycline *on page 392*

Terramycin® w/Polymyxin B Ophthalmic Ointment *see* oxytetracycline and polymyxin b *on page 392*

Tesamone® Injection *see* testosterone *on this page*

Teslac® *see* testolactone *on this page*

tespa *see* thiotepa *on page 517*

Tessalon® Perles *see* benzonatate *on page 61*

Testoderm® Transdermal System *see* testosterone *on this page*

testolactone (tes toe LAK tone)
Brand Names Teslac®
Therapeutic Category Androgen
Use Palliative treatment of advanced disseminated breast carcinoma
Usual Dosage Adults: Females: Oral: 250 mg 4 times/day for at least 3 months; desired response may take as long as 3 months
Dosage Forms Tablet: 50 mg

Testopel® Pellet *see* testosterone *on this page*

testosterone (tes TOS ter one)
Synonyms aqueous testosterone; testosterone cypionate; testosterone enanthate; testosterone propionate
Brand Names Androderm® Transdermal System; Andro-L.A.® Injection; Andropository® Injection; Delatest® Injection; Delatestryl® Injection; depAndro® Injection; Depotest® Injection; Depo®-Testosterone Injection; Duratest® Injection; Durathate® Injection; Everone® Injection; Histerone® Injection; Tesamone® Injection; Testoderm® Transdermal System; Testopel® Pellet
Therapeutic Category Androgen
Controlled Substance C-III
Use Androgen replacement therapy in the treatment of delayed male puberty; male hypogonadism
Usual Dosage I.M.:
Delayed puberty: Children: 40-50 mg/m^2/dose (cypionate or enanthate) monthly for 6 months
Male hypogonadism: 50-400 mg every 2-4 weeks
Initiation of pubertal growth: 40-50 mg/m^2/dose (cypionate or enanthate) monthly until the growth rate falls to prepubertal levels (~5 cm/year)
During terminal growth phase: 100 mg/m^2/dose (cypionate or enanthate) monthly until growth ceases
Maintenance virilizing dose: 100 mg/m^2/dose (cypionate or enanthate) twice monthly or 50-400 mg/dose every 2-4 weeks
Inoperable breast cancer: Adults: 200-400 mg every 2-4 weeks
Hypogonadism: Adults:
Testosterone or testosterone propionate: 10-25 mg 2-3 times/week
Testosterone cypionate or enanthate: 50-400 mg every 2-4 weeks
Postpubertal cryptorchism: Testosterone or testosterone propionate: 10-25 mg 2-3 times/week
Transdermal system: Males: Place the patch on clean, dry, scrotal skin; dry-shaved scrotal hair for optimal skin contact, do not use chemical depilatories; patients should start therapy with 6 mg/day system applied daily; if scrotal area is inadequate, use a 4 mg/day system; the system should be worn for 22-24 hours
Dosage Forms
Injection:
Aqueous suspension: 25 mg/mL (10 mL, 30 mL); 50 mg/mL (10 mL, 30 mL); 100 mg/mL (10 mL, 30 mL)
In oil, as cypionate: 100 mg/mL (1 mL, 10 mL); 200 mg/mL (1 mL, 10 mL)
In oil, as enanthate: 100 mg/mL (5 mL, 10 mL); 200 mg/mL (5 mL, 10 mL)
(Continued)

testosterone *(Continued)*

In oil, as propionate: 50 mg/mL (10 mL, 30 mL); 100 mg/mL (10 mL, 30 mL)
Pellet: 75 mg (1 pellet per vial)
Transdermal system: 2.5 mg/day; 4 mg/day; 6 mg/day

testosterone and estradiol *see* estradiol and testosterone *on page 203*

testosterone cypionate *see* testosterone *on previous page*

testosterone enanthate *see* testosterone *on previous page*

testosterone propionate *see* testosterone *on previous page*

Testred® *see* methyltestosterone *on page 343*

tetanus and diphtheria toxoid *see* diphtheria and tetanus toxoid *on page 174*

tetanus antitoxin (TET a nus an tee TOKS in)

Synonyms tat

Therapeutic Category Antitoxin

Use Tetanus prophylaxis or treatment of active tetanus only when tetanus immune globulin (TIG) is not available

Usual Dosage
Prophylaxis: I.M., S.C.:
Children <30 kg: 1500 units
Children and Adults >30 kg: 3000-5000 units
Treatment: Children and Adults: Inject 10,000-40,000 units into wound; administer 40,000-100,000 units I.V.

Dosage Forms Injection, equine: Not less than 400 units/mL (12.5 mL, 50 mL)

tetanus immune globulin (human)

(TET a nus i MYUN GLOB yoo lin, HYU man)

Synonyms tig

Brand Names Hyper-Tet®

Therapeutic Category Immune Globulin

Use Passive immunization against tetanus; tetanus immune globulin is preferred over tetanus antitoxin for treatment of active tetanus; part of the management of an unclean, nonminor wound in a person whose history of previous receipt of tetanus toxoid is unknown or who has received less than three doses of tetanus toxoid

Usual Dosage I.M.:
Prophylaxis of tetanus:
Children: 4 units/kg; some recommend administering 250 units to small children
Adults: 250 units
Treatment of tetanus:
Children: 500-3000 units; some should infiltrate locally around the wound
Adults: 3000-6000 units

Dosage Forms Injection: 250 units/mL

tetanus toxoid (adsorbed) (TET a nus TOKS oyd, ad SORBED)

Therapeutic Category Toxoid

Use Active immunization against tetanus

Usual Dosage Adults: I.M.:
Primary immunization: 0.5 mL; repeat 0.5 mL at 4-8 weeks after first dose and at 6-12 months after second dose
Routine booster doses are recommended only every 5-10 years

Dosage Forms Injection, adsorbed:
Tetanus 5 Lf units per 0.5 mL dose (0.5 mL, 5 mL)
Tetanus 10 Lf units per 0.5 mL dose (0.5 mL, 5 mL)

tetanus toxoid (fluid) (TET a nus TOKS oyd FLOO id)
Synonyms tetanus toxoid plain
Therapeutic Category Toxoid
Use Active immunization against tetanus in adults and children
Usual Dosage Inject 3 doses of 0.5 mL I.M. or S.C. at 4- to 8-week intervals with fourth dose administered only 6-12 months after third dose
Dosage Forms Injection, fluid:
Tetanus 4 Lf units per 0.5 mL dose (7.5 mL)
Tetanus 5 Lf units per 0.5 mL dose (0.5 mL, 7.5 mL)

tetanus toxoid plain *see* tetanus toxoid (fluid) *on this page*

tetracaine (TET ra kane)
Synonyms amethocaine hydrochloride; tetracaine hydrochloride
Brand Names Pontocaine®
Therapeutic Category Local Anesthetic
Use Local anesthesia in the eye for various diagnostic and examination purposes; spinal anesthesia; topical anesthesia for local skin disorders; local anesthesia for mucous membranes
Usual Dosage
Children: Safety and efficacy have not been established
Adults:
Ophthalmic (not for prolonged use):
Ointment: Apply ½" to 1" to lower conjunctival fornix
Solution: Instill 1-2 drops
Spinal anesthesia 1% solution:
Subarachnoid injection: 5-20 mg
Saddle block: 2-5 mg; a 1% solution should be diluted with equal volume of CSF before administration
Topical mucous membranes (2% solution): Apply as needed; dose should not exceed 20 mg
Topical for skin: Apply to affected areas as needed
Dosage Forms
Cream, as hydrochloride: 1% (28 g)
Injection, as hydrochloride: 1% [10 mg/mL] (2 mL)
With dextrose 6%: 0.2% [2 mg/mL] (2 mL); 0.3% [3 mg/mL] (5 mL)
Ointment, as hydrochloride:
Ophthalmic: 0.5% [5 mg/mL] (3.75 g)
Topical: 0.5% [5 mg/mL] (28 g)
Powder for injection, as hydrochloride: 20 mg
Solution, as hydrochloride:
Ophthalmic: 0.5% [5 mg/mL] (1 mL, 2 mL, 15 mL, 59 mL)
Topical: 2% [20 mg/mL] (30 mL, 118 mL)

tetracaine and dextrose (TET ra kane & DEKS trose)
Brand Names Pontocaine® With Dextrose Injection
Therapeutic Category Local Anesthetic
Use Spinal anesthesia (saddle block)
Usual Dosage Dose varies with procedure, depth of anesthesia, duration desired and physical condition of patient
Dosage Forms Injection: Tetracaine hydrochloride 0.2% and dextrose 6% (2 mL); tetracaine hydrochloride 0.3% and dextrose 6% (5 mL)

tetracaine hydrochloride *see* tetracaine *on this page*
tetracosactide *see* cosyntropin *on page 139*

tetracycline (tet ra SYE kleen)

Synonyms tcn; tetracycline hydrochloride

Brand Names Achromycin® Ophthalmic; Achromycin® Topical; Sumycin® Oral; Topicycline® Topical

Therapeutic Category Antibiotic, Ophthalmic; Antibiotic, Topical; Tetracycline Derivative

Use

Children, Adolescents, and Adults: Treatment of Rocky mountain spotted fever caused by susceptible Rickettsia or brucellosis

Adolescents and Adults: Presumptive treatment of chlamydial infection in patients with gonorrhea

Older Children, Adolescents, and Adults: Treatment of Lyme disease, mycoplasmal disease or *Legionella*

Usual Dosage

Children >8 years:

Oral: 25-50 mg/kg/day in divided doses every 6 hours; not to exceed 3 g/day

Ophthalmic:

Suspension: Instill 1-2 drops 2-4 times/day or more often as needed

Ointment: Instill every 2-12 hours

Adults:

Oral: 250-500 mg/dose every 6 hours

Ophthalmic:

Suspension: Instill 1-2 drops 2-4 times/day or more often as needed

Ointment: Instill every 2-12 hours

Topical: Apply to affected areas 1-4 times/day

Dosage Forms

Capsule, as hydrochloride: 100 mg, 250 mg, 500 mg

Ointment:

Ophthalmic: 1% [10 mg/mL] (3.5 g)

Topical, as hydrochloride: 3% [30 mg/mL] (14.2 g, 30 g)

Solution, topical: 2.2 mg/mL (70 mL)

Suspension:

Ophthalmic: 1% [10 mg/mL] (0.5 mL, 1 mL, 4 mL)

Oral, as hydrochloride: 125 mg/5 mL (60 mL, 480 mL)

Tablet, as hydrochloride: 250 mg, 500 mg

tetracycline hydrochloride *see* tetracycline *on this page*

tetrahydroaminoacrine *see* tacrine *on page 502*

tetrahydrocannabinol *see* dronabinol *on page 185*

tetrahydrozoline (tet ra hye DROZ a leen)

Synonyms tetrahydrozoline hydrochloride; tetryzoline

Brand Names Collyrium Fresh® Ophthalmic [OTC]; Eyesine® Ophthalmic [OTC]; Geneye® Ophthalmic [OTC]; Mallazine® Eye Drops [OTC]; Murine® Plus Ophthalmic [OTC]; Optigene® Ophthalmic [OTC]; Tetrasine® Extra Ophthalmic [OTC]; Tetrasine® Ophthalmic [OTC]; Tyzine® Nasal; Visine® Extra Ophthalmic [OTC]

Therapeutic Category Adrenergic Agonist Agent

Use Symptomatic relief of nasal congestion and conjunctival congestion

Usual Dosage

Nasal congestion:

Children 2-6 years: Instill 2-3 drops of 0.05% solution every 4-6 hours as needed

Children >6 years and Adults: Instill 2-4 drops or 0.1% spray nasal mucosa every 4-6 hours as needed

Conjunctival congestion: Adults: Instill 1-2 drops in each eye 2-3 times/day

Dosage Forms Solution, as hydrochloride:

Nasal: 0.05% (15 mL), 0.1% (30 mL, 473 mL)

Ophthalmic: 0.05% (15 mL)

tetrahydrozoline hydrochloride *see* tetrahydrozoline *on previous page*

Tetramune® *see* diphtheria, tetanus toxoids, whole-cell pertussis, and *haemophilus* b conjugate vaccine *on page 176*

Tetrasine® **Extra Ophthalmic [OTC]** *see* tetrahydrozoline *on previous page*

Tetrasine® **Ophthalmic [OTC]** *see* tetrahydrozoline *on previous page*

tetryzoline *see* tetrahydrozoline *on previous page*

tg *see* thioguanine *on page 515*

6-tg *see* thioguanine *on page 515*

T/Gel® **[OTC]** *see* coal tar *on page 132*

T-Gen® *see* trimethobenzamide *on page 534*

T-Gesic® *see* hydrocodone and acetaminophen *on page 266*

tha *see* tacrine *on page 502*

Thalitone® *see* chlorthalidone *on page 120*

THAM-E® **Injection** *see* tromethamine *on page 538*

THAM® **Injection** *see* tromethamine *on page 538*

thc *see* dronabinol *on page 185*

Theo-24® *see* theophylline *on this page*

Theobid® *see* theophylline *on this page*

Theochron® *see* theophylline *on this page*

Theoclear-80® *see* theophylline *on this page*

Theoclear® **L.A.** *see* theophylline *on this page*

Theo-Dur® *see* theophylline *on this page*

Theolair™ *see* theophylline *on this page*

theophylline (thee OF i lin)

Brand Names Aerolate III®; Aerolate JR®; Aerolate SR®; Aquaphyllin®; Asmalix®; Bronkodyl®; Elixomin®; Elixophyllin®; Lanophyllin®; Quibron®-T; Quibron®-T/SR; Respbid®; Slo-bid™; Slo-Phyllin®; Sustaire®; Theo-24®; Theobid®; Theochron®; Theoclear-80®; Theoclear® L.A.; Theo-Dur®; Theolair™; Theo-Sav®; Theospan®-SR; Theostat-80®; Theovent®; Theo-X®; T-Phyl®; Uni-Dur®; Uniphyl®

Therapeutic Category Theophylline Derivative

Use Treatment of symptoms and reversible airway obstruction due to chronic asthma, chronic bronchitis, or COPD; for treatment of idiopathic apnea of prematurity in neonates

Usual Dosage
Apnea: Dosage should be determined by plasma level monitoring; each 0.5 mg/kg of theophylline administered as a loading dose will result in a 1 mcg/mL increase in serum theophylline concentration

Loading dose: 5 mg/kg; dilute dose in 1 hour I.V. fluid via syringe pump over one hour
Maintenance: 2 mg/kg every 8-12 hours or 1-3 mg/kg/dose every 8-12 hours; administer I.V. push 1 mL/minute (2 mg/minute)

Treatment of acute bronchospasm in older patients: (>6 months of age): Loading dose (in patients not currently receiving theophylline): 6 mg/kg (based on aminophylline) administered I.V. over 20-30 minutes; 4.7 mg/kg (based on theophylline) administered I.V. over 20-30 minutes; administration rate should not exceed 20 mg (1 mL)/minute (theophylline) or 25 mg (1 mL)/minute (aminophylline)

Approximate maintenance dosage for treatment of acute bronchospasm:
Children: 6 months to 9 years of age: 1.2 mg/kg/hour (aminophylline); 0.95 mg/kg/hour (theophylline); 9-16 years and young adult smokers: 1 mg/kg/hour (aminophylline); 0.79 mg/kg/hour (theophylline)
(Continued)

theophylline *(Continued)*

Adults (healthy, nonsmoking): 0.7 mg/kg/hour (aminophylline); 0.55 mg/kg/hour (theophylline)

Older patients and patients with cor pulmonale: 0.6 mg/kg/hour (aminophylline); 0.47 mg/kg/hour (theophylline)

Patients with CHF or liver failure: 0.5 mg/kg/hour (aminophylline); 0.39 mg/kg/hour (theophylline)

Chronic therapy: Slow clinical titration is generally preferred. Initial dose: 16 mg/kg/24 hours or 400 mg/24 hours, whichever is less; increasing dose: the above dosage may be increased in approximately 25% increments at 2- to 3-day intervals so long as the drug is tolerated or until the maximum dose is reached. Monitor serum levels.

Exercise caution in younger children who cannot complain of minor side effects. Older adults and those with cor pulmonale. CHF or liver disease may have unusually low dosage requirements.

Dosage Forms

Capsule:

Immediate release (Bronkodyl®, Elixophyllin®): 100 mg, 200 mg

Timed release:

8-12 hours (Aerolate®): 65 mg [III]; 130 mg [JR], 260 mg [SR]

8-12 hours (Slo-Bid™): 50 mg, 75 mg, 100 mg, 125 mg, 200 mg, 300 mg

8-12 hours (Slo-Phyllin® Gyrocaps®): 60 mg, 125 mg, 250 mg

12 hours (Theobid® Duracaps®): 260 mg

12 hours (Theoclear® L.A.): 130 mg, 260 mg

12 hours (Theospan®-SR): 130 mg, 260 mg

12 hours (Theovent®): 125 mg, 250 mg

24 hours (Theo-24®): 100 mg, 200 mg, 300 mg

Elixir (Asmalix®, Elixomin®, Elixophyllin®, Lanophyllin®): 80 mg/15 mL (15 mL, 30 mL, 480 mL, 4000 mL)

Infusion, in D_5W: 0.4 mg/mL (1000 mL); 0.8 mg/mL (500 mL, 1000 mL); 1.6 mg/mL (250 mL, 500 mL); 2 mg/mL (100 mL); 3.2 mg/mL (250 mL); 4 mg/mL (50 mL, 100 mL);

Solution, oral:

Theolair™: 80 mg/15 mL (15 mL, 18.75 mL, 30 mL, 480 mL)

Syrup:

Aquaphyllin®, Slo-Phyllin®, Theoclear-80®, Theostat-80®: 80 mg/15 mL (15 mL, 30 mL, 500 mL)

Accurbron®: 150 mg/15 mL (480 mL)

Tablet: Immediate release:

Slo-Phyllin®: 100 mg, 200 mg

Theolair™: 125 mg, 250 mg

Quibron®-T: 300 mg

Tablet:

Controlled release (Theo-X®): 100 mg, 200 mg, 300 mg

Timed release:

12-24 hours: 100 mg, 200 mg, 300 mg, 450 mg

8-12 hours (Quibron®-T/SR): 300 mg

8-12 hours (Respbid®): 250 mg, 500 mg

8-12 hours (Sustaire®): 100 mg, 300 mg

8-12 hours (T-Phyl®): 200 mg

12-24 hours (Theochron®): 100 mg, 200 mg, 300 mg

8-24 hours (Theo-Dur®): 100 mg, 200 mg, 300 mg, 450 mg

8-24 hours (Theo-Sav®): 100 mg, 200 mg, 300 mg

24 hours (Theolair™-SR): 200 mg, 250 mg, 300 mg, 500 mg

24 hours (Uni-Dur®): 400 mg, 600 mg

24 hours (Uniphyl®): 400 mg

theophylline and guaifenesin (thee OF i lin & gwye FEN e sin)

Brand Names Bronchial®; Glycerol-T®; Quibron®; Slo-Phyllin GG®

Therapeutic Category Theophylline Derivative

Use Symptomatic treatment of bronchospasm associated with bronchial asthma, chronic bronchitis and pulmonary emphysema

Usual Dosage Adults: Oral: 1-2 capsules every 6-8 hours

Dosage Forms

Capsule: Theophylline 150 mg and guaifenesin 90 mg; theophylline 300 mg and guaifenesin 180 mg

Elixir: Theophylline 150 mg and guaifenesin 90 mg per 15 mL (480 mL)

theophylline, ephedrine, and hydroxyzine

(thee OF i lin, e FED rin, & hye DROKS i zeen)

Brand Names Hydrophed®; Marax®

Therapeutic Category Theophylline Derivative

Use Possibly effective for controlling bronchospastic disorders

Usual Dosage Oral:

Children:

2-5 years: 1/2 tablet 2-4 times/day or 2.5 mL 3-4 times/day

>5 years: 1/2 tablet 2-4 times/day or 5 mL 3-4 times/day

Adults: 1 tablet 2-4 times/day

Dosage Forms

Syrup, dye free: Theophylline 32.5 mg, ephedrine 6.25 mg, and hydroxyzine 2.5 mg per 5 mL

Tablet: Theophylline 130 mg, ephedrine 25 mg, and hydroxyzine 10 mg

theophylline, ephedrine, and phenobarbital

(thee OF i lin, e FED rin, & fee noe BAR bi tal)

Brand Names Tedral®

Therapeutic Category Theophylline Derivative

Use Prevention and symptomatic treatment of bronchial asthma; relief of asthmatic bronchitis and other bronchospastic disorders

Usual Dosage Oral:

Children >60 lb: 1 tablet or 5 mL every 4 hours

Adults: 1-2 tablets or 10-20 mL every 4 hours

Dosage Forms

Suspension: Theophylline 65 mg, ephedrine sulfate 12 mg, and phenobarbital 4 mg per 5 mL

Tablet: Theophylline 118 mg, ephedrine sulfate 25 mg, and phenobarbital 11 mg; theophylline 130 mg, ephedrine sulfate 24 mg, and phenobarbital 8 mg

theophylline ethylenediamine see aminophylline on page 25

Theo-Sav® see theophylline on page 511

Theospan®-SR see theophylline on page 511

Theostat-80® see theophylline on page 511

Theovent® see theophylline on page 511

Theo-X® see theophylline on page 511

Thera-Combex® H-P Kapseals® [OTC] see vitamin b complex with vitamin c on page 553

TheraCys™ see bcg vaccine on page 55

Theraflu® Non-Drowsy Formula Maximum Strength [OTC] see acetaminophen, dextromethorphan, and pseudoephedrine on page 6

Thera-Flur® see fluoride on page 228

Thera-Flur-N® see fluoride on page 228

Theragran® [OTC] see vitamins, multiple (oral, adult) on page 556

Theragran® Hematinic® see vitamins, multiple (oral, adult) on page 556

Theragran® Liquid [OTC] see vitamins, multiple (oral, adult) on page 556

Theragran-M® [OTC] *see* vitamins, multiple (oral, adult) *on page 556*

Thera-Hist® Syrup [OTC] *see* chlorpheniramine and phenylpropanolamine *on page 114*

Theramin® Expectorant [OTC] *see* guaifenesin and phenylpropanolamine *on page 249*

Theraplex Z® [OTC] *see* pyrithione zinc *on page 454*

Thermazene® *see* silver sulfadiazine *on page 479*

Theroxide® Wash [OTC] *see* benzoyl peroxide *on page 61*

thiabendazole (thye a BEN da zole)

Synonyms tiabendazole
Brand Names Mintezol®
Therapeutic Category Anthelmintic
Use Treatment of strongyloidiasis, cutaneous larva migrans, visceral larva migrans, dracunculosis, trichinosis, and mixed helminthic infections
Usual Dosage Children and Adults: Oral: 50 mg/kg/day divided every 12 hours (maximum dose: 3 g/day)
Strongyloidiasis: For 2 consecutive days
Cutaneous larva migrans: For 2-5 consecutive days
Visceral larva migrans: For 5-7 consecutive days
Trichinosis: For 2-4 consecutive days
Dracunculosis: 50-75 mg/kg/day divided every 12 hours for 3 days
Dosage Forms
Suspension, oral: 500 mg/5 mL (120 mL)
Tablet, chewable (orange flavor): 500 mg

thiamazole *see* methimazole *on page 336*

thiamine (THYE a min)

Synonyms aneurine hydrochloride; thiamine hydrochloride; thiaminium chloride hydrochloride; vitamin b_1
Therapeutic Category Vitamin, Water Soluble
Use Treatment of thiamine deficiency including beriberi, Wernicke's encephalopathy syndrome, and peripheral neuritis associated with pellagra; alcoholic patients with altered sensorium; various genetic metabolic disorders
Usual Dosage Dietary supplement (depends on caloric or carbohydrate content of the diet):
Infants: 0.3-0.5 mg/day
Children: 0.5-1 mg/day
Adults: 1-2 mg/day
Note: The above doses can be found as a combination in multivitamin preparations
Children:
Noncritically ill thiamine deficiency: Oral: 10-50 mg/day in divided doses every day for 2 weeks followed by 5-10 mg/day for one month
Beriberi: I.M.: 10-25 mg/day for 2 weeks, then 5-10 mg orally every day for one month (oral as therapeutic multivitamin)
Adults:
Wernicke's encephalopathy: I.M., I.V.: 50 mg as a single dose, then 50 mg I.M. every day until normal diet resumed
Noncritically ill thiamine deficiency: Oral: 10-50 mg/day in divided doses
Beriberi: I.M., I.V.: 10-30 mg 3 times/day for 2 weeks, then switch to 5-10 mg orally every day for one month (oral as therapeutic multivitamin)
Dosage Forms
Injection, as hydrochloride: 100 mg/mL (1 mL, 2 mL, 10 mL, 30 mL); 200 mg/mL (30 mL)
Tablet, as hydrochloride: 50 mg, 100 mg, 250 mg, 500 mg
Enteric coated: 20 mg

thiamine hydrochloride *see* thiamine *on previous page*

thiaminium chloride hydrochloride *see* thiamine *on previous page*

thiethylperazine (thye eth il PER a zeen)
Synonyms thiethylperazine maleate
Brand Names Norzine®; Torecan®
Therapeutic Category Phenothiazine Derivative
Use Relief of nausea and vomiting
Usual Dosage Children >12 years and Adults:
Oral, I.M., rectal: 10 mg 1-3 times/day as needed
I.V. and S.C. routes of administration are not recommended
Dosage Forms
Injection, as maleate: 5 mg/mL (2 mL)
Suppository, rectal, as maleate: 10 mg
Tablet, as maleate: 10 mg

thiethylperazine maleate *see* thiethylperazine *on this page*

thimerosal (thye MER oh sal)
Brand Names Aeroaid® [OTC]; Mersol® [OTC]; Merthiolate® [OTC]
Therapeutic Category Antibacterial, Topical
Use Organomercurial antiseptic with sustained bacteriostatic and fungistatic activity
Usual Dosage Apply 1-3 times/day
Dosage Forms
Ointment, ophthalmic: 0.02% [0.2 mg/mL] (3.5 g)
Solution, topical: 0.1% [1 mg/mL = 1:1000] (120 mL, 480 mL, 4000 mL)
Spray, antiseptic: 0.1% [1 mg/mL = 1:1000] with alcohol 2% (90 mL)
Tincture: 0.1% [1 mg/mL = 1:1000] with alcohol 50% (120 mL, 480 mL, 4000 mL)

thioguanine (thye oh GWAH neen)
Synonyms 2-amino-6-mercaptopurine; tg; 6-tg; 6-thioguanine; tioguanine
Therapeutic Category Antineoplastic Agent
Use Remission induction in acute myelogenous (nonlymphocytic) leukemia; treatment of chronic myelogenous leukemia and acute lymphocytic leukemia
Usual Dosage Refer to individual protocols. Oral:
Infants <3 years: Combination drug therapy for acute nonlymphocytic leukemia: 3.3 mg/kg/day in divided doses twice daily for 4 days
Children and Adults: 2-3 mg/kg/day calculated to nearest 20 mg or 75-200 mg/m^2/day in 1-2 divided doses for 5-7 days or until remission is attained
Dosage Forms Tablet, scored: 40 mg

6-thioguanine *see* thioguanine *on this page*

Thiola™ *see* tiopronin *on page 520*

thiopental (thye oh PEN tal)
Synonyms thiopental sodium
Brand Names Pentothal® Sodium
Therapeutic Category Barbiturate
Controlled Substance C-III
Use Induction of anesthesia; adjunct for intubation in head injury patients; control of convulsive states; treatment of elevated intracranial pressure
Usual Dosage I.V.:
Induction anesthesia:
Infants: 5-8 mg/kg
Children 1-12 years: 5-6 mg/kg
Adults: 3-5 mg/kg
(Continued)

thiopental *(Continued)*

Maintenance anesthesia:
  Children: 1 mg/kg as needed
  Adults: 25-100 mg as needed
Increased intracranial pressure: Children and Adults: 1.5-5 mg/kg/dose; repeat as needed to control intracranial pressure
Seizures:
  Children: 2-3 mg/kg/dose, repeat as needed
  Adults: 75-250 mg/kg/dose, repeat as needed
Rectal administration: (Patient should be NPO for no less than 3 hours prior to administration)
  Suggested initial doses of thiopental rectal suspension are:
  <3 months: 15 mg/kg/dose
  >3 months: 25 mg/kg/dose
  Note: The age of a premature infant should be adjusted to reflect the age that the infant would have been if full-term (eg, an infant, now age 4 months, who was 2 months premature should be considered to be a 2-month old infant).
  Doses should be rounded downward to the nearest 50 mg increment to allow for accurate measurement of the dose
  Inactive or debilitated patients and patients recently medicated with other sedatives, (eg, chloral hydrate, meperidine, chlorpromazine, and promethazine), may require smaller doses than usual
If the patient is not sedated within 15-20 minutes, a single repeat dose of thiopental can be administered; the single repeat doses are:
  <3 months of age: <7.5 mg/kg/dose
  >3 months of age: 15 mg/kg/dose
  Adults weighing >90 kg should not receive >3 g as a total dose (initial plus repeat doses)
  Children weighing >34 kg should not receive >1 g as a total dose (initial plus repeat doses)
  Neither adults nor children should receive more than one course of thiopental rectal suspension (initial dose plus repeat dose) per 24-hour period
Dosage Forms
  Injection, as sodium: 250 mg, 400 mg, 500 mg, 1 g, 2.5 g, 5 g
  Suspension, rectal, as sodium: 400 mg/g (2 g)

thiopental sodium *see* thiopental *on previous page*

thioridazine *(thye oh RID a zeen)*

Synonyms thioridazine hydrochloride
Brand Names Mellaril®; Mellaril-S®
Therapeutic Category Phenothiazine Derivative
Use Management of psychotic disorders; depressive neurosis; dementia in elderly; severe behavioral problems in children
Usual Dosage Oral:
  Children >2 years: Range: 0.5-3 mg/kg/day in 2-3 divided doses; usual: 1 mg/kg/day; maximum: 3 mg/kg/day
  Behavior problems: Initial: 10 mg 2-3 times/day, increase gradually
  Severe psychoses: Initial: 25 mg 2-3 times/day, increase gradually
  Adults:
  Psychoses: Initial: 50-100 mg 3 times/day with gradual increments as needed and tolerated; maximum daily dose: 800 mg/day in 2-4 divided doses
  Depressive disorders, dementia: Initial: 25 mg 3 times/day; maintenance dose: 20-200 mg/day
Dosage Forms
  Concentrate, oral: 30 mg/mL (120 mL); 100 mg/mL (3.4 mL, 120 mL)
  Suspension, oral: 25 mg/5 mL (480 mL); 100 mg/5 mL (480 mL)
  Tablet: 10 mg, 15 mg, 25 mg, 50 mg, 100 mg, 150 mg, 200 mg

thioridazine hydrochloride *see* thioridazine *on previous page*

thiotepa (thye oh TEP a)

Synonyms tespa; triethylenethiophosphoramide; tspa

Therapeutic Category Antineoplastic Agent

Use Treatment of superficial tumors of the bladder; palliative treatment of adenocarcinoma of breast or ovary; lymphomas and sarcomas; meningeal neoplasms; control pleural, pericardial or peritoneal effusions caused by metastatic tumors; high-dose regimens with autologous bone marrow transplantation

Usual Dosage Refer to individual protocols

Children: Sarcomas: I.V.: 25-65 mg/m^2 as a single dose every 21 days

Adults:

I.M., I.V., S.C.: 8 mg/m^2 daily for 5 days or 30-60 mg/m^2 once per week

High dose therapy for bone marrow transplant: I.V.: 500 mg/m^2

Intracavitary: 0.6-0.8 mg/kg or 60 mg in 60 mL SWI instilled into the bladder at 1- to 4-week intervals

Intrathecal: Doses of 1-10 mg/m^2 administered 1-2 times/week in concentrations of 1 mg/mL diluted with preservative free sterile water for injection

Dosage Forms Powder for injection: 15 mg

thiothixene (thye oh THIKS een)

Synonyms thiothixene hydrochloride; tiotixene

Brand Names Navane®

Therapeutic Category Thioxanthene Derivative

Use Management of psychotic disorders

Usual Dosage

Children <12 years: Oral: Not well established; 0.25 mg/kg/24 hours in divided doses

Children >12 years and Adults:

Oral: Initial: 2 mg 3 times/day, up to 20-30 mg/day; maximum: 60 mg/day

I.M. (administer undiluted injection): 4 mg 2-4 times/day, increase dose gradually; usual: 16-20 mg/day; maximum: 30 mg/day; change to oral dose as soon as able

Dosage Forms

Capsule: 1 mg, 2 mg, 5 mg, 10 mg, 20 mg

Powder for injection, as hydrochloride: 5 mg/mL (2 mL)

thiothixene hydrochloride *see* thiothixene *on this page*

Thorazine® *see* chlorpromazine *on page 119*

Thrombate III™ *see* antithrombin III *on page 38*

Thrombinar® *see* thrombin, topical *on this page*

thrombin, topical (THROM bin, TOP i kal)

Brand Names Thrombinar®; Thrombogen®; Thrombostat®

Therapeutic Category Hemostatic Agent

Use Hemostasis whenever minor bleeding from capillaries and small venules is accessible

Usual Dosage Use 1000-2000 units/mL of solution where bleeding is profuse; apply powder directly to the site of bleeding or on oozing surfaces; use 100 units/mL for bleeding from skin or mucosal surfaces

Dosage Forms Powder: 1000 units, 5000 units, 10,000 units, 20,000 units, 50,000 units

Thrombogen® *see* thrombin, topical *on this page*

Thrombostat® *see* thrombin, topical *on this page*

Thypinone® **Injection** *see* protirelin *on page 448*

Thyrar® *see* thyroid *on next page*

Thyro-Block® *see* potassium iodide *on page 430*

thyroid (THYE royd)

Synonyms desiccated thyroid; thyroid extract
Brand Names Armour® Thyroid; S-P-T; Thyrar®; Thyroid Strong®
Therapeutic Category Thyroid Product
Use Replacement or supplemental therapy in hypothyroidism
Usual Dosage Adults: Oral: Start at 30 mg/day and titrate by 30 mg/day in increments of 2- to 3-week intervals; usual maintenance dose: 60-120 mg/day
Dosage Forms
Capsule, pork source in soybean oil (S-P-T): 60 mg, 120 mg, 180 mg, 300 mg
Tablet:
Armour® Thyroid: 15 mg, 30 mg, 60 mg, 90 mg, 120 mg, 180 mg, 240 mg, 300 mg
Thyrar® (bovine source): 30 mg, 60 mg, 120 mg
Thyroid Strong® (60 mg is equivalent to 90 mg thyroid USP):
Regular: 30 mg, 60 mg, 120 mg
Sugar coated: 30 mg, 60 mg, 120 mg, 180 mg
Thyroid USP: 15 mg, 30 mg, 60 mg, 120 mg, 180 mg, 300 mg

thyroid extract see thyroid on this page

thyroid-stimulating hormone see thyrotropin on this page

Thyroid Strong® see thyroid on this page

Thyrolar® see liotrix on page 310

thyrotropin (thye roe TROE pin)

Synonyms thyroid-stimulating hormone; tsh
Brand Names Thytropar®
Therapeutic Category Diagnostic Agent
Use Diagnostic aid to determine subclinical hypothyroidism or decreased thyroid reserve, to differentiate between primary and secondary hypothyroidism and between primary hypothyroidism and euthyroidism in patients receiving thyroid replacement
Usual Dosage I.M., S.C.: 10 units/day for 1-3 days; follow by a radioiodine study 24 hours past last injection, no response in thyroid failure, substantial response in pituitary failure
Dosage Forms Injection: 10 units

Thytropar® see thyrotropin on this page

tiabendazole see thiabendazole on page 514

Tiamate® see diltiazem on page 170

Tiazac® see diltiazem on page 170

Ticar® see ticarcillin on this page

ticarcillin (tye kar SIL in)

Synonyms ticarcillin disodium
Brand Names Ticar®
Therapeutic Category Penicillin
Use Treatment of infections such as septicemia, acute and chronic respiratory tract infections, skin and soft tissue infections, and urinary tract infections due to susceptible strains of Pseudomonas, Proteus, Escherichia coli, and Enterobacter
Usual Dosage I.V. (ticarcillin is generally administered I.M. only for the treatment of uncomplicated urinary tract infections):
Infants and Children: 200-300 mg/kg/day in divided doses every 4-6 hours; maximum dose: 24 g/day
Adults: 1-4 g every 4-6 hours
Dosage Forms Powder for injection, as disodium: 1 g, 3 g, 6 g, 20 g, 30 g

ticarcillin and clavulanate potassium
(tye kar SIL in & klav yoo LAN ate poe TASS ee um)

Synonyms clavulanic acid and ticarcillin; ticarcillin and clavulanic acid

Brand Names Timentin®

Therapeutic Category Penicillin

Use Treatment of infections caused by susceptible organisms involving the lower respiratory tract, urinary tract, skin and skin structures, bone and joint, and septicemia. Clavulanate expands activity of ticarcillin to include beta-lactamase producing strains of *S. aureus*, *H. influenzae*, *Branhamella catarrhalis*, *B. fragilis*, *Klebsiella*, and *Proteus* species

Usual Dosage I.V.:
Children: 200-300 mg of ticarcillin/kg/day in divided doses every 4-6 hours
Adults: 3.1 g (ticarcillin 3 g plus clavulanic acid 0.1 g) every 4-6 hours; maximum: 18-24 g/day; for urinary tract infections: 3.1 g every 6-8 hours

Dosage Forms
Infusion, premixed (frozen): Ticarcillin disodium 3 g and clavulanate potassium 0.1 g (100 mL)
Powder for injection: Ticarcillin disodium 3 g and clavulanate potassium 0.1 g (3.1 g, 31 g)

ticarcillin and clavulanic acid *see* ticarcillin and clavulanate potassium *on this page*

ticarcillin disodium *see* ticarcillin *on previous page*

TICE® BCG *see* bcg vaccine *on page 55*

Ticlid® *see* ticlopidine *on this page*

ticlopidine (tye KLOE pi deen)
Synonyms ticlopidine hydrochloride

Brand Names Ticlid®

Therapeutic Category Antiplatelet Agent

Use Platelet aggregation inhibitor that reduces the risk of thrombotic stroke in patients who have had a stroke or stroke precursors

Usual Dosage Adults: Oral: 1 tablet twice daily with food

Dosage Forms Tablet, as hydrochloride: 250 mg

ticlopidine hydrochloride *see* ticlopidine *on this page*

Ticon® *see* trimethobenzamide *on page 534*

tig *see* tetanus immune globulin (human) *on page 508*

Tigan® *see* trimethobenzamide *on page 534*

Tilade® Inhalation Aerosol *see* nedocromil sodium *on page 366*

tiludronate (tye LOO droe nate)
Synonyms tiludronate disodium

Brand Names Skelid®

Therapeutic Category Bisphosphonate Derivative

Use Paget's disease of the bone

Usual Dosage Adults: Oral: 400 mg (2 tablets) [tiludronic acid] daily

Dosage Forms Tablet, as disodium: 240 mg [tiludronic acid 200 mg]; dosage is expressed in terms of tiludronic acid.

tiludronate disodium *see* tiludronate *on this page*

Timentin® *see* ticarcillin and clavulanate potassium *on this page*

timolol (TYE moe lole)

Synonyms timolol hemihydrate; timolol maleate

Brand Names Betimol® Ophthalmic; Blocadren® Oral; Timoptic® Ophthalmic; Timoptic-XE® Ophthalmic

Therapeutic Category Beta-Adrenergic Blocker

Use Ophthalmic dosage form used to treat elevated intraocular pressure such as glaucoma or ocular hypertension; orally for treatment of hypertension and angina and for prevention of myocardial infarction and migraine headaches

Usual Dosage

Children and Adults: Ophthalmic: Initial: 0.25% solution, instill 1 drop twice daily; increase to 0.5% solution if response not adequate; decrease to 1 drop/day if controlled; do not exceed 1 drop twice daily of 0.5% solution

Adults: Oral:

Hypertension: Initial: 10 mg twice daily, increase gradually every 7 days, usual dosage: 20-40 mg/day in 2 divided doses; maximum: 60 mg/day

Prevention of myocardial infarction: 10 mg twice daily initiated within 1-4 weeks after infarction

Migraine headache: Initial: 10 mg twice daily, increase to maximum of 30 mg/day

Dosage Forms

Gel, ophthalmic, as maleate (Timoptic-XE®): 0.25% (2.5 mL, 5 mL); 0.5% (2.5 mL, 5 mL)

Solution, ophthalmic:

As hemihydrate (Betimol®): 0.25% (2.5 mL, 5 mL, 10 mL, 15 mL); 0.5% (2.5 mL, 5 mL, 10 mL, 15 mL)

As maleate: 0.25% (2.5 mL, 5 mL, 10 mL, 15 mL); 0.5% (2.5 mL, 5 mL, 10 mL, 15 mL)

Timoptic®: 0.25% (2.5 mL, 5 mL, 10 mL, 15 mL); 0.5% (2.5 mL, 5 mL, 10 mL, 15 mL)

As maleate, preservative free, single use (Timoptic® OcuDose®): 0.25%, 0.5%

Tablet, as maleate (Blocadren®): 5 mg, 10 mg, 20 mg

timolol hemihydrate see timolol on this page

timolol maleate see timolol on this page

Timoptic® Ophthalmic see timolol on this page

Timoptic-XE® Ophthalmic see timolol on this page

Tinactin® [OTC] see tolnaftate on page 523

Tinactin® for Jock Itch [OTC] see tolnaftate on page 523

TinBen® [OTC] see benzoin on page 61

TinCoBen® [OTC] see benzoin on page 61

Tine Test PPD see tuberculin tests on page 539

Ting® [OTC] see tolnaftate on page 523

Tinver® Lotion see sodium thiosulfate on page 488

tioconazole (tye oh KONE a zole)

Brand Names Vagistat-1® Vaginal [OTC]

Therapeutic Category Antifungal Agent

Use Local treatment of vulvovaginal candidiasis

Usual Dosage Vaginal: Insert 1 applicatorful in vagina, just prior to bedtime, as a single dose

Dosage Forms Cream, vaginal: 6.5% with applicator (4.6 g)

tioguanine see thioguanine on page 515

tiopronin (tye oh PROE nin)

Brand Names Thiola™

Therapeutic Category Urinary Tract Product

Use Prevention of kidney stone (cystine) formation in patients with severe homozygous cystinuric who have urinary cystine >500 mg/day who are resistant to treatment with high fluid intake, alkali, and diet modification, or who have had adverse reactions to penicillamine

Usual Dosage Adults: Initial: 800 mg/day; average dose: 1000 mg/day

Dosage Forms Tablet: 100 mg

tiotixene *see* thiothixene *on page 517*

Ti-Screen® [OTC] *see* methoxycinnamate and oxybenzone *on page 339*

Tisit® Blue Gel [OTC] *see* pyrethrins *on page 452*

Tisit® Liquid [OTC] *see* pyrethrins *on page 452*

Tisit® Shampoo [OTC] *see* pyrethrins *on page 452*

tissue plasminogen activator, recombinant *see* alteplase *on page 19*

Titralac® Plus Liquid [OTC] *see* calcium carbonate and simethicone *on page 83*

tizanidine (tye ZAN i deen)

Brand Names Zanaflex®

Therapeutic Category Alpha$_2$-Adrenergic Agonist Agent

Use Intermittent management of increased muscle tone associated with spasticity (eg, multiple sclerosis, spinal cord injury)

Usual Dosage Adults: Oral: Initial dose: 4 mg every 6-8 hours, not to exceed 3 doses/day or 36 mg in a 24-hour period; doses may be increased at 2 mg or 4 mg increments with single doses not exceeding 12 mg

Dosage Forms Tablet: 4 mg

tmp *see* trimethoprim *on page 534*

tmp-smx *see* co-trimoxazole *on page 140*

TobraDex® Ophthalmic *see* tobramycin and dexamethasone *on next page*

tobramycin (toe bra MYE sin)

Synonyms tobramycin sulfate

Brand Names AKTob® Ophthalmic; Nebcin® Injection; Tobrex® Ophthalmic

Therapeutic Category Aminoglycoside (Antibiotic); Antibiotic, Ophthalmic

Use Treatment of documented or suspected infections caused by susceptible gram-negative bacilli including *Pseudomonas aeruginosa*; infection with a nonpseudomonal enteric bacillus which is more sensitive to tobramycin than gentamicin based on susceptibility tests; susceptible organisms in lower respiratory tract infections, septicemia; intra-abdominal, skin, bone, and urinary tract infections; empiric therapy in cystic fibrosis and immunocompromised patients; used topically to treat superficial ophthalmic infections caused by susceptible bacteria

Usual Dosage Dosage should be based on an estimate of ideal body weight

Infants and Children: I.M., I.V.: 2.5 mg/kg/dose every 8 hours
Note: Some patients may require larger or more frequent doses if serum levels document the need (ie, cystic fibrosis or febrile granulocytopenic patients)
Adults: I.M., I.V.: 3-5 mg/kg/day in 3 divided doses

Children and Adults:
Renal dysfunction: 2.5 mg/kg (2-3 serum level measurements should be obtained after the initial dose to measure the half-life in order to determine the frequency of subsequent doses)
Ophthalmic: 1-2 drops every 4 hours; apply ointment 2-3 times/day; for severe infections apply ointment every 3-4 hours, or 2 drops every 30-60 minutes initially, then reduce to less frequent intervals

Dosage Forms
Injection, as sulfate (Nebcin®): 10 mg/mL (2 mL); 40 mg/mL (1.5 mL, 2 mL)
(Continued)

tobramycin *(Continued)*
Ointment, ophthalmic (Tobrex®): 0.3% (3.5 g)
Powder for injection (Nebcin®): 40 mg/mL (1.2 g vials)
Solution, ophthalmic: 0.3% (5 mL)
 AKTob®, Tobrex®: 0.3% (5 mL)

tobramycin and dexamethasone (toe bra MYE sin & deks a METH a sone)
Synonyms dexamethasone and tobramycin
Brand Names TobraDex® Ophthalmic
Therapeutic Category Antibiotic/Corticosteroid, Ophthalmic
Use Treatment of external ocular infection caused by susceptible gram-negative bacteria and steroid responsive inflammatory conditions of the palpebral and bulbar conjunctiva, lid, cornea, and anterior segment of the globe
Usual Dosage Ophthalmic: Adults:
Ointment: Apply 1.25 cm (½") every 3-4 hours to 2-3 times/day
Suspension: Instill 1-2 drops every 4-6 hours (first 24-48 hours may increase frequency to every 2 hours until signs of clinical improvement are seen); apply every 30-60 minutes for severe infections
Dosage Forms
Ointment, ophthalmic: Tobramycin 0.3% and dexamethasone 0.1% (3.5 g)
Suspension, ophthalmic: Tobramycin 0.3% and dexamethasone 0.1% (2.5 mL, 5 mL)

tobramycin sulfate *see* tobramycin *on previous page*

Tobrex® Ophthalmic *see* tobramycin *on previous page*

tocainide (toe KAY nide)
Synonyms tocainide hydrochloride
Brand Names Tonocard®
Therapeutic Category Antiarrhythmic Agent, Class I-B
Use Suppress and prevent symptomatic ventricular arrhythmias
Usual Dosage Adults: Oral: 1200-1800 mg/day in 3 divided doses
Dosage Forms Tablet, as hydrochloride: 400 mg, 600 mg

tocainide hydrochloride *see* tocainide *on this page*

tocophersolan (toe kof er SOE lan)
Synonyms TPGS
Brand Names Liqui-E®
Therapeutic Category Vitamin, Fat Soluble
Use Treatment of vitamin E deficiency resulting from malabsorption due to prolonged cholestatic hepatobiliary disease
Usual Dosage Dietary supplement: Oral: 15 mg (400 units) every day
Dosage Forms Liquid: 26.6 units/mL

Tofranil® *see* imipramine *on page 280*

Tofranil-PM® *see* imipramine *on page 280*

tolazamide (tole AZ a mide)
Brand Names Tolinase®
Therapeutic Category Antidiabetic Agent (Oral)
Use Adjunct to diet for the management of mild to moderately severe, stable, noninsulin-dependent (type II) diabetes mellitus
Usual Dosage Adults: Oral: 100-1000 mg/day
Dosage Forms Tablet: 100 mg, 250 mg, 500 mg

tolazoline (tole AZ oh leen)
Synonyms benzazoline hydrochloride; tolazoline hydrochloride
Brand Names Priscoline®
Therapeutic Category Alpha-Adrenergic Blocking Agent
Use Persistent pulmonary hypertension of the newborn (PPHN), also known as persistent fetal circulation (PFC); peripheral vasospastic disorders
Usual Dosage
Neonates: Initial: I.V.: 1-2 mg/kg over 10-15 minutes via scalp vein or upper extremity; maintenance: 1-2 mg/kg/hour; use lower maintenance doses in patients with decreased renal function. Also used in neonates for acute vasospasm "cath toes" at 0.25 mg/kg/hour (no load)
Adults: Peripheral vasospastic disorder: I.M., I.V., S.C.: 10-50 mg 4 times/day
Dosage Forms Injection, as hydrochloride: 25 mg/mL (4 mL)

tolazoline hydrochloride *see* tolazoline *on this page*

tolbutamide (tole BYOO ta mide)
Synonyms tolbutamide sodium
Brand Names Orinase® Diagnostic Injection; Orinase® Oral
Therapeutic Category Antidiabetic Agent (Oral)
Use Adjunct to diet for the management of mild to moderately severe, stable, noninsulin-dependent (type II) diabetes mellitus
Usual Dosage Adults:
Oral: 250-2000 mg/day
I.V. bolus: 20 mg/kg
Dosage Forms
Injection, diagnostic, as sodium: 1 g (20 mL)
Tablet: 250 mg, 500 mg

tolbutamide sodium *see* tolbutamide *on this page*

Tolectin® *see* tolmetin *on this page*

Tolectin® DS *see* tolmetin *on this page*

Tolinase® *see* tolazamide *on previous page*

tolmetin (TOLE met in)
Synonyms tolmetin sodium
Brand Names Tolectin®; Tolectin® DS
Therapeutic Category Analgesic, Non-narcotic; Nonsteroidal Anti-Inflammatory Agent (NSAID)
Use Treatment of inflammatory and rheumatoid disorders, including juvenile rheumatoid arthritis
Usual Dosage Oral:
Children ≥2 years: Anti-inflammatory: Initial: 20 mg/kg/day in 3 divided doses, then 15-30 mg/kg/day in 3 divided doses; maximum dose: 30 mg/kg/day
Adults: 400 mg 3 times/day; usual dose: 600 mg to 1.8 g/day; maximum: 2 g/day
Dosage Forms
Capsule, as sodium: 400 mg
Tolectin® DS: 400 mg
Tablet, as sodium: 200 mg, 600 mg
Tolectin®: 200 mg, 600 mg

tolmetin sodium *see* tolmetin *on this page*

tolnaftate (tole NAF tate)
Brand Names Absorbine® Antifungal [OTC]; Absorbine® Jock Itch [OTC]; Absorbine Jr.® Antifungal [OTC]; Aftate® for Athlete's Foot [OTC]; Aftate® for Jock Itch [OTC]; Blis-To-Sol® [OTC]; Breezee® Mist Antifungal [OTC]; Dr Scholl's Athlete's Foot [OTC]; Dr (Continued)

tolnaftate *(Continued)*

Scholl's Maximum Strength Tritin [OTC]; Genaspor® [OTC]; NP-27® [OTC]; Quinsana Plus® [OTC]; Tinactin® [OTC]; Tinactin® for Jock Itch [OTC]; Ting® [OTC]; Zeasorb-AF® Powder [OTC]

Therapeutic Category Antifungal Agent

Use Treatment of tinea pedis, tinea cruris, tinea corporis, tinea manuum caused by *Trichophyton rubrum, T. mentagrophytes, T. tonsurans, M. canis, M. audouinii,* and *E. floccosum*; also effective in the treatment of tinea versicolor infections due to *Malassezia furfur*

Usual Dosage Children and Adults: Topical: Wash and dry affected area; apply 1-2 drops of solution or a small amount of cream or powder and rub into the affected areas twice daily for 2-4 weeks

Dosage Forms
Aerosol, topical:
Liquid: 1% (59.2 mL, 90 mL, 120 mL)
Powder: 1% (56.7 g, 100 g, 105 g, 150 g)
Cream: 1% (15 g, 30 g)
Gel, topical: 1% (15 g)
Powder, topical: 1% (45 g, 90 g)
Solution, topical: 1% (10 mL)

Tolu-Sed® DM [OTC] *see* guaifenesin and dextromethorphan *on page 248*

Tomocat® *see* radiological/contrast media (ionic) *on page 457*

Tonocard® *see* tocainide *on page 522*

Tonopaque® *see* radiological/contrast media (ionic) *on page 457*

Topamax® *see* topiramate *on this page*

Topicort® *see* desoximetasone *on page 155*

Topicort®-LP *see* desoximetasone *on page 155*

Topicycline® Topical *see* tetracycline *on page 510*

topiramate *(toe PYE ra mate)*

Brand Names Topamax®
Therapeutic Category Anticonvulsant
Use Adjunctive therapy for partial onset seizures in adults
Usual Dosage Adults: Oral: 200 mg twice daily (400 mg/day)
Dosage Forms Tablet: 25 mg, 100 mg, 200 mg

TOPO *see* topotecan *on this page*

Toposar® Injection *see* etoposide *on page 213*

topotecan *(toe poe TEE kan)*

Synonyms Hycamptamine; SKF 104864; TOPO; topotecan hydrochloride; TPT
Brand Names Hycamtin®
Therapeutic Category Antineoplastic Agent
Use Treatment of ovarian cancer after failure of first-line chemotherapy
Usual Dosage
Children: A phase I study in pediatric patients by CCSG determined the recommended phase II dose to be 5.5 mg/m² as a 24-hour continuous infusion
Adults: Most phase II studies currently utilize topotecan at 1.5-2.0 mg/m²/day for 5 days, repeated every 21-28 days. Alternative dosing regimens evaluated in phase I studies have included 21-day continuous infusion (recommended phase II dose: 0.53-0.7 mg/m²/day) and weekly 24-hour infusions (recommended phase II dose: 1.5 mg/m²/week). Dose modifications: Dosage modification may be required for toxicity
Dosage Forms Powder for injection, as hydrochloride, lyophilized: 4 mg (base)

topotecan hydrochloride *see* topotecan *on previous page*

Toprol XL® *see* metoprolol *on page 346*

topv *see* poliovirus vaccine, live, trivalent, oral *on page 423*

Toradol® **Injection** *see* ketorolac tromethamine *on page 297*

Toradol® **Oral** *see* ketorolac tromethamine *on page 297*

Torecan® *see* thiethylperazine *on page 515*

Tornalate® *see* bitolterol *on page 69*

torsemide (TOR se mide)

Brand Names Demadex®

Therapeutic Category Diuretic, Loop

Use Management of edema associated with congestive heart failure and hepatic or renal disease; used alone or in combination with antihypertensives in treatment of hypertension

Usual Dosage Adults:

Oral: 5-10 mg once daily; if ineffective, may double dose until desired effect is achieved

I.V.: 10-20 mg/dose repeated in 2 hours as needed with a doubling of the dose with each succeeding dose until desired diuresis is achieved

Continues to be effective in patients with cirrhosis, no apparent change in dose is necessary

Dosage Forms

Injection: 10 mg/mL (2 mL, 5 mL)

Tablet: 5 mg, 10 mg, 20 mg, 100 mg

Totacillin® *see* ampicillin *on page 33*

Totacillin®**-N** *see* ampicillin *on page 33*

Touro Ex® *see* guaifenesin *on page 247*

Touro LA® *see* guaifenesin and pseudoephedrine *on page 250*

t-PA *see* alteplase *on page 19*

TPGS *see* tocophersolan *on page 522*

T-Phyl® *see* theophylline *on page 511*

TPT *see* topotecan *on previous page*

Trace-4® *see* trace metals *on this page*

trace metals (trase MET als)

Synonyms chromium injection; copper injection; manganese injection; molybdenum injection; neonatal trace metals; zinc injection

Brand Names Chroma-Pak®; Iodopen®; Molypen®; M.T.E.-4®; M.T.E.-5®; M.T.E.-6®; MulTE-PAK-4®; MulTE-PAK-5®; Neotrace-4®; PedTE-PAK-4®; Pedtrace-4®; P.T.E.-4®; P.T.E.-5®; Sele-Pak®; Selepen®; Trace-4®; Zinca-Pak®

Therapeutic Category Trace Element

Use Prevent and correct trace metal deficiencies

Dosage Forms

Chromium: Injection: 4 mcg/mL, 20 mcg/mL

Copper: Injection: 0.4 mg/mL, 2 mg/mL

Manganese: Injection: 0.1 mg/mL (as chloride or sulfate salt)

Molybdenum: Injection: 25 mcg/mL

Selenium: Injection: 40 mcg/mL

Zinc: Injection: 1 mg/mL (sulfate); 1 mg/mL (chloride); 5 mg/mL (sulfate)

Tracrium® *see* atracurium *on page 46*

tramadol (TRA ma dole)
Synonyms tramadol hydrochloride
Brand Names Ultram®
Therapeutic Category Analgesic, Non-narcotic
Use Relief of moderate to moderately severe pain
Usual Dosage Adults: Oral: 50-100 mg every 4-6 hours, not to exceed 400 mg/day
Dosage Forms Tablet, as hydrochloride: 50 mg

tramadol hydrochloride *see* tramadol *on this page*

Trandate® *see* labetalol *on page 299*

trandolapril (tran DOE la pril)
Brand Names Mavik®
Therapeutic Category Angiotensin-Converting Enzyme (ACE) Inhibitors
Use Management of hypertension alone or in combination with other antihypertensive agents

Unlabeled use: As a class, ACE inhibitors are recommended in the treatment of systolic congestive heart failure
Usual Dosage Adults:
Non-Black patients: 0.5-1 mg for those not receiving diuretics; increase dose at 0.5-1 mg increments at 1- to 2-week intervals; maximum dose: 4 mg/day
Black patients: Initiate doses of 1-2 mg; maximum dose: 4 mg/day
Dosage Forms Tablet: 1 mg, 2 mg, 4 mg

trandolapril and verapamil (tran DOE la pril & ver AP a mil)
Brand Names Tarka®
Therapeutic Category Antihypertensive, Combination
Use Combination drug for the treatment of hypertension
Dosage Forms Tablet:
Trandolapril 1 mg and verapamil hydrochloride 240 mg
Trandolapril 2 mg and verapamil hydrochloride 180 mg
Trandolapril 2 mg and verapamil hydrochloride 240 mg
Trandolapril 4 mg and verapamil hydrochloride 240 mg

tranexamic acid (tran eks AM ik AS id)
Brand Names Cyklokapron®
Therapeutic Category Antihemophilic Agent
Use Short-term use (2-8 days) in hemophilia patients during and following tooth extraction to reduce or prevent hemorrhage
Usual Dosage Children and Adults: I.V.: 10 mg/kg immediately before surgery, then 25 mg/kg/dose orally 3-4 times/day for 2-8 days

Alternatively:
Oral: 25 mg/kg 3-4 times/day beginning 1 day prior to surgery
I.V.: 10 mg/kg 3-4 times/day in patients who are unable to take oral
Dosage Forms
Injection: 100 mg/mL (10 mL)
Tablet: 500 mg

transamine sulphate *see* tranylcypromine *on next page*

Transdermal-NTG® Patch *see* nitroglycerin *on page 376*

Transderm-Nitro® Patch *see* nitroglycerin *on page 376*

Transderm Scop® Patch *see* scopolamine *on page 475*

Trans-Ver-Sal® AdultPatch [OTC] *see* salicylic acid *on page 472*

Trans-Ver-Sal® PediaPatch [OTC] *see* salicylic acid *on page 472*

Trans-Ver-Sal® PlantarPatch [OTC] *see* salicylic acid *on page 472*

Tranxene® *see* clorazepate *on page 131*

tranylcypromine (tran il SIP roe meen)
Synonyms transamine sulphate; tranylcypromine sulfate
Brand Names Parnate®
Therapeutic Category Antidepressant, Monoamine Oxidase Inhibitor
Use Symptomatic treatment of depressed patients refractory to or intolerant to tricyclic antidepressants or electroconvulsive therapy; has a more rapid onset of therapeutic effect than other MAO inhibitors, but causes more severe hypertensive reactions
Usual Dosage Adults: Oral: 10 mg twice daily, increase by 10 mg increments at 1- to 3-week intervals; maximum: 60 mg/day
Dosage Forms Tablet, as sulfate: 10 mg

tranylcypromine sulfate *see* tranylcypromine *on this page*

Trasylol® *see* aprotinin *on page 40*

trazodone (TRAZ oh done)
Synonyms trazodone hydrochloride
Brand Names Desyrel®
Therapeutic Category Antidepressant, Triazolopyridine
Use Treatment of depression
Usual Dosage Oral:
Adolescents: Initial: 25-50 mg/day; increase to 100-150 mg/day in divided doses
Adults: Initial: 150 mg/day in 3 divided doses (may increase by 50 mg/day every 3-7 days); maximum: 600 mg/day
Dosage Forms Tablet, as hydrochloride: 50 mg, 100 mg, 150 mg, 300 mg

trazodone hydrochloride *see* trazodone *on this page*

Trecator®-SC *see* ethionamide *on page 211*

Trental® *see* pentoxifylline *on page 405*

tretinoin (oral) (TRET i noyn, oral)
Synonyms All-*trans*-Retinoic Acid
Brand Names Vesanoid®
Therapeutic Category Antineoplastic Agent
Use Acute promyelocytic leukemia (APL): Induction of remission in patients with APL, French American British (FAB) classification M3 (including the M3 variant), characterized by the presence of the t(15;17) translocation or the presence of the PML/RARα gene who are refractory to or who have relapsed from anthracycline chemotherapy, or for whom anthracycline-based chemotherapy is contraindicated. Tretinoin is for the induction of remission only. All patients should receive an accepted form of remission consolidation or maintenance therapy for APL after completion of induction therapy with tretinoin.
Usual Dosage Oral:
Children: There are limited clinical data on the pediatric use of tretinoin. Of 15 pediatric patients (age range: 1-16 years) treated with tretinoin, the incidence of complete remission was 67%. Safety and efficacy in pediatric patients <1 year of age have not been established. Some pediatric patients experience severe headache and pseudotumor cerebri, requiring analgesic treatment and lumbar puncture for relief. Increased caution is recommended. Consider dose reduction in children experiencing serious or intolerable toxicity; however, the efficacy and safety of tretinoin at doses <45 mg/m^2/day have not been evaluated.
Adults: 45 mg/m^2/day administered as two evenly divided doses until complete remission is documented. Discontinue therapy 30 days after achievement of complete remission or after 90 days of treatment, whichever occurs first. If after initiation of treatment
(Continued)

tretinoin (oral) *(Continued)*

the presence of the t(15;17) translocation is not confirmed by cytogenetics or by polymerase chain reaction studies and the patient has not responded to tretinoin, consider alternative therapy.

Note: Tretinoin is for the induction of remission only. Optimal consolidation or maintenance regimens have not been determined. All patients should, therefore, receive a standard consolidation or maintenance chemotherapy regimen for APL after induction therapy with tretinoin unless otherwise contraindicated.

Dosage Forms Capsule: 10 mg

tretinoin (topical) (TRET i noyn, TOP i kal)

Synonyms retinoic acid; vitamin a acid

Brand Names Avita®; Retin-A™ Micro Topical; Retin-A™ Topical

Therapeutic Category Retinoic Acid Derivative

Use Treatment of acne vulgaris, photodamaged skin, and some skin cancers

Usual Dosage Children >12 years and Adults: Topical: Apply once daily before retiring; if stinging or irritation develop, decrease frequency of application

Dosage Forms

Cream:

Retin-A™: 0.025% (20 g, 45 g); 0.05% (20 g, 45 g); 0.1% (20 g, 45 g)

Avita®: 0.025% (20 g, 45 g)

Gel, topical:

Retin-A™: 0.01% (15 g, 45 g); 0.025% (15 g, 45 g)

Retin-A™ Micro: 0.1% (20 g, 45 g)

Liquid, topical (Retin-A™): 0.05% (28 mL)

Triacet® *see* triamcinolone *on this page*

triacetin (trye a SEE tin)

Synonyms glycerol triacetate

Brand Names Ony-Clear® Nail

Therapeutic Category Antifungal Agent

Use Fungistat for athlete's foot and other superficial fungal infections

Usual Dosage Topical: Apply twice daily, cleanse areas with dilute alcohol or mild soap and water before application; continue treatment for 7 days after symptoms have disappeared

Dosage Forms

Cream: With cetylpyridinium chloride and chloroxylenol (30 g)

Liquid: With cetylpyridinium chloride and chloroxylenol (30 mL)

Solution: With cetylpyridinium chloride, chloroxylenol, and benzalkonium chloride in an oil base (15 mL)

Spray, aerosol: With cetylpyridinium chloride, chloroxylenol, and benzalkonium chloride (45 mL, 60 mL)

triacetyloleandomycin *see* troleandomycin *on page 537*

Triacin-C® *see* triprolidine, pseudoephedrine, and codeine *on page 537*

triaconazole *see* terconazole *on page 505*

Triam-A® *see* triamcinolone *on this page*

triamcinolone (trye am SIN oh lone)

Synonyms triamcinolone acetonide; triamcinolone diacetate; triamcinolone hexacetonide

Brand Names Amcort®; Aristocort®; Aristocort® A; Aristocort® Forte; Aristocort® Intralesional; Aristospan® Intra-Articular; Aristospan® Intralesional; Atolone®; Azmacort™; Delta-Tritex®; Flutex®; Kenacort®; Kenaject-40®; Kenalog®; Kenalog-10®; Kenalog-40®; Kenalog® H; Kenalog® in Orabase®; Kenonel®; Nasacort®; Nasacort® AQ; Tac™-3;

Tac™-40; Triacet®; Triam-A®; Triam Forte®; Triderm®; Tri-Kort®; Trilog®; Trilone®; Tristoject®

Therapeutic Category Adrenal Corticosteroid; Corticosteroid, Topical

Use Severe inflammation or immunosuppression; nasal spray for symptoms of seasonal and perennial allergic rhinitis

Usual Dosage In general, single I.M. dose of 4-7 times oral dose will control patient from 4-7 days up to 3-4 weeks.

Children 6-12 years:
Inhalation: 1-2 inhalations 3-4 times/day, not to exceed 12 inhalations/day
I.M.: Acetonide or hexacetonide: 0.03-0.2 mg/kg at 1- to 7-day intervals

Children >12 years and Adults:
Intranasal: 2 sprays in each nostril once daily; may increase after 4-7 days up to 4 sprays once daily or 1 spray 4 times/day in each nostril
Topical: Apply a thin film 2-3 times/day
Oral: 4-100 mg/day
I.M.: Acetonide or hexacetonide: 60 mg (of 40 mg/mL), additional 20-100 mg doses (usual: 40-80 mg) may be administered when signs and symptoms recur, best at 6-week intervals to minimize HPA suppression
Oral inhalation: 2 inhalations 3-4 times/day, not to exceed 16 inhalations/day
Intra-articularly, intrasynovially, intralesionally: 2.5-40 mg as diacetate salt or acetonide salt, dose may be repeated when signs and symptoms recur
Intra-articularly: Hexacetonide: 2-20 mg every 3-4 weeks as hexacetonide salt
Intralesional (use 10 mg/mL): Diacetate or acetonide: 1 mg/injection site, may be repeated one or more times/week depending upon patients response; maximum; 30 mg at any one time; may use multiple injections if they are more than 1 cm apart
Intra-articular, intrasynovial, and soft-tissue injection (use 10 mg/mL or 40 mg/mL): Diacetate or acetonide: 2.5-40 mg depending upon location, size of joints, and degree of inflammation; repeat when signs and symptoms recur
Sublesionally (as acetonide): Up to 1 mg per injection site and may be repeated one or more times weekly; multiple sites may be injected if they are 1 cm or more apart, not to exceed 30 mg

Dosage Forms
Aerosol:
Oral inhalation: 100 mcg/metered spray (2 oz)
Nasal: 55 mcg per actuation (15 mL)
Topical, as acetonide: 0.2 mg/2 second spray (23 g, 63 g)
Cream, as acetonide: 0.025% (15 g, 60 g, 80 g, 240 g, 454 g); 0.1% (15 g, 30 g, 60 g, 80 g, 90 g, 120 g, 240 g); 0.5% (15 g, 20 g, 30 g, 240 g)
Injection:
As acetonide: 10 mg/mL (5 mL); 40 mg/mL (1 mL, 5 mL, 10 mL)
As diacetate: 25 mg/mL (5 mL); 40 mg/mL (1 mL, 5 mL, 10 mL)
As hexacetonide: 5 mg/mL (5 mL); 20 mg/mL (1 mL, 5 mL)
Lotion, as acetonide: 0.025% (60 mL); 0.1% (15 mL, 60 mL)
Ointment:
Oral: 0.1% (5 g)
Topical, as acetonide: 0.025% (15 g, 30 g, 60 g, 80 g, 120 g, 454 g); 0.1% (15 g, 30 g, 60 g, 80 g, 120 g, 240 g, 454 g); 0.5% (15 g, 20 g, 30 g, 240 g)
Spray, nasal, as acetonide: 55 mcg per actuation in aqueous base (16.5 g)
Syrup: 2 mg/5 mL (120 mL); 4 mg/5 mL (120 mL)
Tablet: 1 mg, 2 mg, 4 mg, 8 mg

triamcinolone acetonide *see* triamcinolone *on previous page*

triamcinolone and nystatin *see* nystatin and triamcinolone *on page 381*

triamcinolone diacetate *see* triamcinolone *on previous page*

triamcinolone hexacetonide *see* triamcinolone *on previous page*

Triam Forte® *see* triamcinolone *on previous page*

Triaminic® Allergy Tablet [OTC] *see* chlorpheniramine and phenylpropanolamine on page 114

Triaminic® AM Decongestant Formula [OTC] *see* pseudoephedrine on page 449

Triaminic® Cold Tablet [OTC] *see* chlorpheniramine and phenylpropanolamine on page 114

Triaminic® Expectorant [OTC] *see* guaifenesin and phenylpropanolamine on page 249

Triaminicol® Multi-Symptom Cold Syrup [OTC] *see* chlorpheniramine, phenyl-propanolamine, and dextromethorphan on page 117

Triaminic® Oral Infant Drops *see* pheniramine, phenylpropanolamine, and pyrilamine on page 409

Triaminic® Syrup [OTC] *see* chlorpheniramine and phenylpropanolamine on page 114

triamterene (trye AM ter een)
Brand Names Dyrenium®
Therapeutic Category Diuretic, Potassium Sparing
Use Alone or in combination with other diuretics to treat edema and hypertension; decreases potassium excretion caused by kaliuretic diuretics
Usual Dosage Oral:
Children: 2-4 mg/kg/day in 1-2 divided doses; maximum: 300 mg/day
Adults: 100-300 mg/day in 1-2 divided doses; maximum dose: 300 mg/day
Dosage Forms Capsule: 50 mg, 100 mg

triamterene and hydrochlorothiazide *see* hydrochlorothiazide and triamterene on page 265

Triapin® *see* butalbital compound and acetaminophen on page 78

Triavil® *see* amitriptyline and perphenazine on page 27

triazolam (trye AY zoe lam)
Brand Names Halcion®
Therapeutic Category Benzodiazepine
Controlled Substance C-IV
Use Short-term treatment of insomnia
Usual Dosage Oral (onset of action is rapid, patient should be in bed when taking medication):
Children <18 years: Dosage not established
Adults: 0.125-0.25 mg at bedtime
Dosage Forms Tablet: 0.125 mg, 0.25 mg

Triban® *see* trimethobenzamide on page 534

tribavirin *see* ribavirin on page 464

Tri-Chlor® *see* trichloroacetic acid on next page

trichlormethiazide (trye klor meth EYE a zide)
Brand Names Metahydrin®; Naqua®
Therapeutic Category Diuretic, Thiazide
Use Management of mild to moderate hypertension; treatment of edema in congestive heart failure and nephrotic syndrome
Usual Dosage Oral:
Children >6 months: 0.07 mg/kg/24 hours or 2 mg/m^2/24 hours
Adults: 1-4 mg/day
Dosage Forms Tablet: 2 mg, 4 mg

trichloroacetaldehyde monohydrate *see* chloral hydrate on page 107

trichloroacetic acid (trye klor oh a SEE tik AS id)
Brand Names Tri-Chlor®
Therapeutic Category Keratolytic Agent
Use Debride callous tissue
Usual Dosage Apply to verruca, cover with bandage for 5-6 days, remove verruca, reapply as needed
Dosage Forms Liquid: 80% (15 mL)

Trichophyton skin test (trye koe FYE ton skin test)
Brand Names Dermatophytin®
Therapeutic Category Diagnostic Agent
Use Assess cell-mediated immunity
Usual Dosage 0.1 mL intradermally, examine reaction site in 24-48 hours; induration of ≥5 mm in diameter is a positive reaction
Dosage Forms Injection:
Diluted: 1:30 V/V (5 mL)
Undiluted: 5 mL

Tri-Clear® Expectorant [OTC] *see* guaifenesin and phenylpropanolamine *on page 249*

Triderm® *see* triamcinolone *on page 528*

Tridesilon® Topical *see* desonide *on page 155*

tridihexethyl (trye dye heks ETH il)
Synonyms tridihexethyl chloride
Brand Names Pathilon®
Therapeutic Category Anticholinergic Agent
Use Adjunctive therapy in peptic ulcer treatment
Usual Dosage Adults: Oral: 1-2 tablets 3-4 times/day before meals and 2 tablets at bedtime
Dosage Forms Tablet, as chloride: 25 mg

tridihexethyl chloride *see* tridihexethyl *on this page*

Tridil® Injection *see* nitroglycerin *on page 376*

Tridione® *see* trimethadione *on page 533*

trientine (TRYE en teen)
Synonyms trientine hydrochloride
Brand Names Syprine®
Therapeutic Category Chelating Agent
Use Treatment of Wilson's disease in patients intolerant to penicillamine
Usual Dosage Oral (administer on an empty stomach):
Children <12 years: 500-750 mg/day in divided doses 2-4 times/day; maximum: 1.5 g/day
Adults: 750-1250 mg/day in divided doses 2-4 times/day; maximum daily dose: 2 g
Dosage Forms Capsule, as hydrochloride: 250 mg

trientine hydrochloride *see* trientine *on this page*

triethanolamine polypeptide oleate-condensate
(trye eth a NOLE a meen pol i PEP tide OH lee ate-KON den sate)
Brand Names Cerumenex® Otic
Therapeutic Category Otic Agent, Cerumenolytic
Use Removal of ear wax (cerumen)
Usual Dosage Children and Adults: Otic: Fill ear canal, insert cotton plug; allow to remain 15-30 minutes; flush ear with lukewarm water
(Continued)

triethanolamine polypeptide oleate-condensate *(Continued)*
Dosage Forms Solution, otic: 6 mL, 12 mL

triethanolamine salicylate (trye eth a NOLE a meen sa LIS i late)
Brand Names Myoflex® [OTC]; Sportscreme® [OTC]
Therapeutic Category Analgesic, Topical
Use Relief of pain of muscular aches, rheumatism, neuralgia, sprains, arthritis on intact skin
Usual Dosage Topical: Apply to area as needed
Dosage Forms Cream: 10% in a nongreasy base

triethylenethiophosphoramide *see* thiotepa *on page 517*

Trifed-C® *see* triprolidine, pseudoephedrine, and codeine *on page 537*

trifluoperazine (trye floo oh PER a zeen)
Synonyms trifluoperazine hydrochloride
Brand Names Stelazine®
Therapeutic Category Phenothiazine Derivative
Use Treatment of psychoses and management of anxiety
Usual Dosage
  Children 6-12 years: Psychoses:
    Oral: Hospitalized or well supervised patients: Initial dose: 1 mg 1-2 times/day, gradually increase until symptoms are controlled or adverse effects become troublesome; maximum: 15 mg/day
    I.M.: 1 mg twice daily
  Adults:
    Psychoses:
      Outpatients: Oral: 1-2 mg twice daily
      Hospitalized or well supervised patients: Initial dose: 2-5 mg twice daily with optimum response in the 15-20 mg/day range; do not exceed 40 mg/day
      I.M.: 1-2 mg every 4-6 hours as needed up to 10 mg/24 hours maximum
      Nonpsychotic anxiety: Oral: 1-2 mg twice daily; maximum: 6 mg/day; therapy for anxiety should not exceed 12 weeks; do not exceed 6 mg/day for longer than 12 weeks when treating anxiety; agitation, jitteriness or insomnia may be confused with original neurotic or psychotic symptoms
Dosage Forms
  Concentrate, oral, as hydrochloride: 10 mg/mL (60 mL)
  Injection, as hydrochloride: 2 mg/mL (10 mL)
  Tablet, as hydrochloride: 1 mg, 2 mg, 5 mg, 10 mg

trifluoperazine hydrochloride *see* trifluoperazine *on this page*

trifluorothymidine *see* trifluridine *on next page*

triflupromazine (trye floo PROE ma zeen)
Synonyms triflupromazine hydrochloride
Brand Names Vesprin®
Therapeutic Category Phenothiazine Derivative
Use Treatment of psychoses, nausea, vomiting, and intractable hiccups
Usual Dosage
  Children: I.M.: 0.2-0.25 mg/kg
  Adults:
    I.M.: 5-15 mg every 4 hours
    I.V.: 1 mg
Dosage Forms Injection, as hydrochloride: 20 mg/mL (1 mL)

triflupromazine hydrochloride *see* triflupromazine *on this page*

trifluridine (trye FLURE i deen)
Synonyms f₃t; trifluorothymidine
Brand Names Viroptic® Ophthalmic
Therapeutic Category Antiviral Agent
Use Treatment of primary keratoconjunctivitis and recurrent epithelial keratitis caused by herpes simplex virus types I and II
Usual Dosage Adults: Ophthalmic: Instill 1 drop into affected eye every 2 hours while awake, to a maximum of 9 drops/day, until re-epithelialization of corneal ulcer occurs; then use 1 drop every 4 hours for another 7 days; do **not** exceed 21 days of treatment
Dosage Forms Solution, ophthalmic: 1% (7.5 mL)

triglycerides, medium chain *see* medium chain triglycerides *on page 325*

Trihexy® *see* trihexyphenidyl *on this page*

trihexyphenidyl (trye heks ee FEN i dil)
Synonyms benzhexol hydrochloride; trihexyphenidyl hydrochloride
Brand Names Artane®; Trihexy®
Therapeutic Category Anticholinergic Agent; Anti-Parkinson's Agent
Use Adjunctive treatment of Parkinson's disease; also used in treatment of drug-induced extrapyramidal effects and acute dystonic reactions
Usual Dosage Oral:
Parkinsonism: Initial: Administer 1-2 mg the first day; increase by 2 mg increments at intervals of 3-5 days, until a total of 6-10 mg is administered daily. Many patients derive maximum benefit from a total daily dose of 6-10 mg; however, postencephalitic patients may require a total daily dose of 12-15 mg in 3-4 divided doses
Concomitant use with levodopa: 3-6 mg/day in divided doses is usually adequate
Drug-induced extrapyramidal disorders: Start with a single 1 mg dose; daily dosage usually ranges between 5-15 mg in 3-4 divided doses
Dosage Forms
Capsule, as hydrochloride, sustained release: 5 mg
Elixir, as hydrochloride: 2 mg/5 mL (480 mL)
Tablet, as hydrochloride: 2 mg, 5 mg

trihexyphenidyl hydrochloride *see* trihexyphenidyl *on this page*

Tri-Immunol® *see* diphtheria, tetanus toxoids, and whole-cell pertussis vaccine *on page 175*

Tri-K® *see* potassium acetate, potassium bicarbonate, and potassium citrate *on page 426*

Tri-Kort® *see* triamcinolone *on page 528*

Trilafon® *see* perphenazine *on page 407*

Tri-Levlen® *see* ethinyl estradiol and levonorgestrel *on page 208*

Trilisate® *see* choline magnesium trisalicylate *on page 121*

Trilog® *see* triamcinolone *on page 528*

Trilone® *see* triamcinolone *on page 528*

Trimazide® *see* trimethobenzamide *on next page*

trimethadione (trye meth a DYE one)
Synonyms troxidone
Brand Names Tridione®
Therapeutic Category Anticonvulsant
Use Control absence (petit mal) seizures refractory to other drugs
Usual Dosage Oral:
Children: Initial: 25-50 mg/kg/24 hours in 3-4 equally divided doses every 6-8 hours
Adults: Initial: 900 mg/day in 3-4 equally divided doses, increase by 300 mg/day at weekly intervals until therapeutic results or toxic symptoms appear
(Continued)

trimethadione *(Continued)*
Dosage Forms
Capsule: 300 mg
Solution: 40 mg/mL (473 mL)
Tablet, chewable: 150 mg

trimethaphan camsylate (trye METH a fan KAM si late)
Brand Names Arfonad® Injection
Therapeutic Category Alpha-Adrenergic Blocking Agent
Use Hypertensive emergencies; controlled hypotension during surgery
Usual Dosage I.V.:
Children: 50-150 mcg/kg/minute
Adults: Initial: 0.5-2 mg/minute; titrate to effect; usual dose: 0.3-6 mg/minute
Dosage Forms Injection: 50 mg/mL (10 mL)

trimethobenzamide (trye meth oh BEN za mide)
Synonyms trimethobenzamide hydrochloride
Brand Names Arrestin®; Pediatric Triban®; Tebamide®; T-Gen®; Ticon®; Tigan®; Triban®; Trimazide®
Therapeutic Category Anticholinergic Agent; Antiemetic
Use Control of nausea and vomiting (especially for long term antiemetic therapy)
Usual Dosage Rectal use: Contraindicated in neonates and premature infants
Children:
Oral, rectal: 15-20 mg/kg/day or 400-500 mg/m^2/day divided into 3-4 doses
I.M.: Not recommended
Adults:
Oral: 250 mg 3-4 times/day
I.M., rectal: 200 mg 3-4 times/day
Dosage Forms
Capsule, as hydrochloride: 100 mg, 250 mg
Injection, as hydrochloride: 100 mg/mL (2 mL, 20 mL)
Suppository, rectal, as hydrochloride: 100 mg, 200 mg

trimethobenzamide hydrochloride *see* trimethobenzamide *on this page*

trimethoprim (trye METH oh prim)
Synonyms tmp
Brand Names Proloprim®; Trimpex®
Therapeutic Category Antibiotic, Miscellaneous
Use Treatment and prophylaxis of urinary tract infections; in combination with other agents for treatment of *Pneumocystis carinii* pneumonia
Usual Dosage Adults: Oral: 100 mg every 12 hours or 200 mg every 24 hours
Dosage Forms Tablet: 100 mg, 200 mg

trimethoprim and polymyxin b (trye METH oh prim & pol i MIKS in bee)
Synonyms polymyxin b and trimethoprim
Brand Names Polytrim® Ophthalmic
Therapeutic Category Antibiotic, Ophthalmic
Use Treatment of surface ocular bacterial conjunctivitis and blepharoconjunctivitis
Usual Dosage Ophthalmic: Instill 1-2 drops in eye(s) every 4-6 hours
Dosage Forms Solution, ophthalmic: Trimethoprim sulfate 1 mg and polymyxin B sulfate 10,000 units per mL (10 mL)

trimethoprim and sulfamethoxazole *see* co-trimoxazole *on page 140*
trimethylpsoralen *see* trioxsalen *on next page*

trimetrexate glucuronate (tri me TREKS ate gloo KYOOR oh nate)

Brand Names Neutrexin™ Injection

Therapeutic Category Antibiotic, Miscellaneous

Use Alternative therapy for the treatment of moderate-to-severe *Pneumocystis carinii* pneumonia (PCP) in immunocompromised patients, including patients with acquired immunodeficiency syndrome (AIDS), who are intolerant of, or are refractory to, co-trimoxazole therapy or for whom co-trimoxazole is contraindicated

Usual Dosage Adults: I.V.: 45 mg/m^2 once daily over 60 minutes for 21 days; it is necessary to reduce the dose in patients with liver dysfunction, although no specific recommendations exist

Dosage Forms Powder for injection: 25 mg

trimipramine (trye MI pra meen)

Synonyms trimipramine maleate

Brand Names Surmontil®

Therapeutic Category Antidepressant, Tricyclic (Tertiary Amine)

Use Treatment of various forms of depression, often in conjunction with psychotherapy

Usual Dosage Oral: 50-150 mg/day as a single bedtime dose

Dosage Forms Capsule, as maleate: 25 mg, 50 mg, 100 mg

trimipramine maleate *see* trimipramine *on this page*

Trimox® *see* amoxicillin *on page 30*

Trimpex® *see* trimethoprim *on previous page*

Trinalin® *see* azatadine and pseudoephedrine *on page 50*

Tri-Nefrin® Extra Strength Tablet [OTC] *see* chlorpheniramine and phenylpropanolamine *on page 114*

Tri-Norinyl® *see* ethinyl estradiol and norethindrone *on page 209*

Triofed® Syrup [OTC] *see* triprolidine and pseudoephedrine *on next page*

Triostat™ Injection *see* liothyronine *on page 309*

Triotann® Tablet *see* chlorpheniramine, pyrilamine, and phenylephrine *on page 118*

trioxsalen (trye OKS a len)

Synonyms trimethylpsoralen

Brand Names Trisoralen®

Therapeutic Category Psoralen

Use In conjunction with controlled exposure to ultraviolet light or sunlight for repigmentation of idiopathic vitiligo; increasing tolerance to sunlight with albinism; enhance pigmentation

Usual Dosage Children >12 years and Adults: Oral: 10 mg/day as a single dose, 2-4 hours before controlled exposure to UVA or sunlight

Dosage Forms Tablet: 5 mg

Tripedia® *see* diphtheria, tetanus toxoids, and acellular pertussis vaccine *on page 175*

tripelennamine (tri pel EN a meen)

Synonyms tripelennamine citrate; tripelennamine hydrochloride

Brand Names PBZ®; PBZ-SR®

Therapeutic Category Antihistamine

Use Perennial and seasonal allergic rhinitis and other allergic symptoms including urticaria

Usual Dosage Oral:

Infants and Children: 5 mg/kg/day in 4-6 divided doses, up to 300 mg/day maximum

(Continued)

tripelennamine *(Continued)*

Adults: 25-50 mg every 4-6 hours, extended release tablets 100 mg morning and evening up to 100 mg every 8 hours

Dosage Forms

Elixir, as citrate: 37.5 mg/5 mL [equivalent to 25 mg hydrochloride] (473 mL)

Tablet, as hydrochloride: 25 mg, 50 mg

Tablet, extended release, as hydrochloride: 100 mg

tripelennamine citrate *see* tripelennamine *on previous page*

tripelennamine hydrochloride *see* tripelennamine *on previous page*

Triphasil® *see* ethinyl estradiol and levonorgestrel *on page 208*

Tri-Phen-Chlor® *see* chlorpheniramine, phenyltoloxamine, phenylpropanolamine, and phenylephrine *on page 117*

Triphenyl® Expectorant [OTC] *see* guaifenesin and phenylpropanolamine *on page 249*

Triphenyl® Syrup [OTC] *see* chlorpheniramine and phenylpropanolamine *on page 114*

Triple Antibiotic® Topical *see* bacitracin, neomycin, and polymyxin b *on page 53*

triple sulfa *see* sulfabenzamide, sulfacetamide, and sulfathiazole *on page 496*

Triple X® Liquid [OTC] *see* pyrethrins *on page 452*

Triposed® Syrup [OTC] *see* triprolidine and pseudoephedrine *on this page*

Triposed® Tablet [OTC] *see* triprolidine and pseudoephedrine *on this page*

triprolidine and pseudoephedrine

(trye PROE li deen & soo doe e FED rin)

Synonyms pseudoephedrine and triprolidine

Brand Names Actagen® Syrup [OTC]; Actagen® Tablet [OTC]; Allercon® Tablet [OTC]; Allerfrin® Syrup [OTC]; Allerfrin® Tablet [OTC]; Allerphed Syrup [OTC]; Aprodine® Syrup [OTC]; Aprodine® Tablet [OTC]; Cenafed® Plus Tablet [OTC]; Genac® Tablet [OTC]; Silafed® Syrup [OTC]; Triofed® Syrup [OTC]; Triposed® Syrup [OTC]; Triposed® Tablet [OTC]

Therapeutic Category Antihistamine/Decongestant Combination

Use Temporary relief of nasal congestion, running nose, sneezing, itching of nose or throat and itchy, watery eyes due to common cold, hay fever or other upper respiratory allergies

Usual Dosage May dose according to **pseudoephedrine** component (4 mg/kg/day in divided doses 3-4 times/day) Oral:

Children:

4 months to 2 years: 1.25 mL 3-4 times/day

2-4 years: 2.5 mL 3-4 times/day

4-6 years: 3.75 mL 3-4 times/day

6-12 years: 5 mL or ½ tablet 3-4 times/day, not to exceed 2 tablets/day

Children >12 years and Adults: 10 mL or 1 tablet 3-4 times/day, not to exceed 4 tablets/day

Dosage Forms

Capsule: Triprolidine hydrochloride 2.5 mg and pseudoephedrine hydrochloride 60 mg

Extended release: Triprolidine hydrochloride 5 mg and pseudoephedrine hydrochloride 120 mg

Syrup: Triprolidine hydrochloride 1.25 mg and pseudoephedrine hydrochloride 30 mg per 5 mL

Tablet: Triprolidine hydrochloride 2.5 mg and pseudoephedrine hydrochloride 60 mg

triprolidine, pseudoephedrine, and codeine
(trye PROE li deen, soo doe e FED rin, & KOE deen)
Brand Names Actagen-C®; Allerfrin® w/Codeine; Aprodine® w/C; Triacin-C®; Trifed-C®
Therapeutic Category Antihistamine/Decongestant/Antitussive
Controlled Substance C-V
Use Symptomatic relief of cough
Usual Dosage Oral:
Children:
2-6 years: 2.5 mL 4 times/day
7-12 years: 5 mL 4 times/day
Children >12 years and Adults: 10 mL 4 times/day
Dosage Forms Syrup: Triprolidine hydrochloride 1.25 mg, pseudoephedrine hydrochloride 30 mg, and codeine phosphate 10 mg per 5 mL with alcohol 4.3%

TripTone® Caplets® [OTC] *see* dimenhydrinate *on page 171*

tris buffer *see* tromethamine *on next page*

tris(hydroxymethyl)aminomethane *see* tromethamine *on next page*

Trisoralen® *see* trioxsalen *on page 535*

Tri-Statin® II Topical *see* nystatin and triamcinolone *on page 381*

Tristoject® *see* triamcinolone *on page 528*

trisulfapyrimidines *see* sulfadiazine, sulfamethazine, and sulfamerazine *on page 498*

Tri-Tannate Plus® *see* chlorpheniramine, ephedrine, phenylephrine, and carbetapentane *on page 115*

Tri-Tannate® Tablet *see* chlorpheniramine, pyrilamine, and phenylephrine *on page 118*

Tritec® *see* ranitidine bismuth citrate *on page 459*

Tri-Vi-Flor® *see* vitamin, multiple (pediatric) *on page 554*

Trobicin® *see* spectinomycin *on page 490*

Trocaine® [OTC] *see* benzocaine *on page 59*

Trocal® [OTC] *see* dextromethorphan *on page 160*

troglitazone (TROE gli to zone)
Brand Names Rezulin®
Therapeutic Category Thiazolidinedione Derivative
Use Use in patients with type II diabetes currently on insulin therapy whose hyperglycemia is not controlled (HbA$_{1c}$ >8.5%) despite insulin therapy of over 30 units/day given as multiple infections
Usual Dosage Adults: Oral: 200 mg once daily with a meal; for patients on insulin therapy (continue current insulin dose); dose may be increased to 400 mg/day after 2-4 weeks in those who are not responding adequately; maximum recommended dose: 600 mg/day; it is recommended that the insulin dose should be reduced by 10% to 25% when fasting plasma glucose concentrations decrease to <120 mg/dL in those patients receiving concomitant insulin
Dosage Forms Tablet: 200 mg, 400 mg

troleandomycin (troe lee an doe MYE sin)
Synonyms triacetyloleandomycin
Brand Names Tao®
Therapeutic Category Macrolide (Antibiotic)
Use Adjunct in the treatment of severe corticosteroid-dependent asthma due to its steroid-sparing properties; obsolete antibiotic with spectrum of activity similar to erythromycin
(Continued)

troleandomycin (Continued)

Usual Dosage Oral:
Children: 25-40 mg/kg/day divided every 6 hours
Adjunct in corticosteroid-dependent asthma: 14 mg/kg/day in divided doses every 6-12 hours not to exceed 250 mg every 6 hours; dose is tapered to once daily then alternate day dosing
Adults: 250-500 mg 4 times/day
Dosage Forms Capsule: 250 mg

tromethamine (troe METH a meen)

Synonyms tris buffer; tris(hydroxymethyl)aminomethane
Brand Names THAM-E® Injection; THAM® Injection
Therapeutic Category Alkalinizing Agent
Use Correction of metabolic acidosis associated with cardiac bypass surgery or cardiac arrest; to correct excess acidity of stored blood that is preserved with acid citrate dextrose (ACD); to prime the pump-oxygenator during cardiac bypass surgery; indicated in severe metabolic acidosis in patients in whom sodium or carbon dioxide elimination is restricted [eg, infants needing alkalinization after receiving maximum sodium bicarbonate (8-10 mEq/kg/24 hours)]
Usual Dosage Dose depends on buffer base deficit; when deficit is known: tromethamine mL of 0.3 M solution = body weight (kg) x base deficit (mEq/L); when base deficit is not known: 3-6 mL/kg/dose I.V. (1-2 mEq/kg/dose)

Metabolic acidosis with cardiac arrest:
I.V.: 3.5-6 mL/kg (1-2 mEq/kg/dose) into large peripheral vein; 500-1000 mL if needed in adults
I.V. continuous drip: Infuse slowly by syringe pump over 3-6 hours
Excess acidity of ACD priming blood: 14-70 mL of 0.3 molar solution added to each 500 mL of blood
Dosage Forms Injection:
THAM®: 18 g [0.3 molar] (500 mL)
THAM-E®: 36 g with sodium 30 mEq, potassium 5 mEq, and chloride 35 mEq (1000 mL)

Tronolane® [OTC] see pramoxine on page 432

Tropicacyl® see tropicamide on this page

tropicamide (troe PIK a mide)

Synonyms bistropamide
Brand Names Mydriacyl®; Opticyl®; Tropicacyl®
Therapeutic Category Anticholinergic Agent
Use Short-acting mydriatic used in diagnostic procedures; as well as preoperatively and postoperatively; treatment of some cases of acute iritis, iridocyclitis, and keratitis
Usual Dosage Children and Adults: Ophthalmic:
Cycloplegia: 1-2 drops (1%); may repeat in 5 minutes
Mydriasis: 1-2 drops (0.5%) 15-20 minutes before exam; may repeat every 30 minutes as needed
Dosage Forms Solution, ophthalmic: 0.5% (2 mL, 15 mL); 1% (2 mL, 3 mL, 15 mL)

troxidone see trimethadione on page 533

Truphylline® see aminophylline on page 25

Trusopt® see dorzolamide on page 182

trypsin, balsam peru, and castor oil

(TRIP sin, BAL sam pe RUE , & KAS tor oyl)
Brand Names Granulex
Therapeutic Category Protectant, Topical

Use Treatment of decubitus ulcers, varicose ulcers, debridement of eschar, dehiscent wounds and sunburn

Usual Dosage Topical: Apply a minimum of twice daily or as often as necessary

Dosage Forms Aerosol, topical: Trypsin 0.1 mg, balsam Peru 72.5 mg, and castor oil 650 mg per 0.82 mL (60 g, 120 g)

Trysul® *see* sulfabenzamide, sulfacetamide, and sulfathiazole *on page 496*

tsh *see* thyrotropin *on page 518*

tspa *see* thiotepa *on page 517*

T-Stat® **Topical** *see* erythromycin, topical *on page 201*

tuberculin tests (too BER kyoo lin)

Synonyms Mantoux; old tuberculin; ppd; purified protein derivative

Brand Names Aplisol®; Aplitest®; Tine Test PPD; Tubersol®

Therapeutic Category Diagnostic Agent

Use Skin test in diagnosis of tuberculosis, to aid in assessment of cell-mediated immunity; routine tuberculin testing is recommended at 12 months of age and at every 1-2 years thereafter, before the measles vaccination

Usual Dosage Children and Adults: Intradermally: 0.1 mL approximately 4" below elbow; use ¼" to ½" or 26- or 27-gauge needle; significant reactions are ≥5 mm in diameter

Dosage Forms Injection:
First test strength: 1 TU/0.1 mL (1 mL)
Intermediate test strength: 5 TU/0.1 mL (1 mL, 5 mL, 10 mL)
Second test strength: 250 TU/0.1 mL (1 mL)
Tine: 5 TU each test

Tubersol® *see* tuberculin tests *on this page*

tubocurarine (too boe kyoor AR een)

Synonyms d-tubocurarine chloride; tubocurarine chloride

Therapeutic Category Skeletal Muscle Relaxant

Use Adjunct to anesthesia to induce skeletal muscle relaxation

Usual Dosage Children and Adults: I.V.: 0.2-0.4 mg/kg as a single dose; maintenance: 0.04-0.2 mg/kg/dose as needed to maintain paralysis
Alternative adult dose: 6-9 mg once daily, then 3-4.5 mg as needed to maintain paralysis

Dosage Forms Injection, as chloride: 3 mg/mL [3 units/mL] (5 mL, 10 mL, 20 mL)

tubocurarine chloride *see* tubocurarine *on this page*

Tucks® **[OTC]** *see* witch hazel *on page 557*

Tuinal® *see* amobarbital and secobarbital *on page 29*

Tums® **[OTC]** *see* calcium carbonate *on page 82*

Tums® **E-X Extra Strength Tablet [OTC]** *see* calcium carbonate *on page 82*

Tums® **Extra Strength Liquid [OTC]** *see* calcium carbonate *on page 82*

Tusibron® **[OTC]** *see* guaifenesin *on page 247*

Tusibron-DM® **[OTC]** *see* guaifenesin and dextromethorphan *on page 248*

Tussafed® **Drops** *see* carbinoxamine, pseudoephedrine, and dextromethorphan *on page 91*

Tussafin® **Expectorant** *see* hydrocodone, pseudoephedrine, and guaifenesin *on page 268*

Tuss-Allergine® **Modified T.D. Capsule** *see* caramiphen and phenylpropanolamine *on page 88*

Tussar® **SF Syrup** *see* guaifenesin, pseudoephedrine, and codeine *on page 251*

Tuss-DM® **[OTC]** *see* guaifenesin and dextromethorphan *on page 248*

Tussigon® *see* hydrocodone and homatropine *on page 267*

Tussionex® *see* hydrocodone and chlorpheniramine *on page 266*

Tussi-Organidin® **DM NR** *see* guaifenesin and dextromethorphan *on page 248*

Tussi-Organidin® **NR** *see* guaifenesin and codeine *on page 247*

Tuss-LA® *see* guaifenesin and pseudoephedrine *on page 250*

Tussogest® **Extended Release Capsule** *see* caramiphen and phenylpropanolamine *on page 88*

Tusstat® **Syrup** *see* diphenhydramine *on page 173*

Twice-A-Day® **Nasal [OTC]** *see* oxymetazoline *on page 390*

Twilite® **Oral [OTC]** *see* diphenhydramine *on page 173*

Twin-K® *see* potassium citrate and potassium gluconate *on page 429*

Two-Dyne® *see* butalbital compound and acetaminophen *on page 78*

Tylenol® **[OTC]** *see* acetaminophen *on page 3*

Tylenol® **Cold Effervescent Medication Tablet [OTC]** *see* chlorpheniramine, phenylpropanolamine, and acetaminophen *on page 117*

Tylenol® **Cold No Drowsiness [OTC]** *see* acetaminophen, dextromethorphan, and pseudoephedrine *on page 6*

Tylenol® **Extended Relief [OTC]** *see* acetaminophen *on page 3*

Tylenol® **Flu Maximum Strength [OTC]** *see* acetaminophen, dextromethorphan, and pseudoephedrine *on page 6*

Tylenol® **Sinus, Maximum Strength [OTC]** *see* acetaminophen and pseudoephedrine *on page 5*

Tylenol® **With Codeine** *see* acetaminophen and codeine *on page 3*

Tylox® *see* oxycodone and acetaminophen *on page 390*

Typhim Vi® *see* typhoid vaccine *on this page*

typhoid vaccine (TYE foid vak SEEN)

Synonyms typhoid vaccine live oral ty21a

Brand Names Typhim Vi®; Vivotif Berna™ Oral

Therapeutic Category Vaccine, Inactivated Bacteria

Use Promotes active immunity to typhoid fever for patients exposed to typhoid carrier or foreign travel to typhoid fever endemic area

Usual Dosage

Oral: Adults:

Primary immunization: 1 capsule on alternate days (day 1, 3, 5, and 7)

Booster immunization: Repeat full course of primary immunization every 5 years

S.C.:

Children 6 months to 10 years: 0.25 mL; repeat in ≥4 weeks (total immunization is 2 doses)

Children >10 years and Adults: 0.5 mL; repeat dose in ≥4 weeks (total immunization is 2 doses)

Booster: 0.25 mL every 3 years for children 6 months to 10 years and 0.5 mL every 3 years for adults and children >10 years

Dosage Forms

Capsule, enteric coated (Vivotif Berna®): Viable *S. typhi* Ty21a Colony-forming units 2-6 x 10^9 and nonviable *S. typhi* Ty21a Colony-forming units 50 x 10^9 with sucrose, ascorbic acid, amino acid mixture, lactose and magnesium stearate

Injection, suspension (H-P): Heat- and phenol-inactivated, killed Ty-2 strain of *S. typhi* organisms; provides 8 units/mL, ≤1 billion/mL and ≤35 mcg nitrogen/mL (5 mL, 10 mL)

Injection (Typhim Vi®): Purified Vi capsular polysaccharide 25 mcg/0.5 mL (0.5 mL)

Powder for suspension (AKD): 8 units/mL ≤1 billion/mL, acetone inactivated dried (50 doses)

typhoid vaccine live oral ty21a *see* typhoid vaccine *on previous page*

Tyzine® Nasal *see* tetrahydrozoline *on page 510*

U-90152S *see* delavirdine *on page 152*

UAD Otic® *see* neomycin, polymyxin b, and hydrocortisone *on page 369*

UCB-P071 *see* cetirizine *on page 105*

Ucephan® *see* sodium phenylacetate and sodium benzoate *on page 486*

uk *see* urokinase *on page 543*

Ulcerease® [OTC] *see* phenol *on page 410*

ULR-LA® *see* guaifenesin and phenylpropanolamine *on page 249*

Ultane® *see* sevoflurane *on page 478*

Ultiva® *see* remifentanil *on page 461*

Ultram® *see* tramadol *on page 526*

Ultra Mide® Topical *see* urea *on next page*

Ultrase® MT12 *see* pancrelipase *on page 394*

Ultrase® MT20 *see* pancrelipase *on page 394*

Ultra Tears® Solution [OTC] *see* artificial tears *on page 42*

Ultravate™ *see* halobetasol *on page 255*

Unasyn® *see* ampicillin and sulbactam *on page 33*

undecylenic acid and derivatives (un de sil EN ik AS id & dah RIV ah tivs)

Synonyms zinc undecylenate

Brand Names Caldesene® Topical [OTC]; Fungoid® AF Topical Solution [OTC]; Pedi-Pro Topical [OTC]

Therapeutic Category Antifungal Agent

Use Treatment of athlete's foot (tinea pedis), ringworm (except nails and scalp), prickly heat, jock itch (tinea cruris), diaper rash and other minor skin irritations due to superficial dermatophytes

Usual Dosage Children and Adults: Topical: Apply as needed twice daily after cleansing the affected area for 2-4 weeks

Dosage Forms
Cream: Total undecylenate 20% (15 g, 82.5 g)
Foam, topical: Undecylenic acid 10% (42.5 g)
Liquid, topical: Undecylenic acid 10% (42.5 g)
Ointment, topical: Total undecylenate 22% (30 g, 60 g, 454 g); total undecylenate 25% (60 g, 454 g)
Powder, topical: Calcium undecylenate 10% (45 g, 60 g, 120 g); total undecylenate 22% (45 g, 54 g, 81 g, 90 g, 105 g, 165 g, 454 g)
Solution, topical: Undecylenic acid 25% (29.57 mL)

Unguentine® [OTC] *see* benzocaine *on page 59*

Uni-Ace® [OTC] *see* acetaminophen *on page 3*

Uni-Bent® Cough Syrup *see* diphenhydramine *on page 173*

Unicap® [OTC] *see* vitamins, multiple (oral, adult) *on page 556*

Uni-Decon® *see* chlorpheniramine, phenyltoloxamine, phenylpropanolamine, and phenylephrine *on page 117*

Uni-Dur® *see* theophylline *on page 511*

Unilax® [OTC] *see* docusate and phenolphthalein *on page 180*

Unipen® Injection *see* nafcillin *on page 361*

Unipen® Oral *see* nafcillin *on page 361*

Uniphyl® *see* theophylline *on page 511*

Uniretic® *see* moexipril and hydrochlorothiazide *on page 354*

Unitrol® **[OTC]** *see* phenylpropanolamine *on page 413*

Uni-tussin® **[OTC]** *see* guaifenesin *on page 247*

Uni-tussin® **DM [OTC]** *see* guaifenesin and dextromethorphan *on page 248*

Univasc® *see* moexipril *on page 354*

Unna's boot *see* zinc gelatin *on page 561*

Unna's paste *see* zinc gelatin *on page 561*

Uracel® *see* sodium salicylate *on page 488*

uracil mustard (YOOR a sil MUS tard)

Therapeutic Category Antineoplastic Agent

Use Palliative treatment in symptomatic chronic lymphocytic leukemia; non-Hodgkin's lymphomas

Usual Dosage Oral:

Children: 0.3 mg/kg in a single weekly dose for 4 weeks

Adults: 0.15 mg/kg in a single weekly dose for 4 weeks

Thrombocytosis: 1-2 mg/day for 14 days

Dosage Forms Capsule: 1 mg

urea (yoor EE a)

Synonyms carbamide

Brand Names Amino-Cerv™ Vaginal Cream; Aquacare® Topical [OTC]; Carmol® Topical [OTC]; Gormel® Creme [OTC]; Lanaphilic® Topical [OTC]; Nutraplus® Topical [OTC]; Rea-Lo® [OTC]; Ultra Mide® Topical; Ureacin®-20 Topical [OTC]; Ureacin®-40 Topical; Ureaphil® Injection

Therapeutic Category Diuretic, Osmotic; Topical Skin Product

Use Reduce intracranial pressure and intraocular pressure (30%); promotes hydration and removal of excess keratin in hyperkeratotic conditions and dry skin; mild cervicitis

Usual Dosage

Children: I.V. slow infusion:

<2 years: 0.1-0.5 g/kg

>2 years: 0.5-1.5 g/kg

Adults:

I.V. infusion: 1-1.5 g/kg by slow infusion (1-2$^1/_2$ hours); maximum: 120 g/24 hours

Topical: Apply 1-3 times/day

Vaginal: 1 applicatorful in vagina at bedtime for 2-4 weeks

Dosage Forms

Cream:

Topical: 2% [20 mg/mL] (75 g); 10% [100 mg/mL] (75 g, 90 g, 454 g); 20% [200 mg/mL] (45 g, 75 g, 90 g, 454 g); 30% [300 mg/mL] (60 g, 454 g); 40% (30 g)

Vaginal: 8.34% [83.4 mg/g] (82.5 g)

Injection: 40 g/150 mL

Lotion: 2% (240 mL); 10% (180 mL, 240 mL, 480 mL); 15% (120 mL, 480 mL); 25% (180 mL)

urea and hydrocortisone (yoor EE a & hye droe KOR ti sone)

Synonyms hydrocortisone and urea

Brand Names Carmol-HC® Topical

Therapeutic Category Corticosteroid, Topical

Use Inflammation of corticosteroid-responsive dermatoses

Usual Dosage Topical: Apply thin film and rub in well 1-4 times/day

Dosage Forms Cream, topical: Urea 10% and hydrocortisone acetate 1% in a water-washable vanishing cream base (30 g)

Ureacin®**-20 Topical [OTC]** *see* urea *on this page*

Ureacin®-40 Topical *see* urea *on previous page*

urea peroxide *see* carbamide peroxide *on page 90*

Ureaphil® Injection *see* urea *on previous page*

Urecholine® *see* bethanechol *on page 66*

Urex® *see* methenamine *on page 336*

Urispas® *see* flavoxate *on page 223*

Urobak® *see* sulfamethoxazole *on page 498*

Urocit®-K *see* potassium citrate *on page 428*

Urodine® *see* phenazopyridine *on page 408*

urofollitropin (yoor oh fol li TROE pin)

Brand Names Fertinex® Injection; Metrodin® Injection

Therapeutic Category Ovulation Stimulator

Use Induction of ovulation in patients with polycystic ovarian disease and to stimulate the development of multiple oocytes

Usual Dosage Adults: Female: I.M.: 75 units/day for 7-12 days, used with hCG may repeat course of treatment 2 more times

Dosage Forms Injection: 0.83 mg [75 units FSH activity] (2 mL); 1.66 mg [150 units FSH activity]

Urogesic® *see* phenazopyridine *on page 408*

urokinase (yoor oh KIN ase)

Synonyms uk

Brand Names Abbokinase® Injection

Therapeutic Category Thrombolytic Agent

Use Treatment of recent severe or massive deep vein or arterial thrombosis, pulmonary emboli, and occluded arteriovenous cannulas

Usual Dosage

Children and Adults: Deep vein thrombosis: I.V.: Loading: 4400 units/kg over 10 minutes, then 4400 units/kg/hour for 12 hours

Adults:

Myocardial infarction: Intracoronary: 750,000 units over 2 hours (6000 units/minute over up to 2 hours)

Occluded I.V. catheters:

5000 units (use only Abbokinase® Open Cath) in each lumen over 1-2 minutes, leave in lumen for 1-4 hours, then aspirate; may repeat with 10,000 units in each lumen if 5000 units fails to clear the catheter; **do not infuse into the patient**; volume to instill into catheter is equal to the volume of the catheter

I.V. infusion: 200 units/kg/hour in each lumen for 12-48 hours at a rate of at least 20 mL/hour

Dialysis patients: 5000 units is administered in each lumen over 1-2 minutes; leave urokinase in lumen for 1-2 days, then aspirate

Clot lysis (large vessel thrombi): Loading: I.V.: 4400 units/kg over 10 minutes, increase to 6000 units/kg/hour; maintenance: 4400-6000 units/kg/hour adjusted to achieve clot lysis or patency of affected vessel; doses up to 50,000 units/kg/hour have been used. **Note:** Therapy should be initiated as soon as possible after diagnosis of thrombi and continued until clot is dissolved (usually 24-72 hours).

Acute pulmonary embolism: Three treatment alternatives: 3 million unit dosage

Alternative 1: 12-hour infusion: 4400 units/kg (2000 units/lb) bolus over 10 minutes followed by 4400 units/kg/hour (2000 units/lb); begin heparin 1000 units/hour approximately 3-4 hours after completion of urokinase infusion or when PTT is <100 seconds

Alternative 2: 2-hour infusion: 1 million unit bolus over 10 minutes followed by 2 million units over 110 minutes; begin heparin 1000 units/hour approximately 3-4 hours after completion of urokinase infusion or when PTT is <100 seconds

(Continued)

urokinase *(Continued)*

Alternative 3: Bolus dose only: 15,000 units/kg over 10 minutes; begin heparin 1000 units/hour approximately 3-4 hours after completion of urokinase infusion or when PTT is <100 seconds
Dosage Forms
Powder for injection: 250,000 units (5 mL)
Catheter clear: 5000 units (1 mL)

Uro-KP-Neutral® *see* potassium phosphate and sodium phosphate *on page 431*

Urolene Blue® *see* methylene blue *on page 342*

Urovist Cysto® *see* radiological/contrast media (ionic) *on page 457*

Urovist® **Meglumine** *see* radiological/contrast media (ionic) *on page 457*

Urovist® **Sodium 300** *see* radiological/contrast media (ionic) *on page 457*

ursodeoxycholic acid *see* ursodiol *on this page*

ursodiol (ER soe dye ole)

Synonyms ursodeoxycholic acid
Brand Names Actigall™
Therapeutic Category Gallstone Dissolution Agent
Use Gallbladder stone dissolution
Usual Dosage Oral: 8-10 mg/kg/day in 2-3 divided doses
Dosage Forms Capsule: 300 mg

Vagistat-1® **Vaginal [OTC]** *see* tioconazole *on page 520*

Vagitrol® *see* sulfanilamide *on page 498*

valacyclovir (val ay SYE kloe veer)

Brand Names Valtrex®
Therapeutic Category Antiviral Agent
Use Treatment of herpes zoster (shingles) in immunocompetent patients
Usual Dosage Adults: Oral: 1000 mg 3 times/day for 7 days
Dosage Forms Caplets: 500 mg

Valergen® **Injection** *see* estradiol *on page 202*

Valertest No.1® **Injection** *see* estradiol and testosterone *on page 203*

Valisone® *see* betamethasone *on page 64*

Valium® *see* diazepam *on page 162*

valproic acid and derivatives (val PROE ik AS id & dah RIV ah tives)

Synonyms dipropylacetic acid; divalproex sodium; dpa; 2-propylpentanoic acid; 2-propylvaleric acid
Brand Names Depacon®; Depakene®; Depakote®
Therapeutic Category Anticonvulsant
Use Management of simple and complex absence seizures; mixed seizure types; myoclonic and generalized tonic-clonic (grand mal) seizures; prevent migraine headaches in adults (Depakote®); mania associated with bipolar disorder; may be effective in partial seizures and infantile spasms; Depakote® can be used for the treatment of complex partial seizures; Depacon® is indicated as a temporary intravenous alternative when oral administration is not possible
Usual Dosage Children and Adults:
Oral: Initial: 10-15 mg/kg/day in 1-3 divided doses; increase by 5-10 mg/kg/day at weekly intervals until therapeutic levels are achieved; maintenance: 30-60 mg/kg/day in 2-3 divided doses
Children receiving more than 1 anticonvulsant (ie, polytherapy) may require doses up to 100 mg/kg/day in 3-4 divided doses

I.V.: Administer as a 60 minute infusion (≤20 mg/min) with the same frequency as oral products; switch patient to oral products as soon as possible

Rectal: Dilute syrup 1:1 with water for use as a retention enema; loading dose: 17-20 mg/kg one time; maintenance: 10-15 mg/kg/dose every 8 hours

Dosage Forms

Capsule, sprinkle, as divalproex sodium (Depakote® Sprinkle®): 125 mg

As valproic acid (Depakene®): 250 mg

Injection, as sodium valproate (Depacon®): 100 mg/mL (5 mL)

Syrup, as sodium valproate (Depakene®): 250 mg/5 mL (5 mL, 50 mL, 480 mL)

Tablet, delayed release, as divalproex sodium (Depakote®): 125 mg, 250 mg, 500 mg

valsartan (val SAR tan)

Brand Names Diovan®

Therapeutic Category Angiotensin II Antagonists

Use Treatment of hypertension alone or in combination with other antihypertensives

Dosage Forms Capsule: 80 mg, 160 mg

Valtrex® see valacyclovir *on previous page*

Vancenase® AQ Inhaler see beclomethasone *on page 56*

Vancenase® Nasal Inhaler see beclomethasone *on page 56*

Vanceril® Oral Inhaler see beclomethasone *on page 56*

Vancocin® see vancomycin *on this page*

Vancoled® see vancomycin *on this page*

vancomycin (van koe MYE sin)

Synonyms vancomycin hydrochloride

Brand Names Lyphocin®; Vancocin®; Vancoled®

Therapeutic Category Antibiotic, Miscellaneous

Use Treatment of patients with the following infections or conditions: treatment of infections due to documented or suspected methicillin-resistant *S. aureus* or beta-lactam resistant coagulase negative *Staphylococcus*; treatment of serious or life-threatening infections (ie, endocarditis, meningitis, osteomyelitis) due to documented or suspected staphylococcal or streptococcal infections in patients who are allergic to penicillins and/ or cephalosporins; empiric therapy of infections associated with central lines, VP shunts, hemodialysis shunts, vascular grafts, prosthetic heart valves; used orally for staphylococcal enterocolitis or for antibiotic-associated pseudomembranous colitis produced by *C. difficile*

Usual Dosage I.V. (initial dosage recommendation):

Infants >1 month and Children: 40 mg/kg/day in divided doses every 6 hours

Infants >1 month and Children with staphylococcal central nervous system infection: 60 mg/kg/day in divided doses every 6 hours

Adults: With normal renal function: 0.5 g every 6 hours or 1 g every 12 hours

Intrathecal:

Children: 5-20 mg/day

Adults: 20 mg/day

Oral:

Children: 10-50 mg/kg/day in divided doses every 6-8 hours; not to exceed 2 g/day

Adults: 0.5-2 g/day in divided doses every 6-8 hours

Pseudomembranous colitis produced by *C. difficile*:

Children: 40 mg/kg/day in divided doses, added to fluids

Adults: 500 mg to 2 g/day administered in 3 or 4 divided doses for 7-10 days

Dosage Forms

Capsule, as hydrochloride: 125 mg, 250 mg

Powder:

For oral solution, as hydrochloride: 1 g, 10 g

For injection, as hydrochloride: 500 mg, 1 g, 2 g, 5 g, 10 g

vancomycin hydrochloride *see* vancomycin *on previous page*

Vanoxide® [OTC] *see* benzoyl peroxide *on page 61*

Vanoxide-HC® *see* benzoyl peroxide and hydrocortisone *on page 62*

Vansil™ *see* oxamniquine *on page 387*

Vantin® *see* cefpodoxime *on page 99*

varicella virus vaccine (var i SEL a VYE rus vak SEEN)

Synonyms chicken pox vaccine; varicella-zoster virus (VZV) vaccine

Brand Names Varivax®

Therapeutic Category Vaccine, Live Virus

Use The American Association of Pediatrics recommends that the chickenpox vaccine should be given to all healthy children between 12 months and 18 years; children between 12 months and 13 years who have not been immunized or who have not had chickenpox should receive 1 vaccination while children 13-18 years of age require 2 vaccinations 4-8 weeks apart; the vaccine has been added to the childhood immunization schedule for infants 12-28 months of age and children 11-12 years of age who have not been vaccinated previously or who have not had the disease; it is recommended to be given with the measles, mumps, and rubella (MMR) vaccine

Usual Dosage S.C.:

Children 12 months to 12 years: 0.5 mL

Children 12 years to Adults: 2 doses of 0.5 mL separated by 4-8 weeks

Dosage Forms Powder for injection, lyophilized powder, preservative free: 1350 plaque forming units (PFU)/0.5 mL (0.5 mL single-dose vials)

varicella-zoster immune globulin (human)

(var i SEL a- ZOS ter i MYUN GLOB yoo lin HYU man)

Synonyms vzig

Therapeutic Category Immune Globulin

Use Passive immunization of susceptible immunodeficient patients after exposure to varicella; most effective if begun within 96 hours of exposure

VZIG supplies are limited, restrict administration to those meeting the following criteria:

One of the following underlying illnesses or conditions:

Neoplastic disease (eg, leukemia or lymphoma)

Congenital or acquired immunodeficiency

Immunosuppressive therapy with steroids, antimetabolites or other immunosuppressive treatment regimens

Newborn of mother who had onset of chickenpox within 5 days before delivery or within 48 hours after delivery

Premature (≥28 weeks gestation) whose mother has no history of chickenpox

Premature (<28 weeks gestation or ≤1000 g VZIG) regardless of maternal history

One of the following types of exposure to chickenpox or zoster patient(s):

Continuous household contact

Playmate contact (>1 hour play indoors)

Hospital contact (in same 2-4 bedroom or adjacent beds in a large ward or prolonged face-to-face contact with an infectious staff member or patient)

Susceptible to varicella-zoster

Age of <15 years; administer to immunocompromised adolescents and adults and to other older patients on an individual basis

An acceptable alternative to VZIG prophylaxis is to treat varicella, if it occurs, with high-dose I.V. acyclovir

Usual Dosage High-risk susceptible patients who are exposed again more than 3 weeks after a prior dose of VZIG should receive another full dose; there is no evidence VZIG modifies established varicella-zoster infections.

I.M.: Administer by deep injection in the gluteal muscle or in another large muscle mass. Inject 125 units/10 kg (22 lb); maximum dose: 625 units (5 vials); minimum dose: 125 units; do not administer fractional doses. Do not inject I.V.

Dosage Forms Injection: 125 units of antibody in single dose vials

varicella-zoster virus (VZV) vaccine *see* varicella virus vaccine *on previous page*

Varivax® *see* varicella virus vaccine *on previous page*

Vascor® *see* bepridil *on page 63*

Vascoray® *see* radiological/contrast media (ionic) *on page 457*

Vaseretic® 10-25 *see* enalapril and hydrochlorothiazide *on page 193*

Vasocidin® Ophthalmic *see* sulfacetamide sodium and prednisolone *on page 497*

VasoClear® Ophthalmic [OTC] *see* naphazoline *on page 364*

Vasocon-A® [OTC] Ophthalmic *see* naphazoline and antazoline *on page 365*

Vasocon Regular® Ophthalmic *see* naphazoline *on page 364*

Vasodilan® *see* isoxsuprine *on page 293*

vasopressin (vay soe PRES in)

Synonyms antidiuretic hormone; 8-arginine vasopressin

Brand Names Pitressin® Injection

Therapeutic Category Hormone, Posterior Pituitary

Use Treatment of diabetes insipidus; prevention and treatment of postoperative abdominal distention; differential diagnosis of diabetes insipidus; adjunct in the treatment of acute massive hemorrhage of GI tract or esophageal varices

Usual Dosage

Diabetes insipidus:

I.M., S.C.:

Children: 2.5-5 units 2-4 times/day as needed

Adults: 5-10 units 2-4 times/day as needed (dosage range 5-60 units/day)

Intranasal: Administer on cotton pledget or nasal spray

Abdominal distention Adults: I.M.: 5 mg stat, 10 mg every 3-4 hours

GI hemorrhage: I.V.: Administer in a peripheral vein; dilute aqueous in NS or D_5W to 0.1-1 unit/mL and infuse at 0.2-0.4 unit/minute and progressively increase to 0.9 unit/minute if necessary; I.V. infusion administration requires the use of an infusion pump and should be administered in a peripheral line to minimize adverse reactions on coronary arteries

Dosage Forms Injection, aqueous: 20 pressor units/mL (0.5 mL, 1 mL)

Vasosulf® Ophthalmic *see* sulfacetamide sodium and phenylephrine *on page 496*

Vasotec® *see* enalapril *on page 192*

Vasotec® I.V. *see* enalapril *on page 192*

Vasoxyl® *see* methoxamine *on page 339*

vcr *see* vincristine *on page 550*

V-Dec-M® *see* guaifenesin and pseudoephedrine *on page 250*

Vectrin® *see* minocycline *on page 351*

vecuronium (ve KYOO roe nee um)

Synonyms ORG NC 45

Brand Names Norcuron®

Therapeutic Category Skeletal Muscle Relaxant

Use Adjunct to anesthesia, to facilitate endotracheal intubation, and provide skeletal muscle relaxation during surgery or mechanical ventilation

(Continued)

vecuronium *(Continued)*

Usual Dosage I.V.:
Infants >7 weeks to 1 year: Initial: 0.08-0.1 mg/kg/dose; maintenance: 0.05-0.1 mg/kg/ every hour as needed
Children >1 year and Adults: Initial: 0.08-0.1 mg/kg/dose; maintenance: 0.05-0.1 mg/kg/ every hour as needed; may be administered as a continuous infusion at 0.1 mg/kg/hour

Note: Children may require slightly higher initial doses and slightly more frequent supplementation
Dosage Forms Powder for injection: 10 mg (5 mL, 10 mL)

Veetids® *see* penicillin v potassium *on page 402*

Velban® *see* vinblastine *on page 550*

Velosef® *see* cephradine *on page 104*

Velosulin® **Human** *see* insulin preparations *on page 284*

venlafaxine (VEN la faks een)

Brand Names Effexor®
Therapeutic Category Antidepressant, Phenethylamine
Use Treatment of depression
Usual Dosage Adults: Oral: 75 mg/day, administered in 2 or 3 divided doses with food; dose may be increased to 150 mg/day up to 225-375 mg/day
Dosage Forms Tablet: 25 mg, 37.5 mg, 50 mg, 75 mg, 100 mg

Venoglobulin®**-I** *see* immune globulin, intravenous *on page 281*

Venoglobulin®**-S** *see* immune globulin, intravenous *on page 281*

Ventolin® *see* albuterol *on page 14*

Ventolin® **Rotocaps**® *see* albuterol *on page 14*

VePesid® **Injection** *see* etoposide *on page 213*

VePesid® **Oral** *see* etoposide *on page 213*

verapamil (ver AP a mil)

Synonyms iproveratril hydrochloride; verapamil hydrochloride
Brand Names Calan®; Calan® SR; Covera-HS®; Isoptin®; Isoptin® SR; Verelan®
Therapeutic Category Antiarrhythmic Agent, Class IV; Calcium Channel Blocker
Use Angina, hypertension; I.V. for supraventricular tachyarrhythmias (PSVT, atrial fibrillation, atrial flutter)
Usual Dosage
Children: I.V.:
0-1 year: 0.1-0.2 mg/kg/dose, repeated after 30 minutes as needed
1-16 years: 0.1-0.3 mg/kg over 2-3 minutes; maximum: 5 mg/dose, may repeat dose once in 30 minutes if adequate response not achieved; maximum for second dose: 10 mg/dose
Children: Oral (dose not well established):
4-8 mg/kg/day in 3 divided doses **or** 1-5 years: 40-80 mg every 8 hours
>5 years: 80 mg every 6-8 hours
Adults:
Oral: 240-480 mg/24 hours divided 3-4 times/day
I.V.: 5-10 mg (0.075-0.15 mg/kg); may repeat 10 mg (0.15 mg/kg) 15-30 minutes after the initial dose if needed and if patient tolerated initial dose
Dosage Forms
Capsule, as hydrochloride, sustained release (Verelan®): 120 mg, 180 mg, 240 mg, 360 mg
Injection, as hydrochloride: 2.5 mg/mL (2 mL, 4 mL)
Isoptin®: 2.5 mg/mL (2 mL, 4 mL)
Tablet, as hydrochloride: 40 mg, 80 mg, 120 mg

Calan®, Isoptin®: 40 mg, 80 mg, 120 mg
Tablet, as hydrochloride, sustained release: 180 mg, 240 mg
Calan® SR, Isoptin® SR: 120 mg, 180 mg, 240 mg
Covera-HS®: 180 mg, 240 mg

verapamil hydrochloride *see* verapamil *on previous page*

Verazinc® Oral [OTC] *see* zinc sulfate *on page 561*

Verelan® *see* verapamil *on previous page*

Vergon® [OTC] *see* meclizine *on page 324*

Vermizine® *see* piperazine *on page 419*

Vermox® *see* mebendazole *on page 324*

Verrex-C&M® *see* podophyllin and salicylic acid *on page 422*

Versacaps® *see* guaifenesin and pseudoephedrine *on page 250*

Versed® *see* midazolam *on page 349*

Vesanoid® *see* tretinoin (oral) *on page 527*

Vesprin® *see* triflupromazine *on page 532*

Vexol® Ophthalmic Suspension *see* rimexolone *on page 467*

Vibramycin® Injection *see* doxycycline *on page 184*

Vibramycin® Oral *see* doxycycline *on page 184*

Vibra-Tabs® *see* doxycycline *on page 184*

Vicks® 44D Cough & Head Congestion *see* pseudoephedrine and dextromethorphan *on page 450*

Vicks® 44E [OTC] *see* guaifenesin and dextromethorphan *on page 248*

Vicks® 44 Non-Drowsy Cold & Cough Liqui-Caps [OTC] *see* pseudoephedrine and dextromethorphan *on page 450*

Vicks Children's Chloraseptic® [OTC] *see* benzocaine *on page 59*

Vicks Chloraseptic® Sore Throat [OTC] *see* benzocaine *on page 59*

Vicks® DayQuil® Allergy Relief 4 Hour Tablet [OTC] *see* brompheniramine and phenylpropanolamine *on page 73*

Vicks® DayQuil® Sinus Pressure & Congestion Relief [OTC] *see* guaifenesin and phenylpropanolamine *on page 249*

Vicks Formula 44® [OTC] *see* dextromethorphan *on page 160*

Vicks Formula 44® Pediatric Formula [OTC] *see* dextromethorphan *on page 160*

Vicks® Pediatric Formula 44E [OTC] *see* guaifenesin and dextromethorphan *on page 248*

Vicks Sinex® Nasal Solution [OTC] *see* phenylephrine *on page 411*

Vicodin® *see* hydrocodone and acetaminophen *on page 266*

Vicodin® ES *see* hydrocodone and acetaminophen *on page 266*

Vicodin® HP *see* hydrocodone and acetaminophen *on page 266*

Vicon-C® [OTC] *see* vitamin b complex with vitamin c *on page 553*

Vicon Forte® *see* vitamins, multiple (oral, adult) *on page 556*

Vicon® Plus [OTC] *see* vitamins, multiple (oral, adult) *on page 556*

Vicoprofen® *see* hydrocodone and ibuprofen *on page 267*

vidarabine (vye DARE a been)

Synonyms adenine arabinoside; ara-a; arabinofuranosyladenine; vidarabine monohydrate

(Continued)

549

vidarabine *(Continued)*

Brand Names Vira-A® Ophthalmic
Therapeutic Category Antiviral Agent
Use Treatment of acute keratoconjunctivitis and epithelial keratitis due to herpes simplex virus; herpes simplex encephalitis; neonatal herpes simplex virus infections; disseminated varicella-zoster in immunosuppressed patients
Usual Dosage Children and Adults: Ophthalmic: Keratoconjunctivitis: 1/2" of ointment in lower conjunctival sac 5 times/day every 3 hours while awake until complete re-epithelialization has occurred, then twice daily for an additional 7 days
Dosage Forms Ointment, ophthalmic, as monohydrate: 3% [30 mg/mL = 28 mg/mL base] (3.5 g)

vidarabine monohydrate *see vidarabine on previous page*

Vi-Daylin® [OTC] *see vitamin, multiple (pediatric) on page 554*

Vi-Daylin/F® *see vitamin, multiple (pediatric) on page 554*

Videx® *see didanosine on page 166*

vinblastine *(vin BLAS teen)*

Synonyms vinblastine sulfate; vincaleukoblastine; vlb
Brand Names Alkaban-AQ®; Velban®
Therapeutic Category Antineoplastic Agent
Use Palliative treatment of Hodgkin's disease; advanced testicular germinal-cell cancers; non-Hodgkin's lymphoma, histiocytosis, and choriocarcinoma
Usual Dosage Refer to individual protocol. Varies depending upon clinical and hematological response. Administer at intervals of at least 7 days and only after leukocyte count has returned to at least 4000/mm^3; maintenance therapy should be titrated according to leukocyte count. Dosage should be reduced in patients with recent exposure to radiation therapy or chemotherapy; single doses in these patients should not exceed 5.5 mg/m^2.

Children and Adults: I.V.: 4-12 mg/m^2 every 7-10 days **or** 5-day continuous infusion of 1.4-1.8 mg/m^2/day **or** 0.1-0.5 mg/kg/week
Dosage Forms
Injection, as sulfate: 1 mg/mL (10 mL)
Powder for injection, as sulfate: 10 mg

vinblastine sulfate *see vinblastine on this page*

vincaleukoblastine *see vinblastine on this page*

Vincasar® PFS™ Injection *see vincristine on this page*

vincristine *(vin KRIS teen)*

Synonyms lcr; leurocristine; vcr; vincristine sulfate
Brand Names Oncovin® Injection; Vincasar® PFS™ Injection
Therapeutic Category Antineoplastic Agent
Use Treatment of leukemias, Hodgkin's disease, neuroblastoma, malignant lymphomas, Wilms' tumor, and rhabdomyosarcoma
Usual Dosage Refer to individual protocol as dosages vary with protocol used. Adjustments are made depending upon clinical and hematological response and upon adverse reactions

Children: I.V.:
≤10 kg or BSA <1 m^2: 0.05 mg/kg once weekly
2 mg/m^2; may repeat every week
Adults: I.V.: 0.4-1.4 mg/m^2, up to 2 mg maximum; may repeat every week
Dosage Forms Injection, as sulfate: 1 mg/mL (1 mL, 2 mL, 5 mL)

vincristine sulfate *see vincristine on this page*

vinorelbine (vi NOR el been)
Synonyms vinorelbine tartrate
Brand Names Navelbine®
Therapeutic Category Antineoplastic Agent
Use Treatment of nonsmall cell lung cancer (as a single agent or in combination with cisplatin)
Unlabeled use: Breast cancer, ovarian carcinoma (cisplatin-resistant), Hodgkin's disease
Usual Dosage Varies depending upon clinical and hematological response (refer to individual protocols)

Adults: I.V.: 30 mg/m^2 every 7 days

Dosage adjustment in hematological toxicity (based on granulocyte counts):
Granulocytes ≥1500 cells/mm^3 on day of treatment: Administer 30 mg/m^2
Granulocytes 1000-1499 cells/mm^3 on day of treatment: Administer 15 mg/m^2
Granulocytes <1000 cells/mm^3 on day of treatment: Do not administer. Repeat granulocyte count in one week; if 3 consecutive doses are held because granulocyte count is <1000 cells/mm^3, discontinue vinorelbine

For patients who, during treatment, have experienced fever or sepsis while granulocytopenic or had 2 consecutive weekly doses held due to granulocytopenia, subsequent doses of vinorelbine should be:
22.5 mg/m^2 for granulocytes ≥1,500 cells/mm^3
11.25 mg/m^2 for granulocytes 1000-1499 cells/mm^3
Dosage Forms Injection, as tartrate: 10 mg/mL (1 mL, 5 mL)

vinorelbine tartrate *see* vinorelbine *on this page*

Vioform® [OTC] *see* clioquinol *on page 128*

Viokase® *see* pancrelipase *on page 394*

viosterol *see* ergocalciferol *on page 197*

Vira-A® Ophthalmic *see* vidarabine *on page 549*

Viracept® *see* nelfinavir *on page 367*

Viramune® *see* nevirapine *on page 372*

Virazole® Aerosol *see* ribavirin *on page 464*

Virilon® *see* methyltestosterone *on page 343*

Viroptic® Ophthalmic *see* trifluridine *on page 533*

Viscoat® *see* chondroitin sulfate-sodium hyaluronate *on page 122*

Visine® Extra Ophthalmic [OTC] *see* tetrahydrozoline *on page 510*

Visine® L.R. Ophthalmic [OTC] *see* oxymetazoline *on page 390*

Visken® *see* pindolol *on page 418*

Vistacon® *see* hydroxyzine *on page 275*

Vistaject-25® *see* hydroxyzine *on page 275*

Vistaject-50® *see* hydroxyzine *on page 275*

Vistaquel® *see* hydroxyzine *on page 275*

Vistaril® *see* hydroxyzine *on page 275*

Vistazine® *see* hydroxyzine *on page 275*

Vistide® *see* cidofovir *on page 123*

Vita-C® [OTC] *see* ascorbic acid *on page 42*

VitaCarn® Oral *see* levocarnitine *on page 304*

Vital HN® [OTC] *see* enteral nutritional products *on page 194*

vitamin a (VYE ta min aye)
Synonyms oleovitamin a
Brand Names Aquasol A®; Del-Vi-A®; Palmitate-A® 5000 [OTC]
Therapeutic Category Vitamin, Fat Soluble
Use Treatment and prevention of vitamin A deficiency; supplementation in patients with measles
Usual Dosage
RDA:
0-3 years: 400 mcg•
4-6 years: 500 mcg•
7-10 years: 700 mcg•
>10 years: 800-1000 mcg•
•mcg retinol equivalent (0.3 mcg retinol = 1 unit vitamin A)

Supplementation in measles: Children: Oral:
<1 year: 100,000 units/day for 2 days
>1 year: 200,000 units/day for 2 days
Severe deficiency with xerophthalmia:
Children 1-8 years:
 Oral: 5000-10,000 units/kg/day for 5 days or until recovery occurs
 I.M.: 5000-15,000 units/day for 10 days
Children >8 years and Adults:
 Oral: 500,000 units/day for 3 days, then 50,000 units/day for 14 days, then 10,000-20,000 units/day for 2 months
 I.M.: 50,000-100,000 units/day for 3 days, 50,000 units/day for 14 days
Deficiency (without corneal changes): Oral:
Infants <1 year: 10,000 units/kg/day for 5 days, then 7500-15,000 units/day for 10 days
Children 1-8 years: 5000-10,000 units/kg/day for 5 days, then 17,000-35,000 units/day for 10 days
Children >8 years and Adults: 100,000 units/day for 3 days then 50,000 units/day for 14 days
Malabsorption syndrome (prophylaxis): Children >8 years and Adults: Oral: 10,000-50,000 units/day of water miscible product
Dietary supplement: Oral:
Infants up to 6 months: 1500 units/day
Children:
 6 months to 3 years: 1500-2000 units/day
 4-6 years: 2500 units/day
 7-10 years: 3300-3500 units/day
 Children >10 years and Adults: 4000-5000 units/day
Dosage Forms
Capsule: 10,000 units [OTC], 25,000 units, 50,000 units
Drops, oral (water miscible) [OTC]: 5000 units/0.1 mL (30 mL)
Injection: 50,000 units/mL (2 mL)
Tablet [OTC]: 5000 units

vitamin a acid *see* tretinoin (topical) *on page 528*

vitamin a and vitamin d (VYE ta min aye & VYE ta min dee)
Synonyms cod liver oil
Brand Names A and D™ Ointment [OTC]
Therapeutic Category Protectant, Topical
Use Temporary relief of discomfort due to chapped skin, diaper rash, minor burns, abrasions, as well as irritations associated with ostomy skin care
Usual Dosage
Oral, oil: Dietary supplement: 2.5 mL/day
Topical: Apply locally with gentle massage as needed
Dosage Forms Ointment, topical: In a lanolin-petrolatum base (60 g)

vitamin b₁ *see* thiamine *on page 514*

vitamin b₂ *see* riboflavin *on page 465*

vitamin b₃ *see* niacin *on page 372*

vitamin b₅ *see* pantothenic acid *on page 395*

vitamin b₆ *see* pyridoxine *on page 453*

vitamin b₁₂ *see* cyanocobalamin *on page 142*

vitamin b₁₂ₐ *see* hydroxocobalamin *on page 272*

vitamin b complex (VYE ta min bee KOM pleks)

Brand Names Apatate® [OTC]; Gevrabon® [OTC]; Lederplex® [OTC]; Lipovite® [OTC]; Mega B® [OTC]; Megaton™ [OTC]; Mucoplex® [OTC]; NeoVadrin® B Complex [OTC]; Orexin® [OTC]; Surbex® [OTC]

Therapeutic Category Vitamin, Water Soluble

Usual Dosage Dosage is usually 1 tablet or capsule/day; please refer to package insert

Dosage Forms
Capsule
Solution: 5 mL, 360 mL

vitamin b complex with vitamin c

(VYE ta min bee KOM pleks with VYE ta min see)

Brand Names Allbee® With C [OTC]; Surbex-T® Filmtabs® [OTC]; Surbex® with C Filmtabs® [OTC]; Thera-Combex® H-P Kapseals® [OTC]; Vicon-C® [OTC]

Therapeutic Category Vitamin, Water Soluble

Use Supportive nutritional supplementation in conditions in which water-soluble vitamins are required like GI disorders, chronic alcoholism, pregnancy, severe burns, and recovery from surgery

Usual Dosage Adults: Oral: 1 tablet/capsule every day

Dosage Forms Actual vitamin content may vary slightly depending on product used
Tablet/capsule: Vitamin B_1 10-15 mg, vitamin B_2 10 mg, vitamin B_3 100 mg, vitamin B_5 20 mg, vitamin B_6 2-5 mg, vitamin B_{12} 6-10 mg, vitamin C 300-500 mg

vitamin b complex with vitamin c and folic acid

(VYE ta min bee KOM pleks with VYE ta min see & FOE lik AS id)

Brand Names Berocca®; Nephrocaps®

Therapeutic Category Vitamin, Water Soluble

Use Supportive nutritional supplementation in conditions in which water-soluble vitamins are required like GI disorders, chronic alcoholism, pregnancy, severe burns, and recovery from surgery

Usual Dosage Adults: Oral: 1 capsule every day

Dosage Forms Capsule

vitamin c *see* ascorbic acid *on page 42*

vitamin d₂ *see* ergocalciferol *on page 197*

vitamin e (VYE ta min ee)

Synonyms *d*-alpha tocopherol; *dl*-alpha tocopherol

Brand Names Amino-Opti-E® [OTC]; Aquasol E® [OTC]; E-Complex-600® [OTC]; E-Vitamin® [OTC]; Vita-Plus® E Softgels® [OTC]; Vitec® [OTC]; Vite E® Creme [OTC]

Therapeutic Category Vitamin, Fat Soluble; Vitamin, Topical

Use Prevention and treatment of vitamin E deficiency

Usual Dosage
RDA: Oral:
Premature infants ≤3 months: 25 units/day
Infants:
≤6 months: 4.5 units/day
(Continued)

vitamin e *(Continued)*

6-12 months: 6 units/day
Children:
1-3 years: 9 units/day
4-10 years: 10.5 units/day
Adults >11 years:
Female: 12 units/day
Male: 15 units/day

Prevention of vitamin E deficiency: Neonates, premature, low birthweight (results in normal levels within 1 week): Oral: 25-50 units/24 hours until 6-10 weeks of age or 125-150 units/kg total in 4 doses on days 1, 2, 7, and 8 of life

Vitamin E deficiency treatment: Adults: Oral: 50-200 units/24 hours for 2 weeks

Topical: Apply a thin layer over affected areas as needed

Dosage Forms
Capsule: 100 units, 200 units, 330 mg, 400 units, 500 units, 600 units, 1000 units
 Water miscible: 73.5 mg, 147 mg, 165 mg, 330 mg, 400 units
Cream: 50 mg/g (15 g, 30 g, 60 g, 75 g, 120 g, 454 g)
Drops, oral: 50 mg/mL (12 mL, 30 mL)
Liquid, topical: 10 mL, 15 mL, 30 mL, 60 mL
Lotion: 120 mL
Oil: 15 mL, 30 mL, 60 mL
Ointment, topical: 30 mg/g (45 g, 60 g)
Tablet: 200 units, 400 units

vitamin g *see* riboflavin *on page 465*

vitamin k₁ *see* phytonadione *on page 416*

vitamin, multiple (injectable)

Brand Names M.V.C.® 9 + 3; M.V.I.®-12; M.V.I.® Concentrate; M.V.I.® Pediatric
Therapeutic Category Vitamin
Usual Dosage I.V.:
Children:
≤5 kg: 10 mL/1000 mL TPN (M.V.I.® Pediatric)
5.1 kg to 11 years: 5 mL/one TPN bag/day (M.V.I.® Pediatric)
Children >11 years and Adults: 5 mL of vials 1 and 2 (M.V.I.®-12)/one TPN bag/day
Dosage Forms See Multivitamins table.

vitamin, multiple (pediatric)

Synonyms children's vitamins; multivitamins/fluoride
Brand Names Adeflor®; Florvite®; LKV-Drops® [OTC]; Multi Vit® Drops [OTC]; Poly-Vi-Flor®; Poly-Vi-Sol® [OTC]; Tri-Vi-Flor®; Vi-Daylin® [OTC]; Vi-Daylin/F®
Therapeutic Category Vitamin
Use Nutritional supplement, vitamin deficiency
Usual Dosage Oral: 0.6 mL or 1 mL/day; please refer to package insert
Dosage Forms See Multivitamins table.

vitamin, multiple (prenatal)

Synonyms prenatal vitamins
Brand Names Chromagen® OB [OTC]; Filibon® [OTC]; Natabec® [OTC]; Natabec® FA [OTC]; Natabec® Rx; Natalins® [OTC]; Natalins® Rx; NeoVadrin® [OTC]; Niferex®-PN; Pramet® FA; Pramilet® FA; Prenavite® [OTC]; Secran®; Stuartnatal® 1+1; Stuart Prenatal® [OTC]
Therapeutic Category Vitamin
Use Nutritional supplement, vitamin deficiency
Usual Dosage Oral: 1 tablet or capsule daily; please refer to package insert

Multivitamin Products Available

Product	Content Given Per	A IU	D IU	E IU	C mg	FA mg	B₁ mg	B₂ mg	B₃ mg	B₆ mg	B₁₂ mcg	Other
Theragran®	5 mL liquid	10,000	400		200		10	10	100	4.1	5	B₅ 21.4 mg
Vi-Daylin®	1 mL drops	1500	400	4.1	35		0.5	0.6	8	0.4	1.5	Alcohol <0.5%
Vi-Daylin® Iron	1 mL	1500	400	4.1	35		0.5	0.6	8	0.4		Fe 10 mg
Albee® with C	tablet				300		15	10.2		5		Niacinamide 50 mg, pantothenic acid 10 mg
Vitamin B complex	tablet					400 mcg	1.5	1.7		2	6	Niacinamide 20 mg
Hexavitamin	cap/tab	5000	400		75		2	3	20			
Iberet-Folic-500®	tablet				500	0.8	6	6	30	5	25	B₅ 10 mg, Fe 105 mg
Stuartnatal® 1+1	tablet	4000	400	11	120	1	1.5	3	20	10	12	Cu, Zn 25 mg, Fe 65 mg, Ca 200 mg
Theragran-M®	tablet	5000	400	30	90	0.4	3	3.4	30	3	9	Cl, Cr, I, K, B₅ 10 mg, Mg, Mn, Mo, P, Se, Zn 15 mg, Fe 27 mg, biotin 30 mcg, beta-carotene 1250 IU
Vi-Daylin®	tablet	2500	400	15	60	0.3	1.05	1.2	13.5	1.05	4.5	B₅ 15 mg, biotin 60 mcg
M.V.I.®-12 injection	5 mL	3300	200	10	100	0.4	3	3.6	40	4	5	
M.V.I.®-12 unit vial	20 mL											
M.V.I.® pediatric powder	5 mL	2300	400	7	80	0.14	1.2	1.4	17	1	1	B₅ 5 mg, biotin 20 mcg, vitamin K 200 mcg

vitamins, multiple (oral, adult)

Brand Names Becotin® Pulvules®; Cefol® Filmtab®; Eldercaps® [OTC]; Iberet-Folic-500®; Mega-B® [OTC]; Stresstabs® 600 Advanced Formula Tablets [OTC]; Theragran® [OTC]; Theragran® Hematinic®; Theragran® Liquid [OTC]; Theragran-M® [OTC]; Unicap® [OTC]; Vicon Forte®; Vicon® Plus [OTC]; Z-Bec® [OTC]

Therapeutic Category Vitamin

Use Dietary supplement

Usual Dosage
Infants 1.5-3 kg: I.V.: 3.25 mL/24 hours (M.V.I.® Pediatric)
Children:
Oral:
≤2 years: Drops: 1 mL/day (premature infants may get 0.5-1 mL/day)
>2 years: Chew 1 tablet/day
≥4 years: 5 mL/day liquid
I.V.: >3 kg and <11 years: 5 mL/24 hours (M.V.I.® Pediatric)
Adults:
Oral: 1 tablet/day or 5 mL/day liquid
I.V.: >11 years: 5 mL of vials 1 and 2 (M.V.I.®-12)/one TPN bag/day
I.V. solutions: 10 mL/24 hours (M.V.I.®-12)

Dosage Forms See Multivitamins table.

Vitaneed™ [OTC] *see* enteral nutritional products *on page 194*

Vita-Plus® E Softgels® [OTC] *see* vitamin e *on page 553*

Vitec® [OTC] *see* vitamin e *on page 553*

Vite E® Creme [OTC] *see* vitamin e *on page 553*

Vitrasert® *see* ganciclovir *on page 237*

Vivactil® *see* protriptyline *on page 449*

Viva-Drops® Solution [OTC] *see* artificial tears *on page 42*

Vivelle™ Transdermal *see* estradiol *on page 202*

Vivonex® [OTC] *see* enteral nutritional products *on page 194*

Vivonex® T.E.N. [OTC] *see* enteral nutritional products *on page 194*

Vivotif Berna™ Oral *see* typhoid vaccine *on page 540*

V-Lax® [OTC] *see* psyllium *on page 451*

vlb *see* vinblastine *on page 550*

vm-26 *see* teniposide *on page 504*

Volmax® *see* albuterol *on page 14*

Voltaren® Ophthalmic *see* diclofenac *on page 164*

Voltaren® Oral *see* diclofenac *on page 164*

Voltaren-XR® Oral *see* diclofenac *on page 164*

Vontrol® *see* diphenidol *on page 174*

VōSol® HC Otic *see* acetic acid, propylene glycol diacetate, and hydrocortisone *on page 7*

VōSol® Otic *see* acetic acid *on page 7*

vp-16 *see* etoposide *on page 213*

Vumon Injection *see* teniposide *on page 504*

V.V.S.® *see* sulfabenzamide, sulfacetamide, and sulfathiazole *on page 496*

Vytone® Topical *see* iodoquinol and hydrocortisone *on page 287*

vzig *see* varicella-zoster immune globulin (human) *on page 546*

warfarin (WAR far in)
Synonyms warfarin sodium
Brand Names Coumadin®
Therapeutic Category Anticoagulant
Use Prophylaxis and treatment of venous thromboembolic disorders; prevention of arterial thromboembolism in patients with prosthetic heart valves or atrial fibrillation; prevention of death, venous thromboembolism, and recurrent MI after acute MI
Usual Dosage
Oral:
Infants and Children: 0.05-0.34 mg/kg/day; infants <12 months of age may require doses at or near the high end of this range; consistent anticoagulation may be difficult to maintain in children <5 years of age
Adults: 5-15 mg/day for 2-5 days, then adjust dose according to results of prothrombin time; usual maintenance dose ranges from 2-10 mg/day
I.V. (administer as a slow bolus injection): 2-5 mg/day
Dosage Forms
Powder for injection, as sodium, lyophilized: 2 mg, 5 mg
Tablet, as sodium: 1 mg, 2 mg, 2.5 mg, 4 mg, 5 mg, 7.5 mg, 10 mg

warfarin sodium *see* warfarin *on this page*

Wart-Off® [OTC] *see* salicylic acid *on page 472*

4-Way® Long Acting Nasal Solution [OTC] *see* oxymetazoline *on page 390*

Wellbutrin® *see* bupropion *on page 77*

Wellbutrin® SR *see* bupropion *on page 77*

Wellcovorin® *see* leucovorin *on page 302*

Westcort® *see* hydrocortisone *on page 268*

Whitfield's Ointment [OTC] *see* benzoic acid and salicylic acid *on page 61*

whole root rauwolfia *see* rauwolfia serpentina *on page 460*

Wigraine® *see* ergotamine *on page 198*

40 Winks® [OTC] *see* diphenhydramine *on page 173*

WinRho SD® *see* rh$_o$(D) immune globulin (intravenous-human) *on page 463*

Winstrol® *see* stanozolol *on page 491*

witch hazel (witch HAY zel)
Synonyms hamamelis water
Brand Names Tucks® [OTC]
Therapeutic Category Astringent
Use After-stool wipe to remove most causes of local irritation; temporary management of vulvitis, pruritus ani and vulva; help relieve the discomfort of simple hemorrhoids, anorectal surgical wounds, and episiotomies
Usual Dosage Apply to anorectal area as needed
Dosage Forms
Cream: 50% (40 g)
Gel: 50% with glycerin (19.8 g)
Pads: 50% with glycerin, water and methylparaben (40/jar)

Wolfina® *see* rauwolfia serpentina *on page 460*

wood sugar *see* d-xylose *on page 187*

Wyamine® Sulfate Injection *see* mephentermine *on page 329*

Wycillin® *see* penicillin g procaine *on page 401*

Wydase® Injection *see* hyaluronidase *on page 263*

Wygesic® *see* propoxyphene and acetaminophen *on page 445*

Wymox® *see* amoxicillin *on page 30*

Wytensin® *see* guanabenz *on page 252*

Xalatan® *see* latanoprost *on page 302*

Xanax® *see* alprazolam *on page 18*

X-Prep® Liquid [OTC] *see* senna *on page 477*

X-seb® T [OTC] *see* coal tar and salicylic acid *on page 133*

Xylocaine® *see* lidocaine *on page 307*

Xylocaine® With Epinephrine *see* lidocaine and epinephrine *on page 308*

xylometazoline (zye loe met AZ oh leen)
Synonyms xylometazoline hydrochloride
Brand Names Otrivin® Nasal [OTC]
Therapeutic Category Adrenergic Agonist Agent
Use Symptomatic relief of nasal and nasopharyngeal mucosal congestion
Usual Dosage
   Children <12 years: 2-3 drops (0.05%) in each nostril every 8-10 hours
   Children >12 years and Adults: 2-3 drops or sprays (0.1%) in each nostril every 8-10 hours
Dosage Forms Solution, nasal, as hydrochloride: 0.05% [0.5 mg/mL] (20 mL); 0.1% [1 mg/mL] (15 mL, 20 mL)

xylometazoline hydrochloride *see* xylometazoline *on this page*

Xylo-Pfan® [OTC] *see* d-xylose *on page 187*

Yeast-Gard® Medicated Douche *see* povidone-iodine *on page 431*

yellow fever vaccine (YEL oh FEE ver vak SEEN)
Brand Names YF-VAX®
Therapeutic Category Vaccine, Live Virus
Use Active immunization against yellow fever
Usual Dosage Single-dose S.C.: 0.5 mL
Dosage Forms Injection: Not less than 5.04 Log_{10} Plaque Forming Units (PFU) per 0.5 mL

yellow mercuric oxide *see* mercuric oxide *on page 330*

YF-VAX® *see* yellow fever vaccine *on this page*

Yocon® *see* yohimbine *on this page*

Yodoxin® *see* iodoquinol *on page 287*

yohimbine (yo HIM bine)
Synonyms yohimbine hydrochloride
Brand Names Aphrodyne™; Dayto Himbin®; Yocon®; Yohimex™
Therapeutic Category Miscellaneous Product
Use No FDA sanctioned indications
Usual Dosage Adults: Oral: 1 tablet 3 times/day
Dosage Forms Tablet, as hydrochloride: 5.4 mg

yohimbine hydrochloride *see* yohimbine *on this page*

Yohimex™ *see* yohimbine *on this page*

Yutopar® *see* ritodrine *on page 467*

zafirlukast (za FIR loo kast)
Brand Names Accolate®
Therapeutic Category Leukotriene Receptor Antagonist

Use Prophylaxis and chronic treatment of asthma in adults and children ≥12 years

Usual Dosage Adults: Oral: 20 mg twice daily; take 1 hour before food or 2 hours after food

Dosage Forms Tablet: 20 mg

Zagam® *see* sparfloxacin *on page 490*

zalcitabine (zal SITE a been)

Synonyms ddc; dideoxycytidine

Brand Names Hivid®

Therapeutic Category Antiviral Agent

Use Treatment of HIV infections as monotherapy (in patients intolerant to zidovudine or with disease progression while on zidovudine) or in combination with zidovudine in patients with advanced HIV disease (adult CD4 cell count of 150-300 cells/mm^3)

Usual Dosage

Safety and efficacy in children <13 years of age have not been established

Adults: Oral (dosed in combination with zidovudine): Daily dose: 0.750 mg every 8 hours, administered together with 200 mg of zidovudine (ie, total daily dose: 2.25 mg of zalcitabine and 600 mg of zidovudine)

Dosage Forms Tablet: 0.375 mg, 0.75 mg

Zanaflex® *see* tizanidine *on page 521*

Zanosar® *see* streptozocin *on page 493*

Zantac® *see* ranitidine hydrochloride *on page 460*

Zantac® 75 [OTC] *see* ranitidine hydrochloride *on page 460*

Zarontin® *see* ethosuximide *on page 211*

Zaroxolyn® *see* metolazone *on page 345*

Z-Bec® [OTC] *see* vitamins, multiple (oral, adult) *on page 556*

Zeasorb-AF® Powder [OTC] *see* miconazole *on page 348*

Zeasorb-AF® Powder [OTC] *see* tolnaftate *on page 523*

Zebeta® *see* bisoprolol *on page 68*

Zefazone® *see* cefmetazole *on page 97*

Zemuron® *see* rocuronium *on page 468*

Zephiran® [OTC] *see* benzalkonium chloride *on page 59*

Zephrex® *see* guaifenesin and pseudoephedrine *on page 250*

Zephrex LA® *see* guaifenesin and pseudoephedrine *on page 250*

Zerit® *see* stavudine *on page 492*

Zestoretic® *see* lisinopril and hydrochlorothiazide *on page 311*

Zestril® *see* lisinopril *on page 311*

Zetar® [OTC] *see* coal tar *on page 132*

Ziac™ *see* bisoprolol and hydrochlorothiazide *on page 68*

zidovudine (zye DOE vyoo deen)

Synonyms azidothymidine; azt; compound s

Brand Names Retrovir®

Therapeutic Category Antiviral Agent

Use Management of patients with HIV infections who have had at least one episode of *Pneumocystis carinii* pneumonia or who have CD4 cell counts (cells/mm^3) of ≤500 in children >6 years and adults, <750 in children 2-6 years, <1000 in children 1-2 years, and <1750 for children <1 year; patients who have HIV-related symptoms or who are asymptomatic with abnormal laboratory values indicating HIV-related immunosuppression; prevention of maternal-fetal HIV transmission

(Continued)

zidovudine *(Continued)*

Usual Dosage
Children 3 months to 12 years:
Oral: 90-180 mg/m^2/dose every 6 hours; maximum: 200 mg every 6 hours
I.V. continuous infusion: 0.5-1.8 mg/kg/hour
I.V. intermittent infusion: 100 mg/m^2/dose every 6 hours
Adults:
Oral:
Asymptomatic infection: 100 mg every 4 hours while awake (500 mg/day)
Symptomatic HIV infection: Initial: 200 mg every 4 hours (1200 mg/day), then after 1 month, 100 mg every 4 hours (600 mg/day)
I.V.: 1-2 mg/kg/dose every 4 hours
Dosage Forms
Capsule: 100 mg
Injection: 10 mg/mL (20 mL)
Syrup (strawberry flavor): 50 mg/5 mL (240 mL)
Tablet: 300 mg

zidovudine and lamivudine

Synonyms AZT + 3TC
Brand Names Combivir®
Therapeutic Category Antiviral Agent
Use Combivir® given twice a day, provides an alternative regimen to lamivudine 150 mg twice a day plus zidovudine 600 mg per day in divided doses; this drug form reduces capsule/tablet intake for these two drugs to two per day instead of up to eight
Dosage Forms Tablet: Zidovudine 300 mg and lamivudine 150 mg

Zilactin-B® Medicated [OTC] *see* benzocaine *on page 59*

Zilactin-L® [OTC] *see* lidocaine *on page 307*

ZilaDent® [OTC] *see* benzocaine *on page 59*

zileuton *(zye LOO ton)*

Brand Names Zyflo®
Therapeutic Category 5-Lipoxygenase Inhibitor
Use Prophylaxis and chronic treatment of asthma in adults and children ≥12 years of age
Usual Dosage Children ≥12 years and Adults: Oral: 1 tablet 4 times/day, may be taken with meals and at bedtime
Dosage Forms Tablet: 600 mg

Zinacef® Injection *see* cefuroxime *on page 101*

Zinca-Pak® *see* trace metals *on page 525*

Zincate® Oral *see* zinc sulfate *on next page*

zinc chloride *(zingk KLOR ide)*

Therapeutic Category Trace Element
Use Cofactor for replacement therapy to different enzymes helps maintain normal growth rates, normal skin hydration and senses of taste and smell
Usual Dosage Clinical response may not occur for up to 6-8 weeks
Supplemental to I.V. solutions:
Premature Infants <1500 g, up to 3 kg: 300 mcg/kg/day
Full-term Infants and Children ≤5 years: 100 mcg/kg/day
Adults:
Stable with fluid loss from small bowel: 12.2 mg zinc/liter TPN or 17.1 mg zinc/kg (added to 1000 mL I.V. fluids) of stool or ileostomy output
Metabolically stable: 2.5-4 mg/day, add 2 mg/day for acute catabolic states
Dosage Forms Injection: 1 mg/mL (10 mL)

Zincfrin® Ophthalmic [OTC] *see* phenylephrine and zinc sulfate *on page 413*

zinc gelatin (zingk JEL ah tin)
Synonyms Unna's boot; Unna's paste
Brand Names Gelucast®
Therapeutic Category Protectant, Topical
Use Protectant and to support varicosities and similar lesions of the lower limbs
Usual Dosage Apply externally as an occlusive boot
Dosage Forms Bandage: 3" x 10 yards, 4" x 10 yards

zinc injection *see* trace metals *on page 525*

Zincon® Shampoo [OTC] *see* pyrithione zinc *on page 454*

zinc oxide (zingk OKS ide)
Synonyms Lassar's zinc paste
Therapeutic Category Topical Skin Product
Use Protective coating for mild skin irritations and abrasions; soothing and protective ointment to promote healing of chapped skin, diaper rash
Usual Dosage Infants, Children, and Adults: Topical: Apply several times daily to affected area
Dosage Forms
Ointment, topical: 20% in white ointment (480 g)
Paste, topical: 25% in white petrolatum (480 g)

zinc oxide, cod liver oil, and talc (zingk OKS ide, kod LIV er oyl, & talk)
Brand Names Desitin® [OTC]
Therapeutic Category Protectant, Topical
Use Relief of diaper rash, superficial wounds and burns, and other minor skin irritations
Usual Dosage Topical: Apply thin layer as needed
Dosage Forms Ointment, topical: Zinc oxide, cod liver oil and talc in a petrolatum and lanolin base (30 g, 60 g, 120 g, 240 g, 270 g)

zinc sulfate (zingk SUL fate)
Brand Names Eye-Sed® Ophthalmic [OTC]; Orazinc® Oral [OTC]; Verazinc® Oral [OTC]; Zincate® Oral
Therapeutic Category Electrolyte Supplement
Use Zinc supplement (oral and parenteral); may improve wound healing in those who are deficient
Usual Dosage
RDA: Oral:
Birth to 6 months: 3 mg elemental zinc/day
6-12 months: 5 mg elemental zinc/day
1-10 years: 10 mg elemental zinc/day
≥11 years: 15 mg elemental zinc/day

Zinc deficiency: Oral:
Infants and Children: 0.5-1 mg elemental zinc/kg/day divided 1-3 times/day; somewhat larger quantities may be needed if there is impaired intestinal absorption or an excessive loss of zinc
Adults: 110-220 mg zinc sulfate (25-50 mg elemental zinc)/dose 3 times/day
Dosage Forms
Capsule: 110 mg [elemental zinc 25 mg]; 220 mg [elemental zinc 50 mg]
Injection: 1 mg/mL (10 mL, 30 mL); 4 mg/mL (10 mL); 5 mg/mL (5 mL, 10 mL, 50 mL)
Tablet: 66 mg [elemental zinc 15 mg]; 200 mg [elemental zinc 46 mg]

zinc undecylenate *see* undecylenic acid and derivatives *on page 541*

Zinecard® *see* dexrazoxane *on page 158*

Zithromax™ *see* azithromycin *on page 51*

ZNP® **Bar [OTC]** *see* pyrithione zinc *on page 454*

Zocor® *see* simvastatin *on page 480*

Zofran® *see* ondansetron *on page 383*

Zoladex® **Implant** *see* goserelin *on page 245*

Zolicef® *see* cefazolin *on page 96*

Zoloft™ *see* sertraline *on page 478*

zolpidem (zole PI dem)
    Synonyms zolpidem tartrate
    Brand Names Ambien™
    Therapeutic Category Hypnotic, Nonbarbiturate
    Use Short-term treatment of insomnia
    Usual Dosage Adults: Oral: 10 mg immediately before bedtime
    Dosage Forms Tablet, as tartrate: 5 mg, 10 mg

zolpidem tartrate *see* zolpidem *on this page*

Zonalon® **Topical Cream** *see* doxepin *on page 183*

Zone-A Forte® *see* pramoxine and hydrocortisone *on page 433*

ZORprin® *see* aspirin *on page 44*

Zostrix® **[OTC]** *see* capsaicin *on page 87*

Zostrix-® **HP [OTC]** *see* capsaicin *on page 87*

Zosyn™ *see* piperacillin and tazobactam sodium *on page 419*

Zovia® *see* ethinyl estradiol and ethynodiol diacetate *on page 208*

Zovirax® *see* acyclovir *on page 10*

Zyban® *see* bupropion *on page 77*

Zydone® *see* hydrocodone and acetaminophen *on page 266*

Zyflo® *see* zileuton *on page 560*

Zyloprim® *see* allopurinol *on page 17*

Zymase® *see* pancrelipase *on page 394*

Zyprexa® *see* olanzapine *on page 382*

Zyrtec™ *see* cetirizine *on page 105*

APPENDIX

ABBREVIATIONS & SYMBOLS COMMONLY USED IN MEDICAL ORDERS

Abbreviation	From	Meaning
μga		microgram
μmol		micromole
°C		degrees Celsius (Centigrade)
[		less than
]		greater than
≤		less than or equal to
≥		greater than or equal to
a̅a̅, aa	ana	of each
ABG		arterial blood gas
ac	ante cibum	before meals or food
ACE		angiotensin-converting enzyme
ACLS		adult cardiac life support
ad	ad	to, up to
a.d.	aurio dextra	right ear
ADH		antidiuretic hormone
ad lib	ad libitum	at pleasure
AED		antiepileptic drug
a.l.	aurio laeva	left ear
ALL		acute lymphoblastic leukemia
ALT		alanine aminotransferase (was SGPT)
AM	ante meridiem	morning
AML		acute myeloblastic leukemia
amp		ampul
amt		amount
ANA		antinuclear antibodies
ANC		absolute neutrophil count
ANL		acute nonlymphoblastic leukemia
aq	aqua	water
aq. dest.	aqua destillata	distilled water
APTT		activated partial thromboplastin time
a.s.	aurio sinister	left ear
ASA (class I-IV)		classification of surgical patients according to their baseline health (eg, healthy ASA and II or increased severity of illness ASA III or IV)
ASAP		as soon as possible
AST		aspartate aminotransferase (was SGOT)
a.u.	aures utrae	each ear
A-V		atrial-ventricular
bid	bis in die	twice daily
bm		bowel movement
BMT		bone marrow transplant
bp		blood pressure
BSA		body surface area
BUN		blood urea nitrogen
c	cong	a gallon
c̄	cum	with
cal		calorie
cAMP		cyclic adenosine monophosphate
cap	capsula	capsule
CBC		complete blood count
cc		cubic centimeter
CHF		congestive heart failure
CI		cardiac index
CI_{cr}		creatinine clearance
cm		centimeter
CNS		central nervous system
comp	compositus	compound

(continued)

Abbreviation	From	Meaning
cont		continue
COPD		chronic obstructive pulmonary disease
CSF		cerebral spinal fluid
CT		computed tomography
CVA		cerebral vascular accident
CVP		central venous pressure
d	dies	day
D_5W		dextrose 5% in water
$D_{5/0.45}W$		dextrose 5% in sodium chloride 0.45%
$D_{10}W$		dextrose 10% in water
d/c		discontinue
DIC		disseminated intravascular coagulation
dil	dilue	dilute
disp	dispensa	dispense
div	divide	divide
DNA		deoxyribonucleic acid
dtd	dentur tales doses	give of such a dose
DVT		deep vein thrombosis
EEG		electroencephalogram
EKG		electrocardiogram
elix, el	elixir	elixir
emp		as directed
ESR		erythrocyte sedimentation rate
E.T.		endotracheal
et	et	and
ex aq		in water
f, ft	fac, fiat, fiant	make, let be made
FDA		Food and Drug Administration
$FEV_1 1$		forced expiratory volume
FVC		forced vital capacity
g	gramma	gram
G-6-PD		glucose-6-phosphate dehydrogenase
GA		gestational age
GABA		gamma-aminobutyric acid
GE		gastroesophageal
GI		gastrointestinal
gr	granum	grain
gtt	gutta	a drop
GU		genitourinary
h	hora	hour
HIV		human immunodeficiency virus
HPLC		high performance liquid chromatography
hs	hora somni	at bedtime
IBW		ideal body weight
ICP		intracranial pressure
IgG		immune globulin G
I.M.		intramuscular
INR		international normalized ratio
I.O.		intraosseous
I & O		input and output
IOP		intraocular pressure
I.T.		intrathecal
I.V.		intravenous
IVH		intraventricular hemorrhage
IVP		intravenous push
JRA		juvenile rheumatoid arthritis
kcal		kilocalorie
kg		kilogram
L		liter
LDH		lactate dehydrogenase
LE		lupus erythematosus

(continued)

Abbreviation	From	Meaning
liq	liquor	a liquor, solution
LP		lumbar puncture
M	misce	mix
MAO		monoamine oxidase
MAP		mean arterial pressure
mcg		microgram
m. dict	more dictor	as directed
mEq		milliequivalent
mg		milligram
MI		myocardial infarction
min		minute
mixt	mixtura	a mixture
mL		milliliter
mm		millimeter
mo		month
mOsm		milliosmols
MRI		magnetic resonance image
ND		nasoduodenal
NF		National Formulary
ng		nanogram
no.	numerus	number
noc	nocturnal	in the night
non rep	non repetatur	do not repeat, no refills
NPO		nothing by mouth
NSAID		nonsteroidal anti-inflammatory drug
O, Oct	octarius	a pint
o.d.	oculus dexter	right eye
o.l.	oculus laevus	left eye
O.R.		operating room
o.s.	oculus sinister	left eye
OTC		over-the-counter (nonprescription)
o.u.	oculo uterque	each eye
PALS		pediatric advanced life support
pc, post cib	post cibos	after meals
PCA		postconceptional age
PCP		*Pneumocystis carinii* pneumonia
PCWP		pulmonary capillary wedge pressure
PDA		patent ductus arteriosus
per		through or by
PM	post meridiem	afternoon or evening
PNA		postnatal age
P.O.	per os	by mouth
P.R.	per rectum	rectally
prn	pro re nata	as needed
PSVT		paroxysmal supraventricular tachycardia
PT		prothrombin time
PTT		partial thromboplastin time
PUD		peptic ulcer disease
pulv	pulvis	a powder
PVC		premature ventricular contraction
q		every
qad	quoque alternis die	every other day
qd		every day
qh	quiaque hora	every hour
qid	quater in die	four times a day
qod		every other day
qs	quantum sufficiat	a sufficient quantity
qs ad		a sufficient quantity to make
qty		quantity
qv	quam volueris	as much as you wish
Rx	recipe	take, a recipe

(continued)

Abbreviation	From	Meaning
RAP		right atrial pressure
rep	repetatur	let it be repeated
$\bar{s}$	sine	without
S-A		sino-atrial
sa	secundum artem	according to art
sat	sataratus	saturated
S.C.		subcutaneous
S_{cr}		serum creatinine
SIADH		syndrome of inappropriate antidiuretic hormone
sig	signa	label, or let it be printed
S.L.		sublingual
SLE		systemic lupus erythematosus
sol	solutio	solution
solv		dissolve
$\bar{ss}$, ss	semis	one-half
sos	si opus sit	if there is need
stat	statim	at once, immediately
supp	suppositorium	suppository
SVR		systemic vascular resistance
SVT		supraventricular tachycardia
SWI		sterile water for injection
syr	syrupus	syrup
tab	tabella	tablet
tal		such
tid	ter in die	three times a day
tr, tinct	tincture	tincture
trit		triturate
tsp		teaspoonful
TT		thrombin time
u.d., ut dict	ut dictum	as directed
ung	unguentum	ointment
USAN		United States Adopted Names
USP		United States Pharmacopeia
UTI		urinary tract infection
V_d		volume of distribution
V_{dss}		volume of distribution at steady-state
v.o.		verbal order
w.a.		while awake
x3		3 times
x4		4 times
y		year

NORMAL LABORATORY VALUES FOR ADULTS*

CHEMISTRY

Chemistry, Routine

Albumin		3.5-5.0 g/dL
Bilirubin, conjugated		0-0.2 mg/dL
Bilirubin, total		0.2-1.2 mg/dL
Blood urea nitrogen		8-23 mg/dL
Calcium		8.4-10.3 mg/dL
Creatinine		0.5-1.2 mg/dL
Glucose		65-110 mg/dL
Phosphorus		2.8-4.5 mg/dL
Protein, total		6.0-8.0 g/dL
Uric acid	male	3.5-7.2 mg/dL
	female	2.6-6.5 mg/dL

Electrolytes

Chlorides	100-110 mEq/L
CO_2	23-31 mEq/L
Potassium	3.5-5.0 mEq/L
Sodium	136-146 mEq/L
Anion gap	5-14 mEq/L

Enzymes

Alkaline phosphatase	male	34-110 units/L
	female	24-100 units/L
ALT		5-35 units/L
AST		5-35 units/L
CPK	male	0-206 units/L
	female	0-175 units/L
LDH		50-200 units/L

Thyroid Function

FTI (free thyroxine index)	4.5-12.0
T_3 resin uptake	25%-35%
T_3 (tri-iodothyronine) by RIA	70-200 ng/dL
T_4 (thyroxine) by RIA	4.0-11.0 µg/dL

Others

Ammonia, plasma		20-60 µg/dL
Amylase, serum		44-128 units/L
Calcium, ionized		4.6-5.2 mg/dL
Cholesterol		140-230 mg/dL
Iron, serum		50-170 µg/dL
Lactate, serum		1.4-3.9 mEq/L
Lipase		10-208 units/L
Magnesium		1.5-2.5 mg/dL
Oncotic pressure		22-28 mm Hg
Osmolality		280-300 mOsm/kg
Serum ferritin	male	25-400 ng/mL
	female	10-150 ng/mL
TIBC		270-390 µg/dL
Triglycerides		50-150 mg/dL

---

*The normal ranges for laboratory values vary with different age groups, and may change as new methodologies for the lab tests are used. These values are current for adults (age 17 years or older). **Note:** Normal laboratory values may differ according to laboratory, institution, and analytical technique.

HEMATOLOGY

Hematocrit	male	40%-52%
	female	35%-47%
Hemoglobin	male	13.5-17.5 g/dL
	female	11.5-16.0 g/dL
MCH		27-34 pg
MCV		82-100 fL
Platelet count		150-450 10^3/mm^3
RBC count	male	4.5-5.9 10^6/mm^3
	female	4.0-4.9 10^6/mm^3
Reticulocyte count		0.5%-1.5%
Sed rate (Westergren)	male	0-10 mm/h
	female	0-20 mm/h
WBC count		4.5-11.0 10^3/mm^3
WBC differential		
bands		2%-8%
basophils		0%-2%
eosinophils		0%-4%
lymphocytes		20%-45%
monocytes		2%-8%
neutrophils		40%-70%

BLOOD GASES

	Arterial	Venous
Base excess	-3.0 to +3.0 mEq/L	-5.0 to +5.0 mEq/L
HCO_3	18-25 mEq/L	18-25 mEq/L
O_2 saturation	90%-98%	60%-85%
pCO_2	34-45 mm Hg	35-52 mm Hg
pH	7.35-7.45	7.32-7.42
pO_2	80-95 mm Hg	30-48 mm Hg
TCO_2	23-29 mEq/L	24-30 mEq/L

Weight/Volume Equivalents

1 mg/dL = 10 μg/mL   1 ppm = 1 mg/L

1 mg/dL = 1 mg%   1 μg/mL = 1 mg/L

NORMAL LABORATORY VALUES FOR CHILDREN

CHEMISTRY

Albumin	0-1 y	2-4 g/dL
	1 y - adult	3.5-5.5 g/dL
Ammonia	newborn	90-150 µg/dL
	child	40-120 µg/dL
	adult	18-54 µg/dL
Amylase	newborn	0-60 units/L
	adult	30-110 units/L
Bilirubin, conjugated, direct	newborn	<1.5 mg/dL
	1 mo - adult	0-0.5 mg/dL
Bilirubin, total	0-3 d	2-10 mg/dL
	1 mo - adult	0-1.5 mg/dL
Bilirubin, unconjugated, indirect		0.6-10.5 mg/dL
Calcium	newborn	7-12 mg/dL
	0-2 y	8.8-11.2 mg/dL
	2 y - adult	9-11 mg/dL
Calcium, ionized, whole blood		4.4-5.4 mg/dL
Carbon dioxide, total		23-33 mEq/L
Chloride		95-105 mEq/L
Cholesterol	newborn	45-170 mg/dL
	0-1 y	65-175 mg/dL
	1-20 y	120-230 mg/dL
Creatinine	0-1 y	≤0.6 mg/dL
	1 y - adult	0.5-1.5 mg/dL
Glucose	newborn	30-90 mg/dL
	0-2 y	60-105 mg/dL
	child - adult	70-110 mg/dL
Iron	newborn	110-270 µg/dL
	infant	30-70 µg/dL
	child	55-120 µg/dL
	adult	70-180 µg/dL
Iron binding	newborn	59-175 µg/dL
	infant	100-400 µg/dL
	adult	250-400 µg/dL
Lactic acid, lactate		2-20 mg/dL
Lead, whole blood		<30 µg/dL
Lipase	child	20-140 units/L
	adult	0-190 units/L
Magnesium		1.5-2.5 mEq/L
Osmolality, serum		275-296 mOsm/kg
Osmolality, urine		50-1400 mOsm/kg

Chemistry *(continued)*

Phosphorus	newborn	4.2-9 mg/dL
	6 wk - 19 mo	3.8-6.7 mg/dL
	18 mo - 3 y	2.9-5.9 mg/dL
	3-15 y	3.6-5.6 mg/dL
	>15 y	2.5-5 mg/dL
Potassium, plasma	newborn	4.5-7.2 mEq/L
	2 d - 3 mo	4-6.2 mEq/L
	3 mo - 1 y	3.7-5.6 mEq/L
	1-16 y	3.5-5 mEq/L
Protein, total	0-2 y	4.2-7.4 g/dL
	>2 y	6-8 g/dL
Sodium		136-145 mEq/L
Triglycerides	infant	0-171 mg/dL
	child	20-130 mg/dL
	adult	30-200 mg/dL
Urea nitrogen, blood	0-2 y	4-15 mg/dL
	2 y - adult	5-20 mg/dL
Uric acid	male	3-7 mg/dL
	female	2-6 mg/dL

ENZYMES

Alanine aminotransferase (ALT) (SGPT)	0-2 mo	8-78 units/L
	>2 mo	8-36 units/L
Alkaline phosphatase (ALKP)	newborn	60-130 units/L
	0-16 y	85-400 units/L
	>16 y	30-115 units/L
Aspartate aminotransferase (AST) (SGOT)	infant	18-74 units/L
	child	15-46 units/L
	adult	5-35 units/L
Creatine kinase (CK)	infant	20-200 units/L
	child	10-90 units/L
	adult male	0-206 units/L
	adult female	0-175 units/L
Lactate dehydrogenase (LDH)	newborn	290-501 units/L
	1 mo - 2 y	110-144 units/L
	>16 y	60-170 units/L

BLOOD GASES

	Arterial	Capillary	Venous
pH	7.35-7.45	7.35-7.45	7.32-7.42
pCO_2 (mm Hg)	35-45	35-45	38-52
pO_2 (mm Hg)	70-100	60-80	24-48
HCO_3 (mEq/L)	19-25	19-25	19-25
TCO_2 (mEq/L)	19-29	19-29	23-33
O_2 saturation (%)	90-95	90-95	40-70
Base excess (mEq/L)	-5 to +5	-5 to +5	-5 to +5

THYROID FUNCTION TESTS

T_4 (thyroxine)	1-7 d	10.1-20.9 µg/dL
	8-14 d	9.8-16.6 µg/dL
	1 mo - 1 y	5.5-16 µg/dL
	>1 y	4-12 µg/dL
FTI	1-3 d	9.3-26.6
	1-4 wk	7.6-20.8
	1-4 mo	7.4-17.9
	4-12 mo	5.1-14.5
	1-6 y	5.7-13.3
	>6 y	4.8-14
T_3 by RIA	newborns	100-470 ng/dL
	1-5 y	100-260 ng/dL
	5-10 y	90-240 ng/dL
	10 y - adult	70-210 ng/dL
T_3 uptake		35%-45%
TSH	cord	3-22 µU/mL
	1-3 d	<40 µU/mL
	3-7 d	<25 µU/mL
	>7 d	0-10 µU/mL

HEMATOLOGY VALUES

Complete Blood Count

	Hgb (g/dL)	Hct (%)	MCV (fL)	MCH (pg)	MCHC (%)	RBC (x 10^6/mm^3)	RDW	PLTS (x 10^3/mm^3)
0-3 d	15.0-20.0	45-61	95-115	31-37	29-37	4.0-5.9	<18.0	250-450
1-2 wk	12.5-18.5	39-57	86-110	28-36	28-38	3.6-5.5	<17.0	250-450
1-6 mo	10.0-13.0	29-42	74-96	25-35	30-36	3.1-4.3	<16.5	300-700
7 mo - 2 y	10.5-13.0	33-38	70-84	23-30	31-37	3.7-4.9	<16.0	250-600
2-5 y	11.5-13.0	34-39	75-87	24-30	31-37	3.9-5.0	<15.0	250-550
5-8 y	11.5-14.5	35-42	77-95	25-33	31-37	4.0-4.9	<15.0	250-550
13-18 y	12.0-15.2	36-47	78-96	25-35	31-37	4.5-5.1	<14.5	150-450
Adult male	13.5-16.5	41-50	80-100	26-34	31-37	4.5-5.9	<14.5	150-450
Adult female	12.0-15.0	36-45	80-100	26-34	31-37	4.0-4.9	<14.5	150-450

WBC and Differential

	WBC (x 10^3/mm^3)	Segs	Bands	Eos	Basos	Lymphs	Atypical Lymphs	Monos	# of NRBCs
0-3 d	9.0-35.0	32-62	10-18	0-2	0-1	19-29	0-8	5-7	0-2
1-2 wk	5.0-20.0	14-34	6-14	0-2	0-1	36-45	0-8	6-10	0
1-6 mo	6.0-17.5	13-33	4-12	0-3	0-1	41-71	0-8	4-7	0
7 mo - 2 y	6.0-17.0	15-35	5-11	0-3	0-1	45-76	0-8	3-6	0
2-5 y	5.5-15.5	23-45	5-11	0-3	0-1	35-65	0-8	3-6	0
5-8 y	5.0-14.5	32-54	5-11	0-3	0-1	28-48	0-8	3-6	0
13-18 y	4.5-13.0	34-64	5-11	0-3	0-1	25-45	0-8	3-6	0
Adults	4.5-11.0	35-66	5-11	0-3	0-1	24-44	0-8	3-6	0

Sedimentation rate, Westergren
    Children   0-20 mm/h
    Adult male   0-15 mm/h
    Adult female   0-20 mm/h
Sedimentation rate, Wintrobe
    Children   0-13 mm/h
    Adult male   0-10 mm/h
    Adult female   0-15 mm/h
Reticulocyte count
    Newborn   2%-6%
    1-6 months   0%-2.8%
    Adults   0.5%-1.5%

APOTHECARY/METRIC CONVERSIONS

Liquid Measures

Basic equivalent: 1 fluid ounce = 30 mL

Examples:

1 gallon	.3800 mL	4 fluid ounces	. . .120 mL
1 quart	960 mL	15 minims	1 mL
1 pint	480 mL	10 minims	0.6 mL
8 fluid ounces	240 mL		

1 gallon	128 fluid ounces
1 quart	32 fluid ounces
1 pint	16 fluid ounces

Approximate Household Equivalents

1 teaspoonful . . . . 5 mL   1 tablespoonful . . . .15 mL

Weights

Basic equivalents:

1 ounce = 30 g   15 grains = 1 g

Examples:

4 ounces	120 g	1 grain	.60 mg
2 ounces	60 g	$1/100$ grain	600 µg
10 grains	600 mg	$1/150$ grain	400 µg
7 $1/2$ grains	500 mg	$1/200$ grain	300 µg
16 ounces	1 pound		

Metric Conversions

Basic equivalents:

1 g . . . . .1000 mg   1 mg . . . . 1000 µg

Examples:

5 g	.5000 mg	5 mg	5000 µg
0.5 g	500 mg	0.5 mg	500 µg
0.05 g	50 mg	0.05 mg	.50 µg

Exact Equivalents

1 gram (g) = 15.43 grains	0.1 mg = 1/600 gr
1 milliliter (mL) = 16.23 minims	0.12 mg = 1/500 gr
1 minim = 0.06 milliliter	0.15 mg = 1/400 gr
1 grain (gr) = 64.8 milligrams	0.2 mg = 1/300 gr
1 ounce (oz) = 28.35 grams	0.5 mg = 1/120 gr
1 pound (lb) = 453.6 grams	0.8 mg = 1/80 gr
1 kilogram (kg) = 2.2 pounds	1 mg = 1/65 gr

Solids*

$1/4$ grain = 15 mg
$1/2$ grain = 30 mg
$1 1/2$ grain = 100 mg
5 grains = 300 mg
10 grains = 600 mg

*Use exact equivalents for compounding and calculations requiring a high degree of accuracy.

POUNDS/KILOGRAMS CONVERSION

1 pound = 0.45359 kilograms
1 kilogram = 2.2 pounds

lb	=	kg	lb	=	kg	lb	=	kg
1		0.45	70		31.75	140		63.50
5		2.27	75		34.02	145		65.77
10		4.54	80		36.29	150		68.04
15		6.80	85		38.56	155		70.31
20		9.07	90		40.82	160		72.58
25		11.34	95		43.09	165		74.84
30		13.61	100		45.36	170		77.11
35		15.88	105		47.63	175		79.38
40		18.14	110		49.90	180		81.65
45		20.41	115		52.16	185		83.92
50		22.68	120		54.43	190		86.18
55		24.95	125		56.70	195		88.45
60		27.22	130		58.91	200		90.72
65		29.48	135		61.24			

TEMPERATURE CONVERSION

Centigrade to Fahrenheit = ($^{\circ}$C x 9/5) + 32 = $^{\circ}$F
Fahrenheit to Centigrade = ($^{\circ}$F - 32) x 5/9 = $^{\circ}$C

$^{\circ}$C	=	$^{\circ}$F	$^{\circ}$C	=	$^{\circ}$F	$^{\circ}$C	=	$^{\circ}$F
100.0		212.0	39.0		102.2	36.8		98.2
50.0		122.0	38.8		101.8	36.6		97.9
41.0		105.8	38.6		101.5	36.4		97.5
40.8		105.4	38.4		101.1	36.2		97.2
40.6		105.1	38.2		100.8	36.0		96.8
40.4		104.7	38.0		100.4	35.8		96.4
40.2		104.4	37.8		100.1	35.6		96.1
40.0		104.0	37.6		99.7	35.4		95.7
39.8		103.6	37.4		99.3	35.2		95.4
39.6		103.3	37.2		99.0	35.0		95.0
39.4		102.9	37.0		98.6	0		32.0
39.2		102.6						

ACQUIRED IMMUNODEFICIENCY SYNDROME (AIDS)

This list of tests is not intended in any way to suggest patterns of physician's orders, nor is it complete. These tests may support possible clinical diagnoses or rule out other diagnostic possibilities. Each laboratory test relevant to AIDS is listed and weighted. Two symbols (**) indicate that the test is diagnostic, that is, documents the diagnosis if the expected is found. A single symbol (*) indicates a test frequently used in the diagnosis or management of the disease. The other listed tests are useful on a selective basis with consideration of clinical factors and specific aspects of the case.

Acid-Fast Stain
Acid-Fast Stain, Modified, *Nocardia* Species
Antimicrobial Susceptibility Testing, Fungi
Antimicrobial Susceptibility Testing, Mycobacteria
Arthropod Identification
Babesiosis Serological Test
Bacteremia Detection, Buffy Coat Micromethod
Bacterial Culture, Blood
Bacterial Culture, Bronchoscopy Specimen
Bacterial Culture, Sputum
Bacterial Culture, Stool
Bacterial Culture, Throat
Bacterial Culture, Urine, Clean Catch
Beta$_2$-Microglobulin
Blood and Fluid Precautions, Specimen Collection
Bronchial Washings Cytology
Bronchoalveolar Lavage Cytology
Brushings Cytology
Candida Antigen
Candidiasis Serologic Test
Cat Scratch Disease Serology
CD4/CD8 Enumeration
Cerebrospinal Fluid Cytology
Cryptococcal Antigen Titer
Cryptosporidium Diagnostic Procedures
Cytomegalic Inclusion Disease Cytology
Cytomegalovirus Antibody
Cytomegalovirus Antigen Detection
Cytomegalovirus Culture
Cytomegalovirus DNA Detection
Darkfield Examination, Syphilis
Electron Microscopy
Folic Acid, Serum
Fungal Culture, Biopsy or Body Fluid
Fungal Culture, Blood
Fungal Culture, Cerebrospinal Fluid
Fungal Culture, Sputum
Fungal Culture, Stool
Fungal Culture, Urine
Hemoglobin A$_2$
Hepatitis B Surface Antigen
Herpes Cytology
Herpes Simplex Virus Antigen Detection
Herpes Simplex Virus Culture
Histopathology
Histoplasmosis Antibody
Histoplasmosis Antigen
**HIV-1/HIV-2 Serology

HTLV-I/II Antibody
*Human Immunodeficiency Virus Culture
*Human Immunodeficiency Virus DNA Amplification
India Ink Preparation
Inhibitor, Lupus, Phospholipid Type
KOH Preparation
Leishmaniasis Serological Test
Leukocyte Immunophenotyping
Lymphocyte Transformation Test
Microsporidia Diagnostic Procedures
Mycobacteria by DNA Probe
Mycobacterial Culture, Biopsy or Body Fluid
Mycobacterial Culture, Cerebrospinal Fluid
Mycobacterial Culture, Cutaneous and Subcutaneous Tissue
Mycobacterial Culture, Sputum
Mycobacterial Culture, Stool
Neisseria gonorrhoeae Culture and Smear
Nocardia Culture
Ova and Parasites, Stool
*p24 Antigen
Platelet Count
Pneumocystis carinii Preparation
Pneumocystis Immunofluorescence
Polymerase Chain Reaction
Red Blood Cell Indices
Risks of Transfusion
Skin Biopsy
Sputum Cytology
Toxoplasmosis Serology
VDRL, Serum
Viral Culture
Viral Culture, Blood
Viral Culture, Body Fluid
Viral Culture, Central Nervous System Symptoms
Viral Culture, Dermatological Symptoms
Viral Culture, Tissue
Virus, Direct Detection by Fluorescent Antibody
White Blood Count

FDA Approved Drugs for HIV Infection and AIDS-Related Conditions

amphotericin B lipid complex (Abelcet®, Ambisome®)
    Treatment of aspergillosis
atovaquone (Mepron®)
    Treatment of mild to moderate Pneumocystic carinii pneumonia in patients who are
        intolerant to Bactrim® or Septra®
azithromycin (Zithromax®)
    Prevention of Mycobacterium avium complex (MAC) in persons with advanced HIV
        infection
cidofovir (Vistide®)
    Treatment of AIDS-related cytomegalovirus retinitis
clarithromycin (Biaxin®, Klacid®)
    Treatment of disseminated mycobacterial infections due to Mycobacterium avium-
        intracellulare complex (MAC); approved for prophylaxis of disseminated MAC in
        patients with advanced HIV infection
daunorubicin-liposomal (DaunoXome®)
    Treatment of advanced HIV-related Kaposi's sarcoma

delavirdine mesylate (Rescriptor®)
> In combination with appropriate antiretrovirals when therapy is warranted for treatment of HIV infection

didanosine (Videx®)
> Treatment of adult and pediatric patients with advanced HIV who are intolerant to or deteriorating on AZT; approved for treatment of adult and pediatric patients with advanced HIV previously treated with AZT; approved for treatment of HIV infection when antiretroviral therapy is warranted

doxorubicin hydrochloride-liposomal (Doxil®)
> Treatment of Kaposi's sarcoma in AIDS patients who are intolerant to or have disease progression on prior combination chemotherapy

dronabinol (Marinol®)
> Treatment of anorexia associated with weight loss in patients with AIDS

erythropoietin (Epogen®, Procrit®)
> Treatment of anemia related to AZT therapy in HIV infection

filgrastim [G-CSF] (Neupogen®)
> Treatment of neutropenia due to chemotherapy for cancers, including lymphomas and Kaposi's sarcoma

fluconazole (Diflucan®)
> Treatment of oropharyngeal and esophageal candidiasis and for treatment of cryptococcal meningitis; approved for treatment of pediatric patients with cryptococcal meningitis and candida infections

foscarnet (Foscavir®)
> Treatment of CMV retinitis in patients with AIDS; approved for the treatment of acyclovir-resistant herpes simplex virus

ganciclovir - I.V., oral (Cytovene®)
> Treatment of CMV retinitis in immunocompromised patients; oral approved for maintenance therapy for CMV retinitis in some patients; approved for prophylaxis of CMV disease

ganciclovir [DHPG] - implant (Vitrasert®)
> Treatment of CMV retinitis in patients with AIDS

immune globulin - I.V. (Gamimune N®)
> Prevention of bacterial infections in pediatric HIV infection

indinavir sulfate (Crixivan®)
> For use alone or in combination with nucleoside analogues for treatment of HIV infection in adults

interferon alfa-2a (Roferon-A®)
> Treatment of AIDS-related Kaposi's sarcoma in selected patients

interferon alfa-2b (Intron-A®)
> Treatment of adult AIDS-related Kaposi's sarcoma in selected patients; approved for treatment of chronic non-A, non-B hepatitis

interferon alfa-n3 (Alferon N®)
> Treatment of condyloma acuminata (genital warts)

itraconazole (Sporanox®)
> Treatment of histoplasmosis, blastomycosis, and aspergillosis in immunocompromised and nonimmunocompromised patients

ketoconazole (Nizoral®)
> Treatment of histoplasmosis, blastomycosis, and candidiasis

lamivudine [3TC] (Epivir®)
> Combination use with AZT as a treatment option for HIV infection in adults and pediatric patients ≥3 months of age

megestrol acetate (Megace®, Ovaban®)
> Treatment of anorexia, cachexia, or unexplained significant weight loss in patients with AIDS

nelfinavir mesylate (Viracept®)
> Treatment of HIV infection when antiretroviral therapy is warranted in adults and pediatrics ≥2 years of age

nevirapine (Viramune®)
  Combination use with nucleoside analogues for treatment of HIV-infected adults experiencing clinical and/or immunologic deterioration
para-aminosalicylic acid (Paser®)
  Treatment of tuberculosis in combination with other active agents
pentamidine - I.M., I.V. (Pentam® 300)
  Treatment of *Pneumocystis carinii* pneumonia
pentamidine - aerosolized (NebuPent®)
  Prevention of *Pneumocystis carinii* pneumonia
pyrimethamine [with sulfonamide] (Daraprim®; Fansidar® when combined with sulfadoxine)
  Treatment of toxoplasmosis
rifabutin (Ansamycin®, Mycobutin®)
  Prevention of *Mycobacterium avium* complex in patients with advanced HIV
ritonavir (Norvir®)
  For use alone or in combination with nucleoside analogues for treatment of HIV infection
saquinavir mesylate (Invirase®)
  Combination use with nucleoside analogues for treatment of advanced HIV infection in selected patients
sargramostim [GM-CSF] (Leukine®)
  Treatment of cancer patients with lymphomas or leukemia who are receiving bone marrow transplants
stavudine [d4T] (Zerit®)
  Treatment of adults with advanced HIV infection who are intolerant to or deteriorating on approved therapies; approved for treatment of adults with advanced HIV infection who have undergone prolonged treatment with AZT; approved for the treatment of pediatrics with HIV infection who have undergone prolonged prior AZT therapy
sulfamethoxazole (Bactrim® when combined with trimethoprim; Septra® when combined with trimethoprim)
  Treatment of *Pneumocystis carinii* pneumonia (PCP); approved for prevention of PCP
trimethoprim (Bactrim® when combined with sulfamethoxazole; Septra® when combined with sulfamethoxazole)
  Treatment of *Pneumocystis carinii* pneumonia (PCP); approved for prevention of PCP
trimetrexate (with leucovorin) [TMTX] (Neutrexin®)
  Treatment of moderate to severe *Pneumocystis carinii* pneumonia when intolerant or refractory to TMP/SMX or when TMP/SMX is contraindicated
zalcitabine [ddC] (Hivid®)
  Combination use with AZT for treatment of selected patients with advanced HIV disease; approved for monotherapy treatment of advanced HIV for patients ≥13 years of age who are intolerant to or have disease progression on AZT
zidovudine [AZT] (Retrovir®)
  Treatment of adult AIDS or symptomatic HIV and CD4 ≤200; approved for treatment of adult HIV infection and CD4 ≤500; approved for treatment of pediatric HIV infection (3 months to 12 years of age); approved for prevention of perinatal transmission in HIV-positive pregnant women between 14 and 34 weeks gestation and in newborns of HIV-positive mothers
zidovudine and lamivudine (Combivir®)
  Combination of AZT (zidovudine) and 3TC (lamivudine) for treating AIDS and HIV infection

Drugs Being Studied in HIV/AIDS Clinical Trials

A-007 [antineoplastic]

APPENDIX

acetaminophen (Tylenol®, Panadol®) [analgesic, antipyretic]
acetylcysteine (Mucomyst®, Respaire®) [antiretroviral, mycolytic]
acitretin (Soriatane®) [antipsoriatic]
acyclovir (Zovirax®) [antiviral]
aldesleukin (Proleukin®) [immunomodulator, antineoplastic]
AL 721 [antiviral]
ALVAC-HIV gp 160 MN (vCP125) [vaccine]
ALVAC-HIV MN120TMG (vCP205) [vaccine]
ALVAC-HIV MN120TMGNP (vCP300) [vaccine]
ALVAC-RG rabies glycoprotein (vCP65) [vaccine]
allopurinol (Zyloprim®) [xanthine oxidase inhibitor]
aluminum hydroxide (Amphogel® [adjuvant, immunostimulant]
alvircept sudotox (CD4-pseudomonas exotoxin) [immunomodulator, antiretroviral]
amikacin sulfate (Kanamycin®) [antibacterial]
aminosalicylic acid [antibacterial]
amitriptyline hydrochloride (Elavil®) [antidepressant, analgesic]
amoxicillin (Amoxil®) [antimicrobial]
amphotericin B (Fungizone®) [antifungal]
amphotericin B lipid complex (Abelcet®, Ambisome®) [antifungal]
ampicillin (Omnipen®) [antimicrobial]
ampligen (Atvogen®) [antiretroviral, immunomodulator]
anti-HIV immune serum globulin (HIVIG®) [immunomodulator]
anti-Rh antibodies (Anti-D) [immunomodulator]
APL 400-003 [vaccine]
AS-101 (ammonium trichlorotellurate) [immunomodulator]
atevirdine mesylate (U-87201E) [antiretroviral]
azidodideoxyuridine (AzdU) [antiretroviral]
beclomethasone dipropionate (Beclovent®) [anti-inflammatory]
benztropine mesylate (Cogentin®) [anticholinergic, antiparkinsonian]
bis-POM PMEA [antiretroviral]
bleomycin (Blenoxane®) [antineoplastic]
butyldeoxynojirimicin (SC-48334) [antiretroviral]
capreomycin sulfate (Caprocin®) [antibacterial]
CD4 antigen [antiretroviral]
CD4-IgG [antiretroviral, immunomodulator]
ceftriaxone sodium (Rocephin®) [antimicrobial]
cefuroxime axetil (Ceftin®) [antibiotic]
chimeric anti-TNF monoclonal antibody (Chimeric A2) [immunomodulator]
chlorhexidine gluconate (Peridex®, Hibiclens®) [topical antibacterial, antimicrobial]
cimetidine (Tagamet®) [immunomodulator, histamine receptor antagonist]
ciprofloxacin (Cipro®) [antibacterial]
CI-0694 (Sulfasim®) [immunomodulator]
clavulanate potassium [antibacterial]
clindamycin (Cleocin®) [antibacterial]
clofazimine (Lamprene®) [antimicrobial, antileprotic]
clotrimazole (Lotrimin®, Mycelex®, Femcare®) [antifungal]
Cryptosporidium immune whey protein (bovine anticryptosporidium immunoglobulin)
    [antidiarrheal]
curdlan sulfate [antiviral]
cyclophosphamide (Cytoxan®) [antineoplastic, immunosuppressant]
cycloserine (Seromycin®) [antibacterial]
cysteamine (MEA; mercaptoethylamine) [antiretroviral, antiurolithic]
cytarabine (Cytosar-U®) [antimetabolite, antineoplastic, antiviral, immunosuppressant]
cytomegalovirus immune globulin intravenous (human) (CytoGam®) [immunomodulator]
dacarbazine [antineoplastic]
dapsone [antibacterial]
delavirdine mesylate (U-90152) [antiretroviral]

deoxy-fluorothymidine (FDT) [antiretroviral]
dexamethasone (Decadron®) [anti-inflammatory, immunomodulator, antineoplastic]
dextran sulfate [antiretroviral]
diclazuril [antiprotozoal]
dideoxyadenosine (ddA) [antiretroviral]
diethylhomospermine (DEHSPM) [antidiarrheal]
dinitrochlorobenzene (DNCB) [contact allergen, immunomodulator]
disulfiram (Antabuse®) [alcohol abuse deterrent, immunomodulator, antiretroviral]
ditiocarb sodium (Imuthiol®) [immunomodulator, chelator]
doxorubicin (Adriamycin®, Rubex®) [antineoplastic]
env 2-3 [vaccine]
ethambutol hydrochloride (Myambutol®) [antibacterial]
ethionamide [antibacterial]
etoposide (VePesid®) [antineoplastic]
F105 human monoclonal antibody [immunomodulator]
fiacitabine (FIAC) [antiviral]
fialuridine (FIAU] [antiviral]
flucytosine (Ancobon®) [antifungal]
fluorouracil (5-FU) [antineoplastic]
glutamic acid (Feracid®) [gastric acidifier]
gp-160 (MicroGeneSys®, VaxSyn®) [vaccine]
gp-160 vaccine (Immuno-AG) [vaccine]
guaifenesin (Robitussin®) [expectorant]
HBY 097 [antiretroviral]
hepatitis b vaccine (Engerix-B®, Recombivax HB®) [vaccine]
heptavalent pneumococcal conjugate vaccine [vaccine]
HIV p17/p24: Ty-VLP [vaccine]
HIV-1 C4-V3 polyvalent peptide vaccine [vaccine]
HIVAC-1e [vaccine]
hypericin (VIMRyxn®) [antiretroviral]
ibuprofen (Advil®; Motrin®; Nuprin®) [nonsteroidal anti-inflammatory]
ifosfamide [antineoplastic]
imipramine hydrochloride (Tofranil®) [antidepressant]
inosine pranobex (Isoprinosine®) [antiviral, immunostimulant, antiretroviral]
insulin-like growth factor (Somatomedin C®) [immunomodulator]
interferon alfa-n1 (Wellferon®) [antineoplastic, antiviral, immunomodulator]
interferon alfa-n3 (Alferon N®) [antineoplastic, antiviral, immunomodulator]
interferon beta (Betaseron®) [antineoplastic, antiviral, immunomodulator, antiretroviral]
interferon gamma (Actimmune®) [antineoplastic, antiviral, immunomodulator]
interleukin-3 (IL-3) [immunomodulator, hematopoietic]
interleukin-4 (IL-4) [immunomodulator, antineoplastic]
interleukin-10 (IL-10) [immunomodulator]
ISIS 2922 [antiviral]
isoniazid (INH) [antibacterial]
isotretinoin (Accutane®) [keratolytic]
ketoconazole (Nizoral®) [antifungal, antineoplastic, antiadrenal]
keyhole-limpet hemocyanin [immunomodulator]
kynostatin 272 (KNI-272®) [protease inhibitor, antiretroviral]
lentinan [immunomodulator, antineoplastic]
letrazuril [antiprotozoal]
leucovorin calcium (Wellcovorin®) [antianemic, antidote for folic acid antagonists]
levamisole [immunomodulator]
levocarnitine [antihyperlipoproteinemic]
levofloxacin [antimicrobial, antiretroviral]
liposome - encapsulated monophosphoryl lipid A [adjuvant, immunostimulant]
liposyn III (IV fat emulsion 2%) [nutritional support]
liposyn II (IV fat emulsion 20%) [nutritional support]

lobucavir [antiviral]
lymphocytes, activated [immunomodulator]
L-697, 639 [antiretroviral]
L-697, 661 [antiretroviral]
magnesium sulfate [electrolyte replenisher, anticonvulsant, laxative]
MDL 28574 [antiretroviral]
methadone hydrochloride (Dolophine®) [detoxification maintenance, narcotic analgesic]
methotrexate (MTX) [antineoplastic, folic acid antagonist, anti-inflammatory]
methoxsalen (Oxsoralen-ultra®) [Photochemotherapeutic]
methylprednisolone (Medrol®) [anti-inflammatory, immunosuppressant]
mexiletine hydrochloride (Mexitil®) [analgesic, antiarrhythmic]
MF59 [adjuvant, immunostimulant]
microparticulate monovalent HIV-1 peptide vaccine [vaccine]
mitoguazone dihydrochloride (MGBG) [antineoplastic]
mitoxantrone hydrochloride (Novantrone®) [antineoplastic]
monophosphoryl lipid A [adjuvant, immunostimulant]
MTP-PE/MF59 [immunostimulant, adjuvant emulsion]
multivalent HIV-1 peptide immunogen [vaccine]
nimodipine (Nimotop®) [calcium channel blocker, vasodilator]
nitazoxanide (NTZ) [antiparasitic]
nystatin (Mycostatin®) [antifungal]
octreotide acetate (Sandostatin®) [antidiarrheal]
OPC 14117 [antioxidant]
oxazepam (Serax®) [anxiolytic, minor tranquilizer]
P3C541b lipopeptide [vaccine]
paclitaxel (Taxol®) [antineoplastic]
paromomycin sulfate (Humatin®) [antibiotic, amebicidal, anthelmintic]
PCLUS [vaccine]
penicillin G [antibacterial]
pentosan polysulfate sodium [antineoplastic, antiviral, anticoagulant, anti-inflammatory,
    antiretroviral]
pentoxifylline (Trental®) [antiretroviral, immunomodulator, vasodilator, hemorrheologic]
peptide T [antiretroviral, immunomodulator]
piritrexim isethionate [antifolate, antineoplastic, antiproliferative, antiprotozoal]
PMEA [antiretroviral]
pneumococcal vaccine polyvalent [vaccine]
polyethylene glycolated IL-2 (PEG IL-2) [immunomodulator]
polymyxin B sulfate/bacitracin zinc ointment (Bacitracin®, Polysporin®) [antibacterial]
prednisone [glucocorticoid]
primaquine [antimalarial]
probenecid (Benemid®, ColBenemid®) [renal tubular blocker, uricosuric]
pseudoephedrine (Actifed®, Sudafed®) [decongestant, sympathomimetic]
pyrazinamide [antibacterial]
pyridoxine hydrochloride (vitamin B6) [vitamin (coenzyme)]
QS-21 [adjuvant, immunostimulant]
quinine (Quinidine®) [antimalarial, neuromuscular]
ranitidine hydrochloride (Zantac®) [histamine receptor antagonist, immunomodulator]
recombinant p24 vaccine [vaccine]
rgp 120/HIV-1IIIB [vaccine]
rgp 120/HIV-1MN [vaccine]
rgp 120/HIV 1MN monovalent octameric V3 peptide (SynVac®) [vaccine]
rgp 120/HIV-1SF2 [vaccine]
ribavirin (Virazole®) [antiviral, antiretroviral]
rifampin (Rifadin®, Rimactane®) [antibacterial]
RMP-7 [antifungal]
RO 24-7429 [antiretroviral, *tat* inhibitor]
saccharomyces boulardii [antidiarrheal]

SC-49483 [antiretroviral]

SC-52151 [protease inhibitor, antiretroviral]

SCH 39304 [antifungal]

selegiline hydrochloride (Deprenyl®) [MAO inhibitor, antidyskinetic, antiparkinsonian]

sevirumab (human monoclonal antibody to cytomegalovirus) [antiviral, immunomodulator]

smallpox vaccine (Dryvax®) [vaccine]

somatrem (human growth hormone Protriptin®) [immunomodulator]

sorivudine (Brovavir®) [antiviral]

SP-303T [antiviral]

sparfloxacin [antibacterial]

spiramycin [antibacterial, antiprotozoal]

streptomycin sulfate [antibacterial]

sulfadiazine [antibacterial]

sulfadoxine (Fansidar® when combined with pyrimethamine) [antibacterial]

syntex adjuvant formulation [adjuvant, immunostimulant]

TBC-3B [vaccine]

tecogalan sodium (SP-PG) [angiogenesis inhibitor]

thalidomide (Synovir®) [immunomodulator, sedative, hypnotic]

thioctic acid [antioxidant]

threonyl muramyl dipeptide [adjuvant, immunostimulant]

thymic humoral factor (THF) [immunomodulator]

thymosin alpha 1 [immunomodulator]

thymopentin (Timunox®) [immunomodulator]

TNP-470 [antineoplastic]

tretinoin (retinoic acid) [keratolytic]

trichosanthin (GLQ 223) [antiretroviral, immunosuppressant]

trifluridine (ophthalmic) [antiviral]

tuberculin purified protein derivative (PPD) [diagnostic aid]

tumor necrosis factor (TNF) [antineoplastic, antiretroviral]

tumor necrosis factor soluble receptor - immunoadhesion complex [immunomodulator]

valacyclovir hydrochloride (Valtrex®) [antiviral]

valproic acid (Depakene®) [anticonvulsant]

varicella virus vaccine live (Varivax®) [vaccine]

vesnarinone (OPC-8212) [antiretroviral, cardiotonic]

vidarabine [antiviral]

vinblastine sulfate (Velban®) [antineoplastic]

vincristine (Oncovin®) [antineoplastic]

WF10 [antiretroviral]

wobenzym [immunomodulator]

WR 6026 [antiprotozoal]

524W91 [antiretroviral]

882C87 [antiviral]

935U83 [antiretroviral]

CANCER CHEMOTHERAPY

Acronyms	Used for
7 + 3	Leukemia — acute myeloid leukemia, induction
ABP	Lymphoma — non-Hodgkin's
ABC-P	Multiple myeloma
ABDIC	Lymphoma — Hodgkin's
ABVD	Lymphoma — Hodgkin's
AC	Sarcoma — bony sarcoma
AC	Breast cancer
AC (DC)	Multiple myeloma
ACE	Lung cancer — small cell
ACe	Breast cancer
ACMF	Breast cancer
ACOMLA	Lymphoma — non-Hodgkin's
ADOC	Thymoma (Malignant)
AVM	Breast cancer
m-BACOD	Lymphoma — non-Hodgkin's
BACOP	Lymphoma — non-Hodgkin's
BAP	Multiple myeloma
BAPP	Thymoma (Malignant)
BCDT	Malignant melanoma
BCNU-DAG	Brain tumors
B-CMF	Head and neck cancer
BCVM	Cervical cancer
BCP	Multiple myeloma
BEP	Genitourinary cancer — testicular, induction, good risk
BHD	Malignant melanoma Breast cancer
BMC	Head and neck cancer
B-MOPP	Lymphoma — Hodgkin's
BMVL	Head and neck cancer
BOMP	Cervical cancer
BVCPP	Lymphoma — Hodgkin's
CAF	Breast cancer
CAFVP	Breast cancer
CAM	Genitourinary cancer — prostate
CAMP	Lung cancer — non-small cell
CAP	Genitourinary cancer — bladder Head and neck cancer Lung cancer — non-small cell Adrenal cortical cancer Endometrial cancer
CAP-BOP	Lymphoma — non-Hodgkin's
CAP-M	Genitourinary cancer — bladder
CBM	Head and neck cancer
CC	Ovarian cancer — epithelial
CCCP	Multiple myeloma
CCNU-VP	Lymphoma — Hodgkin's
CCVPP	Lymphoma — Hodgkin's
CD	Leukemia — acute nonlymphoblastic, consolidation Ewing's sarcoma Genitourinary cancer — prostate
CDC	Ovarian cancer — epithelial
CDF	Genitourinary cancer — prostate

Acronyms	Used for
CE	Adrenal cortical cancer
CF	Head and neck cancer
CFM	Breast cancer
CFPT	Breast cancer
CHAP	Ovarian cancer — epithelial
CHL + PRED	Leukemia — chronic lymphocytic leukemia
CHOP	Lymphoma — non-Hodgkin's
CHOP-B (Yale)	Lymphoma — non-Hodgkin's
CHOP-Bleo	Lymphoma — non-Hodgkin's
CHOP (P)	Lymphoma — non-Hodgkin's
CHOR	Lung cancer — small cell
CISCA	Gastric cancer Genitourinary cancer — bladder
Cladribine (2-CdA)	Leukemia — chronic lymphocytic leukemia
CMB	Cervical cancer
CMC-High Dose	Lung cancer — small cell
CMF	Breast cancer
CMFP	Breast cancer
CMFVP (Cooper's)	Breast cancer
C-MOPP	Lymphoma — non-Hodgkin's
CMV	Genitourinary cancer — bladder
COB	Head and neck cancer
CODE	Lung cancer — small cell
COPE	Lung cancer — small cell
COLP	Thymoma (Malignant)
COM	Colon cancer
COMF	Colon cancer
COP-BLAM	Lymphoma — non-Hodgkin's
COP-BLAM III	Lymphoma — non-Hodgkin's
COP-BLAM IV	Lymphoma — non-Hodgkin's
COP	Lymphoma — non-Hodgkin's
COP-BLAM	Lymphoma — non-Hodgkin's
COPP (or "C" MOPP)	Lymphoma — non-Hodgkin's
CP	Ovarian cancer — epithelial
CV	Lung cancer — non-small cell
CVB	Esophageal cancer
CVI	Lung cancer — non-small cell
CVM	Gestational trophoblastic disease
CVP	Leukemia — chronic lymphocytic leukemia Lymphoma — non-Hodgkin's
CYADIC	Sarcoma — soft tissue
CYVADIC	Sarcoma — bony sarcoma Sarcoma — soft tissue
DAFS	Carcinoid (Malignant)
DAT	Leukemia — acute myeloid leukemia, induction Breast cancer
DC	Multiple myeloma
DHAP	Lymphoma — non-Hodgkin's
DMBV	Throid cancer
DMC	Gestational trophoblastic cancer
DS	Genitourinary cancer — prostate
DTIC-ACTD	Malignant melanoma
DVP	Leukemia — acute lymphoblastic, induction
DVPA	Leukemia — acute lymphoblastic, induction

Acronyms	Used for
ELF	Gastric cancer
EMA-CO	Gestational trophoblastic disease
FAC	Breast cancer
FAC-S	Carcinoid (Malignant)
FAM	Gastric cancer
	Lung cancer — non-small cell
	Pancreatic cancer
FAME	Gastric cancer
FAMTX	Gastric cancer
FAP	Gastric cancer
FAP-2	Pancreatic cancer
FCE	Gastric cancer
F-CL	Colon cancer
FDC	Gastric cancer
FL	Genitourinary cancer — prostate
FLe	Colon cancer
Fludarabine	Leukemia — chronic lymphocytic leukemia
FMS (SMF)	Pancreatic cancer
FMV	Colon cancer
FOAM	Breast cancer
FOMi	Lung cancer — non-small cell
FOMi/CAP	Lung cancer — non-small cell
5FU/LDLF	Colon cancer
FU/HU	Colon cancer
FU/LV	Colon cancer
5FU Hurt	Head and neck cancer
5FU/LV (Weekly)	Colon cancer
FL	Genitourinary cancer — prostate
HDAC	Leukemia — acute myeloid leukemia, induction
HDMTX	Sarcoma — bony sarcoma
IC	Leukemia — acute myeloid leukemia, induction
ID	Sarcoma — soft tissue
IMAC	Sarcoma — bony sarcoma
IMF	Breast cancer
IMVP-16	Lymphoma — non-Hodgkin's
LDAC	Leukemia — acute myeloid leukemia, induction
L-VAM	Genitourinary cancer — prostate
M-2	Multiple myeloma
MAC	Genitourinary cancer — bladder Endometrial cancer
MACC	Lung cancer — non-small cell
MACOP-B	Lymphoma — non-Hodgkin's
MAID	Sarcoma — soft tissue
MAP	Head and neck cancer
MBC (MBD)	Head and neck cancer Cervical cancer Esophageal cancer
MBD	Head and neck cancer
MC	Leukemia — acute myeloid leukemia, induction
MeCP	Multiple myeloma
MF	Head and neck cancer Esophageal cancer
MICE (ICE)	Lung cancer — small cell
MINE	Lymphoma — non-Hodgkin's
MM	Leukemia — acute lymphoblastic, maintenance
MMC (MTX + MP + CTX)	Leukemia — acute lymphoblastic, maintenance
MOF-STREP	Colon cancer

Acronyms	Used for
MOP-BAP	Lymphoma — Hodgkin's
MOPP	Lymphoma — Hodgkin's
MOPP/ABV Hybrid	Lymphoma — Hodgkin's
MP	Multiple myeloma
m-PFL	Genitourinary cancer — bladder
MS	Adrenal cortical cancer
MV	Leukemia — acute myeloid leukemia, induction
MVAC	Genitourinary cancer — bladder
MVPP	Lymphoma — Hodgkin's
NFL	Breast cancer
PAC (CAP)	Ovarian cancer — epithelial Endometrial cancer
PE	Genitourinary cancer — testicular, induction, good risk Lung cancer — small cell
PFL	Gastric cancer Head and neck cancer
PFL + IFV	Head and neck cancer
POCC	Lung cancer — small cell
Pro-MACE	Lymphoma — non-Hodgkin's
Pro-MACE-CytaBOM	Lymphoma — non-Hodgkin's
Pro-MACE-MOPP	Lymphoma — non-Hodgkin's
PT	Ovarian cancer — epithelial
SC	Carcinoid (Malignant)
SCAB	Lymphoma — Hodgkin's
SD	Pancreatic cancer
SF	Carcinoid (Malignant)
SMF	Pancreatic cancer
T-9	Ewing's sarcoma
VAB VI	Genitourinary cancer — testicular, induction, salvage
VAC	Ovarian cancer — germ cell Sarcoma — soft tissue Ewing's sarcoma
VAC (CAV) (Induction)	Lung cancer — small cell
VAD	Leukemia — acute lymphoblastic, induction Multiple myeloma
VADRIAC — High Dose	Sarcoma — bony sarcoma
VAIE	Sarcoma — bony sarcoma
VAM	Breast cancer
VAP	Multiple myeloma
VATH	Breast cancer
VBAP	Multiple myeloma
VBC	Malignant melanoma
VBP (PVB)	Genitourinary cancer — testicular, induction, salvage
VC	Lung cancer — small cell
VCAP	Multiple myeloma
VDCP	Endometrial cancer
VDP	Malignant melanoma
VIP	Genitourinary cancer — testicular, induction, poor risk
VIP (Einhorn)	Genitourinary cancer — testicular, induction, poor risk
VP	Leukemia — acute lymphoblastic, induction
VP-L-Asparaginase	Leukemia — acute lymphoblastic, induction
Wayne State	Head and neck cancer

CANCER CHEMOTHERAPY REGIMENS

ADULT REGIMENS

Breast Cancer

AC
Doxorubicin (Adriamycin®), I.V., 45 mg/m², day 1
Cyclophosphamide, I.V., 500 mg/m², day 1

Repeat cycle every 21 days

ACe
Doxorubicin (Adriamycin®), I.V., 40 mg/m², day 1
Cyclophosphamide, P.O., 200 mg/m²/day, days 1-3 or 3-6

Repeat cycle every 21-28 days

CAF
Cyclophosphamide, P.O., 100 mg/m², days 1-14
Doxorubicin (Adriamycin®), I.V., 30 mg/m², days 1 & 8
Fluorouracil, I.V., 400-500 mg/m², days 1 & 8

Repeat cycle every 28 days

or

Cyclophosphamide, I.V., 500 mg/m², day 1
Doxorubicin (Adriamycin®), I.V., 50 mg/m², day 1
Fluorouracil, I.V., 500 mg/m², day 1

Repeat cycle every 21 days

or Dose Intensification of CAF*

Cyclophosphamide, I.V., 600 mg/m², day 1
Doxorubicin (Adriamycin®), I.V., 60 mg/m², day 1
Fluorouracil, I.V., 600 mg/m², day 1
G-CSF, I.V./S.C., 5 mcg/kg/dose

Repeat cycle every 21 days

*Preliminary data presented at ASCO (March, 1992) suggests better response with dose intensification.

CFM
Cyclophosphamide, I.V., 500 mg/m², day 1
Fluorouracil, I.V., 500 mg/m², day 1
Mitoxantrone, I.V., 10 mg/m², day 1

Repeat cycle every 21 days

CFPT
Cyclophosphamide, I.V., 150 mg/m², days 1-5
Fluorouracil, I.V., 300 mg/m², days 1-5
Prednisone, P.O., 10 mg tid, days 1-7
Tamoxifen, P.O., 10 mg bid, days 1-42

Repeat cycle every 42 days

CMF
Cyclophosphamide, P.O., 100 mg/m², days 1-14
Methotrexate, I.V., 40-60 mg/m², days 1 & 8
Fluorouracil, I.V., 400-600 mg/m², days 1 & 8

Repeat cycle every 28 days

or

Cyclophosphamide, I.V., 600 mg/m², days 1 & 8
Methotrexate, I.V., 40-60 mg/m², days 1 & 8
Fluorouracil, I.V., 400-600 mg/m², days 1 & 8

Repeat cycle every 28 days

Breast Cancer *(continued)*
CMFP

Cyclophosphamide, P.O., 100 mg/m^2, days 1-14
Methotrexate, I.V., 40-60 mg/m^2, days 1 & 8
Fluorouracil, I.V., 600-700 mg/m^2, days 1 & 8
Prednisone, P.O., 40 mg (first 3 cycles only), days 1-14

Repeat cycle every 28 days

CMFVP (Cooper's)

Cyclophosphamide, P.O., 2-2.5 mg/kg/day for 9 months
Methotrexate, I.V., 0.7 mg/kg/wk for 8 weeks then every other week for 7 months
Fluorouracil, I.V., 12 mg/kg/wk for 8 weeks then every other week for 7 months
Vincristine, I.V., 0.035 mg/kg (max: 2 mg/wk) for 5 weeks then once monthly
Prednisone, P.O., 0.75 mg/kg/day, taper over next 40 days, discontinue, days 1-10
or
Cyclophosphamide, I.V., 400 mg/m^2, day 1
Methotrexate, I.V., 30 mg/m^2, days 1 & 8
Fluorouracil, I.V., 400 mg/m^2, days 1 & 8
Vincristine, I.V., 1 mg, days 1 & 8
Prednisone, P.O., 20 mg qid, days 1-7

Repeat cycle every 28 days

FAC

Fluorouracil, I.V., 500 mg/m^2, days 1 & 8
Doxorubicin (Adriamycin®), I.V., 50 mg/m^2, day 1
Cyclophosphamide, I.V., 500 mg/m^2, day 1

Repeat cycle every 21 days

IMF

Ifosfamide, I.V., 1.5 g/m^2, days 1 & 8
Mesna, I.V., 20% of ifosfamide dose, give immediately before and 4 and 8 hours after ifosfamide
infusion, days 1 & 8
Methotrexate, I.V., 40 mg/m^2, days 1 & 8
Fluorouracil, I.V., 600 mg/m^2, days 1 & 8

Repeat cycle every 28 days

NFL

Mitoxantrone (Novantrone®), I.V., 12 mg/m^2, day 1
Fluorouracil, I.V., 350 mg/m^2, days 1-3, given after leucovorin calcium
Leucovorin calcium, I.V., 300 mg/m^2, days 1-3
or
Mitoxantrone (Novantrone®), I.V., 10 mg/m^2, day 1
Fluorouracil, I.V., 1000 mg/m^2 continuous infusion, given after leucovorin calcium, days 1-3
Leucovorin calcium, I.V., 100 mg/m^2, days 1-3

Repeat cycle every 21 days

VATH

Vinblastine, I.V., 4.5 mg/m^2, day 1
Doxorubicin (Adriamycin®), I.V., 45 mg/m^2, day 1
Thiotepa, I.V., 12 mg/m^2, day 1
Fluoxymesterone (Halotestin®), P.O., 30 mg qd, days 1-21

Repeat cycle every 21 days

Breast Cancer *(continued)*

Single-Agent Regimens

Doxorubicin, I.V., 60 mg/m^2, every 3 weeks

or

Doxorubicin, I.V., 20 mg/m^2, every week

or

Doxorubicin, I.V., 20 mg/m^2 continuous infusion, days 1-3, every 3 weeks

Mitomycin C, I.V., 8-10 mg/m^2, every 6-8 weeks

Paclitaxel, I.V., 175 mg/m^2 over 3-24 h, every 21 d
Patient must be premedicated with:
Dexamethasone 20 mg P.O., 12 and 6 h prior
Diphenhydramine 50 mg I.V., 30 min prior
Cimetidine 300 mg I.V., or ranitidine 50 mg I.V., 30 min prior

Vinblastine, I.V., 12 mg/m^2, every 3-4 weeks

Colon Cancer

F-CL

Fluorouracil, I.V., 375 mg/m^2, days 1-5
Calcium leucovorin, I.V., 200 mg/m^2, days 1-5

Repeat cycle every 28 days

or

Fluorouracil, I.V., 500 mg/m^2 weekly 1 h after initiating the calcium leucovorin infusion for 6 weeks
Calcium leucovorin, I.V., 500 mg/m^2, over 2 h, weekly for 6 weeks

Two-week break, then repeat cycle

FLe

Fluorouracil, I.V., 450 mg/m^2 for 5 days, then, after a pause of 4 weeks, 450 mg/m^2, weekly for 48 weeks
Levamisole, P.O., 50 mg tid for 3 days, repeated every 2 weeks for 1 year

FMV

Fluorouracil, I.V., 10 mg/kg/day, days 1-5
Methyl-CCNU, P.O., 175 mg/m^2, day 1
Vincristine, I.V., 1 mg/m^2 (max: 2 mg), day 1

Repeat cycle every 35 days

FU/LV

Fluorouracil, I.V., 370-400 mg/m^2/day, days 1-5
Leucovorin calcium, I.V., 200 mg/m^2/day, commence infusion 15 min prior to fluorouracil infusion, days 1-5

Repeat cycle every 21 days

or

Fluorouracil, I.V., 1000 mg/m^2/day by continuous infusion, days 1-4
Leucovorin calcium, I.V., 200 mg/m^2/day, days 1-4

Repeat cycle every 28 days

Weekly 5FU/LV

Fluorouracil, I.V., 600 mg/m^2 over 1 h given after leucovorin, repeat weekly x 6 then 2-week rest period = 1 cycle, days 1, 8, 15, 22, 29, 36
Leucovorin calcium, I.V., 500 mg/m^2 over 2 h, days 1, 8, 15, 22, 29, 36

Repeat cycle every 56 days

Colon Cancer *(continued)*
5FU/LDLF

    Fluorouracil, I.V., 370 mg/m^2/day, days 1-5
    Leucovorin calcium, I.V., 20-25 mg/m^2/day, days 1-5

               Repeat cycle every 28 days

Gastric Cancer

EAP

    Etoposide, I.V., 120 mg/m^2, days 4, 5, 6
    Doxorubicin (Adriamycin®), I.V., 20 mg/m^2, days 1, 7
    Cisplatin (Platinol®), I.V., 40 mg/m^2, days 2, 8

               Repeat cycle every 21 days

ELF

    Etoposide, I.V., 120 mg/m^2, days 1-3
    Leucovorin calcium, I.V., 300 mg/m^2, days 1-3
    Fluorouracil, I.V., 500 mg/m^2, days 1-3

               Repeat cycle every 21-28 days

FAM

    Fluorouracil, I.V., 600 mg/m^2, days 1, 8, 29, & 36
    Doxorubicin (Adriamycin®), I.V., 30 mg/m^2, days 1 & 29
    Mitomycin C, I.V., 10 mg/m^2, day 1

               Repeat cycle every 56 days

FAME

    Fluorouracil, I.V., 350 mg/m^2, days 1-5, 36-40
    Doxorubicin (Adriamycin®), I.V., 40 mg/m^2, days 1 & 36
    Methyl-CCNU, P.O., 150 mg/m^2, day 1

               Repeat cycle every 70 days

FAMTX

    Methotrexate, IVPB, 1500 mg/m^2, day 1
    Fluorouracil, IVPB, 1500 mg/m^2 1 h after methotrexate, day 1
    Leucovorin calcium, P.O., 15 mg/m^2 q6h x 48 h 24 h after methotrexate, day 2
    Doxorubicin (Adriamycin®), IVPB, 30 mg/m^2, day 15

               Repeat cycle every 28 days

FCE

    Fluorouracil, I.V., 900 mg/m^2/day continuous infusion, days 1-5
    Cisplatin, I.V., 20 mg/m^2, days 1-5
    Etoposide, I.V., 90 mg/m^2, days 1, 3, & 5

               Repeat cycle every 21 days

PFL

    Cisplatin (Platinol®), I.V., 25 mg/m^2 continuous infusion, days 1-5
    Fluorouracil, I.V., 800 mg/m^2 continuous infusion, days 2-5
    Leucovorin calcium, I.V., 500 mg/m^2 continuous infusion, days 1-5

               Repeat cycle every 28 days

Genitourinary Cancer

Bladder

CAP

Cyclophosphamide, I.V., 400 mg/m^2, day 1
Doxorubicin (Adriamycin®), I.V., 40 mg/m^2, day 1
Cisplatin (Platinol®), I.V., 60 mg/m^2, day 1

Repeat cycle every 21 days

CISCA

Cisplatin, I.V., 70-100 mg/m^2, day 2
Cyclophosphamide, I.V., 650 mg/m^2, day 1
Doxorubicin (Adriamycin®), I.V., 50 mg/m^2, day 1

Repeat cycle every 21-28 days

CMV

Cisplatin, I.V., 100 mg/m^2 over 4 h start 12 h after MTX, day 2
Methotrexate, I.V., 30 mg/m^2, days 1 & 8
Vinblastine, I.V., 4 mg/m^2, days 1 & 8

Repeat cycle every 21 days

m-PFL

Methotrexate, I.V., 60 mg/m^2, day 1
Cisplatin (Platinol®), I.V., 25 mg/m^2 continuous infusion, days 2-6
Fluorouracil, I.V., 800 mg/m^2 continuous infusion, days 2-6
Leucovorin calcium, I.V., 500 mg/m^2 continuous infusion, days 2-6

Repeat cycle every 28 days for 4 cycles

MVAC

Methotrexate, I.V., 30 mg/m^2, days 1, 15, 22
Vinblastine, I.V., 3 mg/m^2, days 2, 15, 22
Doxorubicin (Adriamycin®), I.V., 30 mg/m^2, day 2
Cisplatin, I.V., 70 mg/m^2, day 2

Repeat cycle every 28 days

Prostate

FL

Flutamide, P.O., 250 mg tid, days 1-28
Leuprolide acetate, S.C., 1 mg qd, days 1-28

Repeat cycle every 28 days

or

Flutamide, P.O., 250 mg tid, days 1-28
Leuprolide acetate depot, I.M., 7.5 mg, day 1

Repeat cycle every 28 days

FZ

Flutamide, P.O., 250 mg tid
Goserelin acetate (Zoladex®), S.C., 3.6 mg implant, every 28 days

L-VAM

Leuprolide acetate, S.C., 1 mg qd, days 1-28
Vinblastine, I.V., 1.5 mg/m^2/day continuous infusion, days 2-7
Doxorubicin (Adriamycin®), I.V., 50 mg/m^2 continuous infusion, day 1
Mitomycin C, I.V., 10 mg/m^2, day 2

Repeat cycle every 28 days

Testicular, Induction, Good Risk

BEP

Bleomycin, I.V., 30 units, days 2, 9, 16
Etoposide, I.V., 100 mg/m^2, days 1-5
Cisplatin (Platinol®), I.V., 20 mg/m^2, days 1-5

Repeat cycle every 21 days

PE

Cisplatin (Platinol®), I.V., 20 mg/m^2, days 1-5
Etoposide, I.V., 100 mg/m^2, days 1-5

Repeat cycle every 21 days

PVB

Cisplatin (Platinol®), I.V., 20 mg/m^2, days 1-5
Vinblastine, I.V., 6 mg/m^2, days 1, 2
Bleomycin, I.V., 30 units, weekly

Repeat cycle every 21-28 days

Genitourinary Cancer *(continued)*

Testicular, Induction, Poor Risk

VIP

Etoposide (VePesid®), I.V., 75 mg/m^2, days 1-5
Ifosfamide, I.V., 1.2 g/m^2, days 1-5
Cisplatin (Platinol®), I.V., 20 mg/m^2, days 1-5
Mesna, I.V., 120 mg/m^2 then 1200 mg/m^2/day continuous infusion, days 1-5

Repeat cycle every 21 days

VIP (Einhorn)

Vinblastine, I.V., 0.11 mg/kg, days 1-2
Ifosfamide, I.V., 1200 mg/m^2, days 1-5
Cisplatin (Platinol®), I.V., 20 mg/m^2, days 1-5
Mesna, I.V., 120 mg/m^2, then 1200 mg/m^2/day continuous infusion, days 1-5

Repeat cycle every 21 days

Testicular, Induction, Salvage

VAB VI

Vinblastine, I.V., 4 mg/m^2, day 1
Dactinomycin (Actinomycin D), I.V., 1 mg/m^2, day 1
Bleomycin, I.V., 30 units push day 1, then 20 units/m^2/day continuous infusion, days 1-3
Cisplatin, I.V., 120 mg/m^2, day 4
Cyclophosphamide, I.V., 600 mg/m^2, day 1

Repeat cycle every 21 days

VBP (PVB)

Vinblastine, I.V., 6 mg/m^2, days 1 & 2
Bleomycin, I.V., 30 units, days 1, 8, 15, (22)
Cisplatin (Platinol®), I.V., 20 mg/m^2, days 1-5

Repeat cycle every 21-28 days

Gestational Trophoblastic Cancer

DMC
Dactinomycin, I.V., 0.37 mg/m^2, days 1-5
Methotrexate, I.V., 11 mg/m^2, days 1-5
Cyclophosphamide, I.V., 110 mg/m^2, days 1-5

Repeat cycle every 21 days

Head and Neck Cancer

CAP
Cyclophosphamide, I.V., 500 mg/m^2, day 1
Doxorubicin (Adriamycin®), I.V., 50 mg/m^2, day 1
Cisplatin (Platinol®), I.V., 50 mg/m^2, day 1

Repeat cycle every 28 days

CF
Cisplatin, I.V., 100 mg/m^2, day 1
Fluorouracil, I.V., 1000 mg/m^2/day continuous infusion, days 1-5

Repeat cycle every 21-28 days

CF
Carboplatin, I.V., 400 mg/m^2, day 1
Fluorouracil, I.V., 1000 mg/m^2/day continuous infusion, days 1-5

Repeat cycle every 21-28 days

COB
Cisplatin, I.V., 100 mg/m^2, day 1
Vincristine (Oncovin®), I.V., 1 mg/m^2, days 2 & 5
Bleomycin, I.V., 30 units/day continuous infusion, days 2-5

Repeat cycle every 21 days

5-FU HURT
Hydroxyurea, P.O., 1000 mg q12h x 11 doses; start PM of admission, give 2 hours prior to
    radiation therapy, days 0-5
Fluorouracil, I.V., 800 mg/m^2/day continuous infusion, start AM after admission, days 1-5
Paclitaxel, I.V., 5-25 mg/m^2/day continuous infusion, start AM after admission; dose escalation
    study — refer to protocol, days 1-5
G-CSF, S.C., 5 mcg/kg/day, days 6-12, start ≥12 hours after completion of 5-FU infusion

5-7 cycles may be administered

MAP
Mitomycin C, I.V., 8 mg/m^2, day 1
Doxorubicin (Adriamycin®), I.V., 40 mg/m^2, day 1
Cisplatin (Platinol®), I.V., 60 mg/m^2, day 1

Repeat cycle every 28 days

MBC (MBD)
Methotrexate, I.M./I.V., 40 mg/m^2, days 1 & 15
Bleomycin, I.M./I.V., 10 units, days 1, 8, 15
Cisplatin, I.V., 50 mg/m^2, day 4

Repeat cycle every 21 days

MF
Methotrexate, I.V., 125-250 mg/m^2, day 1
Fluorouracil, I.V., 600 mg/m^2 beginning 1 h after methotrexate, day 1
Leucovorin calcium, I.V./P.O., 10 mg/m^2 q6h x 5 doses beginning 24 h after methotrexate

Repeat cycle every 7 days

Head and Neck Cancer *(continued)*
PFL
Cisplatin (Platinol®), I.V., 100 mg/m^2, day 1
Fluorouracil, I.V., 600-800 mg/m^2/day continuous infusion, days 1-5
Leucovorin calcium, I.V., 200-300 mg/m^2/day, days 1-5

Repeat cycle every 21 days

PFL+IFN
Cisplatin (Platinol®), I.V., 100 mg/m^2, day 1
Fluorouracil, I.V., 640 mg/m^2/day continuous infusion, days 1-5
Leucovorin calcium, P.O., 100 mg q4h, days 1-5
Interferon alfa-2b, S.C., 2 x 10^6 units/m^2, days 1-6

Wayne State
Cisplatin (Platinol®), I.V., 100 mg/m^2 over 30 minutes, day 1
Fluorouracil, I.V., 1000 mg/m^2 continuous infusion, days 1-4 (or 5)

Repeat cycle every 21 days

Single-Agent Regimens
Carboplatin, I.V., 300-400 mg/m^2, over 2 hours every 21-28 days
Methotrexate, I.V., 40 mg/m^2, every week, escalating day 14 by 5 mg/m^2/wk as tolerated
Cisplatin I.V., 100 mg/m^2, every 28 days divided into 1, 2, or 4 equal doses per month

Leukemias

Acute Lymphoblastic, Induction

DVP
Daunorubicin, I.V., 45 mg/m^2, days 1, 2, 3, 14
Vincristine, I.V., 2 mg/m^2 (max: 2 mg), days 1, 8, 15, 22
Prednisone, P.O., 45 mg/m^2, days 1-28 (35)

DVPA
Daunorubicin, I.V., 50 mg/m^2, days 1-3
Vincristine, I.V., 2 mg, days 1, 8, 15, 22
Prednisone, P.O., 60 mg/m^2, days 1-28
Asparaginase, I.M., 6000 units/m^2, days 17-28

VAD
Vincristine, I.V., 0.4 mg continuous infusion, days 1-4
Doxorubicin (Adriamycin®), I.V., 12 mg/m^2 continuous infusion, days 1-4
Dexamethasone, P.O., 40 mg, days 1-4, 9-12, 17-20

VP
Vincristine, I.V., 2 mg/m^2/wk for 4-6 weeks (max: 2 mg)
Prednisone, P.O., 60 mg/m^2/day in divided doses for 4 weeks, taper weeks 5-7

VP-L-Asparaginase
Vincristine, I.V., 2 mg/m^2/wk for 4-6 wk (max: 2 mg)
Prednisone, P.O., 60 mg/m^2/day for 4-6 wk, then taper
L-asparaginase, I.V., 10,000 units/m^2/day

Leukemias — Acute Lymphoblastic, Induction *(continued)*

no known acronym
Cyclophosphamide, I.V., 1200 mg/m^2, day 1
Daunorubicin, I.V., 45 mg/m^2, days 1-3
Prednisone, P.O., 60 mg/m^2, days 1-21
Vincristine, I.V., 2 mg/m^2, weekly
L-asparaginase, I.V., 6000 units/m^2, 3 times/wk

or

Pegaspargase, I.M./I.V., 2500 units/m^2, every 14 days if patient develops hypersensitivity to native L-asparaginase

Acute Lymphoblastic, Maintenance

MM
Mercaptopurine, P.O., 50-75 mg/m^2, days 1-7
Methotrexate, P.O./I.V., 20 mg/m^2, day 1

Repeat cycle every 7 days

MMC (MTX + MP + CTX)*
Methotrexate, I.V., 20 mg/m^2/wk
Mercaptopurine, P.O., 50 mg/m^2/da
Cyclophosphamide, I.V., 200 mg/m^2/wk

*Continue all 3 drugs until relapse of disease or after 3 years of remission.

Acute Lymphoblastic, Relapse

AVDP
Asparaginase, I.V., 15,000 units/m^2, days 1-5, 8-12, 15-19, 22-26
Vincristine, I.V., 2 mg/m^2 (max: 2 mg), days 8, 15, 22
Daunorubicin, I.V., 30-60 mg/m^2, days 8, 15, 22
Prednisone, P.O., 40 mg/m^2, days 8-12, 15-19, 22-26

Acute Myeloid Leukemia

5+2

Induction
Cytarabine (Ara-C), I.V., 100-200 mg/m^2 continuous infusion, days 1-5
Daunorubicin, I.V., 45 mg/m^2, days 1-2

7+3

Induction
Cytarabine, I.V., 100-200 mg/m^2/day continuous infusion, days 1-7
Daunorubicin, I.V., 45 mg/m^2/day, days 1-3

Modified 7+3 (considerations in elderly patients)
Cytarabine, I.V., 100 mg/m^2/day continuous infusion, days 1-7
Daunorubicin, I.V., 30 mg/m^2/day, days 1-3

D-3+7

Induction
Daunorubicin, I.V., 45 mg/m^2, days 1-3
Cytarabine (Ara-C), I.V., 100-200 mg/m^2 continuous infusion, days 1-7

Leukemias — Acute Myeloid Leukemia *(continued)*
DAT/DCT

Induction
Daunorubicin, I.V., 60 mg/m^2/day, days 1-3
Cytarabine (Ara-C), I.V., 200 mg/m^2/day continuous infusion, days 1-5
Thioguanine, P.O., 100 mg/m^2 q12h, days 1-5

Modified DAT (considerations in elderly patients)
Daunorubicin, I.V., 50 mg/m^2, day 1
Cytarabine (Ara-C), S.C., 100 mg/m^2/day q12h, days 1-5
Thioguanine, P.O., 100 mg/m^2 q12h, days 1-5

HDAC

Induction
Cytarabine, I.V., 3 g/m^2 I.V. over 2-3 h q12h x 12 doses, days 1-6

Modified (considerations in elderly patients)
Cytarabine, I.V., 2 g/m^2 I.V. over 2-3 h q12h x 12 doses, days 1-6

HiDAC

Consolidation
Cytarabine (Ara-C), I.V., 3000 mg/m^2 q12h, days 1-6
or
Cytarabine (Ara-C), I.V., 3000 mg/m^2 q12h, days 1, 3, 5

I-3+7

Induction
Idarubicin, I.V., 12 mg/m^2, days 1-3
Cytarabine (Ara-C), I.V., 100 mg/m^2 continuous infusion, days 1-7

IC

Induction
Idarubicin (Idamycin®), I.V., 12 mg/m^2/day, days 1-3
Cytarabine, I.V., 100-200 mg/m^2/day continuous infusion, days 1-7

LDAC

Considerations in Elderly Patients
Cytarabine, S.C., 10 mg/m^2 bid, days 10-21

MC

Induction
Mitoxantrone, I.V., 12 mg/m^2/day, days 1-3
Cytarabine, I.V., 100-200 mg/m^2/day continuous infusion, days 1-7

Consolidation
Mitoxantrone, I.V., 12 mg/m^2, days 1-2
Cytarabine (Ara-C), I.V., 100 mg/m^2 continuous infusion, days 1-5

Repeat cycle every 28 days

MV

Induction
Mitoxantrone, I.V., 10 mg/m^2/day, days 1-5
Etoposide (VePesid®), I.V., 100 mg/m^2/day, days 1-3

Acute Nonlymphoblastic, Consolidation

CD
Cytarabine, I.V., 3000 mg/m^2 q12h, days 1-6
Daunorubicin, I.V., 30 mg/m^2/day, days 7-9

Chronic Lymphocytic Leukemia

CHL + PRED
Chlorambucil, P.O., 0.4 mg/kg/day for 1 day every other week
Prednisone, P.O., 100 mg/day for 2 days every other week; adjust dosage according to blood
   counts every 2 weeks prior to therapy; increase initial dose of 0.4 mg/kg by 0.1 mg/kg every 2
   weeks until toxicity or disease control is achieved

CVP
Cyclophosphamide, P.O., 400 mg/m^2/day, days 1-5
Vincristine (Oncovin®), I.V., 1.4 mg/m^2 (max: 2 mg), day 1
Prednisone, P.O., 100 mg/m^2, days 1-5

Repeat cycle every 21 days

Fludarabine, I.V., 25-30 mg/m^2 over 30 min, days 1-5

Repeat cycle every 28 days

Cladribine (2-CdA) for fludarabine resistant, I.V., 0.1 mg/kg/day continuous infusion, days 1-7
Repeat cycle every 28 days

Lung Cancer

Small Cell

ACE/CAE
Doxorubicin (Adriamycin®), I.V., 45 mg/m^2, day 1
Cyclophosphamide, I.V., 1000 mg/m^2, day 1
Etoposide, I.V., 50 mg/m^2/day, days 1-5

Repeat cycle every 21 days

CAV
Cyclophosphamide, I.V., 1000 mg/m^2, day 1
Doxorubicin (Adriamycin®), I.V., 50 mg/m^2, day 1
Vincristine, I.V., 1.4 mg/m^2 (max: 2 mg), day 1

Repeat cycle every 3 weeks

CAVE
Cyclophosphamide, I.V., 750 mg/m^2, day 1
Doxorubicin (Adriamycin®), I.V., 50 mg/m^2, day 1
Vincristine, I.V., 1.4 mg/m^2 (max: 2 mg), day 1
Etoposide, I.V., 60-100 mg/m^2, days 1-3

Repeat cycle every 3 weeks

CHOR*
Cyclophosphamide, I.V., 750 mg/m^2/day, days 1 & 22
Doxorubicin (Adriamycin®), I.V., 50 mg/m^2/day, days 1 & 22
Vincristine, I.V., 1 mg, days 1, 8, 15, 22
Radiation, total dose 3000 rad, 10 daily fractions over 2 weeks beginning with day 36, days 1, 8,
   15, 22

Lung Cancer — Small Cell *(continued)*

CMC-High Dose*

Cyclophosphamide, I.V., 1000 mg/m^2/day, days 1 & 29
Methotrexate, I.V., 15 mg/m^2/day twice weekly for 6 weeks, days 1 & 29
Lomustine (CCNU), P.O., 100 mg/m^2, day 1

*If disease responds, proceed to maintenance therapy.

CODE

Cisplatin, I.V., 25 mg/m^2, every week for 9 weeks
Vincristine (Oncovin®), I.V., 1 mg/m^2, weeks 1, 2, 4, 6, 8
Doxorubicin, I.V., 25 mg/m^2, weeks 1, 3, 5, 7, 9
Etoposide, I.V., 80 mg/m^2, weeks 1, 3, 5, 7, 9

COPE

Cyclophosphamide, I.V., 750 mg/m^2, day 1
Vincristine (Oncovin®), I.V., 1.4 mg/m^2 (max: 2 mg), day 3
Cisplatin (Platinol®), I.V., 20 mg/m^2, days 1-3
Etoposide, I.V., 100 mg/m^2, days 1-3

Repeat cycle every 21 days

EC

Etoposide, I.V., 60-100 mg/m^2, days 1-3
Carboplatin, I.V., 400 mg/m^2, day 1

Repeat cycle every 28 days

EP

Etoposide, I.V., 75-100 mg/m^2, days 1-3
Cisplatin (Platinol®), I.V., 75-100 mg/m^2, day 1

Repeat cycle every 21-28 days

MICE (ICE)

Mesna uroprotection, I.V. at 20% of ifosfamide doses given immediately before and at 4 and 8
    hours after ifosfamide infusion
Ifosfamide, I.V., 2000 mg/m^2, days 1-3
Carboplatin, I.V., 300-350 mg/m^2, day 1
Etoposide, I.V., 60-100 mg/m^2, day 1

PE

Cisplatin (Platinol®), I.V., 50 mg/m^2, day 1
Etoposide, I.V., 60 mg/m^2, days 1-5

Repeat cycle every 21-28 days

or

Cisplatin (Platinol®), I.V., 75 mg/m^2, day 2
Etoposide, I.V., 125 mg/m^2, days 1, 3, & 5

Repeat cycle every 28 days

or

Cisplatin (Platinol®), I.V., 100 mg/m^2, day 1
Etoposide, I.V., 100 mg/m^2, days 1-3

Repeat cycle every 28 days

POCC

Procarbazine, P.O., 100 mg/m^2/day, days 1-14
Vincristine (Oncovin®), I.V., 2 mg/day (max: 2 mg), days 1 & 8
Cyclophosphamide, I.V., 600 mg/m^2/day, days 1 & 8
Lomustine (CCNU), P.O., 60 mg/m^2, day 1

Repeat cycle every 28 days

Lung Cancer — Small Cell *(continued)*
VAC (CAV) (Induction)
Vincristine, I.V., 2 mg/m^2, day 1
Doxorubicin (Adriamycin®), I.V., 50 mg/m^2, day 1
Cyclophosphamide, I.V., 750 mg/m^2, day 1

Repeat cycle every 21 days x 4 cycles

VC
Etoposide (VePesid®), I.V., 100-200 mg/m^2, days 1-3
Carboplatin, I.V., 50-125 mg/m^2, days 1-3

Repeat cycle every 28 days

Single-Agent Regimen
Etoposide, P.O., 160 mg/m^2, days 1-5

Repeat cycle every 28 days

Nonsmall Cell

CAMP
Cyclophosphamide, I.V., 300 mg/m^2, days 1 & 8
Doxorubicin (Adriamycin®), I.V., 20 mg/m^2, days 1 & 8
Methotrexate, I.V., 15 mg/m^2, days 1 & 8
Procarbazine, P.O., 100 mg/m^2, days 1-10

Repeat cycle every 28 days

CAP
Cyclophosphamide, I.V., 400 mg/m^2, day 1
Doxorubicin (Adriamycin®), I.V., 40 mg/m^2, day 1
Cisplatin (Platinol®), I.V., 60 mg/m^2, day 1

Repeat cycle every 28 days

CV
Cisplatin, I.V., 60-80 mg/m^2, day 1
Etoposide (VePesid®), I.V., 120 mg/m^2, days 4, 6, & 8

Repeat cycle every 21-28 days

CVI
Carboplatin, I.V., 300 mg/m^2, day 1
Etoposide (VePesid®), I.V., 60-100 mg/m^2, day 1
Ifosfamide, I.V., 1.5 g/m^2, days 1, 3 & 5
Mesna, I.V., 20% of ifosfamide dose, given immediately before and 4 and 8 hours after ifosfamide
    infusion, days 1, 3 & 5

Repeat cycle every 28 days

EP
Etoposide, I.V., 75-100 mg/m^2, days 1-3
Cisplatin (Platinol®), I.V., 75-100 mg/m^2, day 1

Repeat cycle every 21-28 days

FAM
Fluorouracil, I.V., 600 mg/m^2, days 1, 8, 28, & 36
Doxorubicin (Adriamycin®), I.V., 30 mg/m^2, days 1 & 28
Mitomycin C, I.V., 10 mg/m^2, day 1

Repeat cycle every 56 days

Lung Cancer — Nonsmall Cell *(continued)*

FOMi*

Fluorouracil, I.V., 300 mg/m²/day, days 1-4
Vincristine (Oncovin®), I.V., 2 mg, day 1
Mitomycin C, I.V., 10 mg/m², day 1

*Repeat at 3-week intervals for 3 courses; thereafter, every 6 weeks.

FOMi/CAP

Fluorouracil, I.V., 300 mg/m², days 1-4
Vincristine, I.V., 2 mg, day 1
Mitomycin C, I.V., 10 mg/m², day 1
Cyclophosphamide, I.V., 400 mg/m², day 28
Doxorubicin (Adriamycin®), I.V., 40 mg/m², day 28
Cisplatin, I.V., 40 mg/m², day 28

Repeat cycle every 56 days

MACC

Methotrexate, I.V., 40 mg/m², day 1
Doxorubicin (Adriamycin®), I.V., 40 mg/m², day 1
Cyclophosphamide, I.V., 400 mg/m², day 1
Lomustine, P.O., 30 mg/m², day 1

Repeat cycle every 21 days

MICE (ICE)

Mesna uroprotection, I.V. at 20% of ifosfamide doses given immediately before and at 4 and 8
  hours after ifosfamide infusion
Ifosfamide, I.V., 2000 mg/m², days 1-3
Carboplatin, I.V., 300-350 mg/m², day 1
Etoposide, I.V., 60-100 mg/m², day 1

MVP

Mitomycin, I.V., 8 mg/m², days 1, 29, 71
Vinblastine, I.V., 4.5 mg/m², days 15, 22, 29, then every 2 weeks
Cisplatin (Platinol®), I.V., 120 mg/m², days 1, 29, then every 6 weeks

PFL

Cisplatin (Platinol®), I.V., 25 mg/m², days 1-5
Fluorouracil, I.V., 800 mg/m² continuous infusion, days 2-5
Leucovorin calcium, I.V., 500 mg/m² continuous infusion, days 1-5

Repeat cycle every 28 days

Single-Agent Regimen

Vinorelbine (Navelbine®), I.V., 30 mg/m², every week

Lymphoma

Hodgkin's

ABVD

Doxorubicin (Adriamycin®), I.V., 25 mg/m², days 1 & 15
Bleomycin, I.V., 10 units/m², days 1 & 15
Vinblastine, I.V., 6 mg/m², days 1 & 15
Dacarbazine, I.V., 150 mg/m², days 1-5

Repeat cycle every 28 days

or

Dacarbazine, I.V., 375 mg/m², days 1 & 15

Lymphoma — Hodgkin's *(continued)*

ChlVPP

Chlorambucil, P.O., 6 mg/m^2, days 1-14 (max: 10 mg/day)
Vinblastine, I.V., 6 mg/m^2, days 1-8 (max: 10 mg dose)
Procarbazine, P.O., 50 mg/m^2, days 1-14 (max: 150 mg/day)
Prednisone, P.O., 40 mg/m^2, days 1-14 (25 mg/m^2 for children)

CVPP

Lomustine (CCNU), P.O., 75 mg/m^2, day 1
Vinblastine, I.V., 4 mg/m^2, days 1, 8
Procarbazine, P.O., 100 mg/m^2, days 1-14
Prednisone, P.O., 30 mg/m^2, days 1-14 (cycles 1 & 4 only)

Repeat cycle every 28 days

DHAP

Dexamethasone, P.O./I.V., 40 mg, days 1-4
Cytarabine (Ara-C), I.V., 2 g/m^2, q12h for 2 doses, day 2
Cisplatin (Platinol®), I.V., 100 mg/m^2 continuous infusion, day 1

Repeat cycle every 3-4 weeks

EVA

Etoposide, I.V., 100 mg/m^2, days 1-3
Vinblastine, I.V., 6 mg/m^2, day 1
Doxorubicin (Adriamycin®), I.V., 50 mg/m^2, day 1

Repeat cycle every 28 days

MOPP

Mechlorethamine, I.V., 6 mg/m^2, days 1 & 8
Vincristine (Oncovin®), I.V., 1.4 mg/m^2 (max: 2.5 mg), days 1 & 8
Procarbazine, P.O., 100 mg/m^2, days 1-14
Prednisone, P.O., 40 mg/m^2 (cycles 1 & 4 only), days 1-14

Repeat cycle every 28 days

MOPP/ABV Hybrid

Mechlorethamine, I.V., 6 mg/m^2, day 1
Vincristine (Oncovin®), I.V., 1.4 mg/m^2 (max: 2 mg), day 1
Procarbazine, P.O., 100 mg/m^2, days 1-7
Prednisone, P.O., 40 mg/m^2, days 1-14
Doxorubicin (Adriamycin®), I.V., 35 mg/m^2, day 8
Bleomycin, I.V., 10 units/m^2, day 8
Vinblastine, I.V., 6 mg/m^2, day 8

Repeat cycle every 28 days

MVPP

Mechlorethamine, I.V., 6 mg/m^2, days 1 & 8
Vinblastine, I.V., 6 mg/m^2, days 1 & 8
Procarbazine, P.O., 100 mg/m^2, days 1-14
Prednisone, P.O., 40 mg/m^2, days 1-14

Repeat cycle every 42 days

NOVP

Mitoxantrone (Novantrone®), I.V., 10 mg/m^2, day 1
Vincristine (Oncovin®), I.V., 2 mg, day 8
Vinblastine, I.V., 6 mg/m^2, day 1
Prednisone, P.O., 100 mg/m^2, days 1-5

Repeat cycle every 21 days

Lymphoma — Hodgkin's *(continued)*
Stanford V
Mechlorethamine, I.V., 6 mg/m^2, weeks 1, 5, 9
Doxorubicin, I.V., 25 mg/m^2, weeks 1, 3, 5, 7, 9, 11
Vinblastine, I.V., 6 mg/m^2, weeks 1, 3, 5, 7, 9, 11
Vincristine, I.V., 1.4 mg/m^2, weeks 2, 4, 6, 8, 10, 12
Bleomycin, I.V., 5 units/m^2, weeks 2, 4, 6, 8, 10, 12
Etoposide, I.V., 60 mg/m^2 x 2, weeks 3, 7, 11
Prednisone, P.O., 40 mg/m^2, daily, dose tapered over the last 15 days

Non-Hodgkin's

BACOP
Bleomycin, I.V., 5 units/m^2, days 15 & 22
Doxorubicin (Adriamycin®), I.V., 25 mg/m^2, days 1 & 8
Cyclophosphamide, I.V., 650 mg/m^2, days 1 & 8
Vincristine (Oncovin®), I.V., 1.4 mg/m^2 (max: 2 mg), days 1 & 8
Prednisone, P.O., 60 mg/m^2, days 15-28

Repeat cycle every 28 days

CHOP
Cyclophosphamide, I.V., 750 mg/m^2, day 1
Doxorubicin (Hydroxydaunomycin), I.V., 50 mg/m^2, day 1
Vincristine (Oncovin®), I.V., 1.4 mg/m^2 (max: 2 mg), day 1
Prednisone, P.O., 100 mg/m^2, days 1-5

Repeat cycle every 21 days

CHOP-Bleo
Cyclophosphamide, I.V., 750 mg/m^2, day 1
Doxorubicin (Hydroxydaunomycin), I.V., 50 mg/m^2, day 1
Vincristine (Oncovin®), I.V., 2 mg, days 1 & 5
Prednisone, P.O., 100 mg, days 1-5
Bleomycin, I.V., 15 units, days 1 & 5

Repeat cycle every 21-28 days

COMLA
Cyclophosphamide, I.V., 1500 mg/m^2, day 1
Vincristine (Oncovin®), I.V., 1.4 mg/m^2 (max: 2.5 mg), days 1, 8, 15
Methotrexate, I.V., 120 mg/m^2, days 22, 29, 36, 43, 50, 57, 64, 71
Leucovorin calcium rescue, P.O., 25 mg/m^2, q6h for 4 doses, beginning 24 hours after each
methotrexate dose
Cytarabine (Ara-C), I.V., 300 mg/m^2, days 22, 29, 36, 43, 50, 57, 64, 71

Repeat cycle every 21 days

COP
Cyclophosphamide, I.V., 800-1000 mg/m^2, day 1
Vincristine (Oncovin®), I.V., 1.4 mg/m^2 (max: 2 mg), day 1
Prednisone, P.O., 60 mg/m^2, days 1-5

Repeat cycle every 21 days

COP-BLAM
Cyclophosphamide, I.V., 400 mg/m^2, day 1
Vincristine (Oncovin®), I.V., 1 mg/m^2, day 1
Prednisone, P.O., 40 mg/m^2, days 1-10
Bleomycin, I.V., 15 mg, day 14
Doxorubicin (Adriamycin®), I.V., 40 mg/m^2, day 1
Procarbazine (Matulane®), P.O., 100 mg/m^2, days 1-10

Lymphoma — Non-Hodgkin's *(continued)*

COPP (or 'C" MOPP)
Cyclophosphamide, I.V., 400-650 mg/m^2, days 1 & 8
Vincristine (Oncovin®), I.V., 1.4-1.5 mg/m^2 (max: 2 mg), days 1 & 8
Procarbazine, P.O., 100 mg/m^2, days 1-14
Prednisone, P.O., 40 mg/m^2, days 1-14

Repeat cycle every 28 days

CVP
Cyclophosphamide, P.O., 400 mg/m^2, days 1-5
Vincristine, I.V., 1.4 mg/m^2 (max: 2 mg), day 1
Prednisone, P.O., 100 mg/m^2, days 1-5

Repeat cycle every 21 days

DHAP
Dexamethasone (Decadron®), I.V., 10 mg q6h, days 1-4
Cytarabine (Ara-C), I.V., 2 g/m^2 q12h x 2 doses, day 2
Cisplatin (Platinol®), I.V., 100 mg/m^2 continuous infusion, day 1

Repeat cycle every 21-28 days

ESHAP
Etoposide, I.V., 60 mg/m^2, days 1-4
Cisplatin, I.V., 25 mg/m^2 continuous infusion, days 1-4
Cytarabine (Ara-C), I.V., 2 g/m^2, immediately following completion of etoposide and cisplatin therapy
Methylprednisolone, I.V., 500 mg/day, days 1-4

Repeat cycle every 21-28 days

IMVP-16
Ifosfamide, I.V., 4 g/m^2 continuous infusion over 24 h, day 1
Mesna, I.V., 800 mg/m^2 bolus prior to ifosfamide, then 4 g/m^2 continuous infusion over 12 hours concurrent w/ifosfamide; then 2.4 g/m^2 continuous infusion over 12 hours after ifosfamide infusion, day 1
Methotrexate, I.V., 30 mg/m^2, days 3 & 10
Etoposide (VePesid®), I.V., 100 mg/m^2, days 1-3

Repeat cycle every 21-28 days

MACOP-B
Methotrexate, I.V., 100 mg/m^2 weeks 2, 6, 10
Doxorubicin (Adriamycin®), I.V., 50 mg/m^2 weeks 1, 3, 5, 7, 9, 11
Cyclophosphamide, I.V., 350 mg/m^2 weeks 1, 3, 5, 7, 9, 11
Vincristine (Oncovin®), I.V., 1.4 mg/m^2 (max: 2 mg) weeks 2, 4, 8, 10, 12
Bleomycin, I.V., 10 units/m^2, weeks 4, 8, 12
Prednisone, P.O., 75 mg/day tapered over 15 d, days 1-15
Leucovorin calcium, P.O., 15 mg q6h x 6 doses 24 h after methotrexate, weeks 2, 6, 10

m-BACOD
Methotrexate, I.V., 200 mg/m^2, days 8 & 15
Leucovorin calcium, P.O., 10 mg/m^2 q6h x 8 doses beginning 24 h after each methotrexate dose, days 8 & 15
Bleomycin, I.V., 4 units/m^2, day 1
Doxorubicin (Adriamycin®), I.V., 45 mg/m^2, day 1
Cyclophosphamide, I.V., 600 mg/m^2, day 1
Vincristine (Oncovin®), I.V., 1 mg/m^2, day 1
Dexamethasone, P.O., 6 mg/m^2, days 1-5

Repeat cycle every 21 days

Lymphoma — Non-Hodgkin's *(continued)*
m-BACOS

    Methotrexate, I.V., 1 g/m^2, day 2
    Bleomycin, I.V., 10 units/m^2, day 1
    Doxorubicin (Adriamycin®), I.V., 50 mg/m^2 continuous infusion, day 1
    Cyclophosphamide, I.V., 750 mg/m^2, day 1
    Vincristine (Oncovin®), I.V., 1.4 mg/m^2 (max: 2 mg), day 1
    Leucovorin calcium rescue, P.O., 15 mg q6h for 8 doses, starting 24 hours after methotrexate
    Methylprednisolone, I.V., 500 mg, days 1-3

                                   Repeat cycle every 21-25 days

MINE

    Mesna, I.V., 1.33 g/m^2/day concurrent with ifosfamide dose, then 500 mg P.O. 4 hours after each ifosfamide infusion, days 1-3
    Ifosfamide, I.V., 1.33 g/m^2/day, days 1-3
    Mitoxantrone (Novantrone®), I.V., 8 mg/m^2, day 1
    Etoposide, I.V., 65 mg/m^2/day, days 1-3

                                   Repeat cycle every 28 days

Pro-MACE

    Prednisone, P.O., 60 mg/m^2, days 1-14
    Methotrexate, I.V., 1.5 g/m^2, day 14
    Leucovorin calcium, I.V., 50 mg/m^2 q6h x 5 doses beginning 24 h after methotrexate dose, day 14
    Doxorubicin (Adriamycin®), I.V., 25 mg/m^2, days 1 & 8
    Cyclophosphamide, I.V., 650 mg/m^2, days 1 & 8
    Etoposide, I.V., 120 mg/m^2, days 1 & 8

                                   Repeat cycle every 28 days

Pro-MACE-CytaBOM

    Prednisone, P.O., 60 mg/m^2, days 1-14
    Doxorubicin (Adriamycin®), I.V., 25 mg/m^2, day 1
    Cyclophosphamide, I.V., 650 mg/m^2, day 1
    Etoposide, I.V., 120 mg/m^2, day 1
    Cytarabine, I.V., 300 mg/m^2, day 8
    Bleomycin, I.V., 5 units/m^2, day 8
    Vincristine (Oncovin®), I.V., 1.4 mg/m^2 (max: 2 mg), day 8
    Methotrexate, I.V., 120 mg/m^2, day 8
    Leucovorin calcium, P.O., 25 mg/m^2 q6h x 4 doses, day 9

                                   Repeat cycle every 21 days

Malignant Melanoma

BCDT

    Carmustine (BCNU), I.V., 150 mg/m^2, day 1
    Cisplatin, I.V., 25 mg/m^2, days 1-3, 21-23
    Dacarbazine, I.V., 220 mg/m^2, days 1-3, 21-23
    Tamoxifen, P.O., 10 mg bid, days 1-42

BHD

    Carmustine (BCNU), I.V., 100-150 mg/m^2, day 1

                                     Repeat cycle every 42 days

    Hydroxyurea, P.O., 1480 mg/m^2, days 1-5
    Dacarbazine, I.V., 100-150 mg/m^2, days 1-5

                                   Repeat cycle every 21 days

Malignant Melanoma *(continued)*

DTIC-ACTD
Dacarbazine, I.V., 750 mg/m^2, day 1
Dactinomycin, I.V., 1 mg/m^2, day 1

Repeat cycle every 28 days

VBC
Vinblastine, I.V., 6 mg/m^2, days 1 & 2
Bleomycin, I.V., 15 units/m^2/day continuous infusion, days 1-5
Cisplatin, I.V., 50 mg/m^2, day 5

Repeat cycle every 28 days

VDP
Vinblastine, I.V., 5 mg/m^2, days 1 & 2
Dacarbazine, I.V., 150 mg/m^2, days 1-5
Cisplatin (Platinol®), I.V., 75 mg/m^2, day 5

Repeat cycle every 21-28 days

Multiple Myeloma

AC (DC)
Doxorubicin (Adriamycin®), I.V., 30 mg/m^2, day 1
Carmustine, I.V., 30 mg/m^2, day 1

Repeat cycle every 21-28 days

BCP
Carmustine (BCNU), I.V., 75 mg/m^2, day 1
Cyclophosphamide, I.V., 400 mg/m^2, day 1
Prednisone, P.O., 75 mg, days 1-7

Repeat cycle every 28 days

EDAP
Etoposide, I.V., 100-200 mg/m^2, days 1-4
Dexamethasone, P.O./I.V., 40 mg/m^2, days 1-5
Cytarabine (Ara-C), 1000 mg, day 5
Cisplatin (Platinol®), I.V., 20 mg continuous infusion, days 1-4

MeCP
Methyl-CCNU, P.O., 100 mg/m^2, day 1

Repeat cycle every 56 days

Cyclophosphamide, I.V., 600 mg/m^2, day 1
Prednisone, P.O., 40 mg/m^2/day, days 1-7

Repeat cycle every 28 days

MP
Melphalan, P.O., 8 mg/m^2, days 1-4
Prednisone, P.O., 40 mg/m^2/day, days 1-7

Repeat cycle every 28 days

M-2
Vincristine, I.V., 0.03 mg/kg (max: 2 mg), day 1
Carmustine, I.V., 0.5 mg/kg, day 1
Cyclophosphamide, I.V., 10 mg/kg, day 1
Melphalan, P.O., 0.25 mg/kg, days 1-4
Prednisone, P.O., 1 mg/kg/day, then taper next 14 days, days 1-7

Repeat cycle every 35 days

Multiple Myeloma *(continued)*

VAD
Vincristine, I.V., 0.4 mg/day continuous infusion, days 1-4
Doxorubicin (Adriamycin®), I.V., 9-10 mg/m^2/day continuous infusion, days 1-4
Dexamethasone, P.O., 40 mg, days 1-4, 9-12, 17-20

Repeat cycle every 25-35 days

VBAP
Vincristine, I.V., 1 mg, day 1
Carmustine (BCNU), I.V., 30 mg/m^2, day 1
Doxorubicin (Adriamycin®), I.V., 30 mg/m^2, day 1
Prednisone, P.O., 100 mg, days 1-4

Repeat cycle every 21 days

VCAP
Vincristine, I.V., 1 mg, day 1
Cyclophosphamide, P.O., 100 mg/m^2, days 1-4
Doxorubicin (Adriamycin®), I.V., 25 mg/m^2, day 2
Prednisone, P.O., 60 mg/m^2, days 1-4

Repeat cycle every 28 days

Single-Agent Regimens

DEX
Dexamethasone, 20 mg/m^2 every morning for 4 days beginning on days 1, 9, and 17, every 14 days for 3 cycles

Interferon alfa-2b, S.C., 3 million units 3 times/week for maintenance therapy in patients with significant response to initial chemotherapy treatment

Ovarian Cancer

Epithelial

CC
Carboplatin, I.V., 300 mg/m^2, day 1
Cyclophosphamide, I.V., 600 mg/m^2, day 1

Repeat cycle every 28 days

CDC
Carboplatin, I.V., 300 mg/m^2, day 1
Doxorubicin, I.V., 40 mg/m^2, day 1
Cyclophosphamide, I.V., 500 mg/m^2, day 1

Repeat cycle every 28 days

CHAP
Cyclophosphamide, I.V., 300-500 mg/m^2, day 1
Hexamethylmelamine, P.O., 150 mg/m^2, days 1-7
Doxorubicin (Adriamycin®), I.V., 30-50 mg/m^2, day 1
Cisplatin (Platinol®), I.V., 50 mg/m^2, day 1

Repeat cycle every 28 days

CP
Cyclophosphamide, I.V., 600 mg/m^2, day 1
Cisplatin (Platinol®), I.V., 75-100 mg/m^2, day 1

Repeat cycle every 21 days

Ovarian Cancer — Epithelial *(continued)*
PAC (CAP)

Cisplatin (Platinol®), I.V., 50 mg/m^2, day 1
Doxorubicin (Adriamycin®), I.V., 50 mg/m^2, day 1
Cyclophosphamide, I.V., 750 mg/m^2, day 1

Repeat cycle every 21 days x 8 cycles

PT

Cisplatin (Platinol®), I.V., 75 mg/m^2 (after Taxol®), day 1
Taxol®, I.V., 135 mg/m^2, day 1

Repeat cycle every 21 days

Single-Agent Regimen

Paclitaxel, I.V., 135 mg/m^2 continuous infusion, over 24 hours
Patient must be premedicated with:
Dexamethasone 20 mg P.O., 12 and 6 h prior
Diphenhydramine 50 mg I.V., 30 min prior
Cimetidine 300 mg I.V., or ranitidine 50 mg I.V., 30 min prior

Germ Cell

BEP

Bleomycin, I.V., 30 units, days 2, 9, 16
Etoposide, I.V., 100 mg/m^2, days 1-5
Cisplatin (Platinol®), I.V., 20 mg/m^2, days 1-5

VAC

Vincristine, I.V., 1.2-1.5 mg/m^2 (max: 2 mg) weekly for 10-12 weeks, or every 2 weeks for 12 doses
Dactinomycin (Actinomycin D), I.V., 0.3-0.4 mg/m^2, days 1-5
Cyclophosphamide, I.V., 150 mg/m^2, days 1-5

Repeat every 28 days

Pancreatic Cancer

FAM

Fluorouracil, I.V., 600 mg/m^2/wk, weeks 1, 2, 5, 6, 9
Doxorubicin (Adriamycin®), I.V., 30 mg/m^2/wk, weeks 1, 5, 9
Mitomycin C, I.V., 10 mg/m^2/wk, weeks 1, 9

FMS (SMF)

Fluorouracil, I.V., 600 mg/m^2, days 1, 8, 29 & 36
Mitomycin C, I.V., 10 mg/m^2, day 1
Streptozocin, I.V., 1 g/m^2, days 1, 8, 29 & 36

Repeat cycle every 56 days

SD

Streptozocin, I.V., 500 mg/m^2, days 1-5
Doxorubicin, I.V., 50 mg/m^2, days 1 & 22

Repeat cycle every 42 days

Renal Cancer

Single-Agent Regimens

Aldesleukin (rIL-2), various dosing regimens — please refer to the literature

Interferon alfa-2b, various dosing regimens — please refer to the literature

Floxuridine, S.C., 0.1 mg/kg, days 1-14

Repeat cycle every 21 days

Vinblastine, I.V., 1.2 mg/m^2 continuous infusion, days 1-4

Sarcoma

Bony Sarcoma

AC
Doxorubicin (Adriamycin®), I.V., 75-90 mg/m^2 96-h continuous infusion
Cisplatin, I.A./I.V., 90-120 mg/m^2, 6 days

Repeat cycle every 28 days

CYVADIC
Cyclophosphamide, I.V., 600 mg/m^2, day 1
Vincristine, I.V., 1.4 mg/m^2 (max: 2 mg) weekly x 6 weeks, then on day 1 of future cycles
Doxorubicin (Adriamycin®), I.V., 15 mg/m^2/day continuous infusion, days 1-4
Dacarbazine (DTIC), I.V., 250 mg/m^2/day continuous infusion, days 1-4

Repeat cycle every 21-28 days

HDMTX
Methotrexate, I.V., 8-12 g/m^2
Leucovorin calcium, I.V./P.O., 15-25 mg q6h for at least 10 doses beginning 24 h after methotrexate dose; courses repeated weekly for 2-4 weeks, alternating with various cancer chemotherapy combination regimens

IMAC
Ifosfamide, I.V., 1.2 g/m^2/day continuous infusion, days 1-5
Mesna, I.V., 400 mg/m^2 bolus prior to ifosfamide infusion day 1, then 1.2 g/m^2/day continuous infusion days 1-5 concurrent with ifosfamide, then 600 mg/m^2 continuous infusion over 12 hours after ifosfamide infusion, days 1-5
Doxorubicin (Adriamycin®), I.V., 15 mg/m^2/day continuous infusion, days 2-5
Cisplatin, I.V./I.A., 120 mg/m^2 continuous infusion over 24 hours, day 7

Repeat cycle every 28 days

VAIE
Vincristine, I.V., 1.5 mg/m^2/day, days 1 & 5
Doxorubicin (Adriamycin®), I.V., 20 mg/m^2/day continuous infusion, days 1-4
Ifosfamide, I.V., 1800 mg/m^2/day, days 1-5
Etoposide, I.V., 50 mg/m^2/day, days 1-5

Repeat cycle every 21 days

VADRIAC — High Dose
Vincristine, I.V., 1.5 mg/m^2/day, days 1 & 5
Cyclophosphamide, I.V., 2.1 g/m^2/day, days 1 & 2
Doxorubicin (Adriamycin®), I.V., 25 mg/m^2/day continuous infusion, days 1-3

Repeat cycle every 21 days

Soft-Tissue Sarcoma

CYADIC
Cyclophosphamide, I.V., 600 mg/m^2, day 1
Doxorubicin (Adriamycin®), I.V., 15 mg/m^2/day continuous infusion, days 1-4
Dacarbazine (DTIC), I.V., 250 mg/m^2/day continuous infusion, days 1-4
Repeat cycle every 21-28 days

CYVADIC
Cyclophosphamide, I.V., 500 mg/m^2, day 1
Vincristine, I.V., 1.4 mg/m^2 (max: 2 mg), days 1 & 5
Doxorubicin (Adriamycin®), I.V., 50 mg/m^2, day 1
Dacarbazine (DTIC), I.V., 250 mg/m^2, days 1-5
Repeat cycle every 21 days

ICE
Ifosfamide, I.V., 2000 mg/m^2, days 1-3
Carboplatin, I.V., 300-600 mg/m^2, day 3
Etoposide, I.V., 100 mg/m^2, days 1-3

ID
Ifosfamide, I.V., 5 g/m^2 continuous infusion over 24 hours, day 1
Mesna, I.V., 1 g/m^2 bolus prior to ifosfamide infusion, then 4 g/m^2 continuous infusion over 32
  hours, day 1
Doxorubicin, I.V., 40 mg/m^2, day 1
Repeat cycle every 21 days

MAID
Mesna, I.V., 500 mg/m^2 bolus 15 min prior to ifosfamide infusion, then q3h x 3, days 1-3
Doxorubicin (Adriamycin®), I.V., 20 mg/m^2 continuous infusion over 24 h, days 1-3
Ifosfamide, I.V., 2500 mg/m^2 over 1 h, days 1-3
Dacarbazine*, I.V., 300 mg/m^2 continuous infusion over 24 h, days 1-3
Repeat cycle every 28 days

*Adriamycin and dacarbazine may be mixed in the same bag.

VAC
Vincristine, I.V., 2 mg/m^2 (max: 2 mg) per week on weeks 1-12
Dactinomycin, I.V., 0.015 mg/kg (max: 0.5 mg) every 3 months for 5-6 courses, days 1-5
Cyclophosphamide, P.O., 2.5 mg/kg/day for 2 years

ALL, Induction

DVP
Daunorubicin, I.V., 25 mg/m^2, days 1, 8
Vincristine, I.V., 1.5 mg/m^2 days 1, 8, 15, 22
Prednisone, P.O., 40 mg/m^2, days 1-29

PVDA
Prednisone, P.O., 40 mg/m^2, days 1-29
Vincristine, I.V., 1.5 mg/m^2, days 1, 8, 15, 22
Daunorubicin, I.V., 25 mg/m^2, days 1, 8
Asparaginase, I.M., 10,000 units/m^2, days 2, 4, 6, 8, 10, 12, 15, 17, 19

VPA
Vincristine, I.V., 1.5 mg/m^2, days 1, 8, 15, 22
Daunorubicin, I.V., 25 mg/m^2, days 1, 8
Asparaginase, I.M., 10,000 units/m^2, days 2, 4, 6, 8, 10, 12, 15, 17, 19

AML, Induction

DA
Daunorubicin, I.V., 45-60 mg/m^2 continuous infusion, days 1-3
Cytarabine (Ara-C), I.V., 100 mg/m^2, q12h for 5-7 days

DAT
Daunorubicin, I.V., 45 mg/m^2 continuous infusion, days 1-3
Cytarabine (Ara-C), I.V., 100 mg/m^2 continuous infusion, days 1-7
Thioguanine, P.O., 100 mg/m^2, days 1-7

DAV
Daunorubicin, I.V., 30 mg/m^2 continuous infusion, days 1-3
Cytarabine (Ara-C), I.V., 250 mg/m^2 continuous infusion, days 1-5
Etoposide (VePesid®), I.V., 200 mg/m^2 continuous infusion, days 5-7

VAPA
Vincristine, I.V., 1.5 mg/m^2, days 1, 5
Doxorubicin (Adriamycin®), I.V., 30 mg/m^2 continuous infusion, days 1, 2, 3
Prednisone, P.O., 40 mg/m^2, days 1-5
Cytarabine (Ara-C), I.V., 100 mg/m^2 continuous infusion, days 1-7

Brain Tumors

CDDP/VP
Cisplatin, I.V., 90 mg/m^2, day 1
Etoposide, I.V., 150 mg/m^2, days 2, 3

MOP
Mechlorethamine (nitrogen mustard), I.V., 6 mg/m^2, days 1, 8
Vincristine (Oncovin®), I.V., 1.4 mg/m^2, days 1, 8
Procarbazine, P.O., 100 mg/m^2, days 1-14

For calculating pediatric doses of chemotherapy agents, as a general rule 1 m^2 corresponds to about 30 kg of ideal body weight. **For children weighing <15 kg or with surface area <0.6 m^2**, the dose per m^2 of an agent listed herein should be divided by 30 and multiplied by the weight of the child (in kg) to obtain the correct dose.

Brain Tumors *(continued)*

PCV

Procarbazine, P.O., 60 mg/m², days 18-21
Methyl-CCNU, P.O., 110 mg/m², day 1
Vincristine, I.V., 1.4 mg/m², days 8-29

POC

Prednisone, P.O., 40 mg/m², days 1-14
Methyl-CCNU, P.O., 100 mg/m², day 2
Vincristine, I.V., 1.5 mg/m², days 1, 8, 15

Repeat cycle every 6 weeks

"8 in 1"

Methylprednisolone, I.V., 300 mg/m², day 1
Vincristine, I.V., 1.5 mg/m², day 1
Methyl-CCNU, P.O., 75 mg/m², day 1
Procarbazine, P.O., 75 mg/m²/day, day 1
Hydroxyurea, P.O., 1500 or 3000 mg/m², day 1
Cisplatin, I.V., 60 or 90 mg/m², day 1
Cytarabine, I.V., 300 mg/m², day 1
Cyclophosphamide, I.V., 300 mg/m² **or**
    dacarbazine (DTIC), I.V., 150 mg/m², day 1

Hodgkin's Lymphoma

ABVD

Doxorubicin (Adriamycin®), I.V., 25 mg/m², days 1, 15
Bleomycin, I.V., 10 units/m², days 1-15
Vinblastine, I.V., 6 mg/m², days 1, 15
Dacarbazine (DTIC), I.V., 375 mg/m², days 1, 15

Repeat cycle every 28 days

COMP

Cyclophosphamide, I.V., 500 mg/m², days 1-8
Vincristine (Oncovin®), I.V., 1.4 mg/m², days 1, 8
Methotrexate, I.V., 40 mg/m², days 1, 2
Prednisone, P.O., 40 mg/m², days 1-15

COPP

Cyclophosphamide, I.V., 500 mg/m², days 1-8
Vincristine (Oncovin®), I.V., 1.4 mg/m², days 1, 8
Procarbazine, P.O., 100 mg/m², days 1-15
Prednisone, P.O., 40 mg/m², days 1-15

MOPP

Mechlorethamine (nitrogen mustard), I.V., 6 mg/m², days 1, 8
Vincristine (Oncovin®), I.V., 1.4 mg/m², days 1, 8
Procarbazine, P.O., 100 mg/m², days 1-15
Prednisone, P.O., 40 mg/m², days 1-15

Repeat cycle every 28 days

OPA

Vincristine (Oncovin®), I.V., 1.5 mg/m², days 1, 8, 15
Prednisone, P.O., 60 mg/m², days 1-15
Doxorubicin (Adriamycin®), I.V., 40 mg/m², days 1, 15

For calculating pediatric doses of chemotherapy agents, as a general rule 1 m² corresponds to about 30 kg of ideal body weight. **For children weighing <15 kg or with surface area <0.6 m²,** the dose per m² of an agent listed herein should be divided by 30 and multiplied by the weight of the child (in kg) to obtain the correct dose.

Hodgkin's Lymphoma *(continued)*
OPPA
    Vincristine (Oncovin®), I.V., 1.5 mg/m^2, days 1, 8, 15
    Procarbazine, P.O., 100 mg/m^2, days 1-15
    Prednisone, P.O., 60 mg/m^2, days 1-15
    Doxorubicin (Adriamycin®), I.V., 40 mg/m^2, days 1, 15

        Repeat cycle every 28 days

Osteosarcoma

HDMTX
    Methotrexate, I.V., 12 g/m^2, weekly for 2-12 weeks
    Leucovorin calcium rescue, P.O./I.V., 15 mg/m^2 q6h for 10 doses beginning 30 hours after the
        beginning of the 4-hour methotrexate infusion
    (serum methotrexate levels must be monitored)

MTXCP-PDAdr
    Methotrexate, I.V., 12 g/m^2, weekly for 2-12 weeks
    Leucovorin calcium rescue, P.O./I.V., 15 mg/m^2 q6h for 10 doses beginning 30 hours after the
        beginning of the 4-hour methotrexate infusion
    (serum methotrexate levels must be monitored)
    Cisplatin (Platinol®), I.V., 100 mg/m^2, day 1
    Doxorubicin (Adriamycin®), I.V., 37.5 mg/m^2, days 2, 3

MTXCP-PDAdrI
    Methotrexate, I.V., 12 g/m^2, weekly for 2-12 weeks
    Leucovorin calcium rescue, P.O./I.V., 15 mg/m^2 q6h for 10 doses beginning 30 hours after the
        beginning of the 4-hour methotrexate infusion
    (serum methotrexate levels must be monitored)
    Cisplatin (Platinol®), I.V., 100 mg/m^2, day 1
    Doxorubicin (Adriamycin®), I.V., 37.5 mg/m^2, days 2, 3
    Ifosfamide, I.V., 1.6 mg/m^2, days 1-5

Sarcomas (Bony and Soft-Tissue)

ICE
    Ifosfamide, I.V., 2 g/m^2, days 2, 3, 4
    Carboplatin, I.V., 300-600 mg/m^2, day 1
    Etoposide, I.V., 100 mg/m^2, days 2, 3, 4

VAC + Adr
    Vincristine, I.V., 1.5 mg/m^2 (max: 2 mg)
    Dactinomycin, I.V., 0.5-1.5 mg/m^2, days 1-5, every other week
    Cyclophosphamide, I.V., 500-1500 mg/m^2
    Doxorubicin (Adriamycin®), I.V., 35-60 mg/m^2

VACAdr-IfoVP
    Vincristine, I.V., 1.5 mg/m^2 (max: 2 mg), weekly
    Dactinomycin, I.V., 1.5 mg/m^2 (max: 2 mg), every other week
    Doxorubicin (Adriamycin®), I.V., 60 mg/m^2 continuous infusion over 24 hours
    Cyclophosphamide, I.V., 1-1.5 g/m^2
    Ifosfamide, I.V., 1.6-2 g/m^2, days 1-5
    Etoposide, I.V., 150 mg/m^2, days 1-5

For calculating pediatric doses of chemotherapy agents, as a general rule 1 m^2 corresponds to about 30 kg of ideal body weight. **For children weighing <15 kg or with surface area <0.6 m^2**, the dose per m^2 of an agent listed herein should be divided by 30 and multiplied by the weight of the child (in kg) to obtain the correct dose.

Sarcomas (Bony and Soft-Tissue) *(continued)*

VAdrC
Vincristine, I.V., 1.5 mg/m^2 (max: 2 mg)
Doxorubicin (Adriamycin®), I.V., 35-60 mg/m^2
Cyclophosphamide, I.V., 500-1500 mg/m^2

Wilms' Tumor

VAD
Vincristine, I.V., 1.5 mg/m^2, every other week
Dactinomycin, I.V., 0.4 mg/m^2, every other week
   alternating with doxorubicin, I.V., 25 mg/m^2, every other week

Repeat for a total of 6 months

VAD2
Vincristine, I.V., 1.5 mg/m^2
Dactinomycin, I.V., 0.15 mg/kg, days 1-5
Doxorubicin, I.V., 20 mg/m^2, days 1-3

HERBS AND COMMON NATURAL AGENTS

The authors have chosen to include this list of natural products and proposed medical claims. However, due to limited scientific investigation to support these claims, this list is not intended to imply that these claims have been scientifically proven.

PROPOSED MEDICINAL CLAIMS

Herb	Medicinal Claim
Agrimony	Treat digestive disorders
Alfalfa	Source of carotene (vitamin A); contains natural fluoride
Aloe	Healing agent
Angelica root	Treat diseases of the lungs and heart; creates distaste for alcoholic beverages
Anise seed	Prevent gas
Arthritis tea	Treat osteoarthritis
Astragalus	Enhance energy reserves; used with ginseng
Barberry bark	Treat halitosis
Basil leaf	Treat vomiting
Bayberry bark	Relieve or prevent varicose veins
Bay leaf	Relieve cramps
Bee pollen	Renewal of enzymes, hormones, vitamins, amino acids, and others
Bergamot herb	Used as sedative
Bilberry leaf	Increases night vision, reduces eye fatigue
Birch bark	Treat urinary problems; used for rheumatism
Blackberry leaf	Treat diarrhea
Black cohosh	Relieve menstrual cramps; same effects as estrogen
Blessed thistle (Holy thistle)	Aids circulation to the brain
Blue Cohosh	Regulate menstrual flow; emergency remedy for allergic reactions to bee stings
Blue flag	Useful in the treatment of skin diseases and constipation
Blue violet	Relieve severe headaches
Boldo leaf	Stimulates digestion; treatment of gallstones
Boneset	Treatment of colds and flu
Borage leaf	Reduces high fevers
Bromelain	Fat melting enzyme; stimulates the metabolism
Buchu leaf	Diuretic; treatment of acute and chronic bladder and kidney disorders
Buckthorn bark	Expels worms and will remove warts
Burdock leaf and root	Treatment of severe skin problems and cases of arthritis
Butternut bark	Treat constipation
Calendula flower	Mending and healing of cuts or wounds
Capsicum (Cayenne)	Normalizes blood pressure; stops bleeding on contact
Caraway seed	Aids digestion
Cascara sagrada bark	Treatment for chronic constipation and gallstones
Catnip	Treat gas or stomach cramps
Celery leaf and seed	Treat incontinence
Centaury	Stimulates the salivary gland
Chamomile flower	Excellent for a nervous stomach; relieve cramping associated with the menstrual cycle
Chervil	Stimulant, mild diuretic, lowers blood pressure
Chickweed	Rich in vitamin C and minerals (calcium, magnesium, and potassium)
Chicory root	Effective in disorders of the kidneys, liver, and urinary canal
Cinnamon bark	Prevents infection and indigestion; helps break down fats during digestion

(continued)

Herb	Medicinal Claim
Cleavers	Treatment of kidney and bladder disorders; useful in obstructions of the urinary organ
Colombo root	Treat colon trouble
Coltsfoot herb and flower	Useful for asthma, bronchitis, and spasmodic cough
Coriander seed	Stomach tonic
Cornsilk	Treat prostate gland enlargement
Cranberry	Treat or prevents bladder or kidney infection
Cubeb berry	Treat chronic bladder trouble; increases flow of urine
Damiana leaf	Treatment for sexual impotency
Dandelion leaf and root	Detoxify poisons in the liver; beneficial in lowering blood pressure
Dong Quai root	Prevents and treat menstrual problems
Echinacea root	Treat strep throat, lymph glands
Fennel seed	Remedies for gas and acid stomach
Fenugreek seed	Treat allergies, coughs, digestion, emphysema, headaches, migraines, intestinal inflammation, ulcers, lungs, mucous membranes, and sore throat
Feverfew herb	Treat migraines; helps reduce inflammation in arthritis joints
Garlic capsules	"Nature's antibiotic"
Gentian	Treatment of digestive organs and improves circulation
Ginger root	Remedy for sore throat
Ginkgo biloba	Improves blood circulation to the brain
Ginseng root, Siberian	Resistance against stress; slows the aging process
Goldenseal	Treatment of bladder infections, cankers, mouth sores, mucous membranes, and ulcers
Gota kola	"Memory herb"; nerve tonic
Gravelroot (Queen of the Meadow)	Remedy for stones in the kidney and bladder
Green barley	Excellent antioxidant
Hawthorn	Strengthens and regulates the heart; relieve insomnia
Hibiscus flower	Stimulant for the intestines and kidneys
Holy thistle (Blessed thistle)	Remedy for migraine headaches
Hops flower	Treat insomnia; used to decrease the desire for alcohol
Horehound	Treat acute or chronic sore throat and coughs
Horsetail (Shavegrass)	Rich in minerals, especially silica; used to develop strong fingernails and hair, good for split ends
Ho shou wu	Rejuvenator
Hydrangea root	Treat backaches
Hyssop	Treat or prevents asthma
Juniper berry	Treat kidney ailments
Kava kava root	Induce sleep and help calm nervousness
Kelp	High contents of natural plant iodine, for proper function of the thyroid; high levels of natural calcium, potassium, and magnesium
Lavender flower	Flavor moderator
Lecithin	Break up cholesterol; prevent arteriosclerosis
Licorice root	Treatment of constipation
Ma-huang	Cleanses respiratory system
Malva flower	Soothes inflammation in the mouth and throat; helpful for earaches
Marjoram	Beneficial for a sour stomach or loss of appetite
Marshmallow leaf	Treat inflammation (anti-inflammatory)
Milk thistle herb	Liver detoxifier
Motherwort	Treat chest cold and nervousness
Mugwort	Used for treatment of rheumatism and gout
Mullein leaf	High in iron, magnesium, and potassium; sinuses; relieve swollen joints

(continued)

Herb	Medicinal Claim
Myrrh gum	Removes bad breath; sinus problems
Nettle leaf	In combination with seawrack, will bring splendid results in weight loss; remedy for dandruff
Nutmeg	Treat symptoms of gas
Oregano leaf	Settles the stomach after meals; helps treat colds
Oregon grape root	Treat rheumatism
Papaya leaf	Digestive stimulant; contains the enzyme papain
Paprika (sweet)	Stimulates the appetite and gastric secretions
Parsley leaf	High in iron
Passion flower	Mild sedative
Pau d'arco	Protects immune system
Pennyroyal	Relieve high fevers and brings on perspiration
Peppermint leaf	Treat headaches
Plantain leaf	Useful for infection, hemorrhoids, and inflammation
Pleurisy root	Treatment of a cold
Prickly ash bark	Increases circulation
Prince's pine	Diuretic; for rheumatism and chronic kidney problems
Psyllium seed	Treat constipation, lubricant to the intestinal tract
Red clover	Purify the blood
Red raspberry leaf	Eases menstrual cramps
Rhubarb root	Treat constipation, powerful laxative
Rose hips	High content of vitamin C
Safflower	Eliminates buildup of uric and lactic acid in the body, the leading cause of gout
Saffron	Natural digestive aid
Sanicle	Cleansing herb
Sarsaparilla root	Remedy for rheumatism and gout; acts as a diuretic; same effects on the body as the male hormone testosterone
Sassafras leaf and root	Stimulates the action of the liver to clear toxins from the body
Saw palmetto berry	Symptomatically treat mucus in the head and nose
Scullcap	Nerve sedative; hangover remedy
Seawrack (Bladderwrack)	Combat obesity
Senna leaf	Treat constipation, splendid laxative
Shepherd's purse	Remedy for diarrhea
Sheep sorrel	Remedy for kidney trouble
Slippery elm bark	Normalize bowel movement; beneficial for hemorrhoids and constipation
Solomon's seal root	Poultice for bruises
Speedwell	Used as a gargle for mouth and throat sores
Spikenard	Skin ailments such as acne, pimples, blackheads, rashes, and general skin problems
Star anise	Promotes appetite and relieve flatulence
St John's wort	Correct irregular menstruation
Strawberry leaf	Prevents diarrhea
Sumac berry and bark	Sores and cankers in the mouth
Summer savory leaf	Treat diarrhea, upset stomach, and sore throat
Thyme leaf	Relief of migraine headaches
Uva-ursi leaf	Digestive stimulant
Valerian root	Promotes sleep
Vervain	Remedy for fevers
White oak bark	Strong astringent
White willow bark	Used for minor aches and pains in the body
Wild alum root	Powerful astringent; used as rinse for sores in mouth and bleeding gums
Wild cherry	Prevent or treat asthma

(continued)

Herb	Medicinal Claim
Wild Oregon grape root	Chronic skin disease
Wild yam root	Helps expel gas
Wintergreen leaf	Valuable for colic and gas in the bowels
Witch hazel bark and leaf	Restores circulation; for stiff joints
Wood betony	Relieve pain in the face and head
Woodruff	Treatment of insomnia and hysteria
Wormwood	Aids bruises and sprains
Yarrow root	Unsurpasses for treatment of flu and fevers
Yerba santa	Treatment of bronchial congestion
Yohimbe	Treat impotency, natural aphrodisiac
Yucca root	Reduces inflammation of the joints

SOUND-ALIKE COMPARISON LIST

The following list contains over 960 pairs of sound-alike drugs accompanied by a subjective pronunciation of each drug name. Any such list can only suggest possible pronunciation or enunciation miscues and is by no means meant to be exhaustive.

New or rarely used drugs are likely to cause the most problems related to interpretation. Healthcare workers should be made aware of the existence of both drugs in a sound-alike pair in order to avoid (or minimize) the potential for error. Drug companies attempt to avoid naming different drugs with similar-sounding names; however, mix-ups do occur. Reading current drug advertisements, professional literature, and drug handbooks is a good way to avert or surely lessen such sound-alike drug errors at all levels of the healthcare industry.

Drug Name	Pronunciation	Drug Name	Pronunciation
Accolate®	(ak′ cue late)	Acutrim®	(ak′ yu trim)
Accutane®	(ak′ yu tane)	Actron®	(ak′ tron)
Accolate®	(ak′ cue late)	Adalat®	(ad′ da lat)
Accupril®	(ak′ yu pril)	Adapin®	(ad′ da pin)
Accubron®	(ak′ cue bron)	Adapin®	(ad′ da pin)
Accutane®	(ak′ yu tane)	Adalat®	(ad′ da lat)
Accupril®	(ak′ cue pril)	Adapin®	(ad′ da pin)
Accolate®	(ak′ cue late)	Adipex-P®	(ad′ di pex pea)
Accupril®	(ak′ cue pril)	Adapin®	(ad′ da pin)
Accutane®	(ak′ yu tane)	Ativan®	(at′ tee van)
Accutane®	(ak′ yu tane)	Adderall®	(ad′ der all)
Accubron®	(ak′ cue bron)	Inderal®	(in′ der al)
Accutane®	(ak′ yu tane)	Adipex-P®	(ad′ di pex pea)
Accolate®	(ak′ cue late)	Adapin®	(ad′ da pin)
Accutane®	(ak′ yu tane)	Adriamycin™	(ade rya mye′ sin)
Accupril®	(ak′ cue pril)	Achromycin®	(ak roe mye′ sin)
Accutane®	(ak′ yu tane)	Adriamycin™	(ade rya mye′ sin)
Acutrim®	(ak′ yu trim)	Idamycin®	(eye da mye′ sin)
acetazolamide	(a set a zole′ a mide)	Aerolone®	(air′ o lone)
acetohexamide	(a set o heks′ a mide)	Aralen®	(air′ a len)
acetohexamide	(a set o heks′ a mide)	Afrin®	(aye′ frin or af′ rin)
acetazolamide	(a set a zole′ a mide)	aspirin	(as′ pir in)
Achromycin®	(ak roe mye′ sin)	Afrinol®	(af′ ree nol)
Adriamycin™	(ade rya mye′ sin)	Arfonad®	(arr′ foe nad)
Achromycin®	(ak roe mye′ sin)	Agoral®	(ag′ a ral)
actinomycin	(ak ti noe mye′ sin)	Argyrol®	(ar′ gee roll)
Actidil®	(ak′ tee dill)	AK-Mycin®	(aye kay mye′ sin)
Actifed®	(ak′ tee fed)	Akne-Mycin®	(ak nee mye′ sin)
Actifed®	(ak′ tee fed)	Akne-Mycin®	(ak nee mye′ sin)
Actidil®	(ak′ tee dill)	AK-Mycin®	(aye kay mye′ sin)
actinomycin	(ak ti noe mye′ sin)	AKTob®	(ak′ tobe)
Achromycin®	(ak roe mye′ sin)	AK-Trol®	(aye′ kay trol)
Actron®	(ak′ tron)	AK-Trol®	(aye′ kay trol)
Acutrim®	(ak′ yu trim)	AKTob®	(ak′ tobe)
Acutrim®	(ak′ yu trim)	Alazide®	(al′ a zide)
Accutane®	(ak′ yu tane)	Alazine®	(al′ a zine)
		Alazine®	(al′ a zine)
		Alazide®	(al′ a zide)

APPENDIX

Drug Name	Pronunciation	Drug Name	Pronunciation
Aldactazide®	(al dak′ ta zide)	Ambien™	(am′ bee en)
Aldactone®	(al′ dak tone)	Ambi 10®	(am′ bee ten′)
Aldactone®	(al′ dak tone)	amiodarone	((a mee′ oh da rone)
Aldactazide®	(al dak′ ta zide)	amrinone	(am′ ri none)
Aldomet®	(al′ doe met)	amitripyline	(a mee trip′ ti leen)
Aldoril®	(al′ doe ril)	imipramine	(im ip′ ra meen)
Aldoril®	(al′ doe ril)	ampicillin	(am pi sil′ in)
Aldomet®	(al′ doe met)	bacampicillin	(ba kam pi sil′ in)
Aldoril®	(al′ doe ril)	hydrochloride	
Elavil®	(el′ a vil)	amrinone	(am′ ri none)
Alfenta®	(al fen′ tah)	amiodarone	((a mee′ oh da rone)
Sufenta®	(sue fen′ tah)	Anafranil®	(a naf′ ra nil)
alfentanil	(al fen′ ta nill)	alfentanil	(al fen′ ta nill)
Anafranil®	(a naf′ ra nil)	Anafranil®	(a naf′ ra nil)
alfentanil	(al fen′ ta nil)	enalapril	(e nal′ a pril)
remifentanil	(rem i fen′ ta nil)	Anaprox®	(an′ a prox)
Alferon®	(al′ fer on)	Anaspaz®	(an′ a spaz)
Alkeran®	(al′ ker an)	Anaspaz®	(an′ a spaz)
Alkeran®	(al′ ker an)	Anaprox®	(an′ a prox)
Alferon®	(al′ fer on)	Anaspaz®	(an′ a spaz)
Allerfrin®	(al′ er frin)	Antispas®	(an′ te spaz)
Allergan®	(al′ er gan)	Anatrast®	(an′ a trast)
Allergan®	(al′ er gan)	Anatuss®	(an′ a tuss)
Allerfrin®	(al′ er frin)	Anatuss®	(an′ a tuss)
Allergan®	(al′ er gan)	Anatrast®	(an′ a trast)
Auralate®	(ahl′ a late)	Ancobon®	(an′ coe bon)
Altace™	(al′ tase)	Oncovin®	(on′ coe vin)
alteplase	(al′ te place)	anistreplase	(a nis′ tre place)
alprazolam	(al pray′ zoe lam)	alteplase	(al′ te place)
triazolam	(trye ay′ zoe lam)	Ansaid®	(an′ said)
alteplase	(al′ te place)	Axid®	(aks′ id)
Altace™	(al′ tase)	Antispas®	(an′ te spaz)
alteplase	(al′ te place)	Anaspaz®	(an′ a spaz)
anistreplase	(a nis′ tre place)	Anturane®	(ann′ chu rane)
Alupent®	(al′ yu pent)	Artane®	(ar′ tane)
Atrovent®	(at′ troe vent)	Aplisol®	(ap′ lee sol)
Alupent®	(al′ yu pent)	A.P.L.®	(aye pee el′)
Atrovent®	(at′ troe vent)	A.P.L.®	(aye pee el′)
amantadine	(a man′ ta deen)	Aplisol®	(ap′ lee sol)
rimantadine	(ri man′ to deen)	Apresoline®	(aye press′ sow leen)
Amaryl®	(am′ ah ril)	Priscoline®	(pris′ coe leen)
Ambenyl®	(am′ ba nil)	AquaTar®	(ah′ kwa tar)
Ambenyl®	(am′ ba nil)	Aquatag®	(ah′ kwa tag)
Amaryl®	(am′ ah ril)	Aquatag®	(ah′ kwa tag)
Ambenyl®	(am′ ba nil)	AquaTar®	(ah′ kwa tar)
Aventyl®	(a ven′ til)	Aralen®	(air′ a len)
Ambi 10®	(am′ bee ten′)	Aerolone®	(air′ o lone)
Ambien™	(am′ bee en)	Aralen®	(air′ a len)
		Arlidin®	(ar′ le din)

620

Drug Name	Pronunciation	Drug Name	Pronunciation
Aramine®	(air' a meen)	Aventyl®	(a ven' til)
Artane®	(ar' tane)	Ambenyl®	(am' ba nil)
Arfonad®	(arr' foe nad)	Aventyl®	(a ven' til)
Afrinol®	(af' ree nol)	Bentyl®	(ben' till)
Argyrol®	(ar' gee roll)	Avitene®	(aye' va teen)
Agoral®	(ag' a ral)	Ativan®	(at' tee van)
Arlidin®	(ar' le din)	Axid®	(aks' id)
Aralen®	(air' a len)	Ansaid®	(an' said)
Arrestin®	(aye res' tin)	Aygestin®	(aye ges' tin)
Aygestin®	(aye ges' tin)	Arrestin®	(aye res' tin)
Artane®	(ar' tane)	Azulfidine'	(ay zul' fi deen)
Anturane®	(an' chu rane)	Augmentin®	(aug men' tin)
Artane®	(ar' tane)	bacampicillin	(ba kam pi sil' in)
Aramine®	(air' a meen)	hydrochloride	
		ampicillin	(am pi sil' in)
Asbron®	(as' bron)		
aspirin	(as' pir in)	baclofen	(bak' loe fen)
		Bactroban®	(bak' troe ban)
aspirin	(as' pir in)		
Afrin®	(aye' frin or af' rin)	baclofen	(bak' loe fen)
		Beclovent®	(bec' lo vent)
aspirin	(as' pir in)		
Asbron®	(as' bron)	Bactocill®	(bak' tow sill)
		Pathocil®	(path' o sill)
Atarax®	(at' a raks)		
Ativan®	(at' tee van)	Bactroban®	(bak' troe ban)
		baclofen	(bak' loe fen)
Atarax®	(at' a raks)		
Marax®	(may' raks)	Banophen®	(ban' o fen)
		Barophen®	(bear' o fen)
Atgam®	(at' gam)		
Ativan®	(at' tee van)	Banthine®	(ban' theen)
		Brethine®	(breath' een)
Ativan®	(at' tee van)		
Adapin®	(add' da pin)	Banthine®	(ban' theen)
		Pro-Banthine®	(pro ban' theen)
Ativan®	(at' tee van)		
Atarax®	(at' a raks)	Barophen®	(bear' o fen)
		Banophen®	(ban' o fen)
Ativan®	(at' tee van)		
Atgam®	(at' gam)	Beclovent®	(bec' lo vent)
		baclofen	(bak' loe fen)
Ativan®	(at' tee van)		
ATnativ®	(aye tee nay' tif)	Beconase®	(beck' o nase)
		Bexophene®	(beks' o feen)
Ativan®	(at' tee van)		
Avitene®	(aye' va teen)	Beminal®	(bem' eh nall)
		Benemid®	(ben' a mid)
ATnativ®	(aye tee nay' tif)		
Ativan®	(at' tee van)	Benadryl®	(ben' a drill)
		Bentyl®	(ben' till)
Atrovent®	(at' troe vent)		
Alupent®	(al' yu pent)	Benemid®	(ben' a mid)
		Beminal®	(bem' eh nall)
Augmentin®	(aug men' tin)		
Azulfidine'	(ay zul' fi deen)	Benoxyl®	(ben ox' ill)
		Brevoxyl®	(brev ox' il)
Auralate®	(ahl' a late)		
Allergan®	(al' er gan)	Bentyl®	(ben' till)
		Aventyl®	(a ven' til)
Auralgan®	(a ral' gan)		
Larylgan®	(la ril' gan)	Bentyl®	(ben' till)
		Benadryl®	(ben' a drill)
Auralgan®	(a ral' gan)		
Ophthalgan®	(opp thal' gan)	Bentyl®	(ben' till)
		Cantil®	(can' til)

APPENDIX

Drug Name	Pronunciation	Drug Name	Pronunciation
Bentyl®	(ben' til)	Buprenex®	(byoo' pre nex)
Trental®	(tren' tal)	Bumex®	(byoo' mex)
Benylin®	(ben' eh lin)	Buminate®	(byoo' mi nate)
Ventolin®	(ven' tow lin)	bumetanide	(byoo met' a nide)
Benza®	(ben' zah)	bupivacaine	(byoo piv' a kane)
Benzac®	(ben' zak)	mepivacaine	(me piv' a kane)
Benzac®	(ben' zak)	butabarbital	(byoo ta bar' bi tal)
Benza®	(ben' zah)	butalbital	(byoo tal' bi tal)
Betadine®	(bay' ta deen)	butalbital	(byoo tal' bi tal)
Betagan®	(bay' ta gan)	butabarbital	(byoo ta bar' bi tal)
Betagan®	(bay' ta gan)	Byclomine®	(bye' clo meen)
Betadine®	(bay' ta deen)	Bydramine®	(bye' dra meen)
Betapace®	(bay' ta pace)	Byclomine®	(bye' clo meen)
Betapen®	(bay' ta pen)	Hycomine®	(hye' coe meen)
Betapen®	(bay' ta pen)	Bydramine®	(bye' dra meen)
Betapace®	(bay' ta pace)	Byclomine®	(bye' clo meen)
Bexophene®	(beks' o feen)	Bydramine®	(bye' dra meen)
Beconase®	(beck' o nase)	Hydramyn®	(hye' dra min)
Bicillin®	(bye sil' lin)	Cepastat®	(sea' pa stat)
V-Cillin K®	(vee sil' lin kay)	Capastat®	(kap' a stat)
Bicillin®	(bye sil' lin)	Cankaid®	(kan' kaid)
Wycillin®	(wye sil' lin)	Enkaid®	(enn' kaid)
bleomycin	(blee o mye' sin)	Cantil®	(can' til)
Cleocin®	(klee' o sin)	Bentyl®	(ben' till)
Bleph®-10	(blef ten')	Capastat®	(kap' a stat)
Blephamide®	(blef' a mide)	Cepastat®	(sea' pa stat)
Blephamide®	(blef' a mide)	Capital®	(kap' i tal)
Bleph®-10	(blef ten')	Capitrol®	(kap' i trol)
Borofax®	(boroe' faks)	Capitrol®	(kap' i trol)
Boropak®	(boroe' pak)	Capital®	(kap' i tal)
Boropak®	(boroe' pak)	Capitrol®	(kap' i trol)
Borofax®	(boroe' faks)	captopril	(kap' toe pril)
Brethine®	(breath' een)	captopril	(kap' toe pril)
Banthine®	(ban' theen)	Capitrol®	(kap' i trol)
Bretylol®	(brett' tee loll)	carboplatin	(kar' boe pla tin)
Brevital®	(brev' i tall)	cisplatin	(sis' pla tin)
Brevital®	(brev' i tall)	Cardio-Green®	(kar' dee yo green')
Bretylol®	(brett' tee loll)	Cardioquin®	(kar' dee yo kwin)
Brevoxyl®	(brev ox' il)	Cardioquin®	(kar' dee yo kwin)
Benoxyl®	(ben ox' ill)	Cardio-Green®	(kar' dee yo green')
Bromfed®	(brom' fed)	Cardura®	(kar dur' ah)
Bromphen®	(brom' fen)	Cordarone®	(kor da rone')
Bromphen®	(brom' fen)	Cardura®	(kar dur' ah)
Bromfed®	(brom' fed)	Cordran®	(kor' dran)
bumetanide	(byoo met' a nide)	Catapres®	(kat' a pres)
Buminate®	(byoo' mi nate)	Catarase®	(kat' a race)
Bumex®	(byoo' mex)	Catapres®	(kat' a pres)
Buprenex®	(byoo' pre nex)	Combipres®	(kom' bee pres)

Drug Name	Pronunciation	Drug Name	Pronunciation
Catapres®	(kat' a pres)	Clinoxide®	(klin ox' ide)
Ser-Ap-Es®	(ser ap' ess)	Clipoxide®	(kleh pox' ide)
Catarase®	(kat' a race)	Clipoxide®	(kleh pox' ide)
Catapres®	(kat' a pres)	Clinoxide®	(klin ox' ide)
cefazolin	(sef a' zoe lin)	Clocort®	(klo' kort)
cephalexin	(sef a leks' in)	Cloderm®	(klo' derm)
cefazolin	(sef a' zoe lin)	Cloderm®	(klo' derm)
cephalothin	(sef a' loe thin)	Clocort®	(klo' kort)
cefotaxime	(sef o taks' eem)	clomiphene	(kloe' mi feen)
cefoxitin	(se fox' i tin)	clomipramine	(kloe mi' pra meen)
cefoxitin	(se fox' i tin)	clomiphene	(kloe' mi feen)
cefotaxime	(sef o taks' eem)	clonidine	(kloe' ni deen)
ceftizoxime	(sef ti zoks' eem)	clomipramine	(kloe mi' pra meen)
cefuroxime	(se fyoor ox' eem)	clomiphene	(kloe' mi feen)
cefuroxime	(se fyoor ox' eem)	clonidine	(kloe' ni deen)
ceftizoxime	(sef ti zoks' eem)	clomiphene	(kloe' mi feen)
cephalexin	(sef a leks' in)	clonidine	(kloe' ni deen)
cefazolin	(sef a' zoe lin)	clozapine	(kloe' za peen)
cephalothin	(sef a' loe thin)	clonidine	(kloe' ni deen)
cefazolin	(sef a' zoe lin)	Klonopin™	(klon' o pin)
cephapirin	(sef a pye' rin)	clonidine	(kloe' ni deen)
cephradine	(sef' ra deen)	Loniten®	(lon' eh ten)
cephradine	(sef' ra deen)	clonidine	(kloe' ni deen)
cephapirin	(sef a pye' rin)	quinidine	(kwin' i deen)
chloroxine	(klor ox' een)	clotrimazole	(kloe trim' a zole)
Choloxin®	(koe lox' in)	co-trimoxazole	(koe-trye moks' a zole)
Choloxin®	(koe lox' in)	Cloxapen®	(klox' a pen)
chloroxine	(klor ox' een)	clozapine	(kloe' za peen)
chlorpropamide	(klor proe' pa mide)	Cozaar®	(koe' zar)
chlorpromazine	(klor proe' ma zeen)	Zocor®	(zoe' cor)
chlorpromazine	(klor proe' ma zeen)	clozapine	(kloe' za peen)
chlorpropamide	(klor proe' pa mide)	clonidine	(kloe' ni deen)
Chorex®	(ko' reks)	clozapine	(kloe' za peen)
Chymex®	(kye' meks)	Cloxapen®	(klox' a pen)
Chymex®	(kye' meks)	Co-Lav®	(koe' lav)
Chorex®	(ko' reks)	Colax®	(koe' laks)
cisplatin	(sis' pla tin)	co-trimoxazole	(koe-trye moks' a zole)
carboplatin	(kar' boe pla tin)	clotrimazole	(kloe trim' a zole)
Citracal®	(sit' tra cal)	CodAphen®	(kod' a fen)
Citrucel®	(sit' tru cel)	Codafed®	(kode' a fed)
Citrucel®	(sit' tru cel)	Codafed®	(kode' a fed)
Citracal®	(sit' tra cal)	CodAphen®	(kod' a fen)
clarithromycin	(kla rith' roe mye sin)	codeine	(koe' deen)
erythromycin	(er ith roe mye' sin)	Cophene®	(koe' feen)
Cleocin®	(klee' o sin)	codeine	(koe' deen)
bleomycin	(blee o mye' sin)	Lodine®	(low' deen)
Cleocin®	(klee' o sin)	Colax®	(koe' laks)
Lincocin®	(link' o sin)	Co-Lav®	(koe' lav)

APPENDIX

Drug Name	Pronunciation	Drug Name	Pronunciation
Colestid®	(koe les′ tid)	Cytoxan®	(sye tox′ an)
colistin	(koe lis′ tin)	Cytotec®	(sye′ toe tek)
colistin	(koe lis′ tin)	dacarbazine	(da kar′ ba zeen)
Colestid®	(koe les′ tid)	Dicarbosil®	(dye kar′ bow sil)
Combipres®	(kom′ bee pres)	dacarbazine	(da kar′ ba zeen)
Catapres®	(kat′ a pres)	procarbazine	(proe kar′ ba zeen)
Congestac®	(kon ges′ tin)	dactinomycin	(dak ti noe mye′ sin)
Congestant®	(kon ges′ tant)	daunorubicin	(daw noe roo′ bi sin)
Congestant®	(kon ges′ tant)	Daranide®	(dare′ a nide)
Congestac®	(kon ges′ tin)	Daraprim®	(dare′ a prim)
Cophene®	(koe′ feen)	Daraprim®	(dare′ a prim)
codeine	(koe′ deen)	Daranide®	(dare′ a nide)
Cordarone®	(kor da rone′)	Daricon®	(dare′ eh kon)
Cardura®	(kar dur′ ah)	Darvon®	(dar′ von)
Cordran®	(kor′ dran)	Darvon®	(dar′ von)
Cardura®	(kar dur′ ah)	Daricon®	(dare′ eh kon)
Cort-Dome®	(kort′ dome)	Darvon®	(dar′ von)
Cortone®	(kor′ tone)	Devrom®	(dev′ rom)
cortisone	(kor′ ti sone)	daunorubicin	(daw noe roo′ bi sin)
Cortizone®	(kor′ ti sone)	dactinomycin	(dak ti noe mye′ sin)
Cortizone®	(kor′ ti sone)	daunorubicin	(daw noe roo′ bi sin)
cortisone	(kor′ ti sone)	doxorubicin	(dox o roo′ bi sin)
Cortone®	(kor′ tone)	Daypro®	(day′ pro)
Cort-Dome®	(kort′ dome)	Deprol®	(deh′ prol)
Coumadin®	(ku′ ma din)	Decadron®	(dek′ a dron)
Kemadrin®	(kem′ a drin)	Decholin®	(dek′ o lin)
Crysticillin®	(kris ta sil′ lin)	Decadron®	(dek′ a dron)
Crystodigin®	(kris toe dig′ in)	Percodan®	(per′ coe dan)
Crystodigin®	(kris toe dig′ in)	Decholin®	(dek′ o lin)
Crysticillin®	(kris ta sil′ lin)	Decadron®	(dek′ a dron)
cycloserine	(sye kloe ser′ een)	Deconal®	(dek′ o nal)
cyclosporine	(sye′ kloe spor een)	Deconsal®	(dek′ on sal)
Cyclospasmol®	(sye kloe spas′ mol)	Deconsal®	(dek′ on sal)
cyclosporine	(sye′ kloe spor een)	Deconal®	(dek′ o nal)
cyclosporine	(sye′ kloe spor een)	Delacort®	(del′ a kort)
Cyclospasmol®	(sye kloe spas′ mol)	Delcort®	(del′ kort)
cyclosporine	(sye′ kloe spor een)	Delcort®	(del′ kort)
Cyklokapron®	(sye kloe kay′ pron)	Delacort®	(del′ a kort)
cyclosporine	(sye′ kloe spor een)	Delfen®	(del′ fen)
cycloserine	(sye kloe ser′ een)	Delsym®	(del′ sim)
Cyklokapron®	(sye kloe kay′ pron)	Delsym®	(del′ sim)
cyclosporine	(sye′ kloe spor een)	Delfen®	(del′ fen)
cytarabine	(sye tare′ a been)	Demadex®	(dem′ a deks)
vidarabine	(vye dare′ a been)	Denorex®	(den′ o reks)
Cytotec®	(sye′ toe tek)	Demerol®	(dem′ eh rol)
Cytoxan®	(sye tox′ an)	dicumarol	(dye koo′ ma role)
Cytotec®	(sye′ toe tek)	Demerol®	(dem′ eh rol)
Sytobex®	(sye′ toe beks)	Dymelor®	(dye′ meh lo)

Drug Name	Pronunciation
Demerol® Temaril®	(dem′ eh rol) (tem′ a ril)
Denorex® Demadex®	(den′ o reks) (dem′ a deks)
Depakene® Depakote®	(dep′ a keen) (dep′ a kote)
Depakote® Depakene®	(dep′ a kote) (dep′ a keen)
Depogen® Depoject®	(dep′ o gen) dep′ o ject)
Depoject® Depogen®	(dep′ o ject) (dep′ o gen)
Depo-Testadiol® Depotestogen®	(dep o tes ta dye′ ol) (dep o tes′ tow gen)
Depogen® Depoject®	(dep′ o gen) (dep′ o ject)
Depoject® Depogen®	(dep′ o ject) (dep′ o gen)
Depotestogen® Depo-Testadiol®	(dep o tes′ tow gen) (dep o tes ta dye′ ol)
Deprol® Daypro®	(deh′ prol) (day′ pro)
Dermacort® DermiCort®	(der′ ma kort) (der′ meh kort)
Dermatop® DermiCort®	(der′ ma top) (der′ meh kort)
DermiCort® Dermacort®	(der′ meh kort) (der′ ma kort)
DermiCort® Dermatop®	(der′ meh kort) (der′ ma top)
deserpidine desipramine	(de ser′ pi deen) (dess ip′ ra meen)
Desferal® Disophrol®	(des′ fer al) (dye′ so frol)
Desferal® desflurane	(des′ fer al) (des flu′ rane)
desflurane Desferal®	(des flu′ rane) (des′ fer al)
desipramine deserpidine	(dess ip′ ra meen) (de ser′ pi deen)
desoximetasone dexamethasone	(des ox i met′ a sone) (deks a meth′ a sone)
Devrom® Darvon®	(dev′ rom) (dar′ von)
dexamethasone desoximetasone	(deks a meth′ a sone) (des ox i met′ a sone)
Diaβeta® Diabinese®	(dye a bay′ tah) (dye ab′ beh neese)

Drug Name	Pronunciation
Diabinese® Diaβeta®	(dye ab′ beh neese) (dye a bay′ tah)
Diamox® Trimox®	(dye′ a moks) (trye′ moks)
Dicarbosil® dacarbazine	(dye kar′ bow sil) (da kar′ ba zeen)
diclofenac Diflucan®	(dye kloe′ fen ak) (dye flu′ can)
dicumarol Demerol®	(dye koo′ ma role) (dem′ eh rol)
Diflucan® diclofenac	(dye flu′ can) (dye kloe′ fen ak)
Diflucan® Diprivan®	(dye flu′ can) (dye′ pri van)
digitoxin digoxin	(di ji tox′ in) (di jox′ in)
digoxin digitoxin	(di jox′ in) (di ji tox′ in)
Dilantin® Dilaudid®	(dye lan′ tin) (dye law′ did)
Dilantin® diltiazem	(dye lan′ tin) (dil tye′ a zem)
Dilantin® Dipentum®	(dye lan′ tin) (dye pen′ tum)
Dilaudid® Dilantin®	(dye law′ did) (dye lan′ tin)
diltiazem Dilantin®	(dil tye′ a zem) (dye lan′ tin)
dimenhydrinate diphenhydramine	(dye men hye′ dri nate) (dye fen hye′ dra meen)
Dimetabs® Dimetapp®	(dime′ tabs) (dime′ tap)
Dimetapp® Dimetabs®	(dime′ tap) (dime′ tabs)
Dipentum® Dilantin®	(dye pen′ tum) (dye lan′ tin)
diphenhydramine dimenhydrinate	(dye fen hye′ dra meen) (dye men hye′ dri nate)
Diphenatol® diphenidiol	(dye fen′ ah tol) (dye fen′ i dole)
diphenidiol Diphenatol®	(dye fen′ i dole) (dye fen′ ah tol)
Diphenylan® dyphenylan	(dye fen′ eh lan) (dye fen′ eh lan)
Diprivan® Diflucan®	(dye′ pri van) (dye flu′ can)
Diprivan® Ditropan®	(dip′ riv an) (di troe′ pan)

APPENDIX

Drug Name	Pronunciation	Drug Name	Pronunciation
dipyridamole	(dye peer id' a mole)	Dymelor®	(dye' meh lo)
disopyramide	(dye soe peer' a mide)	Demerol®	(dem' eh rol)
Disophrol®	(dye' so frol)	Dymelor®	(dye' meh lor)
Desferal®	(des' fer al)	Pamelor®	(pam' meh lor)
disopyramide	(dye soe peer' a mide)	Dynabac®	(dye' na bac)
dipyridamole	(dye peer id' a mole)	Dynapen®	(dye' na pen)
Ditropan®	(di troe' pan)	Dynacin®	(dye' na sin)
Diprivan®	(dip' riv an)	Dyazide®	(dye' a zide)
Ditropan®	(di troe' pan)	Dynacin®	(dye' na sin)
Intropin®	(in troe' pin)	Dynapen®	(dye' ne pen)
Diutensin®	(dye yu ten' sin)	Dynapen®	(dye' na pen)
Salutensin®	(sal yu ten' sin)	Dynabac®	(dye' na bac)
dobutamine	(doe byoo' ta meen)	Dynapen®	(dye' ne pen)
dopamine	(doe' pa meen)	Dynacin®	(dye' na sin)
docusate	(dok' yoo sate)	dyphenylan	(dye fen' eh lan)
Doxinate®	(dox' eh nate)	Diphenylan®	(dye fen' eh lan)
Donnapine®	(don' a peen)	Dyrenium®	(dye ren' e um)
Donnazyme®	(don' a zime)	Pyridium®	(pye rid' dee um)
Donnazyme®	(don' a zime)	Dwelle®	(dwell)
Donnapine®	(don' a peen)	Kwell®	(kwell)
dopamine	(doe' pa meen)	Ecotrin®	(eh' ko trin)
dobutamine	(doe byoo' ta meen)	Edecrin®	(ed' eh crin)
dopamine	(doe' pa meen)	Edecrin®	(ed' eh crin)
Dopram®	(doe' pram)	Ecotrin®	(eh' ko trin)
Dopar®	(doe' par)	Edecrin®	(ed' eh crin)
Dopram®	(doe' pram)	Ethaquin®	(eth' a kwin)
Dopram®	(doe' pram)	Elavil®	(el' a vil)
dopamine	(doe' pa meen)	Aldoril®	(al' doe ril)
Dopram®	(doe' pram)	Elavil®	(el' a vil)
Dopar®	(doe' par)	Eldepryl®	(el' de pril)
doxepin	(dox' e pin)	Elavil®	(el' a vil)
Doxidan®	(dox' e dan)	Equanil®	(eh' kwa nil)
Doxidan®	(dox' e dan)	Elavil®	(el' a vil)
doxepin	(dox' e pin)	Mellaril®	(mel' la ril)
Doxinate®	(dox' eh nate)	Elavil®	(el' a vil)
docusate	(dok' yoo sate)	Oruvail®	(or' yu vale)
doxorubicin	(dox o roo' bi sin)	Eldepryl®	(el' de pril)
daunorubicin	(daw noe roo' bi sin)	Elavil®	(el' a vil)
Duo-Cyp®	(du' o sip)	Elixicon®	(eh lix' i con)
DuoCet™	(du' o set)	Elocon®	(ee' lo con)
DuoCet™	(du' o set)	Elocon®	(ee' lo con)
Duo-Cyp®	(du' o sep)	Elixicon®	(eh lix' i con)
Dura-Gest®	(dur' a gest)	emetine	(em' eh teen)
Duragen®	(dur' a gen)	Emetrol®	(em' eh trol)
Duragen®	(dur' a gen)	Emetrol®	(em' eh trol)
Dura-Gest®	(dur' a gest)	emetine	(em' eh teen)
Dyazide®	(dye' a zide)	enalapril	(e nal' a pril)
Dynacin®	(dye' na sin)	Anafranil®	(a naf' ra nil)

Drug Name	Pronunciation	Drug Name	Pronunciation
Endal®	(en′ dal)	ethosuximide	(eth o sux′ i mide)
Intal®	(in′ tal)	methsuximide	(meth sux′ i mide)
Enduron®	(en′ du ron)	etidocaine	(e ti′ doe kane)
Imuran®	(im′ yu ran)	etidronate	(e ti droe′ nate)
Enduron®	(en′ du ron)	etidronate	(e ti droe′ nate)
Inderal®	(in′ der al)	etidocaine	(e ti′ doe kane)
Enduronyl®	(en dur′ o nil)	etidronate	(e ti droe′ nate)
Inderal®	(in′ der al)	etretinate	(e tret′ i nate)
Enduronyl® Forte	(en dur′ o nil for′ tay)	etretinate	(e tret′ i nate)
Inderal® 40	(in′ der al for′ tee)	etidronate	(e ti droe′ nate)
enflurane	(en′ floo rane)	Eurax®	(yoor′ aks)
isoflurane	(eye soe flure′ ane)	Serax®	(sear′ aks)
Enkaid®	(enn′ kaid)	Eurax®	(yoor′ aks)
Cankaid®	(kan′ kaid)	Urex®	(yu′ eks)
ephedrine	(e fed′ rin)	Factrel®	(fak′ trel)
Epifrin®	(ep′ eh frin)	Sectral®	(sek′ tral)
EpiPen®	(ep′ eh pen)	Feldene®	(fel′ deen)
Epifrin®	(ep′ eh frin)	Seldane®	(sel′ dane)
Epifrin®	(ep′ eh frin)	fenoprofen	(fen o proe′ fen)
ephedrine	(e fed′ rin)	flurbiprofen	(flure bi′ proe fen)
Epifrin®	(ep′ eh frin)	Feosol®	(fee′ o sol)
EpiPen®	(ep′ eh pen)	Fer-In-Sol®	(fehr′ in sol)
Epinal®	(ep′ eh nal)	Feosol®	(fee′ o sol)
Epitol®	(ep′ eh tol)	Festal®	(fes′ tal)
Epitol®	(ep′ eh tol)	Feosol®	(fee′ o sol)
Epinal®	(ep′ eh nal)	Fluosol®	(flu′ o sol)
Equanil®	(eh′ kwa nil)	Fer-In-Sol®	(fehr′ in sol)
Elavil®	(el′ a vil)	Feosol®	(fee′ o sol)
erythromycin	(er ith roe mye′ sin)	Festal®	(fes′ tal)
clarithromycin	(kla rith′ roe mye sin)	Feosol®	(fee′ o sol)
Esimil®	(es′ eh mil)	Feverall™	(fee′ ver all)
Estinyl®	(es′ teh nil)	Fiberall®	(fye′ ber all)
Esimil®	(es′ eh mil)	Fiberall®	(fye′ ber all)
Ismelin®	(is′ meh lin)	Feverall™	(fee′ ver all)
Esimil®	(es′ eh mil)	Fioricet®	(fee oh′ reh set)
F.M.L.®	(ef′ em el)	Lorcet®	(lor′ set)
Estinyl®	(es′ teh nil)	Fiorinal®	(fee or′ reh nal)
Esimil®	(es′ eh mil)	Florinef®	(flor′ eh nef)
Estratab®	(es′ tra tab)	Flaxedil®	(flaks′ eh dil)
Ethatab®	(eth′ a tab)	Flexeril®	(fleks′ eh ril)
Eskalith®	(es′ ka lith)	Flexeril®	(fleks′ eh ril)
Estratest®	(es′ tra test)	Flaxedil®	(flaks′ eh dil)
Estratest®	(es′ tra test)	Flomax™	(flo′ maks)
Eskalith®	(es′ ka lith)	Fosamax®	(fos′ a maks)
Ethaquin®	(eth′ a kwin)	Florinef®	(flor′ eh nef)
Edecrin®	(ed′ eh crin)	Fiorinal®	(fee or′ reh nal)
Ethatab®	(eth′ a tab)	flunisolide	(floo nis′ o lide)
Estratab®	(es′ tra tab)	fluocinonide	(floo o sin′ o nide)

Drug Name	Pronunciation	Drug Name	Pronunciation
fluocinolone	(floo o sin' o lone)	Glucotrol®	(glue' co trol)
fluocinonide	(floo o sin' o nide)	Glucophage®	(glue' co faagsch)
fluocinonide	(floo o sin' o nide)	Glycotuss®	(glye' co tuss)
flunisolide	(floo nis' o lide)	Glytuss®	(glye' tuss)
fluocinonide	(floo o sin' o nide)	Glytuss®	(glye' tuss)
fluocinolone	(floo o sin' o lone)	Glycotuss®	(glye' co tuss)
Fluosol®	(flu' o sol)	gonadorelin	(goe nad o rell' in)
Feosol®	(fee' o sol)	guanadrel	(gwahn' a drel)
flurbiprofen	(flure bi' proe fen)	Gonak™	(gon' ak)
fenoprofen	(fen o proe' fen)	Gonic®	(gon' ik)
F.M.L.®	(ef' em el)	Gonic®	(gon' ik)
Esimil®	(es' eh mil)	Gonak™	(gon' ak)
Fosamax®	(fos' a maks)	guaifenesin	(gwye fen' e sin)
Flomax™	(flo' maks)	guanfacine	(gwahn' fa seen)
Fostex®	(fos' teks)	guanadrel	(gwahn' a drel)
pHisoHex®	(fye' so heks)	gonadorelin	(goe nad o rell' in)
Fulvicin®	(ful' vi sin)	guanethidine	(gwahn eth' i deen)
Furacin®	(fur' a sin)	guanidine	(gwahn' i deen)
Furacin®	(fur' a sin)	guanfacine	(gwahn' fa seen)
Fulvicin®	(ful' vi sin)	guaifenesin	(gwye fen' e sin)
Gamastan®	(gam' a stan)	guanidine	(gwahn' i deen)
Garamycin®	(gar a mye' sin)	guanethidine	(gwahn eth' i deen)
Gantanol®	(gan' ta nol)	Haldol®	(hal' dol)
Gantrisin®	(gan' tri sin)	Halenol®	(hal' e nol)
Gantrisin®	(gan' tri sin)	Haldol®	(hal' dol)
Gantanol®	(gan' ta nol)	Halog®	(hay' log)
Gantrisin®	(gan' tri sin)	Halenol®	(hal' e nol)
Gastrosed™	(gas' troe sed)	Haldol®	(hal' dol)
Garamycin®	(gar a mye' sin)	Halfan®	(hal' fan)
Gamastan®	(gam' a stan)	Halfprin®	(half' prin)
Garamycin®	(gar a mye' sin)	Halfprin®	(half' prin)
kanamycin	(kan a mye' sin)	Halfan®	(hal' fan)
Garamycin®	(gar a mye' sin)	Halfprin®	(half' prin)
Terramycin®	(tehr a mye' sin)	Haltran®	(hal' tran)
Gastrosed™	(gas' troe sed)	Halog®	(hay' log)
Gantrisin®	(gan' tri sin)	Haldol®	(hal' dol)
Genapap®	(gen' a pap)	Halotestin®	(hay lo tes' tin)
Genapax®	(gen' a paks)	Halotex®	(hay' lo teks)
Genapap®	(gen' a pap)	Halotestin®	(hay lo tes' tin)
Genatap®	(gen' a tap)	Halotussin®	(hay lo tus' sin)
Genapax®	(gen' a paks)	Halotex®	(hay' lo teks)
Genapap®	(gen' a pap)	Halotestin®	(hay lo tes' tin)
Genatap®	(gen' a tap)	Halotussin®	(hay lo tus' sin)
Genapap®	(gen' a pap)	Halotestin®	(hay lo tes' tin)
gentamicin	(jen ta mye' sin)	Haltran®	(hal' tran)
kanamycin	(kan a mye' sin)	Halfprin®	(half' prin)
Glucophage®	(glue' co faagsch)	Herplex®	(her' pleks)
Glucotrol®	(glue' co trol)	Hiprex®	(hi' preks)

Drug Name	Pronunciation	Drug Name	Pronunciation
Hespan®	(hes' pan)	HyperHep®	(hye' per hep)
Histaspan®	(his' ta span)	Hyper-Tet®	(hye' per tet)
Hexadrol®	(heks' a drol)	Hyperab®	(hye' per ab)
Hexalol®	(heks' a drol)	HyperHep®	(hye' per hep)
Hexalol®	(heks' a drol)	Hyperstat®	(hye' per stat)
Hexadrol®	(heks' a drol)	Hyper-Tet®	(hye' per tet)
Hiprex®	(hi' preks)	Hyperstat®	(hye' per stat)
Herplex®	(her' pleks)	Nitrostat®	(nye' troe stat)
Histaspan®	(his' ta span)	Hytone®	(hye' tone)
Hespan®	(hes' pan)	Vytone®	(vye' tone)
bp#Hycamtin®	(hye cam' tin)	Idamycin®	(eye da mye' sin)
Hycomine®	(hye' co meen)	Adriamycin™	(ade rya mye' sin)
Hycodan®	(hye' co dan)	imipramine	(im ip' ra meen)
Hycomine®	(hye' co meen)	amitripyline	(a mee trip' ti leen)
Hycodan®	(hye' co dan)	imipramine	(im ip' ra meen)
Vicodin®	(vye' co din)	Norpramin®	(nor pray' min)
Hycomine®	(hye' coe meen)	Imuran®	(im' yu ran)
Byclomine®	(bye' clo meen)	Enduron®	(en' du ron)
Hycomine®	(hye' co meen)	Inapsine®	(i nap' seen)
Hycamtin®	(hye cam' tin)	Nebcin®	(neb' sin)
Hycomine®	(hye' co meen)	Inderal®	(in' der al)
Hycodan®	(hye' co dan)	Adderall®	(ad' der all)
Hydergine®	(hye' der geen)	Inderal®	(in' der al)
Hydramyn®	(hye' dra min)	Enduron®	(en' du ron)
hydralazine	(hye dral' a zeen)	Inderal®	(in' der al)
hydroxyzine	(hye drox' i zeen)	Enduronyl®	(en dur' o nil)
Hydramyn®	(hye' dra min)	Inderal®	(in' der al)
Hydergine®	(hye' der geen)	Isordil®	(eye' sor dil)
Hydramyn®	(hye' dra min)	Inderal®	(in' der al)
Bydramine®	(bye' dra meen)	Medrol®	(meh' drol)
Hydrocet®	(hye' dro set)	Inderal® 40	(in' der al for' tee)
Hydrocil®	(hye' dro sil)	Enduronyl® Forte	(en dur' o nil for' tay)
Hydrocil®	(hye' dro sil)	Indocin®	(in' doe sin)
Hydrocet®	(hye' dro set)	Lincocin®	(lin' coe sin)
hydroxyurea	(hye drox ee yoor ee' a)	Indocin®	(in' doe sin)
hydroxyzine	(hye drox' i zeen)	Minocin®	(min' o sin)
hydroxyzine	(hye drox' i zeen)	Intal®	(in' tal)
hydralazine	(hye dral' a zeen)	Endal®	(en' dal)
hydroxyzine	(hye drox' i zeen)	Intropin®	(in tro' pin)
hydroxyurea	(hye drox ee yoor ee' a)	Isoptin®	(eye sop' tin)
Hygroton®	(hye gro' ton)	Intropin®	(in troe' pin)
Regroton®	(reg' ro ton)	Ditropan®	(di troe' pan)
Hyper-Tet®	(hye' per tet)	Ismelin®	(is' meh lin)
HyperHep®	(hye' per hep)	Esimil®	(es' eh mil)
Hyper-Tet®	(hye' per tet)	Ismelin®	(is' meh lin)
Hyperstat®	(hye' per stat)	Ritalin®	(ri' ta lin)
HyperHep®	(hye' per hep)	isoflurane	(eye soe flure' ane)
Hyperab®	(hye' per ab)	enflurane	(en' floo rane)

Drug Name	Pronunciation	Drug Name	Pronunciation
isoflurane	(eye soe flure' ane)	Lanoxin®	(lan ox' in)
isoflurophate	(eye soe flure' o fate)	Levsinex®	(lev' si neks)
isoflurophate	(eye soe flure' o fate)	Lanoxin®	(lan ox' in)
isoflurane	(eye soe flure' ane)	Mefoxin®	(me fox' in)
Isoptin®	(eye sop' tin)	Larylgan®	(la ril' gan)
Intropin®	(in tro' pin)	Auralgan®	(a ral' gan)
Isoptin®	(eye sop' tin)	Lasix®	(lay' siks)
Isopto® Tears	(eye sop' tow tears)	Lidex®	(lye' deks)
Isopto® Tears	(eye sop' tow tears)	leucovorin	(loo koe vor' in)
Isoptin®	(eye sop' tin)	Leukeran®	(lu' keh ran)
Isordil®	(eye' sor dil)	Leukeran®	(lu' keh ran)
Inderal®	(in' der al)	leucovorin	(loo koe vor' in)
Isordil®	(eye' sor dil)	levodopa	(lee voe doe' pa)
Isuprel®	(eye' sue prel)	methyldopa	(meth ill doe' pa)
Isuprel®	(eye' sue prel)	levothyroxine	(lee voe thye rox' een)
Isordil®	(eye' sor dil)	liothyronine	(lye o thye' roe neen)
K-Lor™	(kay' lor)	Levoxine®	(lev ox een)
Kaochlor®	(kay' o klor)	Lanoxin®	(lan ox' in)
kanamycin	(kan a mye' sin)	Levsinex®	(lev' si neks)
Garamycin®	(gar a mye' sin)	Lanoxin®	(lan ox' in)
kanamycin	(kan a mye' sin)	Lidex®	(lye' deks)
gentamicin	(jen ta mye' sin)	Lasix®	(lay' siks)
Kaochlor®	(kay' o klor)	Lidex®	(lye' deks)
K-Lor™	(kay' lor)	Lidox®	(lye' dox)
Keflex®	(keh' fleks)	Lidex®	(lye' deks)
Keflin®	(keh' flin)	Videx®	(vye' deks)
Keflin®	(keh' flin)	Lidex®	(lye' deks)
Keflex®	(keh' fleks)	Wydase®	(wye' dase)
Kemadrin®	(kem' a drin)	Lidox®	(lye' dox)
Coumadin®	(ku' ma din)	Lidex®	(lye' deks)
Klonopin™	(klon' o pin)	Lincocin®	(link' o sin)
clonidine	(kloe' ni deen)	Cleocin®	(klee' o sin)
Komex®	(koe' meks)	Lincocin®	(lin' coe sin)
Koromex®	(kor' o meks)	Indocin®	(in' doe sin)
Koromex®	(kor' o meks)	Lincocin®	(link' o sin)
Komex®	(koe' meks)	Minocin®	(min' o sin)
Kwell®	(kwell)	Lioresal®	(lye or' reh sal)
Dwelle®	(dwell)	lisinopril	(lyse in' o pril)
Lamictal®	(la mic' tal)	liothyronine	(lye o thye' roe neen)
Lamisil®	(lam' eh sil)	levothyroxine	(lee voe thye rox' een)
Lamisil®	(lam' eh sil)	lisinopril	(lyse in' o pril)
Lamictal®	(la mic' tal)	Lioresal®	(lye or' reh sal)
lamotrigine	(la moe' tri jeen)	Lithane®	(lith' ane)
lamivudine	(la mi' vyoo deen)	Lithonate®	(lith' o nate)
lamivudine	(la mi' vyoo deen)	Lithonate®	(lith' o nate)
lamotrigine	(la moe' tri jeen)	Lithane®	(lith' ane)
Lanoxin®	(lan ox' in)	Lithostat®	(lith' o stat)
Levoxine®	(lev ox een)	Lithotabs®	(lith' o tabs)

Drug Name	Pronunciation	Drug Name	Pronunciation
Lithotabs®	(lith′ o tabs)	Marcaine®	(mar′ kane)
Lithostat®	(lith′ o stat)	Narcan®	(nar′ kan)
Lodine®	(low′ deen)	Marinol®	(mare′ i nole)
codeine	(koe′ deen)	Marnal®	(mar′ nal)
Lomodix®	(lo′ mo dix)	Marnal®	(mar′ nal)
Lovenox®	(lo′ ve nox)	Marinol®	(mare′ i nole)
Loniten®	(lon′ eh ten)	Matulane®	(mat′ chu lane)
clonidine	(kloe′ ni deen)	Modane®	(moe′ dane)
Lopressor®	(lo pres′ sor)	Maxidex®	(maks′ i deks)
Lopurin®	(lo pure′ in)	Maxzide®	(maks′ zide)
Lopurin®	(lo pure′ in)	Maxzide®	(maks′ zide)
Lopressor®	(lo pres′ sor)	Maxidex®	(maks′ i deks)
Lopurin®	(lo pure′ in)	Mebaral®	(meb′ a ral)
Lupron®	(lu′ pron)	Medrol®	(med′ role)
Lorcet®	(lor′ set)	Mebaral®	(meb′ a ral)
Fioricet®	(fee oh′ reh set)	Mellaril®	(mel′ a ril)
Lotrimin®	(low′ tri min)	Mebaral®	(meb′ a ral)
Otrivin®	(oh′ tri vin)	Tegretol®	(teg′ ree tol)
Lovenox®	(lo′ ve nox)	mecamylamine	(mek a mill′ a meen)
Lomodix®	(lo′ mo dix)	mesalamine	(me sal′ a meen)
Luminal®	(lu′ mi nal)	Meclan®	(me′ klan)
Tuinal®	(tu′ i nal)	Meclomen®	(meh′ klo men)
Lupron®	(lu′ pron)	Meclan®	(me′ klan)
Lopurin®	(lo pure′ in)	Mezlin®	(mes′ lin)
Lupron®	(lu′ pron)	Meclomen®	(meh′ klo men)
Nuprin®	(nu′ prin)	Meclan®	(me′ klan)
Maalox®	(may′ loks)	Medrol®	(med′ role)
		Mebaral®	(meb′ a ral)
Maalox®	(may′ loks)	Medrol®	(meh′ drol)
Maox®	(may′ oks)	Inderal®	(in′ der al)
Marax®	(mare′ aks)		
Maalox®	(may′ loks)	Mefoxin®	(me fox′ in)
Monodox®	(mon′ o doks)	Lanoxin®	(lan ox′ in)
Maltsupex®	(malt′ su peks)	Mellaril®	(mel′ la ril)
Manoplax®	(man′ o laks)	Elavil®	(el′ a vil)
Mandol®	(man′ dole)	Mellaril®	(mel′ a ril)
nadolol	(nay doe′ lole)	Mebaral®	(meb′ a ral)
Manoplax®	(man′ o laks)	melphalan	(mel′ fa lan)
Maltsupex®	(malt′ su peks)	Mephyton®	(meh fye′ ton)
Maox®	(may′ oks)	mephenytoin	(me fen′ i toyn)
Maalox®	(may′ loks)	Mephyton®	(meh fye′ ton)
Maox®	(may′ oks)	mephenytoin	(me fen′ i toyn)
Marax®	(may′ raks)	Mesantoin®	(meh san′ toyn)
Marax®	(mare′ aks)	mephenytoin	(me fen′ i toyn)
Maalox®	(may′ loks)	phenytoin	(fen′ i toyn)
Marax®	(may′ raks)	mephobarbital	(me foe bar′ bi tal)
Atarax®	(at′ a raks)	methocarbamol	(meth o kar′ ba mole)
Marax®	(may′ raks)	Mephyton®	(meh fye′ ton)
Maox®	(may′ oks)	melphalan	(mel′ fa lan)

APPENDIX

Drug Name	Pronunciation	Drug Name	Pronunciation
Mephyton®	(meh fye' ton)	metyrapone	(me teer' a pone)
mephenytoin	(me fen' i toyn)	metyrosine	(me tye' roe seen)
Mephyton®	(meh fye' ton)	metyrosine	(me tye' roe seen)
methadone	(meth' a done)	metyrapone	(me teer' a pone)
mepivacaine	(me piv' a kane)	Mexitil®	(meks' i til)
bupivacaine	(byoo piv' a kane)	Mezlin®	(mes' lin)
Meprospan®	(meh' pro span)	Mezlin®	(mes' lin)
Naprosyn®	(na' pro sin)	Meclan®	(me' klan)
mesalamine	(me sal' a meen)	Mezlin®	(mes' lin)
mecamylamine	(mek a mill' a meen)	Mexitil®	(meks' i til)
Mesantoin®	(meh san' toyn)	mezlocillin	(mez loe sill' in)
mephenytoin	(me fen' i toyn)	methicillin	(meth i sill' in)
Mesantoin®	(meh san' toyn)	miconazole	(mi kon' a zole)
Mestinon®	(meh' sti non)	Micronase®	(mye' croe nase)
Mestinon®	(meh' sti non)	Micronase®	(mye' croe nase)
Mesantoin®	(meh san' toyn)	Micronor®	(mye' croe nor)
Metahydrin®	(me ta hye' drin)	Micronase®	(mye' croe nase)
Metandren®	(me tan' dren)	miconazole	(mi kon' a zole)
Metandren®	(me tan' dren)	Micronor®	(mye' croe nor)
Metahydrin®	(me ta hye' drin)	Micronase®	(mye' croe nase)
metaproterenol	(met a proe ter' e nol)	Midrin®	(mid' rin)
metoprolol	(me toe' proe lole)	Mydfrin®	(mid' frin)
metaxalone	(me taks' a lone)	Milontin®	(mi lon' tin)
metolazone	(me tole' a zone)	Miltown®	(mil' town)
methadone	(meth' a done)	Milontin®	(mi lon' tin)
Mephyton®	(meh fye' ton)	Mylanta®	(mye lan' tah)
methazolamide	(meth a zoe' la mide)	Miltown®	(mil' town)
metolazone	(me tole' a zone)	Milontin®	(mi lon' tin)
methenamine	(meth en' a meen)	Minizide®	(min' i zide)
methionine	(me thye' o neen)	Minocin®	(min' o sin)
methicillin	(meth i sill' in)	Minocin®	(min' o sin)
mezlocillin	(mez loe sill' in)	Indocin®	(in' doe sin)
methionine	(me thye' o neen)	Minocin®	(min' o sin)
methenamine	(meth en' a meen)	Lincocin®	(link' o sin)
methocarbamol	(meth o kar' ba mole)	Minocin®	(min' o sin)
mephobarbital	(me foe bar' bi tal)	Minizide®	(min' i zide)
methsuximide	(meth sux' i mide)	Minocin®	(min' o sin)
ethosuximide	(eth o sux' i mide)	Mithracin®	(mith' ra sin)
methyldopa	(meth ill doe' pa)	Minocin®	(min' o sin)
levodopa	(lee voe doe' pa)	niacin	(nye' a sin)
metolazone	(me tole' a zone)	minoxidil	(mi nox' i dill)
metaxalone	(me taks' a lone)	metolazone	(me tole' a zone)
metolazone	(me tole' a zone)	Mithracin®	(mith' ra sin)
methazolamide	(meth a zoe' la mide)	Minocin®	(min' o sin)
metolazone	(me tole' a zone)	mitomycin	(mye toe mye' sin)
minoxidil	(mi nox' i dill)	Mutamycin®	(mute a mye' sin)
metoprolol	(me toe' proe lole)	Moban®	(moe' ban)
metaproterenol	(met a proe ter' e nol)	Modane®	(moe' dane)

Drug Name	Pronunciation
Modane®	(moe' dane)
Matulane®	(mat' chu lane)
Modane®	(moe' dane)
Moban®	(moe' ban)
Modicon®	(mod' i kon)
Mylicon®	(mye' li kon)
moexipril	(mo ex' i pril)
Monopril®	(mon' oh pril)
Monodox®	(mon' o doks)
Maalox®	(may' loks)
Monopril®	(mon' oh pril)
moexipril	(mo ex' i pril)
Mutamycin®	(mute a mye' sin)
mitomycin	(mye toe mye' sin)
Myambutol®	(mya am' byoo tol)
Nembutal®	(nem' byoo tal)
Mycelex®	(mye' si leks)
Myoflex®	(mye' o fleks)
Mycifradin®	(mye ce fray' din)
Mycitracin®	(mye ce tray' sin)
Mycitracin®	(mye ce tray' sin)
Mycifradin®	(mye ce fray' din)
Mydfrin®	(mid' frin)
Midrin®	(mid' rin)
Mylanta®	(mye lan' tah)
Milontin®	(mi lon' tin)
Myleran®	(mye' leh ran)
Mylicon®	(mye' li kon)
Mylicon®	(mye' li kon)
Modicon®	(mod' i kon)
Mylicon®	(mye' li kon)
Myleran®	(mye' leh ran)
Myochrysine®	(mye o kris' seen)
vincristine	(vin kris' teen)
Myoflex®	(mye' o fleks)
Mycelex®	(mye' si leks)
nadolol	(nay doe' lole)
Mandol®	(man' dole)
Naldecon®	(nal' dee kon)
Nalfon®	(nal' fon)
Nalfon®	(nal' fon)
Naldecon®	(nal' dee kon)
Nallpen®	(nall' pen)
Nalspan®	(nal' span)
naloxone	(nal ox' one)
naltrexone	(nal treks' one)
Nalspan®	(nal' span)
Nallpen®	(nall' pen)

Drug Name	Pronunciation
naltrexone	(nal treks' one)
naloxone	(nal ox' one)
Naprosyn®	(na' pro sin)
Meprospan®	(meh' pro span)
Naprosyn®	(na' pro sin)
naproxen	(na prox' en)
Naprosyn®	(na' pro sin)
Natacyn®	(na' ta sin)
Naprosyn®	(na' pro sin)
Nebcin®	(neb' sin)
naproxen	(na prox' en)
Naprosyn®	(na' pro sin)
Narcan®	(nar' kan)
Marcaine®	(mar' kane)
Nardil®	(nar' dil)
Norinyl®	(nor' eh nil)
Nasacort®	(nay' sa cort)
Nasalcrom®	(nay' sal crome)
Nasalcrom®	(nay' sal crome)
Nasacort®	(nay' sa cort)
Natacyn®	(na' ta sin)
Naprosyn®	(na' pro sin)
Navane®	(nav' ane)
Norvasc®	(nor' vask)
Nebcin®	(neb' sin)
Inapsine®	(i nap' seen)
Nebcin®	(neb' sin)
Naprosyn®	(na' pro sin)
nelfinavir	(nel fin' a vir)
nevirapine	(ne vir' a peen)
Nembutal®	(nem' byoo tal)
Myambutol®	(mya am' byoo tol)
Neptazane®	(nep' ta zane)
Nesacaine®	(nes' a kane)
Nesacaine®	(nes' a kane)
Neptazane®	(nep' ta zane)
Neupogen®	(nu' po gen)
Nutramigen®	(nu' tra gen)
nevirapine	(ne vir' a peen)
nelfinavir	(nel fin' a vir)
niacin	(nye' a sin)
Minocin®	(min' o sin)
nicardipine	(nye kar' de peen)
nifedipine	(nye fed' i peen)
Nicobid®	(nye' ko bid)
Nitro-Bid®	(nye' troe bid)
Nicorette®	(nik' o ret)
Nordette®	(nor det')

APPENDIX

Drug Name	Pronunciation	Drug Name	Pronunciation
nifedipine	(nye fed' i peen)	olsalazine sodium	(ole sal' a zeen)
nicardipine	(nye kar' de peen)	olanzapine	(oh lan' za peen)
nifedipine	(nye fed' i peen)	Omnipaque®	(om' ni pak)
nimodipine	(nye moe' di peen)	Omnipen®	(om' ni pen)
nifedipine	(nye fed' i peen)	Omnipen®	(om' ni pen)
nisoldipine	(nye' sole di peen)	Omnipaque®	(om' ni pak)
Nilstat®	(nil' stat)	Omnipen®	(om' ni pen)
Nitrostat®	(nye' troe stat)	Unipen®	(yu' ni pen)
Nimodipine	(nye moe' di peen)	Oncovin®	(on' coe vin)
nifedipine	(nye fed' i peen)	Ancobon®	(an' coe bon)
nisoldipine	(nye' sole di peen)	Ophthaine®	(op' thane)
nifedipine	(nye fed' i peen)	Ophthetic®	(op thet' ik)
Nitro-Bid®	(nye' troe bid)	Ophthalgan®	(opp thal' gan)
Nicobid®	(nye' ko bid)	Auralgan®	(a ral' gan)
Nitroglycerin	(nye troe gli' ser in)	Ophthetic®	(op thet' ik)
Nitroglyn®	(nye' troe glin)	Ophthaine®	(op' thane)
Nitroglyn®	(nye' troe glin)	Ophthochlor®	(op' tho klor)
nitroglycerin	(nye troe gli' ser in)	Ophthocort®	(op' tho kort)
Nitrostat®	(nye' troe stat)	Ophthocort®	(op' tho kort)
Hyperstat®	(hye' per stat)	Ophthochlor®	(op' tho klor)
Nitrostat®	(nye' troe stat)	Orabase®	(or' a base)
Nilstat®	(nil' stat)	Orinase®	(or' in ase)
Nordette®	(nor det')	Orasol®	(or' a sol)
Nicorette®	(nik' o ret)	Orasone®	(or' a sone)
Norinyl®	(nor' eh nil)	Orasone®	(or' a sone)
Nardil®	(nar' dil)	Orasol®	(or' a sol)
Norlutate®	(nor' lu tate)	Oretic®	(or et' ik)
Norlutin®	(nor lu' tin)	Oreton®	(or' eh ton)
Norlutin®	(nor lu' tin)	Oreton®	(or' eh ton)
Norlutate®	(nor' lu tate)	Oretic®	(or et' ik)
Norpramin®	(nor pray' min)	Orinase®	(or' in ase)
imipramine	(im ip' ra meen)	Orabase®	(or' a base)
Norvasc®	(nor' vask)	Orinase®	(or' in ase)
Navane®	(nav' ane)	Ornade®	(or' nade)
Norvasc®	(nor' vask)	Orinase®	(or' in ase)
Norvir®	(nor' vir)	Tolinase®	(tole' i nase)
Norvir®	(nor' vir)	Ornade®	(or' nade)
Norvasc®	(nor' vask)	Orinase®	(or' in ase)
Novafed®	(nove' a fed)	Otrivin®	(oh' tri vin)
Nucofed®	(nu' co fed)	Lotrimin®	(low' tri min)
Nucofed®	(nu' co fed)	Oruvail®	(or' yu vale)
Novafed®	(nove' a fed)	Elavil®	(el' a vil)
Nuprin®	(nu' prin)	oxymetazoline	(ox i met az' o leen)
Lupron®	(lu' pron)	oxymetholone	(ox i meth' o lone)
Nutramigen®	(nu' tra gen)	oxymetholone	(ox i meth' o lone)
Neupogen®	(nu' po gen)	oxymetazoline	(ox i met az' o leen)
olanzapine	(oh lan' za peen)	oxymetholone	(ox i meth' o lone)
olsalazine sodium	(ole sal' a zeen)	oxymorphone	(ox i mor' fone)

Drug Name	Pronunciation	Drug Name	Pronunciation
oxymorphone	(ox i mor' fone)	PhosLo®	(fos' lo)
oxymetholone	(ox i meth' o lone)	Phos-Flur®	(fos' flur)
Pamelor®	(pam' meh lor)	PhosLo®	(fos' lo)
Dymelor®	(dye' meh lor)	ProSom™	(pro' som)
Pathilon®	(path' i lon)	Phosphaljel®	(fos' fal gel)
Pathocil®	(path' o sil)	Phospholine®	(fos' fo leen)
Pathocil®	(path' o sil)	Phospholine®	(fos' fo leen)
Pathilon®	(path' i lon)	Phosphaljel®	(fos' fal gel)
Pathocil®	(path' o sil)	Phrenilin®	(fren' ni lin)
Placidyl®	(pla' ce dil)	Phenergan®	(fen' er gan)
Pathocil®	(path' o sill)	Phrenilin®	(fren' ni lin)
Bactocill®	(bak' tow sill)	Trinalin®	(tri' na lin)
Pavabid®	(pav' a bid)	physostigmine	(fye zoe stig' meen)
Pavased®	(pav' a sed)	Prostigmin®	(pro stig' min)
Pavased®	(pav' a sed)	physostigmine	(fye zoe stig' meen)
Pavabid®	(pav' a bid)	pyridostigmine	(peer id o stig' meen)
pentobarbital	(pen toe bar' bi tal)	Pitocin®	(pi toe' sin)
phenobarbital	(fee noe bar' bi tal)	Pitressin®	(ph tres' sin)
Percodan®	(per' coe dan)	Pitressin®	(ph tres' sin)
Decadron®	(dek' a dron)	Pitocin®	(ph toe' sin)
Perdiem®	(per dee' em)	Placidyl®	(pla' ce dil)
Pyridium®	(pye rid' dee um)	Pathocil®	(path' o sil)
Persantine®	(per san' teen)	Plaquenil®	(pla' kwe nil)
Pertofrane®	(per' toe frane)	Platinol®	(pla' tee nol)
Pertofrane®	(per' toe frane)	Platinol®	(pla' tee nol)
Persantine®	(per san' teen)	Plaquenil®	(pla' kwe nil)
Phazyme®	(fay' zeem)	Ponstel®	(pon' stel)
Pherazine®	(fer' a zeen)	Pronestyl®	(pro nes' til)
Phenergan®	(fen' er gan)	pralidoxime	(pra li dox' eem)
Phrenilin®	(fren' ni lin)	pramoxine	(pra moks' een)
Phenergan®	(fen' er gan)	pralidoxime	(pra li dox' eem)
Theragran®	(ther' a gran)	pyridoxine	(peer i dox' een)
phenobarbital	(fee noe bar' bi tal)	Pramosone®	(pra' mo sone)
pentobarbital	(pen toe bar' bi tal)	prednisone	(pred' ni sone)
phentermine	(fen' ter meen)	pramoxine	(pra moks' een)
phentolamine	(fen tole' a meen)	pralidoxime	(pra li dox' eem)
phentolamine	(fen tole' a meen)	prazepam	(pra' ze pam)
phentermine	(fen' ter meen)	prazosin	(pra' zoe sin)
phentolamine	(fen tole' a meen)	prazosin	(pra' zoe sin)
Ventolin®	(ven' to lin)	prazepam	(pra' ze pam)
phenytoin	(fen' i toyn)	Precare®	(pre' kare)
mephenytoin	(me fen' i toyn)	Precose®	(pre' kose)
Pherazine®	(fer' a zeen)	Precose®	(pre' kose)
Phazyme®	(fay' zeem)	Precare®	(pre' kare)
pHisoHex®	(fye' so heks)	Predalone®	(pred' a lone)
Fostex®	(fos' teks)	prednisone	(pred' ni sone)
Phos-Flur®	(fos' flur)	prednisolone	(pred nis' o lone)
PhosLo®	(fos' lo)	prednisone	(pred' ni sone)

Drug Name	Pronunciation	Drug Name	Pronunciation
prednisone	(pred' ni sone)	Protopam®	(proe' toe pam)
Pramosone®	(pra' mo sone)	protamine	(proe' ta meen)
prednisone	(pred' ni sone)	Protopam®	(proe' toe pam)
Predalone®	(pred' a lone)	Protropin®	(proe tro' pin)
prednisone	(pred' ni sone)	Protropin®	(proe tro' pin)
prednisolone	(pred nis' o lone)	Protopam®	(proe' toe pam)
prednisone	(pred' ni sone)	Prozac®	(proe' zak)
primidone	(pri' mi done)	Prilosec™	(pre' lo sek)
prilocaine	(pril' o kane)	Prozac®	(proe' zak)
Prilosec™	(pre' lo sek)	ProStep®	(proe' step)
Prilosec™	(pre' lo sek)	Pyridium®	(pye rid' dee um)
Prozac®	(proe' zak)	Dyrenium®	(dye ren' e um)
Prilosec™	(pre' lo sek)	Pyridium®	(pye rid' dee um)
prilocaine	(pril' o kane)	Perdiem®	(per dee' em)
primidone	(pri' mi done)	Pyridium®	(pye rid' dee um)
prednisone	(pred' ni sone)	pyridoxine	(peer i dox' een)
Priscoline®	(pris' coe leen)	Pyridium®	(pye rid' dee um)
Apresoline®	(aye press' sow leen)	pyrithione	(peer i thye' one)
Pro-Banthine®	(pro ban' theen)	pyridostigmine	(peer id o stig' meen)
Banthine®	(ban' theen)	physostigmine	(fye zoe stig' meen)
Pro-Sof®	(proe' sof)	pyridoxine	(peer i dox' een)
ProSom™	(pro' som)	Pyridium®	(pye rid' dee um)
ProSom™	(pro' som)	pyridoxine	(peer i dox' een)
PhosLo®	(fos' lo)	pralidoxime	(pra li dox' eem)
ProSom™	(pro' som)	pyrithione	(peer i thye' one)
Pro-Sof® Plus	(proe' sof)	Pyridium®	(pye rid' dee um)
ProStep®	(proe' step)	quinidine	(kwin' i deen)
Prozac®	(proe' zak)	clonidine	(kloe' ni deen)
procarbazine	(proe kar' ba zeen)	quinidine	(kwin' i deen)
dacarbazine	(da kar' ba zeen)	quinine	(kwye' nine)
promazine	(proe' ma zeen)	quinine	(kwye' nine)
promethazine	(proe meth' a zeen)	quinidine	(kwin' i deen)
Prometh®	(proe' meth)	Reglan®	(reg' lan)
Promit®	(proe' mit)	Regonol®	(reg' o nol)
promethazine	(proe meth' a zeen)	Regonol®	(reg' o nol)
promazine	(proe' ma zeen)	Reglan®	(reg' lan)
Promit®	(proe' mit)	Regonol®	(reg' o nol)
Prometh®	(proe' meth)	Regutol®	(reg' yu tol)
Pronestyl®	(pro nes' til)	Regroton®	(reg' ro ton)
Ponstel®	(pon' stel)	Hygroton®	(hye gro' ton)
Propacet®	(proe' pa set)	Regutol®	(reg' yu tol)
Propagest®	(proe' pa gest)	Regonol®	(reg' o nol)
Propagest®	(proe' pa gest)	remifentanil	(rem i fen' ta nil)
Propacet®	(proe' pa set)	alfentanil	(al fen' ta nil)
Prostigmin®	(pro stig' min)	Repan®	(ree' pan)
physostigmine	(fye zoe stig' meen)	Riopan®	(rye' o pan)
protamine	(proe' ta meen)	Restore®	(res tore')
Protopam®	(proe' toe pam)	Restoril®	(res' tor ril)

Drug Name	Pronunciation	Drug Name	Pronunciation
Restoril®	(res' tor ril)	Rythmol®	(rith' mol)
Restore®	(res tore')	Rhythmin®	(rith' min)
Restoril®	(res' tor ril)	Salacid®	(sal as' sid)
Vistaril®	(vis' tar ril)	Salagen®	(sal' a gen)
Retrovir®	(re' tro vir)	Salagen®	(sal' a gen)
ritonavir	ri ton' o vir)	Salacid®	(sal as' sid)
Revex®	(rev' ex)	Salutensin®	(sal yu ten' sin)
Revia®	(rev' ve ah)	Diutensin®	(dye yu ten' sin)
Revia®	(rev' ve ah)	saquinavir	(sa kwin' a veer)
Revex®	(rev' ex)	Sinequan®	(si' ne kwan)
Rhythmin®	(rith' min)	Seconal™	(sek' o nal)
Rythmol®	(rith' mol)	Sectral®	(sek' tral)
ribavirin	(rye ba vye' rin)	Sectral®	(sek' tral)
riboflavin	(rye' boe flay vin)	Factrel®	(fak' trel)
riboflavin	(rye' boe flay vin)	Sectral®	(sek' tral)
ribavirin	(rye ba vye' rin)	Seconal™	(sek' o nal)
Rifadin®	(rif' a din)	Seldane®	(sel' dane)
Ritalin®	(ri' ta lin)	Feldene®	(fel' deen)
Rimactane®	(ri mak' tane)	Septa®	(sep' tah)
rimantadine	(ri man' to deen)	Septra®	(sep' trah)
rimantadine	(ri man' to deen)	Septra®	(sep' trah)
Rimactane®	(ri mak' tane)	Septa®	(sep' tah)
rimantadine	(ri man' to deen)	Ser-Ap-Es®	(ser ap' ess)
amantadine	(a man' ta deen)	Catapres®	(kat' a pres)
Riobin®	(rye' o bin)	Serax®	(sear' aks)
Riopan®	(rye' o pan)	Eurax®	(yoor' aks)
Riopan®	(rye' o pan)	Serax®	(sear' aks)
Repan	(ree' pan)	Urex®	(yu' eks)
Riopan®	(rye' o pan)	Serax®	(sear' aks)
Riobin®	(rye' o bin)	Zyrtec®	(zir' tec)
Ritalin®	(ri' ta lin)	Serentil®	(su ren' til)
Ismelin®	(is' meh lin)	Surital®	(su' ri tal)
Ritalin®	(ri' ta lin)	Silace®	(sye' lace)
Rifadin®	(rif' a din)	Silain®	(sye' lain)
Ritalin®	(ri' ta lin)	Silain®	(sye' lain)
ritodrine	(ri' toe dreen)	Silace®	(sye' lace)
ritodrine	(ri' toe dreen)	Sinequan®	(si' ne kwan)
Ritalin®	(ri' ta lin)	saquinavir	(sa kwin' a veer)
ritonavir	ri ton' o vir)	Sinequan®	(si' ne kwan)
Retrovir®	(re' tro vir)	Seroquel®	(seer' oh kwel)
Rocephin®	(roe sef' fen)	Seroquel®	(seer' oh kwel)
Roferon®	(roe fer' on)	Sinequan®	(si' ne kwan)
Roferon®	(roe fer' on)	Solarcaine®	(sole' ar kane)
Rocephin®	(roe sef' fen)	Solatene®	(sole' a teen)
Rynatan®	(rye' na tan)	Solatene®	(sole' a teen)
Rynatuss®	(rye' na tuss)	Solarcaine®	(sole' ar kane)
Rynatuss®	(rye' na tuss)	Staphcillin®	(staf sil' lin)
Rynatan®	(rye' na tan)	Staticin®	(stat' i sin)

APPENDIX

Drug Name	Pronunciation	Drug Name	Pronunciation
Staticin®	(stat' i sin)	Tegretol®	(teg' ree tol)
Staphcillin®	(staf sil' lin)	Mebaral®	(meb' a ral)
streptomycin	(strep toe mye' sin)	Tegretol®	(teg' ree tol)
streptozocin	(strep toe zoe' sin)	Tegopen®	(teg' o pen)
streptozocin	(strep toe zoe' sin)	Tegrin®	(teg' rin)
streptomycin	(strep toe mye' sin)	Tegopen®	(teg' o pen)
Sudafed®	(sue' da fed)	Teldrin®	(tel' drin)
Sufenta®	(sue fen' tah)	Tedral®	(ted' ral)
Sufenta®	(sue fen' tah)	Temaril®	(tem' a ril)
Alfenta®	(al fen' tah)	Demerol®	(dem' eh rol)
Sufenta®	(sue fen' tah)	Temaril®	(tem' a ril)
Sudafed®	(sue' da fed)	Tepanil®	(tep' a nil)
sulfasalazine	(sul fa sal' a zeen)	Tenex®	(ten' eks)
sulfisoxazole	(sul fi sox' a zole)	Xanax®	(zan' aks)
sulfisoxazole	(sul fi sox' a zole)	Tepanil®	(tep' a nil)
sulfasalazine	(sul fa sal' a zeen)	Temaril®	(tem' a ril)
Suprax®	(su' prax)	Tepanil®	(tep' a nil)
Surbex®	(sur' beks)	Tofranil®	(toe fray' nil)
Surbex®	(sur' beks)	terbinafine	(ter' bin a feen)
Suprax®	(su' prax)	terfenadine	(ter fen' na deen)
Surbex®	(sur' beks)	terbinafine	(ter' bin a feen)
Surfak®	(sur' fak)	terbutaline	(ter byoo' ta leen)
Surfak®	(sur' fak)	terbutaline	(ter byoo' ta leen)
Surbex®	(sur' beks)	terbinafine	(ter' bin a feen)
Surital®	(su' ri tal)	terbutaline	(ter byoo' ta leen)
Serentil®	(su ren' til)	tolbutamide	(tole byoo' ta mide)
Sytobex®	(sye' toe beks)	terconazole	(ter kone' a zole)
Cytotec®	(sye' toe tek)	tioconazole	(tye o kone' a zole)
Tacaryl®	(tak' a ril)	terfenadine	(ter fen' na deen)
tacrine	(tak' reen)	terbinafine	(ter' bin a feen)
tacrine	(tak' reen)	Terramycin®	(tehr a mye' sin)
Tacaryl®	(tak' a ril)	Garamycin®	(gar a mye' sin)
Tagamet®	(tag' a met)	testolactone	(tess toe lak' tone)
Tegopen®	(teg' o pen)	testosterone	(tess toss' ter one)
Talacen®	(tal' a sen)	testosterone	(tess toss' ter one)
Tegison®	(teg' i son)	testolactone	(tess toe lak' tone)
Talacen®	(tal' a sen)	Theelin®	(thee' lin)
Tinactin®	(tin ak' tin)	Theolair™	(thee' o lare)
Tedral®	(ted' ral)	Theoclear®	(thee' o clear)
Teldrin®	(tel' drin)	Theolair™	(thee' o lare)
Tegison®	(teg' i son)	Theolair™	(thee' o lare)
Talacen®	(tal' a sen)	Theelin®	(thee' lin)
Tegopen®	(teg' o pen)	Theolair™	(thee' o lare)
Tagamet®	(tag' a met)	Theoclear®	(thee' o clear)
Tegopen®	(teg' o pen)	Theolair™	(thee' o lare)
Tegretol®	(teg' ree tol)	Thiola™	(thye oh' la)
Tegopen®	(teg' o pen)	Theolair™	(thee' o lare)
Tegrin®	(teg' rin)	Thyrolar®	(thye' roe lar)

Drug Name	Pronunciation	Drug Name	Pronunciation
Theragran®	(ther′ a gran)	Tobrex®	(toe′ breks)
Phenergan®	(fen′ er gan)	TobraDex®	(toe′ bra deks)
Theramin®	(there′ a min)	Tofranil®	(toe fray′ nil)
thiamine	(thye′ a min)	Tepanil®	(tep′ a nil)
thiamine	(thye′ a min)	tolazamide	(tole az′ a mide)
Theramin®	(there′ a min)	tolazoline	(tole az′ o leen)
Thiola™	(thye oh′ la)	tolazamide	(tole az′ a mide)
Theolair™	(thee′ o lare)	tolbutamide	(tole byoo′ ta mide)
thioridazine	(thye o rid′ a zeen)	tolazoline	(tole az′ o leen)
thiothixene	(thye o thix′ een)	tolazamide	(tole az′ a mide)
thiothixene	(thye o thix′ een)	tolbutamide	(tole byoo′ ta mide)
thioridazine	(thye o rid′ a zeen)	terbutaline	(ter byoo′ ta leen)
Thyrar®	(thyer′ are)	tolbutamide	(tole byoo′ ta mide)
Thyrolar®	(thye′ roe lar)	tolazamide	(tole az′ a mide)
Thyrar®	(thyer′ are)	Tolinase®	(tole′ i nase)
Ticar®	(tye′ kar)	Orinase®	(or′ in ase)
Thyrolar®	(thye′ roe lar)	tolnaftate	(tole naf′ tate)
Theolair™	(thee′ o lare)	Tornalate®	(tor′ na late)
Thyrolar®	(thye′ roe lar)	Tonocard®	(ton′ o kard)
Thyrar®	(thyer′ are)	Torecan®	(tor′ e kan)
Thyrolar®	(thye′ roe lar)	Torecan®	(tor′ e kan)
Thytropar®	(thye′ troe par)	Tonocard®	(ton′ o kard)
Thytropar®	(thye′ troe par)	Tornalate®	(tor′ na late)
Thyrolar®	(thye′ roe lar)	tolnaftate	(tole naf′ tate)
Ticar®	(tye′ kar)	Trandate®	(tran′ date)
Thyrar®	(thyer′ are)	Trendar®	(tren′ dar)
Ticar®	(tye′ kar)	Trandate®	(tran′ date)
Tigan®	(tye′ gan)	Trental®	(tren′ tal)
Ticon®	(tye′ kon)	Trendar®	(tren′ dar)
Tigan®	(tye′ gan)	Trandate®	(tran′ date)
Tigan®	(tye′ gan)	Trental®	(tren′ tal)
Ticar®	(tye′ kar)	Bentyl®	(ben′ til)
Tigan®	(tye′ gan)	Trental®	(tren′ tal)
Ticon®	(tye′ kon)	Tindal®	(tin′ dal)
timolol	(tye′ moe lole)	Trental®	(tren′ tal)
Tylenol®	(tye′ le nole)	Trandate®	(tran′ date)
Timoptic®	(tim op′ tik)	tretinoin	(tret′ i noyn)
Viroptic®	(vir op′ tik)	trientine	(trye′ en teen)
Tinactin®	(tin ak′ tin)	Tri-Levlen®	(trye′ lev len)
Talacen®	(tal′ a sen)	Trilafon®	(tri′ la fon)
Tindal®	(tin′ dal)	triacetin	(trye a see′ tin)
Trental®	(tren′ tal)	Triacin®	(trye′ a sin)
tioconazole	(tye o kone′ a zole)	Triacin®	(trye′ a sin)
terconazole	(ter kone′ a zole)	triacetin	(trye a see′ tin)
TobraDex®	(toe′ bra deks)	triamterene	(trye am′ ter een)
Tobrex®	(toe′ breks)	trimipramine	(trye mi′ pra meen)
tobramycin	(toe bra mye′ sin)	Triapin®	(trye a pin)
Trobicin®	(troe′ bi sin)	Triban®	(trye′ ban)

APPENDIX

Drug Name	Pronunciation	Drug Name	Pronunciation
triazolam	(trye ay′ zoe lam)	Tylenol®	(tye′ le nole)
alprazolam	(al pray′ zoe lam)	Tuinal®	(tu′ i nal)
Triban®	(trye′ ban)	Tylenol®	(tye′ le nole)
Triapin®	(trye a pin)	Tylox®	(tye′ loks)
trientine	(trye′ en teen)	Tylox®	(tye′ loks)
tretinoin	(tret′ i noyn)	Trimox®	(trye′ moks)
Trilafon®	(tri′ la fon)	Tylox®	(tye′ loks)
Tri-Levlen®	(trye′ lev len)	Tylenol®	(tye′ le nole)
trimeprazine	(trye mep′ ra zeen)	Tylox®	(tye′ loks)
trimipramine	(trye mi′ pra meen)	Wymox®	(wye′ moks)
trimethaphan	(trye meth′ a fan)	Uni-Bent®	(yu′ ni bent)
trimethoprim	(trye meth′ o prim)	Unipen®	(yu′ ni pen)
trimethoprim	(trye meth′ o prim)	Unipen®	(yu′ ni pen)
trimethaphan	(trye meth′ a fan)	Uni-Bent®	(yu′ ni bent)
trimipramine	(trye mi′ pra meen)	Unipen®	(yu′ ni pen)
triamterene	(trye am′ ter een)	Omnipen®	(om′ ni pen)
trimipramine	(trye mi′ pra meen)	Urex®	(yu′ eks)
trimeprazine	(trye mep′ ra zeen)	Eurax®	(yoor′ aks)
Trimox®	(trye′ moks)	Urex®	(yu′ eks)
Diamox®	(dye′ a moks)	Serax®	(sear′ aks)
Trimox®	(trye′ moks)	V-Cillin K®	(vee sil′ lin kay)
Tylox®	(tye′ loks)	Bicillin®	(bye sil′ lin)
Trinalin®	(tri′ na lin)	V-Cillin K®	(vee′ sil lin kay)
Phrenilin®	(fren′ ni lin)	Wycillin®	(wye sil′ lin)
Triofed®	(trye′ o fed)	Vamate®	(vam′ ate)
Triostat™	(tree′ o stat)	Vancenase®	(van′ sen ase)
Triostat™	(tree′ o stat)	Vancenase®	(van′ sen ase)
Triofed®	(trye′ o fed)	Vamate®	(vam′ ate)
Trisoralen®	(trye sore′ a len)	Vanceril®	(van′ ser il)
Trysul®	(trye′ sul)	Vansil™	(van′ sil)
Trobicin®	(troe′ bi sin)	Vansil™	(van′ sil)
tobramycin	(toe bra mye′ sin)	Vanceril®	(van′ ser il)
Tronolane®	(tron′ o lane)	Vasocidin®	(vay so sye′ din)
Tronothane®	(tron′ o thane)	Vasodilan®	(vay so di′ lan)
Tronothane®	(tron′ o thane)	Vasodilan®	(vay so di′ lan)
Tronolane®	(tron′ o lane)	Vasocidin®	(vay so sye′ din)
Trysul®	(trye′ sul)	Vasosulf®	(vay′ so sulf)
Trisoralen®	(trye sore′ a len)	Velosef®	(vel′ o sef)
Tuinal®	(tu′ i nal)	VePesid®	(veh′ pe sid)
Luminal®	(lu′ mi nal)	Versed®	(ver′ sed)
Tuinal®	(tu′ i nal)	Velosef®	(vel′ o sef)
Tylenol®	(tye′ le nole)	Vasosulf®	(vay′ so sulf)
Tussafed®	(tus′ a fed)	Ventolin®	(ven′ to lin)
Tussafin®	(tus′ a fin)	phentolamine	(fen tole′ a meen)
Tussafin®	(tus′ a fin)	Ventolin®	(ven′ tow lin)
Tussafed®	(tus′ a fed)	Benylin®	(ben′ eh lin)
Tylenol®	(tye′ le nole)	Verelan®	(ver′ e lan)
timolol	(tye′ moe lole)	Voltaren®	(vo tare′ en)

Drug Name	Pronunciation	Drug Name	Pronunciation
Versed®	(ver' sed)	Wymox®	(wye' moks)
VePesid®	(veh' pe sid)	Tylox®	(tye' loks)
Vicodin®	(vye' co din)	Xanax®	(zan' aks)
Hycodan®	(hye' co dan)	Tenex®	(ten' eks)
vidarabine	(vye dare' a been)	Xanax®	(zan' aks)
cytarabine	(sye tare' a been)	Zantac®	(zan' tak)
Videx®	(vye' deks)	Xalatan®	(za lan' tan)
Lidex®	(lye' deks)	Zarontin®	(za ron' tin)
vinblastine	(vin blas' teen)	Xylo-Pfan®	(zye' lo fan)
vincristine	(vin kris' teen)	Zyloprim®	(zye' lo prim)
vincristine	(vin kris' teen)	Yocon®	(yo' con)
Myochrysine®	(mye o kris' seen)	Zocor®	(zoe' cor)
vincristine	(vin kris' teen)	Zantac®	(zan' tak)
vinblastine	(vin blas' teen)	Xanax®	(zan' aks)
Viroptic®	(vir op' tik)	Zarontin®	(za ron' tin)
Timoptic®	(tim op' tik)	Xalatan®	(za lan' tan)
Visine®	(vye' seen)	Zarontin®	(za ron' tin)
Visken®	(vis' ken)	Zaroxolyn®	(za roks' o lin)
Visken®	(vis' ken)	Zaroxolyn®	(za roks' o lin)
Visine®	(vye' seen)	Zarontin®	(za ron' tin)
Vistaril®	(vis' tar ril)	Zerit®	(zer' it)
Restoril®	(res' tor ril)	Ziac™	(zye' ak)
Voltaren®	(vo tare' en)	Ziac™	(zye' ak)
Verelan®	(ver' e lan)	Zerit®	(zer' it)
Voltaren®	(vo tare' en)	Zocor®	(zoe' cor)
Vontrol®	(von' trole)	Cozaar®	(koe' zar)
Vontrol®	(von' trole)	Zocor®	(zoe' cor)
Voltaren®	(vo tare' en)	Yocon®	(yo' con)
Vytone®	(vye' tone)	Zofran®	(zoe' fran)
Hytone®	(hye' tone)	Zosyn™	(zoe' sin)
Vytone®	(vye' tone)	Zosyn™	(zoe' sin)
Zydone®	(zye' doan)	Zofran®	(zoe' fran)
Wycillin®	(wye sil' lin)	Zydone®	(zye' doan)
Bicillin®	(bye sil' lin)	Vytone®	(vye' tone)
Wycillin®	(wye sil' lin)	Zyloprim®	(zye' lo prim)
V-Cillin K®	(vee' sil lin kay)	Xylo-Pfan®	(zye' lo fan)
Wydase®	(wye' dase)	Zyrtec®	(zir' tec)
Lidex®	(lye' deks)	Serax®	(sear' aks)

WHAT'S NEW

New Drugs Introduced or Approved by the FDA in 1997

Brand Name	Generic Name	Use
Accolate®	zafirlukast	Asthma
Agrylin®	anagrelide	Thrombocythemia
Aldara®	imiquimod	External genital warts
Alphagan®	brimonidine	Glaucoma
Amaryl®	glimepiride	Type II diabetes
Aphthasol®	amlexanox	Aphthous ulcers
Aricept®	donepezil	Alzheimer's disease
Astelin®	azelastine	Antihistamine (allergic rhinitis)
Baycol®	cerivastatin	High cholesterol
Combivir®	zidovudine and lamivudine	HIV infection
Copaxone®	glatiramer acetate	Multiple sclerosis
Cystadane®	betaine anhydrous	Homocystinuria
Denavir®	penciclovir	Cold sores
Diovan®	valsartan	Hypertension
Dostinex®	cabergoline	Hyperprolactinemia
Duract®	bromfenac	Acute pain
Elmiron®	pentosan polysulfate sodium	Interstitial cystitis
Ethyol®	amifostine	Reduction of cumulative renal toxicity associated with administration of cisplatin
Flomax™	tamsulosin	Benign prostatic hyperplasia (BPH)
Glyset®	miglitol	Type II diabetes
IvyBlock®	bentoquatam	Poison ivy
Levaquin®	levofloxacin	Bacterial respiratory tract infection
Lexxel®	enalapril and felodipine	Hypertension
Lipidil®	fenofibrate	High triglyceride
Lipitor®	atorvastatin	High cholesterol
Mentax®	butenafine	Ringworm and other topical fungi
Mirapex®	pramipexole	Parkinson's disease
Monurol™	fosfomycin	Urinary tract infections
Naropin™	ropivacaine	Anesthetic (infiltration)
Nilandron™	nilutamide	Prostate cancer
Normiflo®	ardeparin	Deep vein thrombosis
Norvir®	ritonavir	HIV infection
Orgaran®	danaparoid	Deep vein thrombosis
Patanol™	olopatadine	Allergic conjunctivitis
Posicor®	mibefradil	Hypertension
ProAmatine®	midodrine	Orthostatic hypotension
Requip®	ropinirole	Parkinson's disease
Rescriptor™	delavirdine	HIV infection
Retavase®	reteplase	Acute myocardial infarction
Rezulin®	troglitazone	Type II diabetes
Seroquel®	quetiapine	Antipsychotic
Skelid®	tiludronate	Paget's disease of the bone
Stromectol®	ivermectin	Intestinal parasites (worms)
Tarka®	trandolapril and verapamil	Hypertension
Tazorac®	tazarotene	Psoriasis, acne vulgaris
Teczem®	enalapril and diltiazem	Hypertension
Topamax®	topiramate	Seizures
Viracept®	nelfinavir	HIV infection
Zagam®	sparfloxacin	Community-acquired pneumonia
Zanaflex®	tizanidine	Multiple sclerosis, spinal cord injury
Zyflo®	zileuton	Asthma

(continued)

Brand Name	Generic Name	Use
Pending Drugs or Drugs in Clinical Trials		
Alredase®	tolrestat	Controlling late complications of diabetes
Arkin-Z®	vesnarinone	Congestive heart failure agent
Baypress®	nitrendipine	Calcium channel blocker for hypertension
Berotec®	fenoterol	Beta-2 agonist for asthma
Catatrol®	viloxazine	Bicyclic antidepressant
Cipralan®	cifenline succinate	Antiarrhythmic agent
Decabid®	indecainide hydrochloride	Antiarrhythmic agent
Delaprem®	hexoprenaline sulfate	Tocolytic agent
Dirame®	propiram	Opioid analgesic
Eldisine®	vindesine sulfate	Antineoplastic
Enable®	tenidap sodium	Arthritis
Fareston®	toremifene citrate	Antiestrogen for breast cancer
Freedox®	triliazad mesylate	Prevents progressive neuronal degeneration
Frisium®	clobazam	Benzodiazepine
Gastrozepine®	pirenzepine	Antiulcer drug
Inhibace®	cilazapril	ACE inhibitor
Isoprinosine®	inosiplex	Immunomodulating drug
Lacipil®	lacidipine	Hypertension
Maxicam®	isoxicam	NSAID
Mentane®	velnacrine	Alzheimer's disease agent
Micturin®	terodiline hydrochloride	Agent for urinary incontinence
Mogadon®	nitrazepam	Benzodiazepine
Motilium®	domperidone	Antiemetic
Napa®	acecainide	Antiarrhythmic agent
Pindac®	pinacidil	Antihypertensive
Prothiaden®	dothiepin hydrochloride	Tricyclic antidepressant
Rimadyl®	caprofen	NSAID
Roxiam®	remoxipride	Antipsychotic agent
Sabril®	vigabatrin	Anticonvulsant
Selecor®	celiprolol hydrochloride	Beta-adrenergic blocker
Soriatane®	acitretin	Recalcitrant psoriasis
Spexil®	trospectomycin	Antibiotic, a spectinomycin analog
Targocoid®	teicoplanin	Antibiotic, similar to vancomycin
Unicard®	dilevalol	Beta-adrenergic blocker
Zaditen®	ketotifen	Antiasthmatic

DRUG PRODUCTS NO LONGER AVAILABLE

Brand Name	Generic Name
Achromycin® Parenteral	tetracycline
Achromycin® V Capsule	tetracycline
Achromycin® V Oral Suspension	tetracycline
ACTH-40®	corticotropin
Actidil®	triprolidine
Actifed® Syrup	triprolidine and pseudoephedrine
Actifed® with Codeine	triprolidine, pseudoephedrine, and codeine
Adipex-P®	phentermine (all products)
Adipost®	phendimetrazine tartrate
Adphen®	phendimetrazine tartrate
Adrin®	nylidrin hydrochloride
Aerolate® Oral Solution	theophylline
Aerosporin® Injection	polymyxin B
Agoral® Plain	mineral oil
Arthritis Foundation® Ibuprofen	ibuprofen
Arthritis Foundation® Nighttime	acetaminophen & diphenhydramine
Arthritis Foundation® Pain Reliever, Aspirin Free	acetaminophen
AK-Zol® Tablet	acetazolamide
Akoline® C.B. Tablet	vitamin
Ala-Tet®	tetracycline
Amonidrin® Tablet	guaifenesin
Anacin-3® (All products)	acetaminophen
Anaids® Tablet	alginic acid and sodium bicarbonate
Anergan® 25 Injection	promethazine hydrochloride
Anoxine-AM® Capsule	phentermine hydrochloride
Antinea® Cream	benzoic acid and salicylic acid
Antivert® Chewable Tablet	meclizine hydrochloride
Antrocol® Capsule & Tablet	atropine and belladonna
Apomorphine	apomorphine (now available as an orphan drug only)
Arcotinic® Tablet	iron and liver combination
Argyrol® S.S.	silver protein, Mild
Arlidin®	nylidrin (all drug products)
Arthritis Strength Bufferin®	aspirin (buffered)
Asbron-G® Tablet	theophylline and guaifenesin
Asproject®	sodium thiosalicylate
Atabrine® Tablet	quinacrine hydrochloride
Atropine Soluble Tablet	atropine soluble tablet
Aureomycin®	chlortetracycline
Axotal®	butalbital compound & aspirin
Azlin® Injection	azlocillin
Azo Gantanol®	sulfamethoxazole and phenazopyridine
Azo Gantrisin®	sulfisoxazole and phenazopyridine
Azulfidine® Suspension	sulfasalazine
B-A-C®	butalbital compound with aspirin
Bancap®	butalbital compound with acetaminophen
Banesin®	acetaminophen
Bantron®	lobeline
Baypress®	nitrendipine
Becomject-100®	vitamin B complex
Beesix®	pyridoxine hydrochloride
Bemote®	dicyclomine
Bena-D®	diphenhydramine
Benadryl® 50 mg Capsule	diphenhydramine hydrochloride
Benahist® Injection	diphenhydramine hydrochloride

(continued)

Brand Name	Generic Name
Benoject®	diphenhydramine hydrochloride
Beta-Val® Ointment	betamethasone
Biamine® Injection	thiamine hydrochloride
Bilezyme® Tablet	pancrelipase
Biphetamine®	amphetamine and dextroamphetamine
Blanex® Capsule	chloroxazone and acetaminophen
Bretylol®	bretylium
Bronkephrine®	ethylnorepinephrine hydrochloride
Buffered®, Tri-buffered	aspirin
Bufferin® Extra Strength	aspirin
Bufferin® Arthritis Strength	aspirin
Butace®	butalbital compound
Caladryl® Spray	diphenhydramine and calamine
Calciparine® Injection	heparin calcium
Camalox® Suspension & Tablet	aluminum hydroxide, calcium carbonate, and magnesium hydroxide
Cantharone®	cantharidin
Cantharone Plus®	cantharidin
Caroid®	cascara sagrada & phenolphthalein
Cedilanid-D® Injection	deslanoside
Cenocort® A-40	triamcinolone
Cenocort® Forte	triamcinolone
Centrax® Capsule & Tablet	prazepam
Cerespan®	papaverine hydrochloride
Cetane®	ascorbic acid
Chenix® Tablet	chenodiol
Chlorofon-A® Tablet	chlorzoxazone
Chloromycetin® Cream	chloramphenicol
Chloromycetin® Kapseals®	chloramphenicol
Chloromycetin® Ophthalmic	chloramphenicol
Chloromycetin® Otic	chloramphenicol
Chloromycetin® Palmitate Oral Suspension	chloramphenicol
Chlortab®	chlorpheniramine maleate
Choledyl®	oxtriphylline
Cithalith-S® Syrup	lithium citrate
Cipralan®	cifenline
Citro-Nesia® Solution	magnesium citrate
Clistin® Tablet	carbinoxamine maleate
Clorpactin® XCB Powder	oxychlorosene sodium
Cobalasine® Injection	adenosine phosphate
Codimal® Expectorant	guaifenesin & phenylpropanolamine
Codimal-A® Injection	brompheniramine maleate
Coly-Mycin® S Oral	colistin sulfate
Constant-T® Tablet	theophylline
Control-L®	pyrethrins
Correctol®	docusate and phenolphthalein
Cortaid® Ointment	hydrocortisone
Cortrophin-Zinc®	corticotropin
Crystodigin® 0.05 mg & 0.15 mg Tablet	digitoxin
Cycrin® 10 mg Tablet	medroxyprogesterone acetate
Danex® Shampoo	pyrithione zinc
Dapex-37.5®	phentermine hydrochloride
Darbid® Tablet	isopropamide iodide
Daricon®	oxyphencyclimine (all products)
Darvon® 32 mg Capsule	propoxyphene hydrochloride
Darvon-N® Oral Suspension	propoxyphene napsylate
Datril® Extra Strength	acetaminophen

(continued)

Brand Name	Generic Name
Decadron® 0.25 mg and 6 mg Tablets	dexamethasone
Decaspray®	dexamethasone
Dehist®	brompheniramine maleate
Deltalin® Capsule	ergocalciferol
Deprol®	meprobamate and benactyzine hydrochloride
Dermoxyl® Gel	benzoyl peroxide
Despec® Liquid	guaifenesin, phenylpropanolamine, and phenylephrine
Dexacen® LA-8	dexamethasone
Dexacen-4®	dexamethasone
Dexedrine® Elixir	dextroamphetamine sulfate
Dialose® Capsule	docusate sodium
Diaparene® Cradol®	methylbenzethonium
Dilaudid® 1 mg & 3 mg Tablet	hydromorphone hydrochloride
Dilantin-30® Pediatric Suspension	phenytoin
Dilantin With Phenobarbital	phenytoin with phenobarbital
Dimetane®	brompheniramine maleate
Diupress®	chlorothiazide & reserpine
Dizymes® Tablet	pancreatin
Dommanate® Injection	dimenhydrinate
Donphen® Tablet	hyoscyamine, atropine, scopolamine, and phenobarbital
Dopastat® Injection	dopamine hydrochloride
Doriden® Tablet	glutethimide
Doxinate® Capsule	docusate sodium
Dramamine® Injection	dimenhydrinate
Dramocen®	dimenhydrinate
Dramoject®	dimenhydramine
Dyflex-400® Tablet	dyphylline
Eldepryl® Tablets (Only)	selegiline
Eldoquin® Lotion	hydroquinone
Elixophyllin® SR Capsule	theophylline
E-Lor® Tablet	propoxyphene and acetaminophen
Emete-Con® Injection	benzquinamide
Emetine Hydrochloride	emetine hydrochloride
Endep® 25 mg, 50 mg, 100 mg	amitriptyline hydrochloride
Enduron® 2.5 mg Tablet	methylclothiazide
E.N.T.®	brompheniramine & phenylpropanolamine
Enovid®	mestranol & norethynodrel
Entozyme®	pancreatin
E.P.Mycin® Capsule	oxytetracycline
Ergostat®]	ergotamine
Ergotrate® Maleate	ergonovine maleate
Eridium®	phenazopyridine hydrochloride
Ery-Sol® Topical Solution	erythromycin, topical
Esidrix® 100 mg Tablet	hydrochlorothiazide
Estradurin® Injection	polyestradiol phosphate
Estroject-L.A.® Injection	estradiol
Estroject-2® Injection	estradiol
Estronol® Injection	estrone
Estrovis®	quinestrol
Ethaquin®	ethaverine hydrochloride
Ethatab®	ethaverine hydrochloride
Ethavex-100®	ethaverine hydrochloride
Euthroid® Tablet	liotrix
Fansidar®	sulfadoxine and pyrimethamine
FemCare®	clotrimazole
Fastin®	phentermine (all products)

(continued)

Brand Name	Generic Name
Femstat®	butoconazole nitrate
Fergon Plus®	iron with vitamin B
Fer-In-Sol® Capsule	ferrous sulfate
Fermalox®	ferrous sulfate, magnesium hydroxide, and docusate
Ferndex	dextroamphetamine sulfate
Folex® Injection	methotrexate
Gamastan®	immune globulin, intramuscular
Gammagard® Injection	immune globulin, intravenous
Gammar®	immune globulin, intramuscular
Gantrisin® Ophthalmic	sulfisoxazole
Gantrisin® Pediatric	sulfisoxazole
Gantrisin® Syrup	sulfisoxazole
Gantrisin® Tablet	sulfisoxazole
Gelusil® Liquid	aluminum hydroxide, magnesium hydroxide, and simethicone
Gen-D-phen®	diphenhydramine hydrochloride
Gentian Violet	gentian violet
Grisactin®	griseofulvin
Gynogen® Injection	estradiol
Halazone Tablet	halazone
Halenol® Tablet	acetaminophen
Harmonyl®	deserpidine
HemFe®	iron with vitamins
Hep-B-Gammagee®	hepatitis b immune globulin
Hetrazan®	diethylcarbamazine citrate
Histaject®	brompheniramine maleate
Histamine Phosphate Injection	histamine phosphate
Hydeltra-T.B.A.®	prednisolone
Hydramine®	diphenhydramine hydrochloride
Hydrobexan® Injection	hydroxocobalamin
Hydropres® 25 mg Tablet	hydrochlorothiazide and reserpine
Hydroxacen®	hydroxyzine
Inhibase®	cilazapril
Intal® Inhalation Capsule	cromolyn sodium
Iodo-Niacin® Tablet	potassium iodide and niacinamide hydroiodide
Ionamin®	phentermine (all products)
Iophen®	iodinated glycerol
Iophen-C®	iodinated glycerol and codeine
Iophylline®	iodinated glycerol and theophylline
Iotuss®	iodinated glycerol and codeine
Iotuss-DM®	iodinated glycerol and dextromethorphan
Iso-Bid®	isosorbide dinitrate
Isopto® P-ES	pilocarpine and physostigmine
Isovex®	ethaverine hydrochloride
Isuprel® Glossets®	isoproterenol
Iveegam® Injection	immune globulin, intravenous
Kaopectate® Children's Tablet	attapulgite
Kato® Powder	potassium chloride
Keflin®	cephalothin sodium
Kestrin® Injection	estrone
Koate®-HS Injection	antihemophilic factor (human)
Koate®-HT Injection	antihemophilic factor (human)
Konyne-HT® Injection	factor ix complex (human)
Kolyum® Powder	potassium chloride and potassium gluconate
Kwell®	lindane
Lamprene® 100 mg	clofazimine
Lasan® Topical	anthralin
Lasan® HP-1 Topical	anthralin

(continued)

Brand Name	Generic Name
Ledercillin VK®	penicillin V potassium
Libritabs® 5 mg	chlordiazepoxide
Lorcet®	hydrocodone & acetaminophen
Lorelco®	probucol
Malotuss® Syrup	guaifenesin
Mandelamine® Tablet	methenamine
Mantadil® Cream	chlorcyclizine
Marezine® Injection	cyclizine hydrochloride
Marplan®	isocarboxazid
Materna®	prenatal vitamin
Max-Caro®	beta-carotene
Meclomen®	meclofenamate sodium
Medihaler-Epi®	epinephrine
Medihaler Ergotamine®	ergotamine
Medrapred®	prednisolone and atropine
Medrol® Acetate Topical	methylprednisolone
Melfiat® Tablet	phendimetrazine tartrate
Meprospan®	meprobamate
Metaprel® Aerosol	metaproterenol sulfate
Metaprel® Inhalation Solution	metaproterenol sulfate
Metaprel® Tablet	metaproterenol sulfate
Metizol® Tablet	metronidazole
Metopirone® Tablet	metyrapone tartrate
Metra®	phendimetrazine tartrate
Miflex® Tablet	chlorzoxazone and acetaminophen
Milprem®	meprobamate and conjugated estrogens
Minocin® Tablet	minocycline
Miochol®	acetylcholine
Moisturel® Lotion	dimethicone
Monocete® Topical Liquid	monochloroacetic acid
Moxam® Injection	moxalactam
Mus-Lax®	chlorzoxazone
Mylaxen® Injection	hexafluorenium bromide
Myochrysine®	gold sodium thiomalate
Nalfon® Tablet	fenoprofen calcium
Narcan® 1 mg/mL Injection	naloxone hydrochloride
Nandrobolic® Injection	nandrolone phenpropionate
Navane® Concentrate & Injection	thiothixene
N-B-P® Ointment	bacitracin, neomycin, & polymyxin B
Neo-Castaderm®	resorcinol, boric acid, acetone
Neo-Cortef® Topical	neomycin & hydrocortisone
Neo-Medrol® Acetate Topical	methylprednisolone and neomycin
Neoquess® Injection	dicyclomine hydrochloride
Neoquess® Tablet	hyoscyamine sulfate
Neo-Synalar® Topical	neomycin and fluocinolone
Neo-Synephrine® 12 Hour Nasal Solution	oxymetazoline hydrochloride
Neutra-Phos® Capsule	potassium phosphate and sodium phosphate
Niac®	niacin
Niacels®	niacin
Niclocide®	niclosamide
Nidryl®	diphenhydramine hydrochloride
Niferex Forte®	iron with vitamins
Niloric®	ergoloid mesylates
Nipride® Injection	nitroprusside sodium
Nisaval®	pyrilamine maleate
Nitro-Bid® Oral	nitroglycerin

(continued)

Brand Name	Generic Name
Nitrocine® Oral	nitroglycerin
Nitrostat® 0.15 mg Tablet	nitroglycerin
Noctec®	chloral hydrate
Noludar®	methyprylon
Norlutate®	norethindrone
Norlutin®	norethindrone
Novafed®	pseudoephedrine
Novahistine DMX® Liquid	guaifenesin, pseudoephedrine, & dextromethorphan
Novahistine DH® Liquid	chlorpheniramine, pseudoephedrine, & codeine
Novahistine® Elixir	chlorpheniramine & phenylephrine
Novahistine® Expectorant	guaifenesin, pseudoephedrine, & codeine
Nursoy®	enteral nutritional therapy
Nydrazid® Injection	isoniazid
Obe-Nix® 30	phentermine (all products)
Obephen®	phentermine (all products)
Obermine®	phentermine (all products)
Obestin-30®	phentermine (all products)
Ophthaine®	proparacaine
Ophthocort®	chloramphenicol, polymyxin B, and hydrocortisone
Oradex-C®	dyclonine
Oratect®	benzocaine
Oreticyl®	deserpidine and hydrochlorothiazide
Organidin®	iodinated glycerol
Otic Tridesilon®	desonide and acetic acid
Oxsoralen® Oral	methoxsalen
Panwarfin®	warfarin sodium
Paplex®	salicylic acid
Paradione®	paramethadione
Para-Hist AT®	promethazine, phenylephrine, & codeine
Pargen Fortified®	chlorzoxazone
Par Glycerol®	iodinated glycerol
Parmine®	phentermine hydrochloride
Parsidol®	ethopropazine
Pavabid HP®	papaverine hydrochloride
Pavesed®	papaverine hydrochloride
Pavasule®	papaverine hydrochloride
Pavatym®	papaverine hydrochloride
Pentids® (all forms)	penicillin g potassium, oral (all products)
Pfizerpen-AS®	penicillin G procaine
Phenaphen®	acetaminophen
Phenaphen®/Codeine #4	acetaminophen and codeine
Phenaseptic®	phenol
Phencen-50®	promethazine
Phenetron®	chlorpheniramine
Phentrol®	phentermine (all products)
Phenurone®	phenacemide
Phos-Ex® 62.5	calcium acetate
Phos-Ex® 125	calcium acetate
Phos-Ex® 167	calcium acetate
Phos-Ex® 250	calcium acetate
pHos-pHaid®	ammonium biphosphate, sodium biphosphate, and sodium acid pyrophosphate
Phosphaljel®	aluminum phosphate
Pindac®	pinacidil
Polargen®	dexchlorpheniramine maleate
Poliovax® Injection	poliovirus vaccine, inactivated
Polyflex® Tablet	chlorzoxazone

APPENDIX

(continued)

Brand Name	Generic Name
Polygam® Injection	immune globulin, intravenous
Predaject-50®	prednisolone
Predalone®	prednisolone
Predicort-50®	prednisolone
Preludin®	phenmetrazine hydrochloride
Premarin® Vaginal Cream	conjugated estrogens
Procan SR®	procainamide
Profilate-HP®	antihemophilic factor (human)
Projestaject® Injection	progesterone
Prometh®	promethazine
Pro-Sof®	docusate sodium
Prolamine®	phenylpropanolamine
Prokine® Injection	sargramostim
Proloid®	thyroglobulin
Proplex® SX-T Injection	factor ix complex (human)
Protopam® Tablet	pralidoxime chloride
Provatene®	beta-carotene
Pyridium Plus®	phenazopyridine, hyoscyamine, and butabarbital
Questran® Tablet	cholestyramine resin
Quinamm®	quinine sulfate
Quiphile®	quinine sulfate
Q-vel®	quinine sulfate
Rectacort® suppository	hydrocortisone
Redux®	dexfenfluramine
Regutol®	docusate
Rep-Pred®	methylprednisolone
R-Gen®	iodinated glycerol
Rhesonativ® Injection	Rh_o(D) immune globulin
Rhindecon®	phenylpropanolamine
Rhinolar®	chlorpheniramine, phenylpropanolamine, & methscopolamine
Rhuli® Cream	benzocaine, calamine, & camphor
Robicillin® VK 500 mg	penicillin V potassium
Robitet®	tetracycline
Romycin® Solution	erythromycin, topical
Rondomycin® Capsule	methacycline hydrochloride
Rufen®	ibuprofen
Sclavo - PPD Solution	tuberculin purified protein derivative
Sclavo Test-PPD	tuberculin purified protein derivative
Sebulex®	sulfur & salicylic acid
Sebulon®	pyrithione zinc
Seconal™ Oral	secobarbital sodium
Selecor®	celiprolol
Selestoject®	betamethasone
Serpasil®	reserpine
Siblin®	psyllium
Skelex®	chlorzoxazone
Sodium P.A.S.	aminosalicylate sodium
Sofarin®	warfarin sodium
Solatene®	beta-carotene
Spasmoject®	dicyclomine
Statobex®	phendimetrazine tartrate
Sterapred®	prednisone
Streptomycin	streptomycin
Sucostrin®	succinylcholine chloride
Sudafed® Cough	guaifenesin, pseudoephedrine, & dextromethorphan
Sudafed® Childrens	pseudoephedrine
Sudafed Plus® Liquid	chlorpheniramine and pseudoephedrine

(continued)

Brand Name	Generic Name
Superchar®	charcoal
Superchar® With Sorbitol	charcoal
Surital®	thiamylal sodium
Symmetrel® Capsule	amantadine hydrochloride
Synkayvite®	menadiol sodium
Tabron®	vitamins, multiple
Tacaryl®	methdilazine hydrochloride
Taractan®	chlorprothixene
Teline®	tetracycline
Temaril®	trimeprazine tartrate
Tepanil®	diethylpropion hydrochloride
Tepanil® TenTabs®	diethylpropion hydrochloride
Tes-Tape®	diagnostic aids (*in vitro*), urine
Tetralan®	tetracycline
Tetram®	tetracycline
Theelin® Aqueous Injection	estrone
Theobid® Jr Duracaps®	theophylline
Theo-Dur® Sprinkle®	theophylline
Theo-Organidin®	iodinated glycerol and theophylline
Thiacide®	methenamine and potassium acid phosphate
Tiject-20®	trimethobenzamide
Tindal®	acetophenazine maleate
Tral®	hexocyclium methylsulfate
Travase®	sutilains
Trimox® 500 mg	amoxicillin
Trofan DS®	L-tryptophan
Trofan®	L-tryptophan
Tryptacin®	L-tryptophan
Tusal®	sodium thiosalicylate
Tussi-Organidin®	iodinated glycerol and codeine
Tussi-Organidin® DM	iodinated glycerol and dextromethorphan
Tuss-Ornade®	caramiphen & phenylpropanolamine
Ultralente® U	insulin zinc suspension, extended
Ultrase® MT24	pancrelipase
Unipres®	hydralazine, hydrochlorothiazide, and reserpine
Ureacin®-40 Topical	urea
Uticort®	betamethasone
Valadol®	acetaminophen
Valergen® Injection	estradiol
Valmid® Capsule	ethinamate
Valpin® 50	anisotropine methylbromide
Valrelease®	diazepam
Vanex-LA®	guaifenesin and phenylpropanolamine
Vanseb-T® Shampoo	coal tar, sulfur, and salicylic acid
V-Cillin K®	penicillin V potassium
Velsar® Injection	vinblastine sulfate
Vercyte®	pipobroman
Verr-Canth®	cantharidin
Verrex®	podophyllin & salicylic acid
Verrusol®	salicylic acid, podophyllin, and cantharidin
V-Gan® Injection	promethazine hydrochloride
Vicks® Vatronol®	ephedrine
Vioform®-Hydrocortisone Topical	clioquinol and hydrocortisone
Visine®	tetrahydrozoline hydrochloride
Vistaject-25®	hydroxyzine
Vistaject-50®	hydroxyzine

APPENDIX

(continued)

Brand Name	Generic Name
Wehamine® Injection	dimenhydrinate
Wehdryl®	diphenhydramine
Wesprin® Buffered	aspirin
Wyamycin S®	erythromycin
Zebrax®	clidinium and chlordiazepoxide
Zetran®	diazepam
Zolyse®	chymotrypsin alpha

INDICATION/THERAPEUTIC CATEGORY
INDEX

Antiseborrheic Agent, Topical

Retinoic Acid Derivative

Tetracycline Derivative

Topical Skin Product

ACQUIRED IMMUNODEFICIENCY SYNDROME (AIDS)

Antiviral Agent

ACROMEGALY

Ergot Alkaloid

Somatostatin Analog

ADAMS-STOKES SYNDROME

Adrenergic Agonist Agent

ADDISON'S DISEASE see also ADRENOCORTICAL FUNCTION ABNORMALITIES

Adrenal Corticosteroid

(Continued)

ASPERGILLOSIS

Antifungal Agent

ASPIRATION PNEUMONITIS see RESPIRATORY DISORDERS

ASTHMA see also RESPIRATORY DISORDERS, CHRONIC OBSTRUCTIVE PULMONARY DISEASE (COPD)

Adrenal Corticosteroid

Adrenergic Agonist Agent

Anticholinergic Agent

Leukotriene Receptor Antagonist

(Continued)

Biological Response Modulator

Estrogen and Androgen Combination

Estrogen Derivative

Gonadotropin Releasing Hormone Analog

COLONIC EVACUATION

Laxative

CONDYLOMA ACUMINATUM

Biological Response Modulator

Keratolytic Agent

CONGESTION (NASAL) *see also* RHINITIS

Adrenergic Agonist Agent

(Continued)

Antihistamine/Decongestant Combination

(Continued)

CONJUNCTIVITIS (VIRAL)

Antiviral Agent

CONSTIPATION

Laxative

Laxative/Stool Softner

Stool Softener

COUGH

Antihistamine

Antihistamine/Antitussive

Antihistamine/Decongestant/Antitussive

Antihistamine/Decongestant Combination

(Continued)

INDICATION/THERAPEUTIC CATEGORY INDEX

DIABETES INSIPIDUS

Antidiuretic Hormone Analog

Hormone, Posterior Pituitary

Vasopressin Analog, Synthetic

DIABETES MELLITUS, INSULIN-DEPENDENT (IDDM)

Antidiabetic Agent, Parenteral

DIABETES MELLITUS, NON-INSULIN-DEPENDENT (NIDDM)

Antidiabetic Agent, Oral

DIABETIC GASTRIC STASIS

Gastrointestinal Agent, Prokinetic

DIAPER RASH

Antifungal Agent

Dietary Supplement

Protectant, Topical

Topical Skin Product

DIARRHEA

Analgesic, Narcotic

Anticholinergic Agent

Antidiarrheal

Gastrointestinal Agent, Miscellaneous

Somatostatin Analog

DIVERTICULITIS

Aminoglycoside (Antibiotic)

Antibiotic, Miscellaneous

Carbapenem (Antibiotic)

Cephalosporin (Second Generation)

Penicillin

DIZZINESS see VERTIGO

DRACUNCULIASIS

Amebicide

DRUG DEPENDENCE (OPIOID)

Analgesic, Narcotic

DRY EYES see XEROPHTHALMIA

DRY MOUTH see XEROSTOMIA

DRY SKIN

Topical Skin Product

Vitamin, Topical

DUCTUS ARTERIOSUS (CLOSURE)

Nonsteroidal Anti-Inflammatory Agent (NSAID)

DUCTUS ARTERIOSUS (TEMPORARY MAINTENANCE OF PATENCY)

Prostaglandin

DUODENAL ULCER

Antacid

Diagnostic Agent

Gastric Acid Secretion Inhibitor

Gastrointestinal Agent, Gastric or Duodenal Ulcer Treatment

Histamine H₂ Antagonist

DWARFISM

Growth Hormone

DYSBETALIPOPROTEINEMIA (FAMILIAL)

Antihyperlipidemic Agent, Miscellaneous

Vitamin, Water Soluble

DYSMENORRHEA

Nonsteroidal Anti-Inflammatory Agent (NSAID)

EDEMA

(Continued)

FEVER

Antipyretic

FIBRILLATION see ARRHYTHMIAS

FIBROCYSTIC BREAST DISEASE

Androgen

FIBROMYOSITIS

Antidepressant, Tricyclic (Tertiary Amine)

FOLLICLE STIMULATION

Ovulation Stimulator

(Continued)

HEART BLOCK

HEAT PROSTRATION

HEAVY METAL POISONING

HELICOBACTER PYLORI

HEMATOLOGIC DISORDERS

(Continued)

Analgesic, Topical *(Continued)*
    No Pain-HP® [OTC] 87
    R-Gel® [OTC] 87
    Zostrix® [OTC] 87
    Zostrix-® HP [OTC] 87

Antiviral Agent
    acyclovir 10
    famciclovir 216
    Famvir™ 216
    valacyclovir 544
    Valtrex® 544
    vidarabine 549
    Vira-A® Ophthalmic 549
    Zovirax® 10

HIATAL HERNIA

Antacid
    calcium carbonate and
      simethicone 83
    magaldrate 317
    magaldrate and simethicone
      317
    Riopan® [OTC] 317
    Riopan Plus® [OTC] 317
    Titralac® Plus Liquid [OTC]
      83

HICCUPS

Phenothiazine Derivative
    chlorpromazine 119
    Ormazine 119
    Thorazine® 119
    triflupromazine 532
    Vesprin® 532

HISTOPLASMOSIS

Antifungal Agent
    amphotericin B 31
    Fungizone® 31
    itraconazole 293
    ketoconazole 296
    Nizoral® 296
    Sporanox® 293

HIV *see* ACQUIRED
    IMMUNODEFICIENCY
    SYNDROME (AIDS)

HODGKIN'S DISEASE

Antineoplastic Agent
    Adriamycin PFS™ 183
    Adriamycin RDF™ 183
    Alkaban-AQ® 550
    BiCNU® 93
    Blenoxane® 69
    bleomycin 69
    carmustine 93
    CeeNU® 312
    chlorambucil 107
    cisplatin 125
    cyclophosphamide 144
    Cytoxan® Injection 144
    Cytoxan® Oral 144
    dacarbazine 147
    doxorubicin 183
    DTIC-Dome® 147
    Gliadel® 93

Idamycin® 278
idarubicin 278
Leukeran® 107
lomustine 312
Matulane® 439
mechlorethamine 324
Mustargen® Hydrochloride
    324
Neosar® Injection 144
Oncovin® Injection 550
Platinol® 125
Platinol®-AQ 125
procarbazine 439
Rubex® 183
streptozocin 493
thiotepa 517
Velban® 550
vinblastine 550
Vincasar® PFS™ Injection
    550
vincristine 550
Zanosar® 493

HOMOCYSTINURIA

Urinary Tract Product
    betaine anhydrous 64
    Cystadane® 64

HOOKWORMS

Anthelmintic
    albendazole 13
    Albenza® 13
    Antiminth® [OTC] 451
    mebendazole 324
    Pin-Rid® [OTC] 451
    Pin-X® [OTC] 451
    pyrantel pamoate 451
    Reese's® Pinworm Medicine
      [OTC] 451
    Vermox® 324

HORMONAL IMBALANCE (FEMALE)

Progestin
    Amen® Oral 326
    Aygestin® 378
    Crinone® 440
    Curretab® Oral 326
    Cycrin® Oral 326
    Depo-Provera® Injection 326
    hydroxyprogesterone caproate
      274
    Hylutin® Injection 274
    Hyprogest® 250 Injection 274
    medroxyprogesterone acetate
      326
    Micronor® 378
    norethindrone 378
    NOR-Q.D.® 378
    Progestasert® 440
    progesterone 440
    Provera® Oral 326

HYDATIDIFORM MOLE (BENIGN)

Prostaglandin
    Cervidil® Vaginal Insert 172
    dinoprostone 172
    Prepidil® Vaginal Gel 172

(Continued)

IDIOPATHIC APNEA OF PREMATURITY

Respiratory Stimulant
caffeine, citrated 80

IDIOPATHIC THROMBOCYTOPENIC PURPURA see HEMATOLOGIC DISORDERS

IMMUNODEFICIENCY

Enzyme
Adagen™ 398
pegademase (bovine) 398

Immune Globulin
Gamimune® N 281
Gammagard® 281
Gammagard® S/D 281
Gammar-P® I.V. 281
immune globulin, intravenous
.... 281
Polygam® 281
Polygam® S/D 281
Sandoglobulin® 281
Venoglobulin®-I 281
Venoglobulin®-S 281

IMPETIGO

Antibiotic, Topical
bacitracin, neomycin, and
 polymyxin b 53
Bactroban® 358
Medi-Quick® Topical Ointment
 [OTC] 53
mupirocin 358
Mycitracin® Topical [OTC]
.... 53
Neomixin® Topical [OTC] 53
Neosporin® Topical Ointment
 [OTC] 53
Ocutricin® Topical Ointment
.... 53
Septa® Topical Ointment [OTC]
.... 53
Triple Antibiotic® Topical 53

Penicillin
Beepen-VK® 402
Betapen®-VK 402
Crysticillin® A.S. 401
penicillin g procaine 401
penicillin v potassium 402
Pen.Vee® K 402
Robicillin® VK 402
Veetids® 402
Wycillin® 401

IMPOTENCY

Androgen
Android® 343
methyltestosterone 343
Oreton® Methyl 343
Testred® 343
Virilon® 343

Miscellaneous Product
Aphrodyne™ 558
Dayto Himbin® 558
Yocon® 558

yohimbine 558
Yohimex™ 558

Vasodilator
ethaverine 207

INFERTILITY (FEMALE)

Ergot Alkaloid
bromocriptine................. 72
Parlodel® 72

Gonadotropin
A.P.L.® 122
Chorex® 122
chorionic gonadotropin 122
Choron® 122
Gonic® 122
Humegon® 328
menotropins 328
Pergonal® 328
Pregnyl® 122
Profasi® HP 122
Repronex® 328

Ovulation Stimulator
Clomid® 129
clomiphene 129
Milophene® 129
Serophene® 129

Progestin
Crinone® 440
Progestasert® 440
progesterone 440

INFERTILITY (MALE)

Gonadotropin
A.P.L.® 122
Chorex® 122
chorionic gonadotropin 122
Choron® 122
Gonic® 122
Humegon® 328
menotropins................. 328
Pergonal® 328
Pregnyl® 122
Profasi® HP 122
Repronex® 328

INFLAMMATION (NONRHEUMATIC)

Adrenal Corticosteroid
Acthar® 138
Adlone® Injection 343
A-hydroCort® 268
Amcort® 528
A-methaPred® Injection 343
Aristocort® 528
Aristocort® A 528
Aristocort® Forte 528
Articulose-50® Injection 434
Atolone® 528
betamethasone 64
Celestone® 64
Cortef® 268
corticotropin 138
cortisone acetate............. 139
Cortone® Acetate 139
Decadron® 156
Decadron®-LA 156

(Continued)

Antihistamine/Decongestant Combination

OILY SKIN

Antiseborrheic Agent, Topical

ONYCHOMYCOSIS

Antifungal Agent

OPHTHALMIC DISORDERS

Adrenal Corticosteroid

OPHTHALMIC SURGERY

Nonsteroidal Anti-Inflammatory Agent (NSAID)

OPHTHALMIC SURGICAL AID

Ophthalmic Agent, Miscellaneous

OPIATE WITHDRAWAL (NEONATAL)

Analgesic, Narcotic

OPIOID POISONING

Antidote

OPTIC NEURITIS *see* OPHTHALMIC DISORDERS

ORAL LESIONS

Local Anesthetic

ORGAN TRANSPLANT *see also* TISSUE GRAFT, GRAFT VS HOST DISEASE

Immunosuppressant Agent

(Continued)

Immunosuppressant Agent
(Continued)

ORGANOPHOSPHATE PESTICIDE POISONING

Anticholinergic Agent

Antidote

OSTEOARTHRITIS *see also* RHEUMATIC DISORDERS

Analgesic, Topical

Nonsteroidal Anti-Inflammatory Agent (NSAID)

(Continued)

Reserve Your Copy of
Quick Look Drug Reference 1998!

$49.95 *plus s/h & sales tax*

WIN/WIN95
Compatible

Order NOW for Spring 1998 Delivery
Send No Money Now — 30 Day FREE Trial!

☐ **YES!** Send me _____ copies of *Quick Look Drug Reference* FREE for 30 days.
If I like it, I'll pay $49.95 per copy plus shipping/handling and any applicable sales tax.
Otherwise, I'll return my order in sellable condition, all components intact, and owe
nothing.

Choose Format: ☐ CD-ROM (#40176-9)   ☐ Diskette (#40175-0)

Get Easy, Automatic Delivery for 1999! Same 30-day free trial offer.
And you won't be billed until the product mails to you. Reserve now!

☐ *Quick Look Drug Book 1999* (#40304-4)

☐ *Quick Look Electronic Drug Reference 1999*
    ☐ CD-ROM (#40302-8) ☐ Diskette (#40303-6)

Name
_____

Company
_____

Address
_____

City   State   Zip
(   )   (   )

Day Phone .   Ext.   Fax
        @

E-Mail
_____

Signature
_____

Call: **1-800-527-5597** or Fax: **1-800-447-8438**
or order from our web site: **www.stedmans.com**

Williams & Wilkins
A WAVERLY COMPANY
351 West Camden Street
Baltimore, MD 21201-2436

D7E631

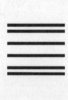

BUSINESS REPLY MAIL

FIRST CLASS   PERMIT NO. 724   BALTIMORE, MD

POSTAGE WILL BE PAID BY ADDRESSEE

WILLIAMS & WILKINS
PROFESSIONAL LEARNING SYSTEMS
PO BOX 1496
BALTIMORE MD 21298-9726

NO POSTAGE
NECESSARY
IF MAILED
IN THE
UNITED STATES

INDICATION/THERAPEUTIC CATEGORY INDEX

INDICATION/THERAPEUTIC CATEGORY INDEX

(Continued)

(Continued)

(Continued)